Adams and Victor's

MANUAL of
NEUROLOGY

Notice

Medicine is an ever-changing science. As new research and clinical experience broaden our knowledge, changes in treatment and drug therapy are required. The editors and the publisher of this work have checked with sources believed to be reliable in their efforts to provide information that is complete and generally in accord with the standards accepted at the time of publication. However, in view of the possibility of human error or changes in medical sciences, neither the editors nor the publisher nor any other party who has been involved in the preparation or publication of this work warrants that the information contained herein is in every respect accurate or complete, and they disclaim all responsibility for any errors or omissions or for the results obtained from use of the information contained in this work. Readers are encouraged to confirm the information contained herein with other sources. For example and in particular, readers are advised to check the product information sheet included in the package of each drug they plan to administer to be certain that the information contained in this work is accurate and that changes have not been made in the recommended dose or in the contraindications for administration. This recommendation is of particular importance in connection with new or infrequently used drugs.

Adams and Victor's

MANUAL of NEUROLOGY

Maurice Victor, M.D.

Professor of Medicine and Neurology
Dartmouth Medical School
Hanover, New Hampshire
Distinguished Physician
*   of the Veterans Administration*
White River Junction, Vermont

Allan H. Ropper, M.D.

Professor and Chairman of Neurology
Tufts University School of Medicine
Chief, Neurology Service
St. Elizabeth's Medical Center
Boston, Massachusetts

McGRAW-HILL

Medical Publishing Division

New York   Chicago   San Francisco   Lisbon   London   Madrid   Mexico City
Milan   New Delhi   San Juan   Seoul   Singapore   Sydney   Toronto

McGraw-Hill

A Division of The **McGraw·Hill** Companies

Adams and Victor's
Manual of Neurology

Copyright © 2002, 1998, 1994, 1991 by *The **McGraw-Hill** Companies, Inc*. All rights reserved. Printed in the United States of America. Except as permitted under the United States Copyright Act of 1976, no part of this publication may be reproduced or distributed in any form or by any means, or stored in a data base or retrieval system, without the prior written permission of the publisher.

1234567890 DOCDOC 0987654321

ISBN 0-07-137351-9

This book was set in Times Roman by Better Graphics, Inc.
The editors were Martin J. Wonsiewicz and Muza Navrozov.
The production supervisor was Catherine H. Saggese.
The index was prepared by Alexandra Nickerson.
R.R. Donnelley & Sons Company was printer and binder.

This book is printed on acid-free paper.

Library of Congress Cataloging in Publication Data

Victor, Maurice—date
    Adams and Victor's manual of neurology / authors, Maurice Victor, Allan H. Ropper.
        p. ; cm.
    Manual to: Adams and Victor's principles of neurology / Maurice Victor, Allan H. Ropper. 7th ed. 2001.
    Includes bibliographical references and index.
    ISBN 0-07-137351-9
    1. Neurology—Handbooks, manuals, etc.   I. Title: Adams and Victor's manual of neurology. II. Ropper, Allan H. III. Victor, Maurice—date. Adams and Victor's manual of neurology. IV. Title.
    [DNLM: 1. Nervous System Diseases—Handbooks. 2. Mental Disorders.—Handbooks.
  WL 39 V644a 2002]
  RC355.V53 2002
  616.8—dc21   2001042560

INTERNATIONAL EDITION ISBN 0-07-115079-X
Copyright © 2002. Exclusive rights by The McGraw-Hill Companies, Inc., for manufacture and export. This book cannot be re-exported from the country to which it is consigned by McGraw-Hill. The International Edition is not available in North America.

Contents

PART V   DISEASES OF PERIPHERAL NERVE AND MUSCLE

PART VI   PSYCHIATRIC DISORDERS

Preface

With each succeeding edition of *Principles of Neurology* and the inevitable growth of its contents, there has been an increasing number of requests from our students and residents for a small companion to our text—a book that could be carried conveniently in a pocket or an instrument bag and provide a quick orientation to a clinical problem when the larger text is not immediately available. It was in response to these requests and with the encouragement of our publisher that we first accepted the challenge of preparing this manual.

Numbering in the hundreds, diseases of the nervous system are too many and varied to be presented without dividing them into categories—traumatic, vascular, neoplastic, infective, metabolic, degenerative, congenital, and so forth. In our textbook, *Principles of Neurology*, we describe the various categories of neurologic disease and the main diseases that constitute each. This subject is introduced by a detailed exposition of the symptoms and signs of disordered nervous function, their anatomic and physiologic bases, and their clinical implications. In addition, a significant portion of the book is allotted to developmental and hereditary metabolic diseases, of particular importance to pediatricians, to muscle diseases, and to common psychiatric illnesses, along with the biologic facts that pertain to these disorders.

Our objectives in this pocket manual version are to provide some guidance in the logic of neurologic case study and the ways in which one reaches a diagnosis; to present briefly the phenomenology or cardinal manifestations of disordered neurologic function; to describe in outline form the clinical approach to each category of neurologic disease, with emphasis on the more frequent and treatable types and on neurologic emergencies; and to satisfy the practical needs of selecting and interpreting the procedures, laboratory tests, and drugs that are used in the investigation and treatment of neurologic disease.

The preparation of the latest (seventh) edition of our larger text has necessitated revision of the smaller one. We have attempted to provide a fresh outlook on all aspects of the texts but in particular an up-to-date presentation of acute neurology.

Although this small volume is patterned after *Principles of Neurology*, the one should not be considered a substitute for the other. The manual is intended to be a companion to the *Principles*, in the sense of satisfying the immediate practical needs of student and resident but turning them to the *Principles* for a more complete and fully referenced account. Concision has been sought at the expense of nuance. We hope that the reader will accept it with these restrictions in mind.

Dr. Raymond Adams, though no longer listed as an active author, has read the entire text and contributed significantly.

My dear friend and mentor Dr. Maurice Victor died during the final stages of preparation of this manual, which he had affectionately called "the little book". For a quarter of a century he diligently crafted and revised the *Principles of Neurology* with Dr. Raymond Adams, a privilege I also shared with Maurice in recent years. He was constantly gauging which material would stand the test of time and justified inclusion in the book, and he had a knack for selecting the perfect turn of phrase to express his ideas on each subject. Through our many hours of writing and discussing every aspect of the book, he imparted insightful lessons regarding neurology, the world of ideas, and the use of the English language. In keeping with his approach, I hope this handbook remains readable and offers a pedagogic perspective that is tempered by personal clinical experience.

A. H. R.

Adams and Victor's
MANUAL of
NEUROLOGY

PART I | APPROACH TO THE PATIENT WITH NEUROLOGIC DISEASE

1 | Case Study in Neurology

Diagnosis of a disorder of the nervous system, like that of any other organ system, begins with a detailed history and a careful examination. However, the symptoms of nervous system disease are much more varied than those of other organ systems, and the physical manifestations are far more numerous and informative. The reason for this diversity is that the nervous system consists not of a single system of uniform function but of multiple systems, each one unique. Moreover, many of the abnormalities of neural function manifest themselves by aberrations of behavior. For these reasons, history taking and examination in patients with neurologic problems is often more time-consuming and demanding than in those without such difficulties.

Once the symptoms and signs have been elicited, they need to be interpreted in terms of anatomy and physiology. This correlation permits *localization* of the disease process; i.e., it provides the *anatomic* or *topographic diagnosis*. For example, paralysis or weakness of the face, arm, and leg on one side, with retained or hyperactive tendon reflexes, incontrovertibly directs attention to the corticospinal tract above its decussation and above the pontine part of the brainstem. Symptoms of diabetes insipidus implicate the anterior hypothalamus and posterior pituitary. As intimated above, this step in case analysis demands certain knowledge of anatomy and physiology. For this reason, each of the following chapters dealing with the motor system, sensory system, and special senses is introduced with a review of the anatomic and physiologic facts that are necessary for understanding the clinical disorders.

The next step in case analysis, that of determining the cause of the lesion(s), requires information of a different order. Here, knowledge of where the lesions lie, coupled with information as to the mode of onset and temporal course of the illness, relevant past and family histories, general medical findings (hypertension, atrial fibrillation, diabetes mellitus, etc.), and the results of appropriate laboratory tests, enables one to deduce the causative disease (*etiologic diagnosis*).

The steps in this clinical method are summarized in Fig. 1-1. Each step follows in logical sequence, and if the first or second step is not secure, the later ones may be misdirected. Thus, if the symptoms or physical signs are misinterpreted—for example, if a localized tremor or choreoathetotic movement (of basal ganglionic origin) is mistaken for partial continuous epilepsy (of cerebral cortical origin)—one would place the lesion incorrectly. One of the most fascinating aspects of neurology is the evident effectiveness and logic of the clinical method in the diagnosis of hundreds of diseases.

TAKING THE HISTORY

An alert, intelligent person should be able to give a coherent account of the problem that brings him* to the physician. There are, however, many

---

*Throughout this text, we follow the traditional practice of using *he*, *his*, or *him* in the generic sense whenever it is not intended to designate the gender of a specific individual.

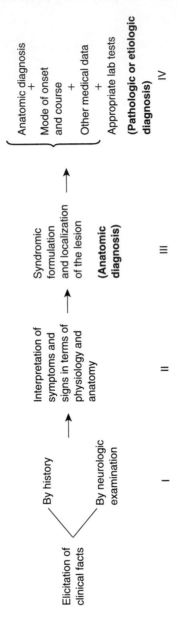

FIG. 1-1   Steps in the diagnosis of neurologic disease.

Elicitation of clinical facts
- By history
- By neurologic examination

I

→ Interpretation of symptoms and signs in terms of physiology and anatomy

II

→ Syndromic formulation and localization of the lesion

(Anatomic diagnosis)

III

→ Anatomic diagnosis
+
Mode of onset and course
+
Other medical data
+
Appropriate lab tests

(Pathologic or etiologic diagnosis)

IV

4

circumstances that may prevent him from doing so. He may have been unconscious when the symptoms had their onset (e.g., as a result of a seizure or concussion). The patient's intellect may be impaired by the very disease under evaluation or by some other one dating from earlier life (e.g., by dementia or mental retardation). The lesion may have affected speech and language mechanisms, preventing communication. Or it may have impaired awareness of a specific neurologic defect, a condition to be described later, under *anosognosia*. Of course, infants and young children lack the ability to make observations concerning their own nervous functioning. A language barrier poses yet another but surmountable problem.

Under these many circumstances, the neurologist must turn to a family member or other witness of the acute event or to a caretaker, parent, or interpreter. Their competence and degree of familiarity with the patient's problems are of critical importance in the first step of case study. *A lack of accurate knowledge of the mode of onset and evolution of the patient's symptoms deprives the physician of the most meaningful diagnostic information.*

THE NEUROLOGIC EXAMINATION

This is an integral part of the general physical examination. With most disease states, the neurologic examination is the last part; in a comatose patient, it immediately follows the recording of vital signs and the cardiopulmonary examination. The type and completeness of the neurologic examination are determined by the nature of the clinical problem. Obviously, it is not necessary to perform a detailed mental status examination in an alert patient with an acute compression of a peroneal nerve. Nevertheless, some assessment of the neurologic status should be part of every general medical examination, and this component of the examination should always be completed in a methodical and uniform manner, to ensure that important aspects of the examination are not omitted. The following are suggestions as to the types of neurologic examination that are pertinent to differing medical situations.

1. The Medical or Surgical Patient without Neurologic Symptoms

Although brevity is desirable, any testing that is performed should be done carefully and recorded accurately in the patient's chart. Assuming that the patient is alert and of normal intelligence, a sufficient examination comprises the following: an assessment of the patient's orientation and grasp of his immediate situation as well as the integrity of speech and language function (all of these are largely evident from conversation with the patient); testing pupillary reactions to light and accommodation, ocular movements, visual and auditory acuity (by questioning), and movements of the face, tongue, and pharynx; observing the bare outstretched arms in the prone and supine postures and during movement (such as touching the nose with the index finger); inquiring about strength and subjective sensory disturbances; eliciting the supinator, biceps, and triceps tendon reflexes; inspecting the legs as the feet and toes are actively flexed and extended; eliciting the patellar, Achilles, and plantar reflexes; testing vibratory and position senses of the fingers and toes; and observing the patient's stance and gait. The entire procedure adds no more than 5 min to the medical examination and sometimes reveals abnormalities of which the patient is unaware. The recording of these data, even negative ones, may be of value in relation to some future illness.

2. Examination of the Patient with Neurologic Disease

Several guides to the examination of the nervous system are available (cf. Ross, Glick, Bickerstaff and Spillane, Staff Members of the Mayo Clinic). They describe innumerable tests in minute detail, but here only the relatively simple and most informative ones are mentioned. Particular forms of testing are considered in subsequent chapters dealing with disorders of consciousness and mentation; cranial nerves; special senses; and motor, sensory, autonomic, and sphincteric functions.

a. Testing of higher cerebral (cortical) functions   In the course of taking the history, one notes the patient's demeanor, emotional state, type of personality, speech, use of language, and capacity for sustained coherent thinking. Attentiveness, speed of response, and ability to remember events also are readily assessed in the course of history taking. This is followed by a systematic inquiry into the patient's orientation, affect, memory, and other cognitive and conative functions (impulse, volition), making due allowance for the patient's level of education and native intelligence. Useful bedside tests are repetition of digits in forward and reverse order, subtraction of 7 serially from 100 or 3 from 30, recalling a brief story or three test items after 5 min, the naming of the last four presidents, and memory of distant facts and events that are appropriate for the patient's age. If there is any suggestion of a speech disorder, one notes the quality of articulation, the choice of words in conversation, and the ability to name various objects and the parts of an object (e.g., the band or stem of a wristwatch), to repeat a spoken sentence, to follow two- and three-step commands, and to read and write. Praxis is tested by asking the patient to perform complex learned acts such as saluting the flag or lighting an imaginary cigarette. Bisecting a line, drawing a clockface, and copying figures are useful tests of visual-spatial and visual-motor functions. Tests of simple arithmetic may demonstrate an impaired ability to concentrate as well as to calculate. In the performance of these tests, the examiner can note the presence or absence of apathy, depression, inattentiveness, and distractibility.

A more complete mental status examination is outlined on pp. 176–177. Abbreviated but systematic surveys (e.g., the Folstein Mini-mental Status Examination) are also useful instruments for the quick assessment of cognitive function (p. 178).

b. Testing of cranial nerves and special senses   Olfaction is tested if the patient complains of impaired smell or taste or if one suspects a lesion of the anterior cranial fossa. It suffices to determine whether the odor of soap, coffee, tobacco, or vanilla can be detected in each nostril. Ammonia and similar pungent substances should not be used because they stimulate trigeminal rather than olfactory nerve endings. Visual acuity in each eye can be assessed by reading newsprint or a Snellen chart. The visual fields should be outlined by confrontation testing and suspected abnormalities checked by computerized perimetry. The size of the pupils and their reactivity to light and accommodation and the range and quality of ocular movements should be noted and the optic fundi (discs, retinae, and blood vessels) carefully inspected.

Sensation over the face is tested with a pin and wisp of cotton and the presence or absence of corneal reflexes noted. Strength of facial muscles is determined by asking the patient to wrinkle his forehead, show his teeth, and forcibly close his eyes and purse his lips. Auditory perception is readily assessed by a number of tuning fork tests and most accurately by formal audiograms. Inspection of the tongue at rest on the floor of the mouth and when protruded may disclose discoloration, loss of papillae, atrophy, fasciculations, tremor, and weakness. Testing of the jaw jerk and buccal and sucking reflexes should not be overlooked, particularly if there is a question of dysarthria and dysphagia or signs of corticospinal tract disease.

Details of these test procedures are described in Chaps. 12 (olfaction and taste), 13 (vision), 14 (ocular movement and pupils), and 15 (hearing and vestibular function).

c. Testing of motor, sensory, and reflex functions A number of simple maneuvers will disclose the strength, coordination, and speed of movements: asking the patient to maintain both arms outstretched or both legs against gravity; alternately touch his nose and the examiner's finger; trace a circle and square with the finger; make rapid alternating movements; button his clothes, open and close a safety pin, and handle common tools; stand and walk on toes and heels; arise from a kneeling and squatting position without help; run the heel down the front of the shin; rhythmically tap the heel on the shin; and touch and follow the examiner's finger with the toe. No examination of motor function is complete without observing the patient's stance and gait and presence or absence of tremor, involuntary movements, and abnormalities of posture and muscle tone; the last is evaluated by passively manipulating the limbs. Peak power of muscular contraction and muscle strength in opposition to that of the examiner is readily assessed and graded. Apraxia, the inability to make requested learned motor acts in the face of preserved strength and sensation, is mentioned above.

The testing of the biceps, triceps, supinator (radial-periosteal), patellar, Achilles, and cutaneous abdominal and plantar reflexes provides an adequate sampling of reflex activity of the spinal cord. Elicitation of a tendon reflex requires a brisk tap on the tendinous insertion of a muscle that is relaxed and partially stretched. Some individuals, particularly those with large muscles, have barely obtainable tendon reflexes that may be reinforced by having the patient pull against interlocked hands (Jendrassic maneuver). When the tendon reflexes are lively, there may be spread to adjacent muscle groups. An extensor plantar reflex (*Babinski sign*) is an unequivocal indicator of corticospinal tract dysfunction; it is elicited by stroking the lateral aspect of the sole with a key or similar object. A positive response consists of dorsiflexion of the large toe, often with slight fanning of the other digits, sometimes with flexion of the leg at knee and hip.

Additional items of the motor examination are considered in Chaps. 3 to 7, which deal with motor paralysis, abnormalities of movement coordination, posture, and disorders of stance and gait, respectively. Particulars of *sensory testing*, the most difficult part of the neurologic examination, are described in the chapters on pain and other forms of somatic sensation (Chaps. 8 and 9). The usual tests are the detection of vibration (using a 128-Hz tuning fork applied to the toes and fingers), touch, pin prick, and joint position sense. The assessment of bladder, bowel, and other autonomic functions is considered in Chap. 26 and meningeal signs in Chaps. 17 and 30.

3. Examination of the Comatose, Psychiatric, and Pediatric Patient

In each of these situations, the neurologic examination, though subject to obvious limitations, may yield considerable information concerning nervous system function. Adaptation of the neurologic examination to the *stuporous or comatose patient* is described in Chap. 17.

In the examination of *patients with psychiatric disorders*, one cannot always rely on the patient's cooperation and must always be critical of his statements and opinions. The depressed patient, for example, may complain of weakness or impairment of memory when neither is present; the sociopath may feign paralysis. Information from a person who knows the patient intimately is mandatory. The special methods of examination of *infants and small children* are summarized in Chap. 28.

PURPOSE OF THE CLINICAL METHOD IN NEUROLOGY

The primary objective of diagnosis is to effect treatment or prevention of disease. Failure to recognize an untreatable disease is a less serious fault than overlooking a treatable one. In general, errors in neurologic diagnosis are traceable to (1) inaccurate history, (2) the misinterpretation of neurologic signs or the overinterpretation of minor and insignificant normal phenomena as symptoms and signs of serious diseases, (3) lack of familiarity with the most common of the almost countless diseases of the nervous system, and (4) the occurrence of unusual variants of well-known diseases.

For a more detailed discussion of this topic, see Victor and Ropper: *Adams and Victor's Principles of Neurology*, 7th ed, pp 3–11.

ADDITIONAL READING

Berg BO (ed): *Principles of Child Neurology*. New York, McGraw-Hill, 1996, pp 5–22.

Bickerstaff ER, Spillane JA: *Neurological Examination in Clinical Practice*, 5th ed. Oxford, Blackwell Scientific, 1989.

Folstein MF, Folstein SE, McHugh PR: "Mini-mental status": A practical method for grading the cognitive state of patients for the clinician. *J Psychiatr Res* 12:189, 1975.

Glick TH: *Neurologic Skills: Examination and Diagnosis*. Boston, Blackwell, 1993.

Holmes G: *Introduction to Clinical Neurology*, 3rd ed. Revised by Bryan Matthews. Baltimore, Williams & Wilkins, 1968.

Mayo Clinic: *Clinical Examinations in Neurology*, 7th ed. St. Louis, Mosby, 1998.

Ross RT: *How to Examine the Nervous System*, 3rd ed. Stamford, CT, Appleton & Lange, 1999.

2 | Special Techniques for Neurologic Diagnosis

Clinical analysis alone may prove adequate for diagnosis, but more often it must be supplemented by one or more ancillary examinations. The frequency with which one resorts to these tests depends in large measure on the type of clinical problem and on the clinical experience and confidence of the physician. In turning to the laboratory for help, the clinician should choose the one or two procedures that are most likely to solve the problem and not blindly subject the patient to one test after another. The thoughtful selection of laboratory procedures is part of the strategy of case study and the intelligent use of medical resources. Their selection should not be dictated by curiosity alone or by a presumed need to protect oneself against litigation.

Without question, the most significant advance in neurology and neurosurgery since the discovery of roentgen rays has been the development of computerized imaging techniques [computed tomography (CT) and magnetic resonance imaging (MRI)]. These techniques permit the visualization of all parts of the brain and spinal cord and much of the vasculature in a living patient as well as many of the lesions residing within them, all accomplished with practically no risk to the patient. A new branch of medical science, *biopathology*, has been created. The older, painful, and potentially dangerous techniques of pneumoencephalography and ventriculography have been eliminated, and the need for conventional angiography and myelography has been greatly reduced. Angiography is now used mainly to expose vascular abnormalities in planning an operation on a vascular tumor or malformation, to quantify the degree of vascular narrowing, and to detect the presence of vasculitis. Plain films of the skull are relied upon only to reveal fractures and certain abnormalities at the craniocervical junction. Even cerebrospinal fluid (CSF) examinations and electroencephalograms (EEGs) are being done less frequently. CSF examinations are used mainly in the diagnosis of infective and noninfective inflammations and tumor invasion of the brain and meninges and in confirming the diagnosis of multiple sclerosis and small subarachnoid hemorrhages; EEGs are used mainly to study seizures and toxic and metabolic disturbances.

The following ancillary procedures have application to a large number of diverse neurologic diseases. Procedures that are pertinent to a particular disease or category of diseases are discussed in the chapters dealing with those entities.

COMPUTED TOMOGRAPHY (CT SCANNING)

In this procedure, the x-ray attenuation of the skull, CSF, cerebral gray and white matter, and blood vessels is measured, with computer assistance, by more than 30,000 beams of x-ray directed successively at several horizontal (axial) or coronal levels of the cranium. The differing densities of bone and the intracranial (or intraspinal) contents are distinguishable in the resulting picture. One can see hemorrhages, arteriovenous malformations, softened and edematous tissue due to infarction or trauma, abscesses, and neoplasms as well as the precise size and position of the ventricles and changes in brain volume. The radiation exposure is equivalent to that from plain skull films.

The latest models of CT scanners yield pictures of great clarity. One can see the cerebral convolutions and sulci, caudate and lenticular nuclei, internal capsules, thalamus and hypothalamus, optic nerves and ocular muscles, and brainstem and cerebellum (Fig. 2-1). Destructive and invasive lesions of these parts are readily localized. Enhancement of CT images by infusion of contrast material demonstrates regions of blood-brain barrier breakdown and small lesions and vascular structures that are not otherwise visualized. Newer techniques (spiral CT contrast angiography) permit even better visualization of blood vessels. The main disadvantages of CT scanning are the obscuration of posterior fossa structures by bony artifacts and the failure to visualize early ischemic infarctions, sometimes for several days.

MAGNETIC RESONANCE IMAGING (MRI)

Like the CT scan, magnetic resonance imaging (MRI) provides images of thin slices of the brain in any plane. The resolution of MR images is higher

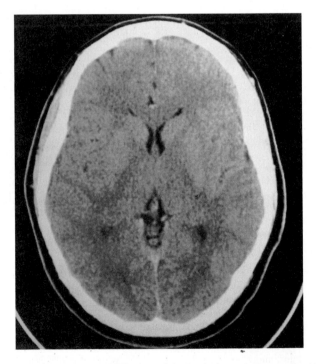

FIG. 2-1   Axial (horizontal) CT scan of the brain through the cerebral hemispheres at the level of the lenticular nuclei. The CSF in the lateral ventricles appears dark. The caudate nuclei and lenticular nuclei appear denser than the internal capsule.

than that of CT. MRI has the additional advantage of using nonionizing energy.

MRI is accomplished by placing the patient within a powerful magnetic field that causes the protons of the tissues and CSF to align themselves in the orientation of the magnetic field. Introducing a specific radio frequency (RF) pulse into the field causes the protons to resonate and to change their axes of alignment. Removal of the RF pulse allows the protons to relax, so to speak, and to resume their original alignment. The RF energy that was absorbed and then emitted is subjected to computer analysis, from which an image is constructed. By varying the RF energy and the method of detecting the energy released by proton relaxation, water, white matter, gray matter, and stagnant or flowing blood can be differentiated (by creating so-called T1, T2, FLAIR, proton-density, diffusion-weighted, and gradient echo images and MR angiography, or MRA).

The images generated by the latest MRI machines are truly remarkable. One can measure the size of all discrete nuclear structures, there being a high degree of contrast between white and gray matter. Deep lesions of the temporal lobe and structures in the posterior fossa and at the cervicomedullary junction and the contents of the spinal canal are seen much better than with CT; all these structures can be displayed in three planes and are unmarred by bony artifact (Fig. 2-2). Demyelinative lesions stand out with

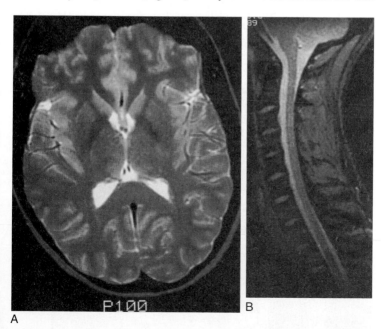

FIG. 2-2   *A.* MRI T2-weighted axial image of the brain at the level of the lenticular nuclei. The gray matter appears brighter than the white matter. The CSF within the lateral and third ventricles is very bright. The caudate nuclei, putamen, and thalamus appear brighter than the internal capsule. *B.* Gradient echo sagittal image of the cervical spine. The bright signal intensity of the CSF provides a "myelographic" effect. The craniocervical junction is clearly defined.

clarity. Unfortunately, at present, the MR images often show alterations of periventricular and central white matter that are uninterpretable, but they will soon be better understood. Each of the products of disintegrated red blood corpuscles—methemoglobin, hemosiderin, and ferritin—can be recognized, and this enables one to estimate the age and observe the resolution of hemorrhages. Infarcts can be seen at an earlier stage than by CT, and certain methods, such as diffusion-weighted imaging (DWI), can disclose infarctions within minutes of their onset. Special techniques are used to visualize the large arteries and veins [MRA (Fig. 2-3) and MR venography, or MRV]. The investigation of developmental defects of the nervous system by MRI is a new and promising field.

ANGIOGRAPHY

The injection of contrast material into cranial arteries permits the visualization of narrowed or occluded arteries and veins, arterial dissections, angiitis, vascular malformations, and saccular aneurysms. Since the advent of CT and MRI, the use of angiography has been more or less limited to the diagnosis of these disorders. The procedure consists of placing a needle in the femoral or brachial artery under local anesthesia; a cannula is threaded through the needle and then along the aorta and the arterial branch (carotid, vertebral) that needs to be visualized. Highly skilled arteriographers can also inject the collateral branches of the spinal arteries and visualize vascular malformations of the spinal cord.

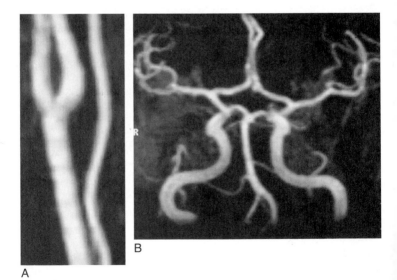

FIG. 2-3   Magnetic resonance angiogram (MRA). *A*. The cervical portions of the common, internal and external carotid and vertebral arteries. *B*. The intracranial circulation showing the circle of Willis and the middle and anterior cerebral and basilar arteries and their main branches.

A refinement of the standard angiographic technique—*digital subtraction angiography*—uses computer processing to improve the images of the major cervical arteries. The advantage of this technique is that the vessels can be visualized with small amounts of dye; the resolution obtained with current machines is comparable to that provided by standard x-ray techniques. Angiography still causes an occasional fatality and a 2.5 percent morbidity, mainly in the form of a worsening of a preexisting vascular lesion or a hematoma or vascular occlusion at the puncture site.

ULTRASOUND SCANNING

This technique, which uses the Doppler shift reflected from flowing blood or sound waves reflected from fixed structures, has been improved to the point where it can be used to insonate the great vessels in the neck (carotid, vertebral), the basal intracranial vessels, and the infant cerebrum. Its main uses are in detecting carotid artery stenosis (discussed in Chap. 34) in the adult and periventricular matrix hemorrhage in the neonate. Transcranial Doppler insonation is used to assess the blood flow and caliber of the large intracranial vessels.

POSITRON EMISSION TOMOGRAPHY (PET) AND SINGLE PHOTON EMISSION COMPUTED TOMOGRAPHY (SPECT)

These techniques utilize radioactive tracers to demonstrate blood flow and brain metabolism. They are used mainly in the special study of certain cerebrovascular diseases and dementias, to localize epileptogenic lesions, and to distinguish cerebral tumor from adjacent radionecrosis.

LUMBAR PUNCTURE AND EXAMINATION OF CEREBROSPINAL FLUID

The *indications for a lumbar puncture* (LP) are as follows:

1. To obtain pressure measurements and to procure a sample of CSF for cellular, chemical, and bacteriologic examination
2. To administer spinal anesthetics and certain antibiotic and antitumor medications
3. To inject a radiopaque substance, as in myelography, or a radioactive agent, as in scintigraphic cisternography

If, because of a localized mass, the intracranial pressure (ICP) is very high, LP carries a risk of inducing or aggravating a temporal lobe or cerebellar herniation. Therefore, if a high ICP is suspected, the LP should be preceded by CT or MRI, which with clinical data may yield sufficient diagnostic information to obviate the need for an LP. Cisternal puncture and high cervical subarachnoid puncture are also safe procedures but should be done only by someone skilled in their performance.

The technique of lumbar puncture is described in *Adams and Victor's Principles of Neurology*, 7th ed. (p. 13). CSF pressure should be measured with the patient relaxed in a horizontal lateral decubitus position. Normally it ranges from 80 to 180 mmH$_2$O and, if the needle is properly placed, small pulse and respiratory excursions are seen. If the pressure is very high (>300 mmH$_2$O), one should obtain the smallest needed sample of fluid and then, according to the suspected disease and patient's condition, administer mannitol and watch the pressure in the manometer until it falls.

The gross appearance of the CSF is noted, and samples are sent to the laboratory for some or all of the following examinations, depending on the nature of the clinical problem: number and types of cells and presence of microorganisms; protein and glucose content (with simultaneous blood glucose measurement); exfoliative cytology using a Millipore-filtered or ultracentrifuged specimen; protein electrophoresis and immunoelectrophoresis for determination of gamma globulin, other protein fractions, oligoclonal bands, and the IgG-albumin index; biochemical tests for pigments, lactate, NH_3, pH, CO_2, enzymes, etc.; and bacteriologic cultures and virus isolation.

If the fluid is hazy or has a yellow-red coloration (xanthochromia), it should be centrifuged immediately in a tube with a conical bottom to detect the presence of red blood cells. If the supernatant is clear, one may assume that any blood in the fluid was the result of a traumatic tap. However, a large bleed, spontaneous or traumatic, may contain sufficient serum to impart a yellow tint to the supernatant, as will hyperbilirubinemia. Certain viruses and other organisms that are difficult to isolate from the CSF (herpes simplex, Mycobacteria, prions, etc.) can now be detected by molecular amplification techniques.

The CSF examination is essential in detecting meningeal inflammation (meningitis), subarachnoid hemorrhage, and metastatic tumors in the meninges. An LP carries virtually no risk if the CT or MRI shows no mass lesion and papilledema is absent. Persistent leakage and low pressure of CSF may give rise to headache on sitting or standing. It usually subsides in a few days, but if not, it may be treated by the injection of 5 to 10 ml of autologous blood into the lumbar epidural space (blood patch, p. 257). Transient weakness of one or both lateral rectus muscles is another less frequent but alarming complication of LP.

RADIOPAQUE MYELOGRAPHY

By injecting 5 to 25 mL of a water-soluble dye through a lumbar puncture needle and then tilting the patient, one can visualize the entire spinal subarachnoid space. The procedure is almost as harmless as the lumbar puncture. In combination with CT scanning, myelography is a particularly useful method for visualizing the cervical spinal canal and exposing ruptured intervertebral discs, exostoses, and tumors. Although this procedure is gradually being replaced by MRI, it still finds use in complicated cases.

ELECTROENCEPHALOGRAPHY

This is an essential technique for the study of patients with epilepsy and those with suspected seizure disorders. It is also helpful in evaluating the cerebral effects of toxic and metabolic diseases, in studying sleep disorders, and in identifying certain unique disorders such as subacute spongiform encephalopathy (Chap. 33).

The instrument for recording electrical activity of the brain, the *electroencephalograph*, comprises 8 to 16 or more separate amplifying units capable of recording from many areas of the scalp at the same time. The electrical brain rhythms passing through cranial bones and scalp are amplified to the point where they are strong enough to move pens, producing a waveform activity in the range of 0.5 to 30 Hz (cycles per second) on a paper moving at 3 cm/s. Increasingly, pen recordings are being replaced by digital techniques that can be viewed on a computer and stored more efficiently than paper records. The resulting trace, or *electroencephalogram (EEG)*—in reality a voltage-versus-time graph—appears as a number of parallel wavy lines, as many as there are amplifying units or "channels." Electrodes, which usually are solder or silver-silver chloride discs 0.5 cm in diameter, are attached to the scalp by means of an adhesive material such as collodion and with conductive paste to improve contact. Patients are usually examined with their eyes closed and while relaxed in a comfortable chair or bed for 30 to 90 min.

In addition to the resting record, it is common practice to use several activating procedures, such as hyperventilation (for 3 min), stroboscopic retinal stimulation (at frequencies of 1 to 20 per second), and induced drowsiness or sleep. Examples of the normal EEG and of EEGs showing seizure discharges, both focal and generalized, hepatic coma with confusion, and brain death are presented in Fig. 2-4. EEGs in the different stages of sleep are described in Chap. 19.

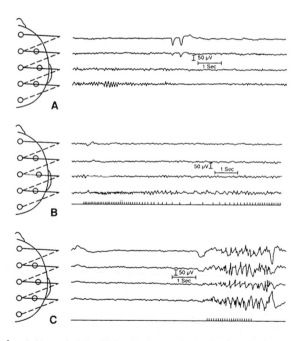

FIG. 2-4 *A.* Normal alpha (9- to 10-per-second) activity is present posteriorly (bottom channel). The top channel contains a large blink artifact. Note the striking reduction of the alpha rhythm with eye opening. *B.* Photic driving. During stroboscopic stimulation of a normal subject, a visually evoked response is seen posteriorly after each flash of light (signaled on the bottom channel). *C.* Stroboscopic stimulation at 14 flashes per second (bottom channel) has produced a photoparoxysmal response in this epileptic patient, evidenced by the spike and slow-wave activity toward the end of the period of stimulation.

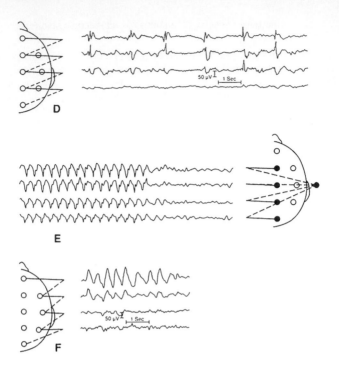

FIG. 2-4 *(continued)* *D.* EEG of patient with focal motor seizures of the left side. Note focal spike discharge in right frontal region (channels 1–3). The activity from the left hemisphere (not shown here) was relatively normal. *E.* Petit mal (absence) epilepsy, showing generalized 3-per-second spike-and-wave discharges. The abnormal activity ends abruptly, and a normal background appears. *F.* Large, slow, irregular delta waves are seen in the right frontal region (channels 1 and 2). In this case, a glioblastoma was found in the right cerebral hemisphere, but the EEG picture does not differ basically from that produced by infarction, abscess, or contusion.

EVOKED POTENTIALS

By the use of computers, one can summate the effects of several thousand visual, auditory, or tactile stimuli and trace them from the periphery to their cerebral terminations. This enables one to detect delays at several points along the course of these sensory pathways, even when there are no clinically manifest sensory symptoms. If visual, auditory, or tactile deficits are present, one can determine at what point the deficit lies. These techniques have found their main use in the diagnosis of multiple sclerosis. Details of the technique of evoked potential testing and the normal interwave latencies are to be found in *Adams and Victor's Principles of Neurology*, 7th ed. (pp. 34–39).

MAGNETIC CORTICAL STIMULATION

A single-pulse high-voltage stimulus applied to the vertex of the skull or over the cervical spine segments can painlessly activate the motor cortex

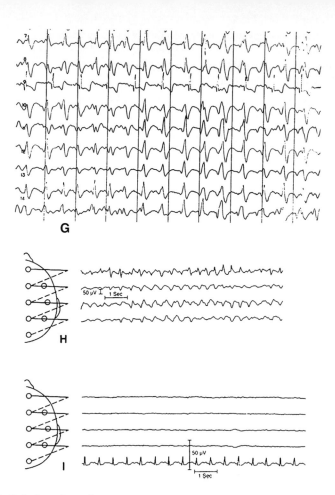

FIG. 2-4 *(continued)* G. Grossly disorganized background activity interrupted by repetitive discharges consisting of large, sharp waves from all leads about once per second. This pattern is characteristic of Creutzfeldt-Jakob disease. *H.* Advanced hepatic coma. Slow (about 2-per-second) waves have replaced the normal activity in all leads. This record demonstrates the triphasic waves sometimes seen in this disorder (channel 1). *I.* Deep coma following cardiac arrest, showing electrocerebral silence. With the highest amplification, ECG and other artifacts may be seen, so that the record is not truly "flat" or isoelectric. However, no cerebral rhythms are visible. Note the ECG (bottom channel).

and corticospinal system. With this method one can detect delays or lack of conduction in descending motor pathways.

ELECTROMYOGRAPHY, NERVE CONDUCTION STUDIES, AND NERVE AND MUSCLE BIOPSY

These are described in Chap. 44. Biopsies of skin, conjunctivum, and brain are sometimes diagnostic and are mentioned in relation to the particular diseases in which they are indicated.

PERIMETRY, AUDIOMETRY, AND TESTS OF LABYRINTHINE FUNCTION

These tests relating to vision, hearing, and balance are described in Chaps. 13 and 15.

PSYCHOMETRY AND NEUROPSYCHOLOGIC TESTING

The measurement of intelligence and the quantification of several aspects of intellectual function, behavior, and emotion are used in the diagnosis of dementia, developmental disorders, and psychiatric diseases (Chaps. 56, 57, and 58).

GENETIC AND OTHER LABORATORY TESTS

Because of rapid advances in molecular genetics, the clinician now has available blood (DNA) testing for the presence of or vulnerability to a number of inherited diseases, such as Huntington chorea, Charcot-Marie-Tooth neuropathy, amyloidosis, certain muscular dystrophies, and the mitochondrial disorders. Testing for these diseases is mentioned in the appropriate chapters.

In addition to these many special laboratory techniques, one often obtains useful information about metabolic and toxic disorders of the brain by analysis of blood samples for O_2, CO_2, glucose, BUN, NH_3, Na, K, Mg, Ca, thyroxin, B_{12}, cortisol, amino acids, and a wide variety of drugs and toxins.

For a more detailed discussion of this topic, see Victor and Ropper: *Adams and Victor's Principles of Neurology*, 7th ed, pp 12–41.

ADDITIONAL READING

Bigner SH: Cerebrospinal fluid (CSF) cytology: Current status and diagnostic applications. *J Neuropathol Exp Neurol* 51:235, 1992.

Chiappa KH (ed): *Evoked Potentials in Clinical Medicine*, 2nd ed. New York, Lippincott-Raven, 1997.

den Hartog Jager WA: *Color Atlas of CSF Cytopathology*. New York, Elsevier/North Holland, 1980.

Fishman RA: *Cerebrospinal Fluid in Diseases of the Nervous System*, 2nd ed. Philadelphia, Saunders, 1992.

Gilman S: Imaging of the brain. *N Engl J Med* 338:812, 889, 1998.

Greenberg JO (ed): *Neuroimaging: A Companion to Adams and Victor's Principles of Neurology*, 2nd ed. New York, McGraw-Hill, 1999.

Latchaw RE (ed): *Computed Tomography of the Head, Neck, and Spine*, 2nd ed. St. Louis, Mosby/Year Book, 1991.

Lee SH, Rao KCVG, Zimmerman RA (eds): *Cranial MRI and CT*, 4th ed. New York, McGraw-Hill, 1999.

Modic MT, Masaryk TJ, Ross JS, et al: *Magnetic Resonance Imaging of the Spine*, 2nd ed. St. Louis, Mosby/Year Book, 1994.

Niedermeyer E, Da Silva FL: *Electroencephalography*, 3rd ed. Baltimore, Urban and Schwarzenberg, 1993.

Osborn AG: *Diagnostic Neuroradiology*. St. Louis, Mosby/Year Book, 1994.

Thompson EJ: Cerebrospinal fluid. *J Neurol Neurosurg Psychiatry* 59:349, 1995.

PART II | CARDINAL MANIFESTATIONS OF NEUROLOGIC DISEASE

3 | Motor Paralysis

The terms *paralysis, plegia,* and *palsy* are used more or less interchange-ably. Customarily, paralysis designates complete or almost complete loss of motor power; *paresis* refers to partial paralysis. On the basis of clinical examination and physiologic study, two types of paralysis or paresis can be recognized: (1) one due to involvement of lower motor neurons and (2) another due to involvement of upper motor neurons (corticospinal and corticobulbar systems).

DISORDERS OF LOWER MOTOR NEURONS

Anatomic and Physiologic Considerations

The *lower motor neurons* include all the anterior horn cells (alpha neurons) of the spinal cord and the somatic motor neurons of the brainstem. Each motor neuron, by way of its axon, innervates from 20 to 1000 or more mus-cle fibers; together, the nerve cell, its axon, and the innervated muscle fibers constitute the *motor unit* and are known physiologically as the *final common pathway*. All variations in force, range, and speed of movement are deter-mined by the number and size of motor units and their rates of discharge. Destruction of the motor nerve cell or its axon paralyzes all the muscle fibers that it innervates regardless of whether they are engaged in reflex or voluntary activity. In some conditions (e.g., motor system disease, ventral root compression), the motor neuron becomes abnormally irritable, resulting in repeated spontaneous contractions of all its muscle fibers. This is mani-fest clinically as coarse twitches or *fasciculations* and, if many units are involved, as cramps or spasms. Fasciculations without weakness, atrophy, or reflex loss are nearly always benign. Fasciculations differ from the smaller independent contractions of individual muscle fibers that have lost their nerve supply (i.e., are denervated); the latter, called *fibrillations*, are generally too small to be observed by the naked eye but are detectable by electromyography.

The axons of many motor nerve cells form the anterior spinal roots and motor parts of the cranial nerves. Many roots intermingle to form plexuses. From the latter emerge individual nerves wherein motor fibers are mixed with sensory and autonomic ones. Each large muscle is supplied by several adjacent roots but usually by only a single nerve. Therefore, the pattern of paralysis following disease of anterior horn cells and roots differs from that following interruption of individual nerves.

Any given movement requires the activity of many muscles, some acting as prime movers or agonists, others as antagonists, fixators, or synergists. These relationships are integrated in the spinal cord or brainstem, an arrangement known as *reciprocal innervation*. Complex motor activities such as flexor withdrawal responses, support reactions, crossed extensor and tonic neck reflexes, the maintenance of tone, posture, stance and gait, and the performance of voluntary and habitual actions depend on intersegmental spinal mechanisms and their integration with corticospinal and other suprasegmental systems.

The *myotatic or tendon reflex* depends on the sudden stretch excitation of the muscle spindles, which lie parallel to muscle fibers (Fig. 3-1). The afferent impulses from the spindles are conducted to the corresponding spinal segments and are transmitted by direct (monosynaptic) connections to the alpha motor neurons. The small gamma motor neurons keep the muscle fibers of the spindle in a proper state of tension. There are also sensory nerve endings in muscle such as Golgi tendon organs, which are sensitive to tension and may induce inhibition. In the spinal cord, this inhibition is mediated by Renshaw cells (1A inhibitory interneurons). Although the muscle spindle and the Golgi tendon organ have different effects on the pool of motor neurons, they are complementary in calibrating the range and force of movements.

A nociceptive or flexor withdrawal reflex is activated by the excitation of A-δ and small-caliber afferent C fibers; this is a polysynaptic reflex in which the afferent volleys excite many anterior horn cells (which flex the limb) and other motor neurons, which inhibit extensor antigravity muscles.

When all or practically all the anterior horn cells or their peripheral motor fibers are interrupted, all voluntary, postural, and reflex movements in the corresponding muscles are lost. The paralyzed muscles become lax and soft and offer little or no resistance to passive stretching. This state is referred to as *flaccidity* and is due to a loss of normal muscle tone (*atonia* or *hypotonia*). Also, the denervated muscles slowly undergo extreme atrophy, losing 70 to 80 percent of their normal bulk over a period of 3 to 4 months. By contrast, in atrophy due to disuse (e.g., limb in a plaster cast), the loss of bulk usually does not exceed 25 to 30 percent. In lower motor neuron paralysis, tendon reflexes are abolished and electrodiagnostic studies demonstrate a reduced amplitude of the muscle action potentials obtained by stimulating the nerve and the presence of fibrillation potentials in the affected muscles. By contrast, nonreflexive contractility in response to a direct tap on the muscle may be preserved (idiomuscular response).

The atrophic, areflexive paralysis of lower motor neuron disease varies with the location of the lesion. If combined with loss of sensory and autonomic function, it indicates disease of the peripheral nerve. If sensory changes are absent, the affliction is usually one of anterior horn cells (*spinal motor neuronopathy*), of anterior roots (*radiculopathy*), or of motor nerve fibers (*motor neuropathy*). The spinal form is exemplified by progressive muscular atrophy, amyotrophic lateral sclerosis, and poliomyelitis (now rare). The most common acute generalized radicular nerve disease, usually with less sensory than motor loss, is the Guillain-Barré syndrome.

Spinal motor neuron activity may under certain circumstances be enhanced, giving rise to muscle cramps, fasciculations, myokymia (continuous rippling activity of muscle), and spasms of diverse type. These phenomena are discussed in Chap. 55.

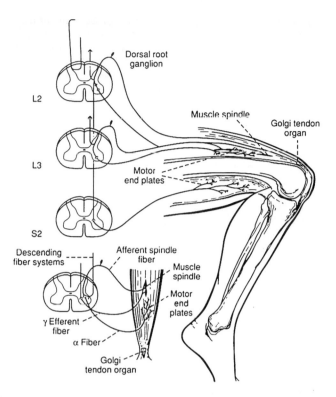

FIG. 3-1   Patellar tendon reflex. The principal receptors are the muscle spindles, which respond to a brisk stretching of the muscle effected by tapping the patellar tendon. Afferent fibers from muscle spindles are shown entering the L3 segment, while afferent fibers from the Golgi tendon organ are shown entering the L2 spinal segment. In this *monosynaptic reflex*, afferent fibers entering segments L2 and L3 and efferent fibers issuing from the anterior horn cells of these and contiguous lower levels complete the reflex arc. Motor fibers, which are shown leaving the S2 spinal segment and passing to the hamstring muscles, illustrate the disynaptic pathway by which inhibitory influences are exerted upon an antagonistic muscle group.

The small diagram illustrates the gamma loop. Gamma efferent fibers pass to the muscle spindle. Contraction of the intrafusal fibers in the polar parts of the spindle stretch the nuclear bag region and cause an afferent impulse to be conducted centrally. The afferent fibers from the spindle synapse with many alpha motor neurons, whose peripheral processes pass to extrafusal muscle fibers, thus completing the loop. Both alpha and gamma motoneurons are influenced by descending fiber systems from supraspinal levels. (*Redrawn, with permission, from Carpenter and Sutin.*)

DISORDERS OF THE CORTICOSPINAL AND OTHER UPPER MOTOR NEURONS

The motor cortex is defined physiologically as the electrically excitable region from which isolated movements can be evoked by stimuli of minimal intensity. Anatomically, this cortical region lies in the posterior part of the frontal lobes and comprises three areas: the precental (area 4), the premotor (area 6), and the supplementary motor area (SMA) on the medial surface of the superior frontal and cingulate convolutions. It is clear, however, that neurons outside these regions, mainly in the postcentral (sensory) gyrus, are capable of eliciting movement.

The descending motor pathways that originate in the motor cortex are designated as *pyramidal*, *corticospinal*, and *upper motor neuron*; the terms are often used interchangeably, but such usage is not completely accurate. Strictly speaking, the pyramidal tract is only the portion of the corticospinal system that passes through the pyramid of the medulla. A destructive lesion confined to the medullary pyramid does not fully reproduce the permanent hemiplegic paralysis that follows corticospinal lesions at higher levels. The direct corticospinal tract has its origin in the Betz cells of the motor cortex (numbering 25,000 to 30,000); in other neurons of the motor, premotor, and supplementary motor cortices; and in cells of several somatosensory regions of the parietal lobe (Brodmann's areas 1, 3, 5, and 7; see Fig. 22-2). The axons of all of these cells descend in the corona radiata and sequentially traverse the posterior limb of the internal capsule, cerebral peduncle, basis pontis, and medullary pyramid (Fig. 3-2). The pyramid contains approximately 1 million fibers, only 60 percent of which originate in the motor cortices. At the junction of the medulla and spinal cord, the majority (70 to 90 percent) of these fibers decussate and descend as the crossed lateral corticospinal pathway, synapsing at various segmental levels of the spinal cord—most with internuncial neurons, which, in turn, project to anterior horn cells; the remainder (20 to 25 percent) synapse directly with anterior horn cells. A smaller contingent of direct corticospinal tract fibers do not decussate and descend as the uncrossed anterior and lateral corticospinal tracts.

In the brainstem, the corticospinal tracts are accompanied by the corticobulbar tracts, which are distributed, after crossing the midline, to the motor nuclei of the cranial nerves. The corticospinal tract is the only direct long-fiber connection between the cerebral cortex and the spinal cord. Offshoots of the corticospinal tracts project to the red nuclei, forming the corticorubrospinal tract, the reticular formations of the brainstem (corticoreticulospinal), the mesencephalic tectum (corticotectospinal), the vestibular nuclei (corticovestibulospinal), and the pontine nuclei and cerebellum (corticopontocerebellar). These *indirect* corticobrainstem-spinal fibers, which do not run in the pyramid, are also involved in volitional as well as reflex and postural movement, supplementing the direct corticospinal system. Ascending sensory systems influence the motor ones at all levels. At the cortical level, motor activity is guided both by the prefrontal cortex (planning and programming of movement) and by sensory projections from the parietal cortex.

In all voluntary movements, the entire motor cortex is activated, but large numbers of neurons can be destroyed without causing weakness or causing only a loss of fine finger control.

Lesions that are restricted to the supplementary motor cortex result in a poverty of movement, akinesia, and mutism; this part, along with the prefrontal region, seems to be involved more in the planning of voluntary movement than in its execution. Lesions confined to the left (dominant) parietal cortex result in apraxia (see further on) and perseveration of move-

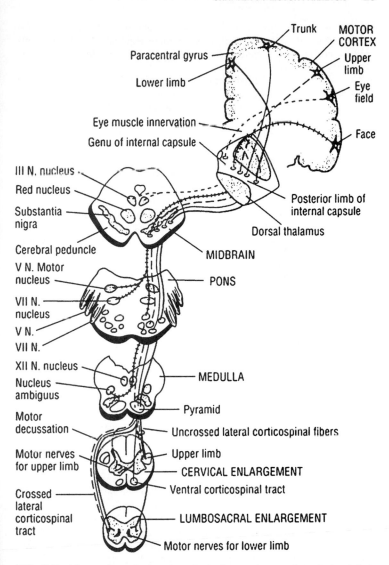

FIG. 3-2   The corticospinal and corticobulbar pathways, from their origin in the cerebral cortex to their nuclei of termination. Variable lines indicate the trajectories from particular parts of the cortex.

ment. With lesions confined to the primary motor area of the cortex there is weakness and hypotonia, without increase in tendon reflexes.

Throughout the corticospinal system the fibers are organized somatotopically. In the motor cortex, neurons innervating facial and pharyngeal muscles are located closest to the Sylvian fissure; those innervating the hand

and arm are located higher on the convexity; and those to the leg, on the medial surface of the frontal lobe. Fibers remain segregated, with those destined for cranial motor neurons lying anteriorly and those for the leg lying posteriorly at all levels.

The corticospinal and corticobulbar tracts (referred to collectively as the *upper motor neuron*) may be interrupted at any point in their course, from motor cortex to spinal cord, and the distribution of the paralysis indicates the level of the lesion. Always a group of muscles is involved, never single ones, and always the paralysis is incomplete, in that most of the reflex, postural, and automatic movements are preserved. A restricted cortical lesion may affect only one limb or even part of a limb. A lesion in the rolandic region of the convexity of the frontal lobe typically affects the hand and lower face. Lesions of the posterior limb of the capsule, where all the descending fibers are collected in a small cross-sectional area, paralyze the lower facial and tongue muscles and those of the arm and leg, always on the opposite side. Lesions below the caudal pons spare the face, tongue, and muscles of speech. The hand and arm are usually affected more severely than the foot and leg. Another general principle is that parts of the body most used for delicate fractionated movements—i.e., the fingers and hand—suffer the most from corticospinal lesions. Muscles that are engaged in bilateral, automatic, and reflexive movements, such as respiration, are hardly affected if at all. Weakness in ipsilateral limb muscles is barely detectable.

With acute lesions of the cerebrum and upper brainstem, the tendon reflexes, which at first are slightly reduced or unchanged, later become more active. There are also *postural changes*. The arm gradually becomes flexed and adducted and the leg extended, and the limbs become spastic. The flexors of hip, leg, and foot and the extensors of arm, hand, and fingers are weaker than their opposing muscles. Attempts at voluntary movement of a hand or foot may increase the tone or cause involuntary contraction of an entire limb (synkinesia). With acute lesions of the cervical or thoracic spinal segments, muscle tone and tendon reflexes may be abolished in the legs for days or weeks, a condition known as *spinal shock* (Chap. 44).

Highly characteristic of upper motor lesions is the phenomenon of *spasticity*, which occasionally may be evident from the time the lesion is incurred but usually becomes evident only after a delay of a week of two. Spasticity is revealed by the patient's attempts at active movement and by passive movement. In passive extension of the spastic arm, for example, there is first a brief nonresistant "free interval," followed by a velocity-dependent catch and rapidly increasing resistance, which gradually yields as the passive stretch is continued (*clasp-knife phenomenon*). In these ways, spasticity differs from the uniform resistance that characterizes *rigidity* (described in the next chapter). A severe hyperreflexive state often gives rise to *clonus*, which is a series of rhythmic involuntary muscular contractions in response to an abruptly applied and sustained passive or active stretching of a muscle group. It is most easily evoked at the ankle, knee, and wrist. The basis of spasticity, hyperreflexia, and clonus is a hyperexcitability of spinal motor neurons, which are released or disinhibited by the corticospinal lesions.

The cutaneomuscular (abdominal and cremasteric) reflexes are abolished, and nocifensor spinal reflexes, of which the Babinski sign is a part, are released. The *Babinski sign* is most consistently elicited by stroking the lateral side of the sole with a key or similar object; but when the spinal reflexes are greatly enhanced, even pinching or touching any part of the foot or leg may evoke the sign, which consists of dorsiflexion of the toes and foot and flexion at the knee and hip. Usually, with a corticospinal lesion, both a Babinski sign and heightened tendon reflexes are present; but since they depend on different mechanisms, they need not appear together in chronic paralysis. With bilateral cerebral lesions, the muscles innervated by the motor nuclei of the brainstem may be paralyzed and their stretch reflexes exaggerated; i.e., jaw and buccal jerks are increased (pseudobulbar palsy, see further on).

Extensive lesions of the motor system liberate a number of abnormalities of posture that are normally under brainstem control. The ones most clearly exposed by disease are decerebrate rigidity and the antigravity support and righting reflexes. In *decerebrate rigidity*, in which the vestibular nuclei are separated from upper brainstem influences and thereby disinhibited, all four limbs or the arm and leg on one side (ipsilateral to a unilateral lesion) are extended and the cervical and thoracolumbar portions of the spine are dorsiflexed; tonic neck reflexes can often be elicited (passive turning of the head results in ipsilateral extension of the limbs and flexion of the opposite arm). Lesions that involve the corticospinal tracts predominantly result not only in paralysis of the contralateral limbs but also in the development of a fixed posture, in which the arm is maintained in flexion and the leg in extension (*decorticate posture*).

While it is clinically convenient to think of motility in terms of upper and lower motor neurons, this is a gross oversimplification. All segments of the spinal cord are integrated in posture and movement, under indirect control of the cerebellar, vestibular, and other brainstem systems, the basal ganglia, and the motor cortices. Some idea of the complexity of the motor system is conveyed by considering the simple act of scratching an insect bite, which involves the action of more than 70 muscles arranged in many patterns, most of them acting involuntarily.

DIAGNOSIS OF PARALYTIC STATES

The term *monoplegia* designates a paralysis of one limb; *hemiplegia*, paralysis of an arm and leg on the same side; *paraplegia* (sometimes referred to as *diplegia*), paralysis of both legs; and *quadriplegia* or *tetraplegia*, paralysis of all four limbs.

Bulbar paralysis, or *palsy*, refers to weakness or paralysis of the muscles innervated by the motor nuclei of the lower brainstem (i.e., muscles of the face, tongue, larynx, and pharynx). The paralysis may be atrophic and flaccid (i.e., lower motor neuron in type), in which case it is most often due to a degeneration of the lower cranial motor nuclei, as occurs in amyotrophic lateral sclerosis. If both right and left corticobulbar pathways are interrupted, voluntary movements of the bulbar musculature are paralyzed, whereas reflexive movements are retained or heightened and muscle atrophy is not evident; this state is referred to as *spastic bulbar* or "*pseudobulbar*" palsy (see also pp. 196 and 205).

An *atrophic monoplegia* with loss of tendon reflexes points to a lesion of the anterior horn cells or, if there are also sensory or autonomic changes, to a lesion of the peripheral nerves. In the absence of atrophy or reflex loss, monoplegia suggests a unilateral spinal cord or, rarely, a restricted cerebral cortical-subcortical lesion.

Hemiplegia with retained or heightened reflexes is the common manifestation of a lesion in the cerebral white matter, internal capsule, cerebral peduncle, basis pontis, or pyramid. Most often it is due to vascular disease, less often to trauma, tumor, or an infective or demyelinative process. If facial muscles are spared, the lesion is in the lower brainstem or high cervical cord. Since brainstem and cord lesions are often bilateral, other motor cranial nerve or nonmotor signs may be added and indicate the level of the corticospinal lesion.

Paraplegia with retained or heightened tendon reflexes indicates involvement of the motor pathways in the thoracic or upper lumbar cord; *quadriplegia*, or *tetraplegia*, points to interruption of motor tracts in the cervical cord, brainstem, or both cerebral hemispheres. *Triplegia* is usually a transitional state in the development of quadriplegia, due most often to lesions at the cervicomedullary junction. Lesions confined to the gray matter of the spinal cord may cause an atrophic, areflexive paralysis of the legs or arms (central cord lesion). Paralysis of individual muscles points to a lesion of anterior horn cells or a peripheral nerve lesion (see above).

One must always remember that *paresis or paralysis may occur in the absence of any disease in the central or peripheral nervous system.* Conditions such as myasthenia gravis, polymyositis, periodic paralysis, severe endocrine and electrolytic disturbances, and botulism constitute this category and are considered in the section on diseases of muscle. Also, paralysis is the most common manifestation of *hysteria* or *malingering.* Usually such a diagnosis is suggested by inconsistencies of voluntary contraction (ability to perform some acts but not others that utilize the same muscles), an obvious lack of effort, lack of reflex changes, and the presence of other symptoms and signs of hysteria (see Chap. 56).

APRAXIA

This term, introduced by Liepmann in 1900, refers to the inability to perform learned patterns of movement in the absence of upper or lower motor neuron signs, ataxia, or extrapyramidal disorder. In Liepmann's view, apraxia could be subdivided into three types—*ideational, ideomotor,* and *kinetic.* In ideational apraxia, there is a failure to conceive or formulate an act, either spontaneously or on command. The anatomic substrate of this activity is thought to be in the dominant parietal lobe. In ideomotor apraxia, the patient may know and remember the planned action but cannot execute it with either hand—presumably because of interruption of connections between the dominant parietal lobe and the supplementary and premotor cortices of both cerebral hemispheres. Kinetic limb apraxia refers to clumsiness of a limb in the performance of a skilled act that cannot be accounted for by paresis, ataxia, or sensory loss. Frontal lobe lesions account for most cases. One tests for apraxia by observing the patient as he engages in tasks such as washing, shaving, and eating. Next the patient is asked to perform a series of symbolic acts—saluting, waving goodbye, blowing a kiss, pretending to comb the hair or brush the teeth. If he fails, he is given the proper utensils with which to perform the act and asked to imitate the examiner. This subject is described further in Chap. 22.

For a more detailed discussion of this topic, see Victor and Ropper: *Adams and Victor's Principles of Neurology*, 7th ed, pp 47–66.

ADDITIONAL READING

Alexander GE, DeLong M: Central mechanisms of initiation and control of movement, in Asbury AK, McKhann GM, McDonald WI (eds): *Diseases of the Nervous System*, 2nd ed. Philadelphia, Saunders, 1992, pp 285–308.

Asanuma H: The pyramidal tract, in Brooks VB (ed): *Handbook of Physiology*, sec 1: *The Nervous System*, vol 2: *Motor Control*. Bethesda, MD, American Physiological Society, 1981, pp 702–733.

Brown P: Pathophysiology of spasticity. *J Neurol Neurosurg Psychiatry* 57:773, 1994.

Carpenter MD, Sutin J: *Human Neuroanatomy*, 8th ed. Baltimore, Williams & Wilkins, 1983.

Ghez C, Krakauer J: The organization of movement, in Kandel ER, Schwartz JH, Jessel TM (eds): *Principles of Neural Science*, 4th ed. New York, Elsevier, 2000, pp 653–673.

Lance JW: The control of muscle tone, reflexes and movement: Robert Wartenburg Lecture. *Neurology* 30:1303, 1980.

Laplane D, Talairach J, Meininger V, et al: Motor consequences of motor area ablations in man. *J Neurol Sci* 31:29, 1977.

Luria AR: *The Working Brain: An Introduction to Neuropsychology*. New York, Basic Books, 1973.

Porter R, Lemon R: *Corticospinal Function and Voluntary Movement*. Oxford, UK, Oxford University Press, 1994.

4 | Abnormalities of Movement and Posture due to Disease of the Basal Ganglia

In this chapter and the next, we consider a second group of motor abnormalities that do not materially reduce muscular power but render it less effective because of rigidity, incoordination, alterations of posture, or the interposition of involuntary movements. These disorders are appropriately subdivided into (1) those due to diseases of the *basal ganglia* (caudate and lenticular nuclei, subthalamic nucleus [also called nucleus of Luys, or corpus Luysii], substantia nigra, red nucleus, and pontomesencephalic reticular formation) and (2) those due to diseases of the *cerebellum*. This chapter deals with the basal ganglionic, or striatonigral, system, disorders of which are called by convention *extrapyramidal movement disorders*. The cerebellar disorders are considered in the following chapter.

In health, the basal ganglionic functions blend with and modulate the corticospinal and corticobulbar motor systems described in Chap. 3. Physiologic studies of primates inform us that in the performance of all planned and learned movements, the basal ganglia and cerebellum, which are partly under cerebral-cortical control, are activated before the corticospinal-corticobulbar systems. Despite these close functional relationships, the division between pyramidal and extrapyramidal motor systems remains a useful if not an essential concept (Table 4-1).

STRIATONIGRAL DISORDERS

As indicated in Figs. 4-1 and 4-2, the prefrontal, premotor, and supplementary motor cortices send fibers to the caudate nucleus and putamen (together referred to as the *striatum*), as do other parts of the cerebral cortex. It is estimated that in each cerebral hemisphere there are 110 million corticostriatal neurons (compared to 1 million corticospinal neurons). The striatal neurons are of many types and sizes and project to the lateral and medial parts of the pallidum (globus pallidus); the lateral, or external, segment has to-and-fro connections with the subthalamic nucleus, which projects in turn to the internal segment of the pallidum and the pars reticulata (nonpigmented part) of the substantia nigra. The putamen and caudate nuclei receive recurrent fibers from the pigmented cells of the substantia nigra. From the pallidum, particularly its medial segment, two bundles of efferent fibers—the ansa and fasciculus lenticularis—sweep medially and caudally to synapse with the ventrolateral and intralaminar thalamic nuclei. The latter nuclei are also the terminus of a major and distinct pathway of fibers from the dentate nuclei of the cerebellum and the red nuclei. Here, in the ventral tier of thalamic nuclei, basal ganglionic and cerebellar impulses are integrated and brought to bear on the corticospinal system. The ventrolateral thalamic nucleus sends fibers to the precentral and supplementary motor cortices (areas 6 and 8). Yet

TABLE 4-1 Clinical Differences between Corticospinal
and Extrapyramidal Syndromes

	Corticospinal	Extrapyramidal
Character of the alteration of muscle tone	Clasp-knife effect (spasticity); ± rigidity	Plastic rigidity throughout passive movement or intermittent (cogwheel rigidity); hypotonia in cerebellar disease
Distribution of hypertonus	Flexors of arms, extensors of legs	Flexors of limbs and trunk (predominantly) or extensors of all four limbs
Involuntary movements	Absent	Presence of tremor, chorea, athetosis, ballismus, dystonia
Tendon reflexes	Increased	Normal or slightly increased
Babinski sign	Present	Absent
Paresis of voluntary movement	Present	Absent or slight

another loop begins in the frontal (premotor) association areas of the cerebral cortex; it projects to the caudate nucleus and thalamus and then back to the prefrontal cortex. In addition, there are several subsidiary loops that involve the centromedian and parafascicular nuclei of the thalamus and the mesencephalic tegmental and subthalamic nuclei. Each structure has to-and-fro modulating connections with all other basal ganglionic structures. The association cortex, via its projecting loops through the basal ganglia, is activated in the initial phases of planned movement.

Physiologically, the basal ganglia have been thought to function as a kind of clearinghouse, in which, during any intended or programmed movement, one set of motor activities is facilitated and other unnecessary ones are suppressed. Thus they are essential in controlling the direction, speed, and amplitude of movement.

Pharmacologic studies have established that dopamine (synthesized from tyrosine and hydroxyphenylalanine) is the nigrostriatal transmitter. Dopamine is elaborated by pigmented nigral cells and has an inhibitory effect on receptors of striatal cells. Acetylcholine, which is formed by large striatal cells, has an excitatory effect. Dopamine and acetylcholine are antagonistic. The inhibitory effects of the pallidum are mediated by gamma aminobutyric acid (GABA) and enkephalin. The main projections from the cortex to the striatum are glutaminergic. The other important transmitters and pathways involved in basal ganglionic function are illustrated in Fig. 4-3.

Clinical Manifestations of Basal Ganglia Disease

In one class of extrapyramidal diseases, exemplified by Parkinson disease, the primary deficit is *akinesia* or *hypokinesia*, terms that refer to a failure of

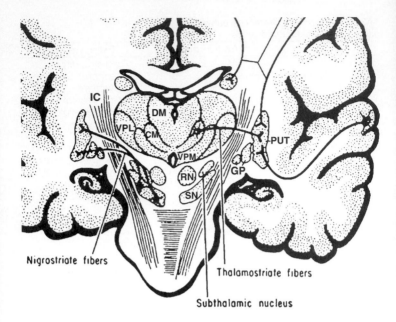

FIG. 4-1   Diagram of the striatal afferent pathways. *Corticostriate* fibers from broad cerebral-cortical areas project to the putamen; from the medial surface of the cortex, fibers project largely to the caudate nucleus. *Nigrostriate* fibers arise from the pars compacta of the substantia nigra. *Thalamostriate* fibers arise from the centromedian-parafascicular complex of the thalamus. CM, centromedial nucleus; DM, dorsomedial nucleus; GP, globus pallidus; IC, internal capsule; PUT, putamen; RN, red nucleus; SN, substantia nigra; VPL, ventral posterolateral nucleus; VPM, ventral posterior medial nucleus.

the patient to engage the limbs in customary activities. The resultant under-activity (*hypokinesia*, or *poverty of movement*) extends to all of the small automatic postural adjustments that are constantly being made by every normal person ("the patient sits still and the face is expressionless"). Also, there is a slight delay in the initiation of volitional and commanded movements (*delayed reaction time*) and slowness in their execution (*bradykinesia*). The basic defect appears to be an inadequacy of rapid (ballistic) movements. Several bursts of activation of agonist muscles are needed to complete the intended action. Alternating movements are particularly hampered. Bradykinesia is regularly accompanied by rigidity but is not caused by it (Table 4-2).

Rigidity is the second component of the parkinsonian syndrome. In contrast to spasticity, the increase in muscle tone is of plastic type, imparting an even resistance in agonists and antagonists from the start of a passive or active movement and throughout its range. There is little loss of muscle power or change in tendon reflexes.

A rhythmic, 3- to 5-per-second *tremor* in repose ("resting" tremor), affecting mainly the fingers, arms, and chin, is the third component of

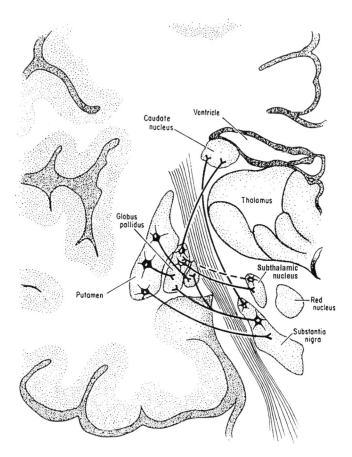

FIG. 4-2   Diagram of the basal ganglia, illustrating main striatal efferents. Also illustrated are the strong to-and-fro connections between the globus pallidus and the subthalamic nucleus.

Parkinson disease and is described in Chap. 6. It is temporarily suppressed by voluntary movements. Passive stretching of the hypertonic muscle exposes a rhythmically interrupted, ratchet-like resistance ("cogwheel phenomenon") and probably represents the superimposition of tremor on rigidity. Other types of tremor attributable to lesions in various parts of the extrapyramidal system are also described in Chap. 6.

These abnormalities are associated with a tendency to flexed postures—head down toward chest, shoulders rounded, and arms and knees slightly flexed. Other important manifestations are a loss of righting reactions and disorders of equilibrium and postural fixation. The standing or sitting patient cannot make appropriate postural adjustments to tilting or falling. These deficits underlie the characteristic abnormality of gait in Parkinson disease,

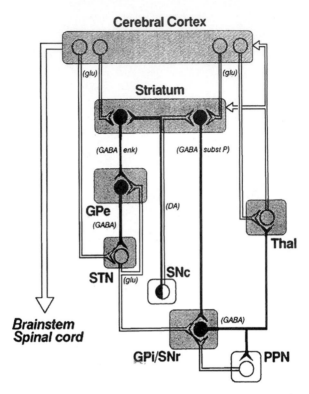

FIG. 4-3 Schematic diagram of the main putative neurotransmitter pathways and their effects in the cortical–basal ganglia–thalamic circuits. The solid circles and lines indicate neurons with excitatory effects, and the white circles and lines indicate inhibitory influences. The internal (medial) segment of the globus pallidus (GPi) and the zona reticulata of the substantia nigra (SNr) are believed to act as one entity that projects via GABA-containing neurons to the thalamus (ventrolateral and ventroanterior nuclei) and to the pedunculopontine nuclei (PPN). Dopaminergic neurons arising in the pars compacta of the substantia nigra (SNc) have an excitatory influence on one portion of the striatum and an inhibitory effect on the portion of the striatum that projects to the external (lateral) pallidum (GPe) and subthalamic nucleus (STN). This scheme is inferred from the effects of pharmacologic agents on the motor and electrophysiologic activities of each structure, but the results of surgical lesions are not always concordant with these principles. Substance P and enkephalin act as modulating neurotransmitters for GABA in pathways that project from the striatum. (glu = glutamine; DA = dopamine.) (*Reprinted with permission from Alexander GE, Crutcher MD: Functional architecture of basal ganglia circuits: Neural substrates of parallel processing.* Trends Neurosci *13:266, 1990.*)

in which the patient makes a series of quickening steps forward or backward, as though chasing his center of gravity (*festination*). Falls often result from the impairment of gait and postural reflexes. Impassivity of facial expression (*hypomimia*) and infrequent blinking complete the clinical picture.

TABLE 4-2 Clinicopathologic Correlations of Extrapyramidal
Motor Disorders

Symptoms	Principal location of lesion(s)
Unilateral plastic rigidity with static tremor (Parkinson syndrome)	Contralateral substantia nigra plus (?) other structures
Unilateral hemiballismus and hemichorea	Contralateral subthalamic nucleus of Luys or luysial-pallidal connections
Chronic chorea of Huntington type	Caudate nucleus and putamen
Athetosis and dystonia	Contralateral striatum; pathology of dystonia musculorum deformans unknown
Cerebellar incoordination, "intention" tremor, and hypotonia (Chap. 5)	Homolateral cerebellar hemi-sphere or middle and inferior cerebellar peduncles or brachium conjunctivum (ipsilateral if below decussation, contralateral if above)
Decerebrate rigidity (extension of arms and legs), opisthotonos	Usually bilateral in tegmentum of upper brainstem, at level of red nucleus or between red and vestibular nuclei
Palatal and facial myoclonus (rhythmic)	Ipsilateral central tegmental tract
Diffuse myoclonus	Neuronal degeneration, usually diffuse or predominating in cerebral or cerebellar cortex and dentate nuclei

The foregoing components of the parkinsonian syndrome are most often manifestations of nigrostriatal lesions; more widespread lesions involving striatum, pallidum, and substantia nigra may be associated with rigidity alone.

Involuntary movements—chorea, ballism, athetosis, and *dystonia*—are the other common signs of basal ganglionic disease.

Chorea refers to arrhythmic movements of a forcible, rapid, jerky type, affecting the fingers, hand, an entire limb, or some other part of the body. Grimacing and respiratory sounds are other expressions of the same disorder. Between movements, the affected limbs tend to be slack. Chorea may be limited to one side of the body (hemichorea); when the movements involve the proximal limb muscles and are unusually violent and flinging, the disorder is referred to as *hemiballismus*. Of all the movement disorders, hemiballismus has the most consistent pathologic anatomy. The lesion in such cases is in or adjacent to the subthalamic nucleus of the opposite side.

Chorea is the major manifestation of Sydenham chorea and chorea gravidarum, both thought to be immune disorders related to rheumatic fever. It is also a feature of Huntington disease, but in the latter the tendency is for the movements to be more confluent, or choreoathetotic. Hemichoreoathetosis may follow partial recovery from hemiplegia. Excessive administration of L-dopa in patients with Parkinson disease results in restricted or generalized choreoathetosis, and the latter is the most common form of tardive dyskinesia due to neuroleptic drugs (Chaps. 43 and 58). Choreoathetosis is also observed in a number of hereditary metabolic diseases (Chap. 37).

Athetosis is the term given to relatively slow, sinuous, patterned involuntary movements that have a tendency to flow into one another. In the limbs, attitudes of flexion-supination alternate with those of extension-pronation. Between movements, the affected limbs may be spastic or rigid, depending on the anatomy of the underlying disease, but often the limb is hypotonic. Cocontraction of agonists and antagonists interferes with effective projected movements, and efforts to contract one agonist group may spread to involve adjacent unneeded muscles (*intention spasm*, or *overflow phenomenon*).

Athetosis may be generalized—as in Huntington disease, double athetosis (due to perinatal hypoxia), chronic hepatic encephalopathy, drug intoxication (phenothiazines, haloperidol, L-dopa), and a variety of degenerative diseases of the basal ganglia (see Chap. 39)—or it may be restricted to one group of cervical or cranial muscles, as in idiopathic oromandibular and tardive dyskinesias and in spasmodic torticollis (see pp. 49 and 366). A rare paroxysmal form of choreoathetosis occurs in certain families. Athetosis and chorea are aggravated by fatigue and emotion and attenuated by repose.

Dystonia, or *torsion spasm*, is manifest as an abnormal contorted posture, classically in one or other of the extremes of athetoid movement, with a predilection for muscles of the trunk and limb girdles or a hand or foot. Dystonic postures also occur without an accompanying athetosis and may at first be reversible or phasic, but later they become fixed. A defining characteristic of dystonia is a cocontraction of corresponding agonist and antagonistic muscles when the affected body part assumes the abnormal posture. Like choreoathetosis, dystonia occurs as a manifestation of many heredodegenerative diseases, as an acute or chronic reaction to certain drugs (phenothiazines, haloperidol), or as a restricted form of extrapyramidal disease affecting facial, oromandibular, tongue, cervical, or hand muscles (see *Adams and Victor's Principles of Neurology*, 7th ed., for details).

Choreic, athetotic, and dystonic movements so often overlap that distinctions between them are probably not fundamental. To compound the difficulty, tremor, myoclonus, and ataxia are added in some cases. Some writers on this subject avoid ambiguities of classification by calling them all *dyskinesias*. The presumed anatomic locations of lesions causing the extrapyramidal movement disorders are summarized in Table 4-2.

Several aspects of the pathophysiology of involuntary movements have now been clarified. In dopamine-evoked choreoathetosis, certain of the putaminal cells appear to be overactive. In monkeys, lesions of the subthalamic nucleus, which normally exerts a strong inhibitory influence upon the globus pallidus and ventral thalamus, produce a "choreoid dyskinesia" of the opposite arm and leg; with removal of this regulatory effect, bursts of irregular choreoid activity are recorded in the intact pallidum, where they are believed to arise. Moreover, the choreoid dyskinesia can be abolished by a second lesion in the pallidum or in pallidofugal fibers or in the ventrolateral nucleus of the thalamus. It is postulated that the choreoathetotic movements of Huntington disease are also pallidal release effects, in this case from lesions in the caudal parts of the striatum.

For a more detailed discussion of this topic, see Victor and Ropper: *Adams and Victor's Principles of Neurology*, 7th ed, pp 67–85.

ADDITIONAL READING

Brodal A: Pathways mediating supraspinal influences on the spinal cord—The basal ganglia, in *Neurological Anatomy in Relation to Clinical Medicine*, 3rd ed. New York, Oxford University Press, 1981, chap 4, pp 180–293

Brooks VB: *The Neural Basis of Motor Control*. New York, Oxford University Press, 1986.

Carpenter MD, Sutin J: The corpus striatum, in *Human Neuroanatomy*, 8th ed. Baltimore, Williams & Wilkins, 1983, pp 579–607.

Marsden CD, Obeso JA: The functions of the basal ganglia and the paradox of stereotaxic surgery in Parkinson's disease. *Brain* 117:877, 1994.

Watts RL, Koller WC (eds): *Movement Disorders. Neurologic Principles and Practice*. New York, McGraw-Hill, 1997.

Young AB, Penny JB Jr: Pharmacologic aspects of motor dysfunction, in Asbury AK, McKhann GM, McDonald WI (eds): *Diseases of the Nervous System*, 2nd ed. Philadelphia, Saunders, 1992, pp 342–352.

5 | Incoordination and Other Disorders of Cerebellar Function

The structure and function of the cerebellum are somewhat less complex and better known than those of other parts of the nervous system. In terms of anatomy and function, the organ can be subdivided into three parts (Fig. 5-1):

1. The *flocculonodular lobe*, which is phylogenetically the oldest part. It is also known as the "vestibulocerebellum," since its main afferent projections are from the vestibular nuclei (via the inferior cerebellar peduncle); it is concerned mainly with the maintenance of equilibrium.
2. The *anterior lobe*, or *paleocerebellum*, consisting essentially of the anterior vermis and paravermian cortex. It is also called the "spinocerebellum," insofar as its afferent projections are from proprioceptors of muscles and tendons of the limbs via the spinocerebellar tracts. The spinocerebellum mainly influences posture and muscle tone and governs the coordination of the lower limbs (gait).
3. The *posterior lobes*, or *neocerebellum*, which consist of the middle portions of the vermis and their large lateral extensions; they form the major portions of the cerebellar hemispheres. The posterior lobes receive afferent fibers from the cerebral cortex via the pontine nuclei and middle cerebellar peduncle (brachium pontis) and are concerned with coordination of skilled movements initiated at a cerebral cortical level. The function of much of the neocerebellum is only partially known.

The efferent connections of the cerebellar cortex, consisting essentially of the axons of Purkinje cells, terminate on the deep cerebellar nuclei (dentate, globose, and fastigial nuclei). These, in turn, project to the cerebral cortex and certain brainstem nuclei (particularly the inferior olives) via three main pathways: (1) The crossed dentatorubrothalamic and dentatothalamic pathways, which together constitute the superior cerebellar peduncle. From the terminus of these pathways, in the ventrolateral thalamic nucleus (in a part different from the terminus of the cortical-striatal-pallidal projection), there is a projection to the pre- and postcentral cortices. (2) The fastigiovestibular pathways to the vestibular and brainstem reticular nuclei. (3) Direct connections with the alpha and gamma neurons in the ventral horns of the spinal cord. Thus, the cerebellum influences spinal motor activity indirectly, through its connections with the motor cortex and brainstem nuclei and their descending pathways, as well as through its direct spinal system. These main pathways are shown in Fig. 5-2. Each of these efferent cerebellar systems has its own chemical transmitter system. The cellular elements of the cerebellum have unique arrangements that allow for rapid integration of motor and sensory information, as discussed in *Adams and Victor's Principles of Neurology*, 7th ed. (pp. 90–93).

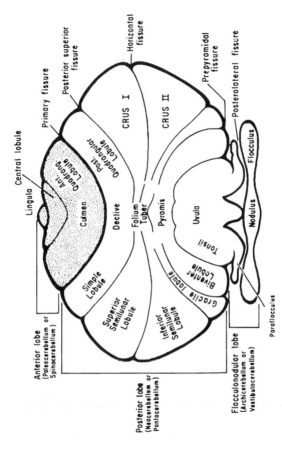

FIG. 5-1 Diagram of the cerebellum, illustrating the major fissures, lobes, and lobules and the major phylogenetic divisions (on the left).

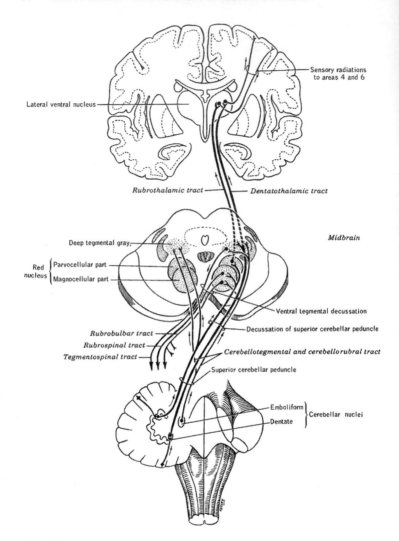

FIG. 5-2   Cerebellar projections to the red nucleus, thalamus, and cerebral cortex. *(Adapted from House EL et al: A Systematic Approach to Neuroscience, 3rd ed. New York, McGraw-Hill, 1979.)*

Thach's studies in primates have shown that the contribution of the cerebellum to the initiation and control of movement entails a corticopontine-cerebellar-thalamocortical circuitry, which functions in large measure before the motor cortex is activated. It is interesting that *planned voluntary activity is prepared by the frontal lobes, basal ganglia, and cerebellum.*

CEREBELLAR SYMPTOMS

Lesions of the cerebellum give rise to (1) incoordination (ataxia) of volitional movement, (2) disorders of equilibrium and gait, (3) a tremor that derives from ataxia and hypotonia, and (4) a reduction in muscle tone. Lesions of the cerebellar peduncles have essentially the same effects as the more extensive hemispheral lesions. Because the efferent cerebellar pathways to the cerebral hemispheres are crossed and the corticospinal system is again crossed, *a unilateral lesion of the cerebellum causes an ipsilateral disorder of movement.*

Incoordination (ataxia) of voluntary movement is the most prominent manifestation of cerebellar disease. It has been designated by a number of descriptive terms (*dysmetria, dyssynergia, dysdiadochokinesia,* etc.), but Holmes's characterization of these disturbances as *abnormalities in the rate, range, and force of movement* is less confusing and more accurate. There may be a slight delay in the initiation of a movement, and the movement itself is slower than normal and irregular. The velocity and force of the movement are not checked in the normal manner. These abnormalities become more prominent in acts requiring rapid alternation of movements. The main result of these disorders is an irregularity in the initiation and accuracy of patterns of movement.

Characteristically, the patient's finger (or toe) oscillates as it approaches a target or moves from side to side on the target itself. This side-to-side movement may assume a pseudorhythmic quality, in which case it is referred to inaccurately as an "intention tremor." The term *ataxic tremor* is more accurate. In addition, movement and attempts at sustained posture may evoke a wide-amplitude, proximal limb action tremor, incorrectly called "rubral tremor" insofar as the lesion is usually in the superior cerebellar peduncle, fibers of which pass through the red nucleus.

Dysarthria following cerebellar lesions may take one of two forms— either a slowing or slurring of speech, like that due to corticobulbar disease, or "scanning speech," in which words are fragmented into syllables, as when a line of poetry is scanned for meter. Each syllable may be uttered with greater or lesser force than is natural. The latter abnormality is uniquely cerebellar. A rhythmic tremor of the head on the trunk at a rate of 3 to 4 per second may accompany midline cerebellar lesions ("titubation"). There are also a variety of abnormalities of ocular movement, including saccadic dysmetria (in which voluntary gaze is accomplished by a series of jerky movements), inability to hold eccentric gaze with drifting of the eyes toward the primary (central) position and the need to make repetitive corrective saccades (gaze-directed nystagmus), and, on occasion, skew (uniocular vertical) deviation (Chap. 14). The *nystagmus* is most prominent with vestibulocerebellar lesions.

Hypotonia of the limbs is more readily demonstrated with acute than with chronic lesions. It can be brought out by tapping the wrists of the outstretched arms, in which case the affected limb(s) will be displaced through a wider range than normal; this represents a failure to fixate the arm at the shoulder. Or a hand or foot may be displaced through an abnormally wide range when the limb is shaken. Pendularity of the knee jerk betrays hypotonicity of the quadriceps and hamstring muscles.

Damage to any of the major efferent or afferent tracts of the cerebellum may produce the main aspects of the cerebellar syndrome. It should be emphasized again that unilateral ataxia is due to a lesion in the ipsilateral cerebellar hemisphere or its corresponding tracts. But it should also be pointed out that a considerable part of a cerebellar hemisphere may suffer damage without recognizable disorder of movement.

Acute lesions may cause a slight weakness and fatigability of the ataxic limbs. Parietal lobe lesions may occasionally give rise to an ataxia that resembles a cerebellar one. However, the absence of sensory deficit and the relative lack of a corrective effect of vision on projected movement distinguish cerebellar ataxia from the sensory type. Certain polyneuropathies that affect large-diameter spinocerebellar fibers may also produce ataxia, tremor, and a gait disorder that simulates closely a cerebellar disease; dysarthria and nystagmus are absent.

Cerebellar disorders of equilibrium and gait are described in Chap. 7.

Table 5-1 summarizes the main disorders that are characterized by generalized cerebellar ataxia, according to their rate of development and the degree of permanence of the ataxia.

TABLE 5-1 Diagnosis of Generalized Cerebellar Ataxia

Mode of development	Causes
Acute-transitory	Intoxication with alcohol, lithium, barbiturate, phenytoin or other anticonvulsants (associated with dysarthria, nystagmus, and sometimes confusion; Chaps. 42, 43). Diamox responsive episodic ataxia (Chap. 37). Childhood hyperammonemias (Chap. 37).
Acute but usually reversible	Postinfectious, with mild inflammatory changes in CSF (Chap. 36). Viral cerebellar encephalitis (Chap. 33).
Acute-enduring	Hyperthermia with coma at onset (Chap. 17). Intoxication with mercury compounds or toluene (glue sniffing; spray painting; Chap. 43).
Subacute (over weeks)	Brain tumors such as medulloblastoma, astrocytoma, hemangioblastoma (usually with headache and papilledema; Chap. 31). Alcoholic-nutritional (Chaps. 41 and 42). Paraneoplastic, often with opsoclonus and anticerebellar antibodies (particularly breast and ovarian carcinoma; Chap. 31). Creutzfeld–Jakob disease (Chap. 33). Abscess (Chap. 32). Rare manifestation of Whipple disease, nontropical sprue, Hashimoto thyroiditis. Idiopathic.
Chronic (months to years)	Friedreich ataxia and other spinocerebellar degenerations; other hereditary cerebellar degenerations [olivopontocerebellar, cerebellar cortical degenerations (Chap. 39)]. Hereditary metabolic diseases, often with myoclonus (Chap. 37). Childhood ataxias, including ataxia telangiectasia, cerebellar agenesis, and dyssynergia cerebellaris myoclonica (Chap. 39).

For a more detailed discussion of this topic, see Victor and Ropper: *Adams and Victor's Principles of Neurology*, 7th ed, pp 86–98.

ADDITIONAL READING

Brooks VB: *The Neural Basis of Motor Control*. New York, Oxford University Press, 1986.

Diener HC, Dichgans J: Pathophysiology of cerebellar ataxia. *Mov Disord* 7:95, 1992.

Ghez C, Thach WT: The cerebellum, in Kandel ER, Schwartz JH, Jessel TM (eds): *Principles of Neural Science*, 4th ed. New York, McGraw-Hill, 2000, pp 832–852.

Gilman S: Cerebellar control of movement. *Ann Neurol* 35:3, 1994.

Holmes G: The cerebellum of man. Hughings Jackson Lecture. *Brain* 62:1, 1939.

Thach WT Jr: The cerebellum, in Mountcastle VB (ed): *Medical Physiology*, 14th ed. St. Louis, Mosby, 1980, vol 1, pp 837–858.

Watts RL, Koller WC (eds): *Movement Disorders. Neurologic Principles and Practice*. New York, McGraw-Hill, 1997, pp 365–417.

6 | Tremor, Myoclonus, Focal Dystonias, and Tics

These disorders of movement are commonly observed in the course of medical practice. Although all of them are manifestations of disease, their clinical significance is quite variable. Moreover, their physiology is not fully understood, and only infrequently is their pathologic basis established. From the clinician's viewpoint, once each of these phenomena has been seen, there is little difficulty in recognizing it on subsequent occasions and assessing its medical implications.

TREMOR

This is defined as a more or less rhythmic oscillation of a part of the body around a fixed point. Tremors are customarily categorized as being of two general types: (1) normal or physiologic and (2) pathologic. *Physiologic tremor* is clinically imperceptible but present in everyone and involves all muscle groups. One element is a fine reverberation from cardiac systole (seen by ballistocardiography), but the more important component is a reflection of incomplete fusion of the twitches of large motor units, which contract at a rate too slow to produce a fused tetanus. It is irregular in both frequency and amplitude; the rate is 8 to 12 Hz or higher and amplitude less than 0.1° at fingers and wrist.

Enhancement of physiologic tremor occurs during hyperadrenergic states (fright, injection of norepinephrine, thyrotoxicosis, use of caffeine, nicotine, and corticosteroids), whereupon it becomes visible when the fingers and hands are outstretched. It is quieted by anxiolytic drugs or when the patient is calm and relaxed.

There are several identifiable types of *pathologic tremor* (Table 6-1), the common ones being essential-familial "action" tremor, parkinsonian tremor, and cerebellar tremors of both the "intention" and the coarse, flapping, or "rubral" types described in the previous chapter, and rhythmic myoclonus.

The *essential or familial action* tremor is the most frequent. Most often it involves the upper extremities, but it may affect the head, jaw and laryngeal muscles (causing quavering voice), and rarely the lower extremities. Its frequency is 5 to 7 Hz and its range may be several millimeters, enough to interfere with writing, eating, etc. A unique characteristic is its appearance only during movement and to a lesser extent during the maintenance of a posture, and its immediate arrest upon relaxation. The tremor increases markedly when the target is approached. For this reason, it is sometimes mistakenly called an intention (ataxic) tremor. A slower type of essential tremor that is most apparent in the act of movement has been termed *kinetic-predominant tremor*. Essential tremor is a common movement abnormality, seen in 400 to 2000 per 100,000 persons. Approximately 50 percent are familial; the inheritance pattern is autosomal dominant. The tremor usually appears during adult years, sometimes first in old age, when it has been

TABLE 6-1 Major Types of Tremor

Type of tremor	Frequency, Hz	Predominant location(s)	Enhancing agents	Attenuating agents
Physiologic	8–13	Hands	Epinephrine, β-adrenergics	Alcohol, β-adrenergic antagonists
Parkinson (rest)	3–5	Hands and forearms, fingers, feet, lips, tongue	Emotional stress	L-Dopa, anticholinergics
Cerebellar (intention, or ataxic)	2–4	Limbs, trunk, head	Emotional stress	Alcohol
Postural, or action	5–8	Hands	Anxiety, fright, β-adrenergics, alcohol withdrawal, xanthines, lithium, exercise	Alcohol, propranolol, primidone
Essential (familial, senile)	4–8	Hands, head, vocal cords	Anxiety, fright, β-adrenergics, alcohol withdrawal, xanthines, lithium, exercise	Alcohol, propranolol, primidone
Essential-kinetic-predominant	3.5–6	Hands, head	Anxiety, fright, β-adrenergics, alcohol withdrawal, xanthines, lithium, exercise	Clonazepam, alcohol, β-adrenergic antagonists, certain anticonvulsants
Orthostatic	4–8, irregular	Legs	Quiet standing	Repose, walking, clonazepam, valproate
Tremor of neuropathy	4–7	Hands	—	
"Palatal myoclonus"	60–100/min (1–2/s)	Palate, sometimes facial, pharyngeal, proximal limb muscles	—	Clonazepam, valproic acid

45

called *senile tremor*. Seldom is it manifest in a child. In a rare form of essential tremor, the lower limbs are involved disproportionately, most prominently during quiet standing (orthostatic tremor).

There is controversy about the mechanism of essential tremor. One view is that it is merely an enhanced physiologic tremor. Young has adduced evidence in favor of a central origin, probably in the brainstem and cerebellum, but no pathologic change has been found in these parts. A similar tremor is produced by placing lesions in the interpositus nucleus of the cerebellum. The tremor can be abolished by an ipsilateral infarct in the cerebellum and by a contralateral ventrolateral thalamic lesion. More puzzling is its enhancement by adrenergic stimulation. The finer, more rapid varieties are due to simultaneous but uneven activation of agonist-antagonist muscles as disclosed by EMG recording. This more common type of fine tremor responds well to propranolol 40 to 80 mg tid and to other beta-adrenergic blocking agents, alcohol, and primidone 25 to 50 mg tid (see Fig. 6-1). The coarser essential tremors are produced by alternating activation of agonist-antagonist muscles in a limb; in our experience, they are not as reliably responsive to these medications. Diazepam, clonazepam, and some of the newer anticonvulsants sometimes prove to be helpful. When such tremors are extreme and disabling, stereotactic thalamotomy may relieve the tremor on the side opposite the lesion.

The *parkinsonian (rest) tremor* has been mentioned in Chap. 4. It is a coarser 3- to 5-Hz tremor that involves the fingers, hands and arms, jaw, lips and tongue, and sometimes the feet. It is present when the limb is in an attitude of repose and disappears momentarily upon voluntary movement. For this reason, it is seldom as disabling as the essential type. It fluctuates in severity, being enhanced by excitement and reduced by relaxation. When studied physiologically, the tremor is seen to correspond with alternating bursts of activity in opposing muscle groups (Fig. 6-1). Often a faster-frequency action tremor is superimposed. Usually the parkinsonian tremor, particularly if unilateral, is a manifestation of Parkinson disease, but it may occur as an isolated phenomenon in an elderly person without akinesia, rigidity, or mask-like facies. Antiparkinson drugs may alleviate the tremor, but they rarely suppress it completely (see Chap. 39). Also, lesions placed in the ventrolateral thalamus or in the subthalamic nucleus will eliminate the tremor in the opposite limbs for a time.

So-called *intention, or ataxic, tremor*, in contrast to the parkinsonian tremor, is absent when the limbs are inactive and during the first part of a voluntary movement. These features distinguish it from essential tremor, as does its conjunction with ataxia. However, as movement continues, and particularly if precision or fine control of the movement is required (e.g., touching the examiner's finger), a slow (2- to 3-Hz), slightly irregular oscillation of the arm occurs. With bilateral cerebellar lesions, a rhythmic oscillation of the head (titubation), trunk, or outstretched arms may also appear. The presence of these types of tremors points to involvement of the cerebellum or its connections, as discussed in Chap. 5.

Another group of coarse rhythmic tremors is more difficult to classify. One type is the wide-ranging tremor of the arms and trunk that occurs whenever these parts are activated. These oscillations may be of several inches in range; they are present from the instant of voluntary contraction and continue until the part is fully relaxed. The limbs are rendered useless; the

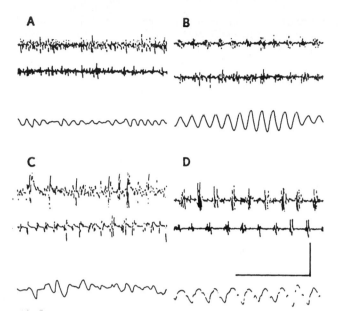

FIG. 6-1   Types of tremor. In each, the lowest trace is an accelerometric recording from the outstretched hand; the upper two traces are surface electromyographs from the wrist extensor (upper) and flexor (middle) muscle groups. *A.* A physiologic tremor; there is no evidence of synchronization of electromyographic (EMG) activity. *B.* Essential-familial tremor of the common fine variety; the movements are very regular, and EMG bursts occur simultaneously in antagonistic muscle groups. *C.* Neuropathic tremor; movements are irregular and EMG bursts vary in timing between the two groups. *D.* Parkinsonian ("rest") tremor; EMG bursts alternate between antagonistic muscle groups. Calibration is 1 s. (*Courtesy of Dr. Robert R. Young.*)

patient may need to sit or lie on his arms to stop the tremor. There may also be ataxia, but movements are so ineffectual that it is difficult to detect. Such a coarse action or kinetic tremor occurs in Wilson disease, in multiple sclerosis, and with vascular and other lesions that involve the dentatorubrothalamic pathway, usually at a mesencephalic level. It has been called rubral tremor, incorrectly, for reasons indicated in Chap. 5. Like the parkinsonian and coarse essential tremors, it can be relieved by stereotactically placed lesions in the contralateral ventrolateral nucleus of the thalamus.

Rhythmic contractions of the uvula and palate (1 or 2 per second), referred to as *palatal myoclonus*, are sometimes associated with coarse rhythmic nystagmus and sometimes with contractions of ocular, facial, or shoulder muscles. It is preferable to classify this as a tremor. But here the lesion (usually vascular but also traumatic, neoplastic, or degenerative) always involves the larger neurons of the lower part of the red nucleus or the central tegmental tract, usually with hypertrophy of the inferior olivary nucleus on one or both sides. An idiopathic variety has also been identified. Clonazepam and valproic acid suppress the disorder.

These several types of tremor must not be confused with myoclonus, asterixis ("negative tremor"), coarse fasciculations, or clonus, which are described below.

ASTERIXIS

This movement disorder consists of brief (35- to 200-ms), coarse arrhythmic lapses of sustained posture, first described by Adams and Foley in patients with hepatic encephalopathy. Asterixis can be elicited in any muscle group that is under sustained contraction but most easily by having the patient hold his arms outstretched with hands and fingers dorsiflexed; the wrists and fingers then undergo abrupt flexion movements at irregular intervals. A fine asterixis of the fingers may simulate an irregular high-frequency tremor, and only EMG can separate them. In most instances, asterixis is a manifestation of a metabolic disorder, such as hepatic failure (hyperammonemia), uremia, hypercapnia, or drug intoxication (e.g., phenytoin). Fluctuations in the severity of asterixis are expected as the metabolic disorder waxes and wanes.

Rarely, asterixis is unilateral, the result of a lesion in the contralateral ventrolateral nucleus of the thalamus or cerebrum.

CLONUS, MYOCLONUS, AND POLYMYOCLONUS

Clonus, myoclonus, and polymyoclonus are symptomatic of a large number of diverse neurologic disorders. Precise usage of these terms is essential if they are to be neurologically meaningful. The following definitions are in common use.

As indicated in Chap. 3, *clonus* refers to a series of *rhythmic*, uniphasic (unidirectional) contraction and relaxation of a group of muscles. These movements involve only an agonist group of muscles and thus differ from tremors, which are diphasic (bidirectional) and involve both agonist muscles and their antagonists. The most common type of *clonus* occurs in relation to corticospinal tract lesions and hyperreflexia, when the spastic muscles are subjected to a rapid sustained stretch.

Myoclonus specifies the *arrhythmic*, shock-like contractions of a muscle or group of muscles, almost always asynchronous and asymmetrical on the two sides of the body. The contractions are extremely brief in duration (36 to 300 ms or less), much briefer than choreic movements. A single contraction or a few repeated contractions of this type are designated as *myoclonus simplex*. *Polymyoclonus* refers to *widespread* lightning-like, arrhythmic contractions of muscles in many parts of the body. This is seen most often after partial recovery from a severe anoxic episode and can be mistaken for tremor (Lance and Adams type). A less intense and more intermittent polymyoclonus occurs with numerous other metabolic derangements, notably acutely after anoxia, with uremia, and with intoxication by haloperidol, lithium, and sometimes anticonvulsants. In the delayed postanoxic variety, the myoclonus is most dramatic with projected movements (action myoclonus), whereas this is not so in the metabolic types.

Polymyoclonus may occur in pure or "essential" form as a benign, nonprogressive familial disease. It may also be combined with epilepsy and dementia as in several types of hereditary metabolic "storage" disease (Lafora-body disease, cherry-red spot–myoclonus syndrome, lipid storage diseases). In spongiform encephalopathy (Creutzfeldt-Jakob disease), an excessive startle response and polymyoclonus are combined with ataxia and dementia. A restricted segmental form of myoclonus, probably of spinal origin, is also known.

A rhythmic palatal movement, incorrectly called *palatal nystagmus* or *palatal myoclonus*, has already been described. *Epilepsia partialis continua* is a special variety of clonus, due to an ongoing focal seizure discharge, in which one group of muscles is involved in a series of rhythmic monophasic contractions that continue for months or even years on end without becoming generalized.

A special form of myoclonus may appear as a single massive flexor spasm of the neck, shoulders, arms, and trunk in West disease, which is one form of infantile or childhood epilepsy ("salaam" seizures). A less severe form of restricted myoclonus, usually appearing in the morning or with sleep deprivation, is part of juvenile myoclonic epilepsy. The latter is a common form of epilepsy that responds well to valproic acid (Chap. 16).

The pathophysiology of polymyoclonus is varied. The frequent association with cerebellar ataxia points to a cerebellar, brainstem, or thalamic localization. Specific sensory evocation—by startle, auditory, visual, and proprioceptive stimuli—suggests a number of different mechanisms centered in the brainstem. Pharmacologic responses are interesting. The massive myoclonic (salaam) seizures of infancy and early childhood respond to adrenocorticotropic hormone (ACTH) and anticonvulsants. Epilepsia partialis continua is sometimes relieved by anticonvulsants. Clonazepam and valproic acid are useful in the treatment of action myoclonus.

SPASMODIC TORTICOLLIS AND LINGUAL, FACIAL, OROMANDIBULAR, AND MANUAL SPASMS (FOCAL DYSTONIAS)

These are involuntary spasms that produce unusual contorted postures of a particular group of muscles. The spasms may be persistent or intermittent and tonic or irregularly clonic, resulting in a turning and retraction of the head, a forceful grimace, closure of the eyelids, protrusion of the tongue, strained voice, pursing of the lips, or so-called writer's cramp. Like all involuntary movements, they are worsened by excitement and emotional upset. Some are observed only with a particular volitional and usually automatic movement, such as writing or playing a musical instrument. The patient cannot inhibit the spasms but usually discovers that certain maneuvers modulate or obscure them. As a rule, these movement disorders appear in midlife or later; once started, they seldom recede spontaneously; only rarely do they extend to other parts of the body. The overactive muscles may undergo "work hypertrophy." Many focal dystonias are accompanied by a small-amplitude tremor of the affected part. Although these disorders were formerly considered by some to be psychogenic, they are now universally understood to represent restricted forms of dystonia, a view supported by the observed cocontraction of agonist and antagonist muscles during the spasm. The following forms of localized spasms or dystonia, which may occur singly or in combination, are recognized:

1. *Blepharospasm*: Involuntary blinking or spasms of orbicularis oculi muscles
2. *Spastic* (better termed *spasmodic*) *dysphonia*: Strained voice due to spasm of laryngeal and respiratory muscles
3. *Meige* or *Brueghel syndrome*: Forceful jaw opening associated with spasms of facial and orbicular muscles (Fig. 6-2)

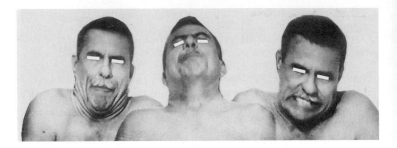

FIG. 6-2 Patient with Meige syndrome, showing spasms of platysma and facial muscles and grimacing combined with retrocollic spasms. (*Courtesy of Dr. Joseph M. Waltz.*)

4. *Spasmodic torticollis*: Rotation and retraction of the head due to contraction of sternocleidomastoid, trapezius, and other neck muscles (Fig. 6-3)
5. *Oromandibular-lingual dyskinesias, often with forced protrusion of the tongue*, most often provoked by neuroleptic drugs ("*tardive dyskinesias*," Chaps. 43 and 58)
6. *Writer's cramp and related occupational spasms*: Contraction of hand and forearm muscles during writing or performance of other skilled motor acts, such as playing a musical instrument

The most successful treatment consists of injecting small amounts of botulinum toxin at the innervatory point in the muscle, which relieves the spasm for several months. The administration of gradually increasing amounts of trihexyphenidyl, until very large dosage is attained, is helpful in some cases (see also Chap. 39). Surgical denervation of affected muscles is a last resort.

TICS

These are quasivoluntary habit spasms; they consist of abrupt, intermittent twitches of a group of muscles, seemingly made to relieve an inner feeling of tension. The patient often concedes that he makes the movements and that he can suppress them by force of will. The most frequent forms are blinking, sniffing, throat clearing, grimacing, hitching a shoulder, or throwing the head to the side or backward.

Children 5 to 10 years old are disposed to the development of tics. Usually, if ignored, they last for only a few weeks or months. Less pressure, more rest, and a calmer environment are thought to be helpful in some. In others, the tics persist into adult life and reappear or worsen whenever the individual is under pressure. If the tics are troublesome and persistent, small doses of pimozide or chlorpromazine may be helpful. Psychotherapy is of questionable value.

A syndrome of multiple tics associated with sniffing, snorting, involuntary vocalization, and the compulsive utterance of obscenities (coprolalia) is the most severe of the tic syndromes (*Gilles de la Tourette syndrome*). The condition persists for months or years. The cause and pathologic basis are

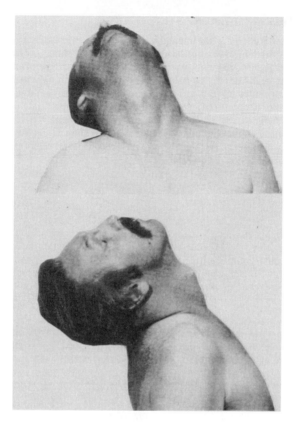

FIG. 6-3   Young adult with severe spasmodic retrocollis. Note hypertrophy of sternocleidomastoid muscles. (*Photos courtesy of Dr. Joseph M. Waltz.*)

not known, but a familial clustering is found in about one-third of the cases. The caudate nuclei have been implicated. There are no consistent psychiatric accompaniments except for a tendency to obsessive-compulsive personality traits. The administration of stimulants to hyperactive boys has preceded the syndrome in some instances. In some series of cases, there has been a higher than expected incidence of "soft neurologic signs" and "organic" impairment of intellect. Haloperidol (Haldol) in gradually increasing doses of 2 to 10 mg/day or pimozide have been the most effective therapies. Benztropine mesylate or other antiparkinsonian drug may also be helpful.

Recently, lesser degrees of tic disorder in children, usually with minor psychiatric or behavioral changes, have been ascribed to a poststreptococcal immune reaction. This association, which is similar to Sydenham chorea, is termed "PANDAS," for pediatric autoimmune neuropsychiatric disorder associated with streptococcal infections.

RHYTHMIAS (MOVEMENT STEREOTYPYS)

In every institution for the mentally retarded, one witnesses a remarkable variety of rhythmic rocking, head-bobbing, hand-waving, eye-rubbing, or other repetitive movements whenever patients are idle. These are reminiscent of the head-banging of babies, but they persist throughout life, seemingly as an outlet for the universal impulse to fidget and squirm during idleness or to derive gratification from rhythmic activity. Some of the most striking examples are the incessant hand-wringing seen in Rett syndrome and the hand-flapping of autism. Their basis is unknown, and the universality of their occurrence in many different types of mental retardation argues against a fixed lesion.

AKATHISIA

This term denotes a state of extreme motor restlessness. The patient cannot sit still; he is constantly squirming, shifting his weight, crossing and uncrossing his legs, standing up, walking in place, and pacing the floor. Originally observed in encephalitic illnesses, akathisia is now observed most often as a complication of neuroleptic drugs—i.e., as a symptom of tardive dyskinesia (see Chap. 43). The restlessness is often accompanied by peculiar ideation. Propranolol and similar drugs may be useful.

STARTLE

This is a natural defensive reaction that, for reasons unknown, may in some families be excessive and insuppressible (hyperexplexia). It is also a cardinal feature, with myoclonus, of the spongiform encephalopathies (Chap. 33).

For a more detailed discussion of this topic, see Victor and Ropper: *Adams and Victor's Principles of Neurology*, 7th ed, pp 99–120.

ADDITIONAL READING

Adams RD, Foley JM: The neurological disorder associated with liver disease. *Res Publ Res Nerv Ment Dis* 32:198, 1953.

Kennedy RH, Bartley GB, Flanagan JC, Waller RR: Treatment of blepharospasm with botulinum toxin. *Mayo Clin Proc* 64:1085, 1989.

Lance JW, Adams RD: The syndrome of intention or action myoclonus as a sequel to hypoxic encephalopathy. *Brain* 87:111, 1963.

Lees AS, Robertson M, Trimble MR, Murray HMF: A clinical study of Gilles de la Tourette syndrome in the United Kingdom. *J Neurol Neurosurg Psychiatry* 47:1, 1984.

Narabayashi H: Surgical approach to tremor, in Marsden CD, Fahn S (eds): *Movement Disorders*. London, Butterworth, 1982, pp 292–299.

Sheehy MP, Marsden CD: Writer's cramp—A focal dystonia. *Brain* 105:461, 1982.

Watts RL, Koller WC: *Movement Disorders: Neurologic Principles and Practice*. New York, McGraw-Hill, 1997.

Young RR: Tremor, in Asbury AK, McKhann GM, McDonald WI (eds): *Diseases of the Nervous System*, 2nd ed. Philadelphia, Saunders, 1992, pp 353–367.

7 | Disorders of Stance and Gait

Normal stance and gait require the execution of patterned alternating limb movements, referred to by physiologists as "central pattern generator activity." In four-footed animals, a locomotor generator resides in the spinal cord, but in humans the control mechanisms are in the brainstem, cerebellum, and basal ganglia, and certainly the cerebral cortex is involved. Also required for normal stance and gait are intact labyrinthine function, proprioception, and vision. A deficit in any one of these control mechanisms alters gait in a predictable way. A blind person or a normal one walking in the dark shortens his steps, holds the body stiffly, and tends to keep his arms forward from the body to prevent collisions. The gait of a person with impaired labyrinthine function is somewhat cautious and unsteady, much more so on turns, slippery or uneven ground, and stairs, where he must hold onto the banister; locomotion in these circumstances is disproportionately dependent on visual cues. Loss of proprioception, if complete, makes upright stance and walking impossible; if the loss is partial, the base is widened, the neck and trunk are flexed slightly, and the steps are irregular and uneven in length and force.

Diseases of the nervous system also disturb stance and gait in predictable ways, and these are often of diagnostic value. But precise diagnosis is at times difficult because the patient tends to compensate for his deficits by enlisting certain common protective mechanisms, such as widening the base, shortening the step, and shuffling (keeping both feet on the floor at all times). These compensatory maneuvers tend to obscure the primary gait disorder.

Stance and gait are best evaluated when the patient does not know that he is being watched, as when entering the examining room. Subsequent testing includes natural walking, running, rising quickly from a chair and stepping out, turning, walking in a circle and in tandem (heel to toe), and standing with feet together and eyes open and then shut (Romberg test).

Tabulated below are the more common disorders of gait, their distinguishing features, and their usual causes.

1. *Cerebellar gait:* Wide base, unsteadiness on standing or sitting, irregularity of steps (erratic placement of feet), and lateral veering (toward side of cerebellar lesion if unilateral) are the main features. On standing with feet together, there is a variable degree of swaying with the eyes open and only slightly more swaying with the eyes closed (Romberg sign is absent). The cerebellar gait is often described as "reeling" or "drunken," but these terms are not entirely apt, for reasons given below.

   The usual causes are multiple sclerosis, cerebellar tumor, hemorrhage, and infarction (particularly those involving the vermis), and cerebellar degenerations, both hereditary and acquired ("alcoholic cerebellar degeneration," paraneoplastic cerebellar degeneration).

2. *Sensory ataxic (tabetic) gait:* Here there is varying difficulty in standing and walking despite retention of muscular power. Leg movements are brusque, erratic in length and height of step, often with an audible stamp. The ground is watched intently. There is loss of position sense in feet and legs, usually of vibration sense as well, and a marked Romberg sign.

The usual causes are multiple sclerosis, spinal cord compression with predominant posterior column involvement (neoplasm or cervical spondylosis), sensory polyneuropathy, tabes dorsalis (now rare), Friedreich ataxia and other spinocerebellar degenerations, and subacute combined degeneration of the spinal cord (vitamin B_{12} deficiency).

3. *Hemiplegic and paraplegic (spastic) gaits:* In *hemiplegia*, the leg is held stiffly with failure of flexion at hip, knee, and ankle; the foot is turned down and inward; the hemiplegic leg advances more slowly than the normal one and may be swung outward, describing a semicircle ("circumduction"). The outer side and toe of the shoe scrape the floor and are worn down. The arm may be flexed and does not swing.

Cerebral infarction or trauma are the common causes, but the disorder may follow any lesion that interrupts the corticospinal tract on one side.

Paraplegic gait: In effect, this is a bilateral hemiplegia; the legs are advanced stiffly and slowly with hyperadduction, yielding a "scissoring" gait. Balance is little affected if sensation is normal.

The usual causes are "cerebral diplegia" (cerebral palsy) due to perinatal anoxic-ischemic injury; chronic spinal cord disease due to multiple sclerosis; amyotrophic lateral sclerosis; subacute combined degeneration; chronic cervical cord compression; heredofamilial degenerations involving the corticospinal tracts; AIDS; and tropical spastic myelopathy.

4. *Parkinsonian gait:* The trunk is bent forward, arms are slightly flexed and do not swing, legs are stiff and slightly bent at the knees, and steps are short and shuffling. With walking, the upper body advances ahead of the lower and steps become increasingly rapid, to the point where the patient may break into a trot, unable to stop (festination).

5. *Steppage or equine gait due to foot drop:* Steps are regular and even; the advancing leg is lifted high so that the foot clears the floor; the foot hangs with toes pointing down and makes a slapping noise as it strikes the floor.

The usual causes are—if unilateral—compression of the common peroneal nerve or damaged anterior horn cells, as in motor neuron disease or poliomyelitis (now rare); if bilateral, chronic acquired or hereditary neuropathy (Charcot-Marie-Tooth), progressive spinal muscular atrophy, and certain types of muscular dystrophy.

6. *Waddling gait:* Alternating excessive lateral movements of the trunk impart a roll or waddle to the gait. This is due to impaired fixation of the weight-bearing hip, usually the result of weakness of gluteal muscles, particularly the gluteus medius. Such patients have difficulty in climbing stairs and arising from a chair.

The usual causes are congenital dislocation of the hips, progressive muscular dystrophy and other myopathies, and chronic forms of spinal muscular atrophy.

7. *Staggering or drunken gait:* This is characteristic of intoxication with alcohol or other sedative drugs or anticonvulsants. The patient totters and reels and with each step threatens to lose his balance. Steps are irregular and variable in length; falling is prevented by facile compensatory movements. Mild degrees resemble the unsteadiness of gait that follows loss of labyrinthine function.

8. *Toppling gait:* This is characterized by tottering and sudden lurches—resulting in a hesitant and uncertain gait and unexpected falls—in the absence of weakness, ataxia, or loss of deep sensation. It is observed in progressive supranuclear palsy, advanced stages of Parkinson disease, and some cases of lateral medullary and inferior cerebellar infarction. In the latter instances, toppling is to one side only.

9. *Gait of normal-pressure hydrocephalus* (Chap. 30): In the absence of significant weakness, rigidity, tremor, or ataxia, the base becomes widened, the gait is slowed, the height and length of each step are diminished, and there is a tendency to shuffle. Difficulty with initiation of gait and a tendency to fall backward are late signs. The body is held stiffly and turns en bloc. There is a mild ataxic element.

10. *Frontal lobe disorder of gait* (less accurately referred to as frontal lobe ataxia or frontal lobe apraxia): Posture is flexed, the base somewhat widened, the gait slow and steps small, hesitant, and eventually shuffling (*marche à petits pas*). Initially, gait may improve with assistance and marching in step with the examiner. Steps shorten progressively, with difficulty in initiating gait and ultimately inability to take a step or to stand (astasia-abasia), sit, or turn over in bed. Final stages are associated with dementia, other frontal lobe signs such as grasping and sucking reflexes, oppositional resistance (*gegenhalten*), and rigid, flexed posture, referred to by Yakovlev as cerebral paraplegia in flexion (Fig. 7-1).

    The stooped, short-stepped, cautious *gait of the elderly* person without overt neurologic disease probably represents a relatively mild degree of the frontal lobe disorder of gait (Fig. 7-2).

11. *Choreoathetotic and dystonic gaits:* The various choreic, athetotic, and dystonic states, described in Chap. 4, are frequently associated with disorders of gait. The legs advance slowly and awkwardly, the result of superimposed involuntary movements and postures—the most characteristic of which are plantar flexion, dorsiflexion or inversion of the foot, momentary suspension of the leg in the air, and twisting of the trunk or pelvis.

12. *Gaits of the mentally retarded:* One observes a wide assortment of gait abnormalities among the mentally handicapped: ungainly stance, body and limbs in ungraceful postures, wide-based gaits with awkward lurches or stomping, unnaturally long or short steps. Often these gait abnormalities are associated with odd stereotyped mannerisms (rhythmias), described in Chap. 6, and failure to acquire the usual age-linked refinements of motor function.

13. *Hysterical gaits:* These do not conform to any of the gait disorders described above. The patient may not lift the leg from the floor but may drag it along or push it in front of him, as though it were on a skate. The patient may walk as though on stilts or lurch wildly in all directions or crumple to the floor (astasia-abasia), sometimes despite the capacity to move the legs normally when not standing (see Chap. 56).

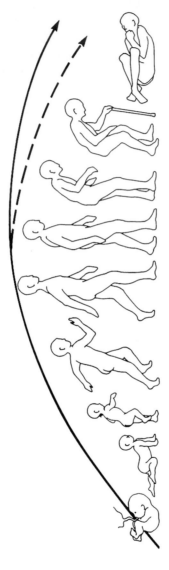

FIG. 7-1 The evolution of erect stance and gait and of paraplegia in flexion of cerebral origin, according to Yakovlev. The ripening forebrain of the infant drives the head and body up and moves the individual forward. When the "driving brain" (frontal lobe, striatum, pallidum) degenerates, the individual curls up again. Lesser degrees of this sequence may account for the nondementing gait of the elderly (upper line).

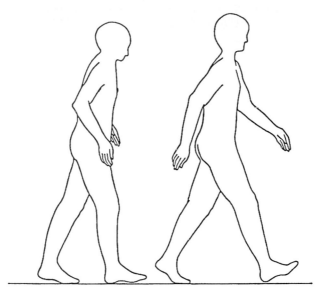

FIG. 7-2   With aging (figure on left) there occurs a decrease in the length of stride, in excursion of the hip, in elevation of the toes of the forward foot and the heel of the rear foot, in shoulder flexion on forward arm swing, and in elbow extension on backward swing. (*Redrawn, with permission, from Murray et al.*)

For a more detailed discussion of this topic, see Victor and Ropper: *Adams and Victor's Principles of Neurology,* 7th ed, pp 121–131.

ADDITIONAL READING

Fisher CM: Hydrocephalus as a cause of disturbances of gait in the elderly. *Neurology* 32:1358, 1982.

Keane JR: Hysterical gait disorders. *Neurology* 39:586, 1989.

Martin JP: The basal ganglia and locomotion. *Ann R Coll Surg Engl* 32:219, 1963.

Masdeu JC, Sudarsky L, Wolfson L (eds): *Gait Disorders of Aging.* Philadelphia, Lippincott-Raven, 1997.

Murray, MP, Kory RC, Clarkson BH: Walking patterns in healthy old men. *J Gerontol* 24:169, 1969.

Nutt JG, Marsden CD, Thompson PD: Human walking and higher-level gait disorders, particularly in the elderly. *Neurology* 43:268, 1993.

Sudarsky L: Geriatrics: Gait disorders in the elderly. *N Engl J Med* 322:1441, 1990.

Sudarsky L, Simon S: Gait disorder in late-life hydrocephalus. *Arch Neurol* 44:263, 1987.

Yakovlev PI: Paraplegia in flexion of cerebral origin. *J Neuropathol Exp Neurol* 13:267, 1954.

8 | Pain

The phenomena to be described in this chapter and the three chapters that follow are more recondite than disorders of motility and are made known to the physician mainly through the statements of the patient. Only to a limited extent can the symptoms of pain, headache, and altered sensation be objectified by clinical examination. Nevertheless, their diagnostic value is undoubted.

Pain is at once the most frequent and worrisome symptom in medicine. Relatively few diseases are without a painful phase, and in most, pain is a characteristic without which the diagnosis often remains in doubt. Because of the ubiquity of this symptom, its anatomy, physiology, and relation to normal sensation assume special importance, for which reason Chaps. 8 and 9 are best read as one unit.

PAIN RECEPTORS AND PERIPHERAL AFFERENT PATHWAYS

Pain receptors are distributed throughout the body—in its integument and deep structures, including the viscera. Two types of afferent fibers have been identified: very fine unmyelinated C fibers (0.4 to 1.1 μm in diameter) and thinly myelinated A-delta (A-δ) fibers (1 to 5 μm in diameter). The terminal receptors of these primary pain afferents are the freely branching nerve endings. Some degree of specialization exists within these nonencapsulated endings and their small fiber afferents. Thermal pain effects are transmitted only by C fibers, whereas mechanical pain effects are transmitted by both A-δ and C fibers. Some unmyelinated afferents are polymodal, responding to both thermal and mechanical stimuli as well as to chemical mediators.

The cell bodies of these afferent fibers lie in the sensory cranial and dorsal root spinal ganglia. Unlike other neurons, they have two axons—a peripheral one and a central one. Distal axons of these cells traverse somatic segmental and splanchnic nerves; central axons traverse the posterior roots and the roots of the trigeminal, facial, glossopharyngeal, and vagal nerves. The *central terminations* of the cranial sensory nerves are the trigeminal and solitarius nuclei. Centrally projecting fibers from the spinal sensory ganglia form the posterior roots of the spinal nerves, which terminate in certain layers or laminae (of Rexed) of the dorsal gray matter of the cord (Fig. 8-1).

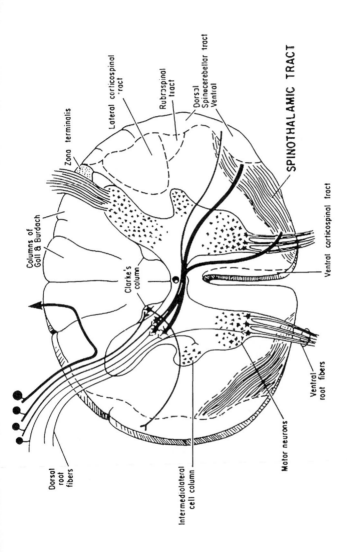

FIG. 8-1 Transverse section of spinal cord, illustrating the course of afferent fibers and major ascending pathways. Fast-conducting pain fibers are not confined to the spinothalamic tract but are also scattered diffusely in the anterolateral funiculus. Several descending tracts are shown as landmarks. (See also Fig. 8-2.)

The main afferent fibers synapse within one or two segments of their entry into the dorsal horn. The second-order neurons project across the midline in the anterior spinal commissure and ascend in the contralateral anterolateral fasciculus, forming the spinothalamic tract, which terminates in thalamic structures, mainly the ventral posterolateral nucleus (VPL). The A-δ pain afferents release several peptide neurotransmitters, of which *substance P* is the most important in exciting secondary dorsal horn neurons. Small neurons in lamina II release inhibitory peptides—*enkephalins*, *endorphins*, and *dynorphins*—which modulate nociceptive transmission to the spinal segments, brainstem, and thalamus. There are also opiate receptors on local circuit neurons in the dorsal horn. One important effect of opiates is to decrease substance P, thus reducing pain as well as pain-evoked spinal reflexes.

ASCENDING AND DESCENDING PAIN PATHWAYS

The main ascending pathway is the *lateral spinothalamic tract*, a fast-conducting pathway that projects directly to the thalamus, mainly to VPL but also to other ventrobasal and posterior nuclei. These thalamic nuclei, in turn, project to the postcentral cortex and to the secondary sensory cortex situated in the inferior parietal lobe. There is also a more slowly conducting, medially placed system, in which sensory projections ascend via short interneuronal chains to the reticular core of the medulla and periaqueductal midbrain and then to the hypothalamus and the medial and intralaminar nuclei of the thalamus. The latter pathway, referred to as *spinoreticulothalamic* or *paleospinothalamic*, projects diffusely to both frontal and limbic lobes. It is believed that the lateral, or direct, spinothalamic pathway subserves the identification and localization of pain sensation, whereas the more slowly conducting polysynaptic medial pathway subserves the affective aspects of pain (i.e., the unpleasant feelings engendered by pain). The somatotopic segmental arrangement of nerve fibers within major tracts is illustrated in Fig. 8-2 and the main somatosensory and reticulothalamic pathways in Figs. 8-3 and 8-4.

In addition, *descending pathways* from brainstem structures have an inhibitory effect on pain. One such pathway, emanating mainly from the periaqueductal region, projects, via a series of brainstem cell stations, to neurons in laminae I and V of the dorsal horns. Other descending pain control systems are derived from noradrenergic and serotoninergic neurons in the dorsolateral pons and rostroventral medulla, respectively (Fig. 8-4).

PHYSIOLOGIC ASPECTS OF PAIN

The usual stimulus for superficial pain is tissue injury—pricking, cutting, crushing, burning, or freezing the skin. In the stomach and intestines, the effective stimuli are inflammation of the mucosa and distention or spasm of smooth muscle; in skeletal and cardiac muscle, it is ischemia; in joints, it is irritation of synovial membranes. In all these circumstances, the receptors may be excited or primed by bradykinins, derived from the circulation, and by histamine, prostaglandins, serotonins, and potassium ions locally from injured tissues.

A complex physiologic arrangement in the dorsal horn of the spinal cord has been postulated to control or modulate incoming pain impulses. Small

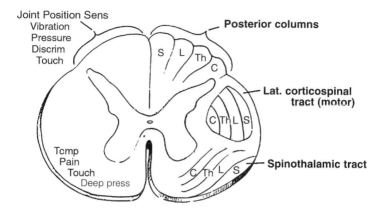

FIG. 8-2   Spinal cord showing topographic and somatotopic lamination of nerve fibers within major tracts. On the left are indicated the sensory modalities mediated by the spinothalamic tract and posterior funiculi: C, cervical; Th, thoracic; L, lumbar; S, sacral. The lateral corticospinal (motor) tract is shown as a landmark.

neurons, believed to be capable of providing an inhibitory gating mechanism, are under the influence of peripheral afferent and descending neuronal systems. Details of the gate-control theory and other theories of pain perception are discussed in *Adams and Victor's Principles of Neurology*, 7th ed.

CLINICAL ASPECTS OF PAIN

Activation of the nerve endings in various tissues and organs induces different types of pain, distinguishable by their quality, location, temporal attributes, and aggravating and alleviating factors. *Skin pain* is of two types: pricking pain, transmitted by A-δ fibers, and stinging or burning pain, transmitted by the slower conducting C fibers. *Deep pain* from visceral and skeletomuscular structures is aching in quality, occasionally knife-like or burning (as in "heartburn"), and poorly localized. It tends to be localized not to skin that overlies the viscera of origin but to other regions that are innervated by the same spinal cord segment(s). This type of pain, projected to a fixed site at a distance from its source, is called *referred pain*. It is explained by the fact that pain afferents from both cutaneous and deep structures converge on the same neurons in lamina V of the dorsal horn, coupled with the facts that superficial afferents are far more numerous than visceral ones and have direct connections with the thalamus. If a receptive pool of neurons in the spinal cord is made hyperactive by a disease of one visceral organ (e.g., of gallbladder), the pain may then be shifted from its usual location (*aberrant reference*) and be attributed to another organ (e.g., the heart).

Neuropathic or *neurogenic pain* are terms that designate painful sensations due to lesions in some part of the sensory system, peripheral or central. There is no demonstrable disease in the innervated organs. Scadding has specified the main attributes of neuropathic pain; it is usually accompanied

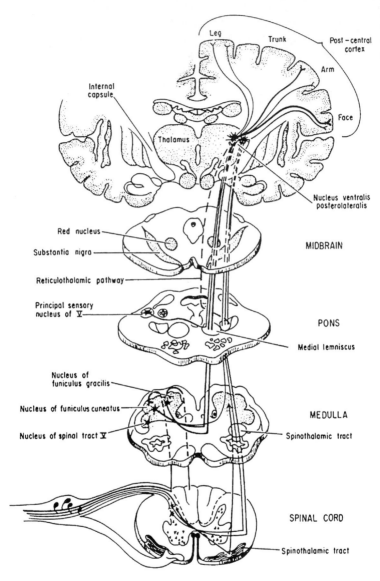

FIG. 8-3 Diagram of the main somatosensory pathways.

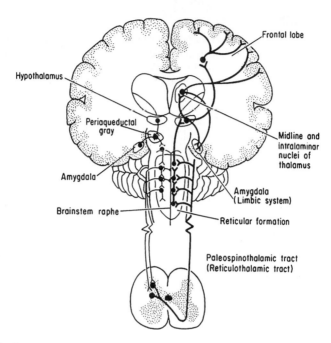

FIG. 8-4 The *paleothalamic* tract is illustrated on the right. This is a slow-conducting multineuron system that mediates poorly localized pain from deep somatic and visceral structures. On the left is the major descending inhibitory pathway, derived mainly from the periaqueductal gray matter and brainstem raphe nuclei. It modulates pain input at the dorsal horn level.

by some degree of sensory deficit; often it is of a burning and aching type, with paroxysms of shooting or stabbing pain; there may be hyperesthesia, hyperalgesia, allodynia, or hyperpathia (these terms are defined below); often there are sudomotor or vasomotor sympathetic changes.

Hyperalgesia refers to an increased sensitivity and a lowered threshold to painful stimuli, as occurs with inflammation or a superficial burn of the skin. With hyperalgesia there may also be *allodynia*, in which pain is produced by stimuli that do not normally induce pain (touch, pressure, warmth, etc.). *Hyperpathia* is a general term for an excessive reaction to painful stimuli, often with a raised threshold or even analgesia. In studying the hyperpathic states, particularly the chronic ones, it becomes apparent that the sensation of pain differs from that of touch, thermal sense, etc. Pain has a dual quality; it is not only a sensory experience (i.e., a sensation evoked by particular stimuli and transmitted along certain pathways) but also an affective one—a mental state intimately linked to emotion. The sensory part may be abolished by a nerve or spinal cord or thalamic lesion, but the patient may be left with the affective component. Conversely, frontal leukotomy and, more specifically, cingulotomy may reduce the patient's reaction to painful stimuli, leaving awareness of the sensation intact.

PAIN SYNDROMES

With a few important exceptions (acute headache and acute pain of spinal or nerve root origin), neurologists are called upon to deal with pain that is chronic or recurrent. The latter forms of pain are essentially of three types: (1) somatic-visceral, originating in an organ; (2) that due to a lesion of the central pain-conducting pathways, thalamus, or sensory cortex; and (3) pain originating from the peripheral nerves, sensory ganglia, or roots. The last two categories are referred to as *neurogenic pain*, as mentioned earlier, but pain from disease of the peripheral nerves is more aptly called *neuropathic*. Painful neuropathies, root compression, partial nerve injury pain, brachial plexitis, and postzoster neuralgia are common examples of the last group. Spinal cord trauma and thalamic infarction with pain are central types of neurogenic pain.

Pain associated with psychiatric disease constitutes a special category (see further on).

Pain with Diseases of the Peripheral Nerves and Roots (Neuropathic Pain)

Diabetic, vasculitic, toxic, and amyloid polyneuropathies are often painful. The pains are described as stabbing, cutting, twisting, and aching and are usually associated with varying degrees of sensory loss. Some patients with alcoholic-nutritional polyneuropathy complain of burning pain in the feet and hands, and these parts are inordinately sensitive to tactile stimulation and superficial pressure ("hyperesthesia" or allodynia). Also, one can usually demonstrate sensory loss in these patients. One hypothetical explanation for the pain is that the larger sensory fibers have been lost, upsetting the balance in favor of the smaller fibers. Dyck and colleagues were unable to identify any single feature of a nerve lesion or the location or pattern of fiber loss that correlated with neuropathic pain except possibly axonal injury. Asbury and Fields attribute the pain in some of these cases to denervation and in others to swelling or edema of nerve, which excites pain endings in the sheaths of the nerves themselves.

Some lesions of nerve are more likely to be painful than others. Avulsion of the cervical roots almost always gives rise to chronic pain. Partial injury of a single nerve in the arm or leg may result in a severe burning type of pain, often involving a region of the limb well beyond the territory supplied by the injured nerve. The pain, once started, may persist for years (*causalgia* or *reflex sympathetic dystrophy*). One widely accepted explanation is that an artificial synapse has been created at the point of nerve injury, permitting the activation of afferent somatic sensory fibers by sympathetic efferent ones (ephaptic transmission). A more likely explanation relates the pain to damaged C-fiber nociceptors, which become hypersensitive and are the source of ectopic impulse generation. After nerve injury, dorsal root ganglion cells and dorsal horn cells become hyperactive. The regenerating axons in a pseudoneuroma, which arises after section of a nerve, are also hypersensitive to adrenergic and mechanical stimulation (Tinel sign), giving rise to chronic pain.

Herpes zoster, especially in the elderly, is often the forerunner of a chronic painful state (Chap. 33). The lesions lie in the spinal ganglia and roots, but severing or blocking the nerve roots often affords little relief, pointing to a central spinal mechanism. An altered state (disinhibition) of secondary spinal neurons due to denervation is the usual postulated mechanism, but there are so many descending modulating and feedback systems that a number of alternative explanations are equally plausible.

Tabes dorsalis, with its lancinating pains and gastric crises, is another (now rare) painful radicular disorder, the spinal ganglia being relatively intact. Diabetes may induce a similar syndrome, for it too may affect small radicular axons.

Probably the most frequent pain syndrome encountered by neurologists is that due to compressive and irritative lesions of the lumbosacral roots and related to *ruptured discs* (see Chap. 11), repeated laminectomies, and focal arachnoiditis. Whether the mechanism is peripheral or central has not been determined.

Reflex Sympathetic Dystrophy and Causalgia

As mentioned above, a special type of severe, chronic pain arises after partial interruption of a nerve, traumatic or surgical. The pain arises in the distal territory of innervation of the nerve after a variable interval; over time, it spreads to adjacent regions. It is burning and aching (causalgia) and the affected part is extremely sensitive to tactile stimulation of any sort. Because of trophic changes and bone resorption developing in the affected hand or foot, the term *reflex sympathetic dystrophy* (RSD) has been used to describe the entire constellation. Treatment is difficult (see Chaps. 11 and 46).

Spinal Cord Pain

Arm, shoulder, and neck pains are distressing symptoms in approximately 30 percent of patients with syringomyelia and traumatic cord damage and, in a few patients, following myelitis. Decompression of the syrinx and the frequently associated Chiari malformation rarely provide relief. Cordotomy for chronic pain in the lower extremity may give rise to intractable pain at the segmental level of the operative site, presumably due to injury of the posterior horn of spinal gray matter.

Other types of unilateral spinal cord injury may give rise to ipsilateral, contralateral, or bilateral burning, stinging, or cramping pain segmentally or below the spinal cord lesion. Usually the spinothalamic tract is implicated. The pain may be aggravated by movement or emotional upset. Some of these pains are referred to regions where sensation is intact (allochiria).

Transection of the spinal cord as a result of trauma, infarction, or myelitis may be a cause of intractable pain, even if all sensory tracts are interrupted. The source of the pain appears to be the sensory neurons in the gray matter in the upper stump of the cord; intrathecal morphine delivered by a catheter or excision of the upper stump may relieve the pain. Complete section of the posterior trigeminal root leaves the patient with pain in the analgesic areas in 10 to 15 percent of cases; this is another example of *analgesia dolorosa*.

Thalamic Pain

This syndrome, almost always the result of infarction, is discussed in the next chapter and in Chap. 34 on cerebrovascular disease.

Pain with Psychiatric Disease

Chronic pain may be the predominant complaint of patients with depression, and most patients with persistent pain are depressed. Differentiating these states is often difficult, and sometimes one must resort to a therapeutic trial of antidepressant medication or even electroconvulsive therapy. If these measures ease the pain, the depression is probably primary. On the other hand, depression that recedes as pain is brought under medical control is probably secondary.

Intractable pain may also be a leading symptom of hysteria. Failure to recognize this association may have dire consequences for the patient, who may become addicted to narcotics or be subjected to repeated unnecessary surgical procedures (see Chap 56).

Hysteria in men (compensation neurosis or malingering) is characterized by complaints of persistent headache, neck pain (whiplash injuries), and low-back pain. Long delay in the settlement of litigation serves only to entrench the symptoms and prolong the disability. An objective appraisal of the injury, an unambiguous statement of the psychiatric diagnosis, and encouragement to settle the legal claims as quickly as possible are the most effective means of dealing with these complaints. Drug addicts may simulate the symptoms of intractable migraine or renal or biliary colic as a means of obtaining drugs.

Chronic Pain of Indeterminate Cause

This is the most problematic type of pain, the type that remains after all medical, neurologic, and psychiatric causes have been excluded by careful and repeated examinations. In some instances, it is difficult to decide whether the pain is nociceptive or neuropathic. Many of the patients in this group are addicted to opioids, and the need for the drug prompts the regular recurrence of pain. Many are also depressed, and compensation for real or imagined injuries may play a part. Hospitalization of the patient and detoxification are the first steps in management, since the ambulatory treatment of addiction almost never succeeds (with the possible exception of some methadone programs) and because pain cannot be assessed in the addicted individual. Settling legal issues, treating the symptoms of depression, training the patient to tolerate the pain, and encouraging him to engage in challenging and satisfying activities are the other methods utilized by centers for the management of difficult pain problems. A number of special procedures such as nerve and root block; epidural and intrathecal infusion of analgesics, steroids, and other drugs; and intravenous bisphosphonates (for RSD) are useful in skilled hands. Also, topically applied irritants (capsaicin), analgesics (lidocaine), and constant low-grade transcutaneous electrical nerve stimulation (TENS) of the skin over the affected region of the spinal cord may be effective in selected patients.

The main medications used in the treatment of chronic pain are listed in Table 8-1. Antidepression drugs, including some of the newer serotoninergic agents and certain anticonvulsants, appear to have an independent effect in ameliorating chronic pain. The use of opiates and other analgesics in the treatment of intractable pain is considered in Chap. 43. When no medical, neurologic, or psychiatric basis for the pain can be found, it is better to be guided by the above-mentioned principles than to prescribe opiates or subject

TABLE 8-1 Common Drugs for the Management of Chronic Pain

Generic name	Oral dose, mg	Interval, h	Comments
Nonopioid analgesics			
Acetylsalicylic acid	650	q4	Enteric-coated preparations available
Acetaminophen	650	q4	Side effects uncommon
Ibuprofen	400	q4–6	
Naproxen	250–500	q12	Delayed effects may be due to long half-life
Ketorolac	10–20	q4–6	Useful postoperatively and for weaning from narcotics
Trisalicylate	1000–1500	q12	Fewer gastrointestinal or platelet effects
Indomethacin	25–50	q8	Gastrointestinal side effects common
Tramadol	50	q6	Potent nonnarcotic with similar side effects but less respiratory depression
Narcotic analgesics			
Codeine	30–60	q4	Nausea common
Oxycodone	5–10	q4–6	Usually available only combined with acetaminophen or aspirin
Morphine	10	q4	
Morphine sustained release	—	q12	Oral slow-release preparation
Hydromorphone	1–2	q4	Shorter-acting than morphine sulfate
Levorphanol	2	q6–8	Longer-acting than morphine sulfate; absorbed well orally
Methadone	10	q6–8	Delayed sedation due to long half-life
Meperidine	75–100	q4	Poorly absorbed orally; normeperidine is a toxic metabolite
Anticonvulsants* and related drugs used for pain control			
Phenytoin	100	q6–8	
Carbamazepine	200–300	q6	
Clonazepam	1	q6	
Mexiletine	150–200	q4–6	
Gabapentin	300–700	q8	

*Total dose for some anticonvulsants may be given once in 24 h.

the patient to ablative neurosurgery. In general, surgical interruption of nerves, roots, spinal tracts, and thalamic nuclei gives only temporary relief from pain and tends to create as many problems as it relieves.

For a more detailed discussion of this topic, see Victor and Ropper: *Adams and Victor's Principles of Neurology*, 7th ed, pp 135–156.

ADDITIONAL READING

Asbury AK, Fields HL: Pain due to peripheral nerve damage: An hypothesis. *Neurology* 34:1587, 1984.

Dyck PJ, Lambert EH, O'Brien PC: Pain in peripheral neuropathy related to rate and kind of fiber degeneration. *Neurology* 26:466, 1976.

Fields HL: *Pain*. New York, McGraw-Hill, 1987.

Gybels JM, Sweet WH: *Neurosurgical Treatment of Chronic Pain: Physiologic and Pathologic Mechanism of Human Pain*. New York, Karger, 1989.

Light AR, Perl ER: Peripheral sensory systems, in Dyck PJ et al (eds): *Peripheral Neuropathy*, 3rd ed. Philadelphia, Saunders, 1993, pp 210–230.

Mountcastle VB: Central nervous mechanisms in sensation, in *Medical Physiology*, 14th ed. St Louis, Mosby, 1980, vol I, part 5, pp 327–605.

Nathan PW: The gate-control theory of pain: A critical review. *Brain* 99:123, 1976.

Sato J, Perl ER: Adrenergic excitation of cutaneous pain receptors induced by peripheral nerve injury. *Science* 251:1608, 1991.

Scadding JW: Neuropathic pain, in Asbury AK, McKhann GM, McDonald WI (eds): *Diseases of the Nervous System*, 2nd ed. Philadelphia, Saunders, 1992, pp 858–872.

9 | General Somatic Sensation

Included under this title are all forms of sensation arising in the skin, muscles, and joints. One form of somatic sensation—pain—has been accorded a chapter of its own because of its clinical importance. Other forms of somatic sensation are touch, pressure, warmth, and cold (which, because of the location of their receptors, are called *cutaneous* or *exteroceptive*). The senses of position, movement, and deep pressure (both painful and painless), which arise from deeper somatic structures, are called *proprioceptive*.

PERIPHERAL SENSORY MECHANISMS

Originally it was thought that each modality of sensation was subserved by a morphologically unique end organ (receptor) that transduced a particular type of stimulus (specificity theory of von Frey). More recent physiologic evidence distinguishes only two functional groups of receptors: (1) encapsulated endings and (2) nonencapsulated, freely branching cutaneous endings. Each of these types of receptor is then classed as a mechanoreceptor, thermoreceptor, or nociceptor, depending on its preferential (but not specific) sensitivity to mechanical, thermal, or noxious stimuli, respectively. Moreover, it has been found that the *quality*, or *modality*, of sensation depends not on the type of ending but on the type of afferent nerve fiber to which it is attached. This specificity is maintained throughout the sensory system, even to the parietal cortex. By contrast, *intensity* of sensation is related to the frequency of stimulation and to recruitment of an increasing number of sensory units (spatial summation). Fibers conveying thermal sensation are unmyelinated or thinly myelinated and slow-conducting, like pain fibers. Touch, pressure, and proprioceptive afferents are larger, myelinated, and fast-conducting. Cutaneous afferent fibers form the superficial sensory nerves, whose only efferent fibers are autonomic. The proprioceptive afferents and postganglionic sympathetic efferents are part of the deep, predominantly muscular nerves. Some deep afferents enter the splanchnic system.

Each afferent channel consists of a cell body located in the dorsal root ganglion and two extensions: (1) a peripheral nerve fiber (axon) with its multiple terminal endings (unitary receptive field) and (2) a central axon connected to the spinal cord or, in the case of a cranial sensory nerve, to a sensory nucleus in the brainstem. The ensemble of the nerve cell body and its peripheral and central axons is called the *primary sensory unit*. The cutaneous area innervated by one unit varies in different parts of the body, and any one area of skin is innervated by many sensory units of multiple modalities. Awareness of the location of a stimulus (*local sign*) is inherent in single sensory units but is given increasing precision by overlapping units.

When a disease affects the peripheral nerves, it nearly always impairs more than one modality of sensation, probably because many fibers of different sizes are implicated. Motor function may or may not be affected. Since proprioceptive afferents travel with muscular nerves, proprioception and motor function are often involved together. As a rule, lesions of proximal parts of nerves affect both sensory and motor fibers. A disease affecting small myelinated and unmyelinated fibers, as would be expected, impairs pain and temperature function as well as postganglionic autonomic function, both of which utilize these small fibers.

When a peripheral nerve to a given area of the skin is severed, all forms of sensation are lost, as are piloerection, sweating, and vasoconstriction. But within days the periphery of the denervated area is invaded by collaterals from adjacent intact pain and thermal sensory units. Tactile units, however, seem to have little capacity for such collateralization. As a result, the zone of tactile loss is larger than that for pain and temperature. In the marginal zone of partially restored sensation, painful stimuli are unpleasant and diffuse and cannot be localized accurately. Observations such as these gave rise to the concept, now considered invalid, of two sensory systems, protopathic and epicritic (for details, see *Adams and Victor's Principles of Neurology*, 7th ed.).

With lesser degrees of dysfunction at any level of the sensory system, there may be positive as well as negative phenomena. These occur with or without overt sensory stimulation. Feelings of tingling (paresthesias) and pressure reflect activity in large myelinated fibers; feelings of warmth, coldness, burning, and itching are positive phenomena associated with dysfunction of small myelinated and unmyelinated fibers. Even the sense of numbness and cramping represents positive phenomena. As to the mechanisms underlying these abnormal sensations, Lindblom and Ochoa have demonstrated sensitization of receptors, spontaneous generation of impulses in axons, changes in central processing, and ephaptic excitation ("crosstalk" between naked axons).

SENSORY PATHWAYS

Each sensory spinal (dorsal) root contains all the fibers from skin, muscles, connective tissue, ligaments, tendons, joints, bones, and viscera that lie within the distribution of a single body segment, or somite. The region of skin innervated by a single sensory root is called a *dermatome*. The distribution of the dermatomes on the surface of the body is illustrated in Fig. 9-1.

It is in the dorsal roots, at their points of entrance into the spinal cord, that sensory fibers are first rearranged according to function (see Figs. 8-1, 8-2, and 8-3). The *larger, heavily myelinated fibers* subserving all sensation but pain and temperature enter the cord just medial to the dorsal horn and divide into descending and ascending branches. Within a few segments of their entrance, the *descending fibers* synapse with nerve cells in the posterior and anterior horns, including large anterior horn cells; these subserve segmental reflexes. Other dorsal root fibers, after synapsing in the dorsal horns, form the spinocerebellar pathways. *Ascending fibers* run uninterrupted in the ipsilateral *posterior columns* of Goll and Burdach (also called gracilis and cuneatus) to the lower medulla, where they synapse in the nuclei of Goll and Burdach and the accessory cuneate nuclei. Fibers from these nuclei cross the midline and form the *medial lemnisci* (see Fig. 8-3). Fibers in the posterior column and the posterior parts of the lateral columns convey sensations of touch, pressure, vibration, perception and direction of movement (position sense), and stereoesthetic sense (whereby one is able to judge the size, shape, and texture of an object by touch).

As described in Chap. 8, a second group of *thinly myelinated or unmyelinated dorsal root fibers* subserving pain and temperature sensation enter the

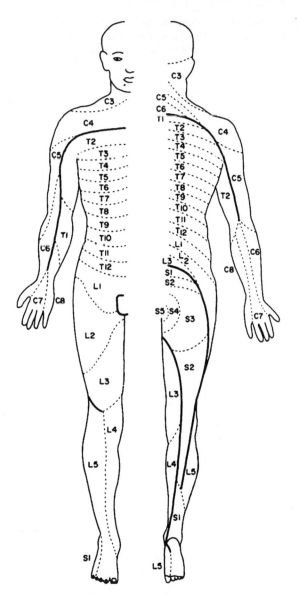

FIG. 9-1 Distribution of the sensory spinal roots on the surface of the body, front and back (dermatomes). (*From Sinclair, with permission.*)

cord on the lateral aspect of the dorsal horn. Within a segment or two of their entry, they synapse with dorsal horn cells; the latter give rise to secondary sensory fibers, most of which decussate and ascend in the anterolateral fasciculus as the lateral and anterior spinothalamic tracts, as illustrated in Fig. 8-3. Yet other sensory fibers are arranged in bilateral multineuronal chains, ascending in the dorsomedial funiculi (see Fig. 8-4).

In the lower brainstem, the medial lemnisci, which are the decussated secondary neurons of the posterior columns, are separated from the spinothalamic tracts. Above the pons, the two pathways merge and are joined by the trigeminothalamic, or quintothalamic, tracts (carrying pain and thermal sensation from the opposite face), and together they terminate in the basal-posterior complex of thalamic nuclei, particularly the ventroposterolateral nucleus (VPL). The thalamic nuclei give rise to a tertiary afferent pathway that projects to the parietal lobe. Some of the pain fibers terminate in the intralaminar thalamic nuclei and project to the limbic cortex (Fig. 8-4).

Cutaneous sensory impulses from the face and anterior scalp pass, via the trigeminal (fifth cranial) nerves, to the pons. Sensory fibers for touch and pressure, after synapsing in the sensory nucleus of cranial nerve V, decussate and join the medial lemniscal fibers, with which they ascend to the thalamus. The pain and temperature fibers descend in a long pathway to the second cervical level and synapse along their course with neurons in the spinal nucleus of the trigeminal nerve; the axons of these secondary neurons decussate and join the lateral spinothalamic tract. Thus, a lesion of the descending trigeminal tract and nucleus can abolish pain and temperature sensation on one side of the face and anterior scalp, leaving touch and pressure senses intact. Afferent fibers concerned with sensation from the pharynx and tonsil travel in the glossopharyngeal and vagus nerves, predominantly the latter, and probably terminate in the spinal trigeminal nucleus.

A regrouping of sensory fibers occurs in the thalamus; those subserving discriminative sensation ascend to the postcentral (primary) and suprasylvian (secondary) sensory cortices. The projecting thalamic nuclei also receive fibers from the sensory cortices. Conscious awareness of sensory stimuli is believed to occur at the thalamic level, for some sensation always remains after complete ablation of the cerebral cortex. The cortex provides the ability to localize stimuli and make other sensory discriminations and to interpret stimuli in terms of previous sensory experience of both cutaneous and visual types.

Finally, one must not conclude from this description of sensory end organs and afferent pathways that perception can be reduced merely to an awareness of sense data. For example, the recognition of an object by touch involves active exploratory movements of the fingers, which continually change the orientation of the sense organs to the physical world. This *stereognosis* requires a synthesis of superficial sensory data with proprioception from muscles and joints. Similarly, the awareness and orientation of the position of our body in space involve a synthesis of vision, proprioception, and vestibular function as one moves about in the environment.

TESTING OF SENSORY FUNCTION

This is the most difficult part of the neurologic examination, demanding, as it does, the close attention and objective attitude of an alert and cooperative patient. Moreover, test procedures are relatively insensitive and their evaluation is difficult, since they depend almost entirely on the patient's interpretation of sensory experiences.

Tactile sensation is conventionally tested with a wisp of cotton. The patient, with eyes closed, is asked to indicate each contact. The light application of the examiner's or the patient's roving fingertips is also a useful method of mapping an area of tactile loss. *Pain* sensation is usually tested by pinpricks delivered about once per second and not over the same spot, the patient being asked to distinguish between blunt and sharp. With more rapid delivery of pinpricks, the effects may summate and obscure a sensory loss. Areas or levels of pain loss are best delineated by proceeding from a region of impaired sensation toward the normal, and the changes are confirmed by dragging a pin lightly over these parts. The evaluation of thermal sense requires that large test objects be used, preferably tubes or flasks containing hot and cold water; the base of each flask is alternately applied to the skin, and the patient is asked to state whether one flask feels warmer or colder than the other. More precise measurements can be made with electronic sensory testing equipment.

Vibration sense is tested by placing a tuning fork with a low frequency and long duration of vibration (128 Hz) over the bony prominences and comparing the point tested with the corresponding opposite part of the patient (if normal) or the corresponding part of the examiner. The perception of passive *movement* and *position sense* is tested most efficiently in the fingers and toes, since the defects are reflected maximally in these parts. The digit is grasped firmly at the sides and moved quickly, and the patient is instructed to report each movement as being "up" or "down" from the previous position.

Discriminative or *"cortical" sensory functions* are assessed by testing the patient's ability to distinguish two points from one (two-point discrimination), to localize cutaneous tactile or painful stimuli, to perceive the direction of stroking the skin, to recognize numbers or letters written on the hands (graphesthesia), and to identify objects such as coins placed in the hand by their shape and size (the primary sense data being relatively intact).

Further details of sensory testing and their implications will be found in *Adams and Victor's Principles of Neurology*, 7th ed.

SENSORY SYNDROMES

The location and pattern of sensory findings are of value in topographic diagnosis and thereby, as stated in Chap. 2, in etiologic diagnosis. The type and location of the sensory changes depend strictly on the anatomy of the lesion. The spinal cord is essentially a segmental structure, each segment innervating its own area of skin and muscles; thus, one need only consult a map, such as the one illustrated in Fig. 9-1, to determine the location of a radicular or segmental spinal cord lesion. Similarly, each peripheral nerve has a more or less constant cutaneous and muscular distribution. Again, it is easier to consult a map, as in Fig. 9-2, than to commit to memory the details of innervation of every part of the body. Useful landmarks are the dorsum of the thumb, C6 (radial nerve); fifth finger, C8 (ulnar nerve), nipple line, T4; umbilicus, T10; large toe, L5 (superficial peroneal nerve); and fifth toe, S1 (tibial nerve).

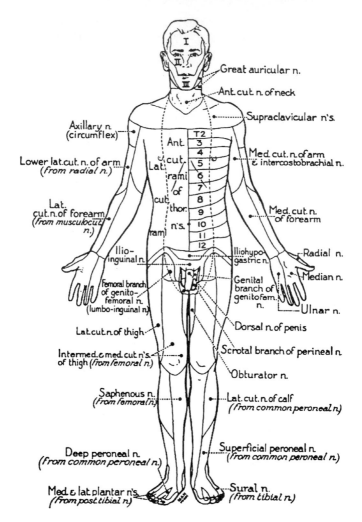

FIG. 9-2   The cutaneous fields of peripheral nerves. (*From W Haymaker, B Woodhall, Peripheral Nerve Injuries, 2nd ed, Philadelphia, Saunders, 1953, with permission.*)

Lesions of Single Peripheral Nerves and Roots

With respect to peripheral nerve lesions, the clinical findings will vary depending on whether the affected nerve is predominantly muscular, cutaneous, or mixed. With interruption of a *cutaneous nerve*, the area of sensory loss is always less than its anatomic distribution because of overlapping innervation from adjacent nerves. Also, for reasons given earlier, loss of tactile sensation is usually a more accurate measure of a cutaneous nerve lesion

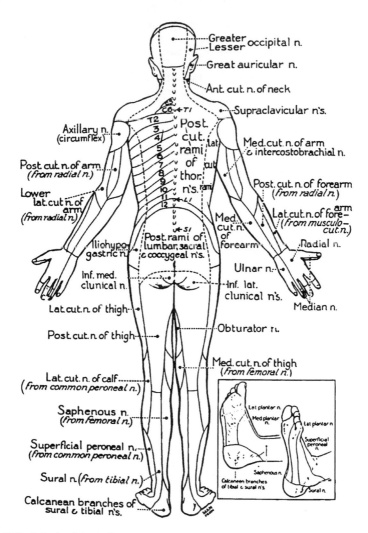

FIG. 9-2 *(continued)*

than is loss of pain and temperature. Sensory nerve fibers of different sizes and degrees of myelination are susceptible to certain pathologic agents and resistant to others. For example, compression may ablate the function of large touch and pressure fibers and spare the small pain, thermal, and autonomic fibers; an opposite effect is produced by ischemia and procaine. Partial nerve lesions, especially after some degree of regeneration, may cause mixtures of hypesthesia, hyperpathic burning pain (causalgia), and reflex sympathetic dystrophy (see Chaps. 8 and 11).

A lesion of a *single sensory root* (e.g., compression by a prolapsed disc) may impair cutaneous sensation in a segmental distribution but never produces a complete loss of sensation because there is considerable overlap of adjacent roots in their cutaneous distribution. Acute changes are more readily demonstrated by pinprick than by touch. In *plexus and peripheral nerve lesions*, all trace of segmental arrangement is lost, because plexuses and nerves are made up of fibers derived from several roots. Sensory changes that characterize the involvement of multiple nerves (polyneuropathy) are described in Chap. 46. Sensory syndromes due to involvement of multiple sensory roots (e.g., tabetic neurosyphilis, some cases of diabetes mellitus) are difficult to distinguish from a posterior column syndrome (see below).

Sensory Neuronopathy (Ganglionopathy)

Widespread disease of the dorsal root ganglia (sensory neuronopathy) produces loss of all modalities of sensation over the trunk, face, and limbs, coupled with severe ataxia and areflexia. The main causes are paraneoplastic and toxic disorders (e.g., cisplatin, pyridoxine excess) and the Sjögren syndrome.

Spinal Sensory Syndromes

The lesions giving rise to these syndromes are shown diagrammatically in Fig. 9-3.

A *complete transverse lesion* of the spinal cord abolishes all motor and sensory functions below the level of the lesion. In a narrow band at the upper level of the analgesic zone, where loss of sensation is only partial, pressing or rubbing the skin lightly may be painful.

A *lesion of one side of the cord* results in a contralateral loss of perception of pain and thermal sense, beginning one to two dermatomes below the level of the lesion, and a loss of vibratory, postural, and discriminatory sensation ipsilaterally. Tactile sense is affected little if at all because it utilizes bilateral pathways (in the posterior parts of the lateral columns). There is also an upper motor neuron paralysis on the side of the lesion. This combination of sensorimotor loss is known as the *Brown-Séquard syndrome*.

Lesions that damage only the *anterior half of the cord* (anterior spinal artery syndrome) cause a bilateral loss of pain and temperature sense, with sparing of posterior column (position and touch) sensation. Contrariwise, *lesions limited to the posterior columns* cause a loss of position and vibratory sense and all types of sensory discrimination, a Romberg sign, a characteristic ataxic or "tabetic" gait (Chap. 7), and, with high cervical lesions, an ataxia of the arms and astereognosis in the hands; tactile sensation is sometimes relatively little affected, and the response to painful and thermal stimuli and to tickle may actually be increased.

Partial lesions of the spinal cord, as would be expected, are expressed by limited sensory deficits. Section of an anterior quadrant (spinothalamic cordotomy) abolishes pain and temperature but not tactile sensation on the opposite side. The loss may recede after some months, when multisynaptic afferent pain neurons in the gray matter of the cord become more active.

Compressive lesions of the cord and intramedullary lesions have variable effects on sensation, depending on their precise location. The sensory fibers

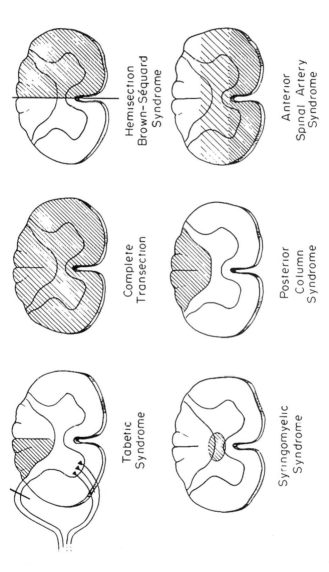

Hemisection
Brown-Séquard
Syndrome

Complete
Transection

Tabetic
Syndrome

Anterior
Spinal Artery
Syndrome

Posterior
Column
Syndrome

Syringomyelic
Syndrome

FIG. 9-3 Some of the sites of lesions that produce characteristic spinal cord syndromes (shaded areas indicate lesions).

in the posterior and lateral columns are laminated, as shown in Fig. 8-2. As new fibers enter the posterior columns at successively ascending levels, fibers from the lower segments are displaced medially and posteriorly. An opposite lamination pertains in the spinothalamic tract; at each ascending segment, crossing fibers for pain and temperature are added to the inner side of the tract so that the longest fibers from the sacral segments come to lie most superficially (Fig. 8-2). Thus, a cord lesion may cause either an ascending or a descending deficit, depending on the direction in which the lesion expands. With lateral compression of the cord, sensory loss begins in the legs and then ascends; an expanding centrally located lesion impairs spinothalamic tract function in the reverse direction, involving the perineum last ("sacral sparing").

Involvement of the posterior horn may cause an ipsilateral radicular sensory loss and pain over one or more segments. Lesions in the anterior commissure that extend over many segments cause a segmental loss of pain and temperature on one or both sides, with sparing of tactile sensation. This type of dissociated sensory loss is characteristic of *syringomyelia* (Chap. 44). Certain lesions of the posterior columns appear to affect some fibers preferentially. It is not unusual to find a loss of vibratory sense with relative preservation of position sense; occasionally the opposite occurs.

Even after extensive lesions, affecting three-quarters of the spinal cord, some tactile and painful sensation remains below the level of injury. Complete transection of the thoracic or cervical cord may leave the patient with intolerable pain in the legs, as described in Chap. 8.

Sensory Loss with Lesions of the Brainstem, Thalamus, and Parietal Lobe

In the lower brainstem (e.g., lateral tegmentum of the medulla), a lesion may involve the descending fibers and nucleus of the trigeminal nerve and the contiguous lateral spinothalamic tract. The result is an ipsilateral loss of pain and temperature sensation over the face and a contralateral loss over the neck, arm, trunk, and leg. The medial lemniscus, which lies more medially, is usually not affected. However, in the upper pons and midbrain, where these tracts merge, a lesion may impair all forms of sensation contralaterally, including tactile sensation.

Lesions of the *ventrolateral thalamus* (usually vascular) abolish all forms of sensation contralaterally. As improvement occurs and the sensory deficit lessens, there may be spontaneous ("thalamic") pain on the affected side, and all stimuli, particularly cold and emotional stress, provoke pain and discomfort of a diffuse, persistent type. The pain may be present even when the threshold for perception of pain and thermal stimuli is raised (*analgesia dolorosa*). A similar state is known to accompany lesions of the parietal white matter. These painful states are also discussed in Chap. 8.

The effects of parietal cortical lesions on the discriminatory qualities of sensation have already been mentioned. Other effects of parietal lesions on sensation and the function of the parietal lobe as a sensory integrating mechanism are discussed in Chap. 22.

For a more detailed discussion of this topic, see Victor and Ropper: *Adams and Victor's Principles of Neurology*, 7th ed, pp 157–174.

ADDITIONAL READING

Brodal A: The somatic afferent pathways, in *Neurological Anatomy*, 3rd ed. New York, Oxford University Press, 1981, pp. 46–147.

Carmon A: Disturbances of tactile sensitivity in patients with unilateral cerebral lesions. *Cortex* 7:83, 1971.

Light AR, Perl ER: Peripheral sensory systems, in Dyck PJ, Thomas PK, et al (eds): *Peripheral Neuropathy*, 3rd ed. Philadelphia, Saunders, 1993, vol I, pp 149–165.

Lindblom U, Ochoa J: Somatosensory function and dysfunction, in Asbury AK, McKhann GM, McDonald W (eds): *Diseases of the Nervous System*, 2nd ed. Philadelphia, Saunders, 1992, pp 213–228.

Nathan PW, Smith MC, Cook AW: Sensory effects in man of lesions in the posterior columns and of some other afferent pathways. *Brain* 109:1003, 1986.

Ochoa JL, Torebjork HE: Paraesthesiae from ectopic impulse generation in human sensory nerves. *Brain* 103:835, 1980.

Sinclair D: *Mechanisms of Cutaneous Sensation*. Oxford, UK, Oxford University Press, 1987.

Trotter W, Davies HM: Experimental studies in the innervation of the skin. *J Physiol* 38:134, 1909.

10 | Headache and Other Craniofacial Pains

Headache is essentially a symptom without a sign. With a few notable exceptions (auscultation of a bruit, palpation of thickened arteries), physical examination of the head during or between headaches yields little useful information. The frequency and multiplicity of causes of headache bring it to the notice of physicians in many specialties. Although usually benign and lacking assignable cause, it is often enough the expression of significant intracranial disease to require consultation with a neurologist or neurosurgeon.

By consensus, headache refers to pain in the cranium. Pains in the face, jaws, throat, and neck are set apart, for they turn attention to a different set of diagnostic possibilities. They are considered briefly in the latter part of this chapter and Chap. 47.

Headache may have its source in a large number of cranial structures, all or most of which are innervated by unmyelinated C fibers and thinly myelinated A-δ fibers contained in the trigeminal, glossopharyngeal, and vagus nerves and first two cervical roots. The pain-sensitive structures include the eye, ear, paranasal sinuses, large extra- and intracranial arteries, dural sinuses, periosteum of the skull, skin, cranial muscles, and upper cervical spine. The pathophysiologic mechanisms whereby pain is evoked on each of these structures vary.

As with all painful states, it is helpful in patients with headache to make careful inquiry about the quality of the headache; its intensity, location, temporal profile, associated symptoms, and clinical course; and the conditions that evoke, intensify, and relieve the pain. Films of the skull and sinuses, computed tomography (CT), magnetic resonance imaging (MRI), electroencephalography (EEG), and examination of the cerebrospinal fluid (CSF) are useful ancillary procedures but are required in only a minority of cases. The art of medicine is to know when to use them.

A large number of people are subject to headache from time to time. It is usually ascribed to ingestion of alcohol or certain foods, lack of sleep, overwork, or nervous tension, and relief is obtained with aspirin, acetaminophen, or other nonsteroidal analgesics. Another type of everyday headache is the frontal-nasal discomfort of upper respiratory infections, the clues to which are nasal blockage and discharge. Only sphenoid sinusitis, which may refer pain to the vertex, and persistence of headache after subsidence of the sinusitis or allergic rhinitis occasionally pose diagnostic problems. Hyperopia (farsightedness) and astigmatism may be associated with pain in the forehead, especially in young people with "eyestrain," but the latter diagnosis is made far more often than the disorder exists. Myopia seldom causes headache. Special importance attaches to the association of ocular pain with glaucoma and iridocyclitis and with temporal arteritis, which, if not recognized, may result in loss of sight (see below). Arthritis of the upper cervical spine may be a source of occipitocervical pain, usually worse after a period

80

of inactivity; its occasional reference to the forehead and other cranial regions is puzzling. Febrile states of all types may be manifest by headache, always raising the specter of meningitis, but viral infections with influenza and the atypical pneumonia agents can cause severe headache without signs of meningeal inflammation.

Depressive illnesses are commonly attended by headache and other chronic head pains.

These generalizations about headache are familiar to every physician and seldom raise problems in diagnosis. Not so are certain instances of intracranial and extracranial disease and migraine, which, because of their subtle variations, may be diagnostically difficult.

In the clinical approach to the patient, it is important to determine whether the headache is a new development, unlike any headache that the patient has experienced before, or merely the recurrence of a frequently experienced headache. Different also is the approach to a patient whose headaches in recent days, weeks, or months have become more frequent, severe, or continuous. In these circumstances, after careful clinical examination, CT scans, MRI, or other investigative measures may be required to reassure the patient (and the physician) that a brain tumor or other intracranial lesion has not been overlooked.

The common types of headache and their clinical features are listed in Table 10-1. Additional features of these and some less common forms of headache are described below.

SEVERE HEADACHE OF ABRUPT ONSET OR RAPID DEVELOPMENT

The important causes are ruptured saccular aneurysm, primary or hypertensive intracerebral hemorrhage, ruptured arteriovenous malformation (AVM), bacterial meningitis, and rarely malignant hypertension or severe hypertension from the autonomic storm of a pheochromocytoma. *These disorders represent medical emergencies, and the headache in each case is notable for its severity.* The hypertensive hemorrhage nearly always progresses to stupor or coma with major neurologic deficit. Subarachnoid hemorrhage from an aneurysm or AVM may leave the patient conscious with few or no focal or lateralizing signs; however, nausea, vomiting, and stiff neck are indicative of intracranial bleeding (Chap. 34). Headaches associated with fever and signs of meningeal irritation, seizures, drowsiness, and confusion are indicative of a bacterial or viral meningitis (Chaps. 32 and 33). Diagnostic difficulty is posed by febrile states with meningismus (stiff neck but normal CSF). Not infrequently a patient presents to an emergency ward with a violent headache following physical exertion or for which no cause is found; CT, MRI, and CSF results are normal. It may be a first attack of migraine or some other headache that will become recurrent. In such patients, close follow-up is essential.

CHRONIC AND RECURRENT HEADACHE
Migraine

Two forms are identifiable clinically: (1) classic or neurologic migraine (migraine with aura) and (2) common migraine (migraine without aura).

TABLE 10-1 Common Types of Headache

Type	Site	Age and sex	Clinical characteristics
Common migraine	Frontotemporal Uni- or bilateral	Children, young to middle-aged adults; more common in women	Throbbing, worse behind one eye or ear; becomes dull ache and generalized; sensitive scalp
Migraine with aura (classic or neurologic migraine)	Hemicranial, sometimes bilateral	Same as above	Same as above; family history frequent
Cluster (histamine headache, migrainous neuralgia)	Orbital-temporal, unilateral	Adolescent and adult males (80–90%)	Intense, nonthrobbing pain
Chronic tension headaches	Generalized, bitemporal	Mainly adults, both sexes, more common in women	Pressure (nonthrobbing), tightness, aching
Meningeal irritation (meningitis, subarachnoid hemorrhage)	Generalized, or bioccipital or bifrontal	Any age, both sexes	Intense, steady deep pain; may be worse in neck
Brain tumor	Unilateral or generalized	Any age, both sexes	Variable intensity; may awaken patient; steady pain
Temporal arteritis	Unilateral or bilateral, usually temporal	More than 60 years, either sex	Throbbing then persistent aching and burning; scalp arteries thickened and tender

Diurnal pattern	Life profile	Provoking factors	Associated features	Treatment
Upon awakening or later in day; lasts hours to 1–2 days	Irregular intervals, weeks to months; tends to decrease in middle age and during pregnancy	Bright light, noise, tension, alcohol; menses; relieved by darkness and sleep	Nausea and often vomiting	Nonsteroidal anti-inflammatory agents; ergotamine or triptans at onset; propranolol or amitriptyline for prevention
Same as above	Same as above	Same as above	Aura of scintillating lights, blindness, and scotomas; other cortical neurologic signs; sometimes vertigo and other brainstem signs (basilar migraine)	Same as above; DHE 0.5–1.5 mg IV with metoclopramide 10 mg for severe headache
Usually nocturnal, one or more hours after falling asleep; occasionally diurnal	Nightly or daily for several weeks to months; recurrence after many months or years	Alcohol in some	Lacrimation, stuffed nostril, rhinorrhea, injected conjunctivum	Ergotamine before anticipated attack; sumatriptan at onset; inhalation of 100% O_2; amitriptyline; corticosteroids and lithium in recalcitrant cases
Continuous, variable intensity for days, weeks, or months	One or more periods of months to years	Fatigue and nervous strain; fear of brain tumor	Depression, worry, anxiety	Antianxiety and antidepression drugs
Rapid evolution—minutes to hours	Single episode	None	Neck stiff on forward bending; Kernig and Brudzinski signs	For meningitis or bleeding (see text)
Lasts minutes to hours; increasing severity	Once in a lifetime: weeks to months	None; prolonged reclining or other position	Papilledema, vomiting, impaired mentation, seizures, focal signs	Corticosteroids, mannitol, treatment of tumor
Intermittent then continuous	Persists for weeks to a few months	None	Loss of vision; polymyalgia rheumatica; fever, weight loss, increased sedimentation rate	Corticosteroids

Both forms occur with great frequency, affecting an estimated 3.5 percent of males and 7.4 percent of females in the general population, and as many as 15 percent of women in their reproductive years.

Criteria that identify *classic migraine* are episodes (lasting hours or a day or longer) of throbbing and usually hemicranial pain of varying degrees of severity, preceded by visual disturbances (sparkles, bright zigzag lines, visual blurring described as "looking through thick or cracked glass," or "wavy lines" interfering with vision, and spreading scotomata) and less often by hemisensory disturbances or hemiparesis, usually on the side opposite the pain, or by aphasia. These prodromata last 5 to 15 min and usually disappear before the headache begins. At its maximal intensity, the headache is associated with nausea, with or without vomiting. Rest in bed and shunning of light and noise are sought if the pain is severe. The scalp may be tender in the region of the headache, and jarring of the head is painful. Sleep tends to alleviate the pain. Unexplained is the brief single stab of cranial pain that is common in migraineurs. Additional criteria are a family history of "sick headaches" and response of the headache to ergot and "triptan" preparations (see "Treatment," below).

Common migraine is similar but occurs without neurologic prodromata. Generalization of the headache is somewhat more frequent than with classic migraine. Occasionally, an attack of classic migraine or, even more rarely, of common migraine is followed by a lasting neurologic deficit—most often a homonymous hemianopia or hemisensory deficit, rarely hemiparesis, aphasia, or oculomotor palsy (*complicated migraine*). In a special form of migraine, the neurologic prodromata suggest a disturbance in the territory of the *basilar artery*; the visual phenomena may occupy all of both visual fields and are accompanied by brainstem signs (vertigo, diplopia, dysarthria, ataxia, etc.), sometimes with stupor. The headache that follows is usually occipital.

The onset of both types of migraine is usually in adolescence, but they may begin in childhood or in early adult or even in midadult life. Attacks usually occur once every month or two, sometimes more frequently, and in some instances the patient lapses into a state of virtually continuous migraine ("decompensated migraine" or "status migrainosus"). Initiation of an attack of migraine by cranial trauma may pose a diagnostic problem. In childhood, the male-to-female ratio for all types of migraine is about equal; later the incidence is twice as high in females. In about 60 percent of women migraineurs, the headaches appear just before the menses. Migraine disappears during pregnancy in about 50 percent of cases, and it is then prudent to discontinue prophylactic medications. Oral contraceptives tend to aggravate migraine and certain ones, particularly those containing high doses of estrogen, may increase the risk of stroke. In later life, migraine may disappear or be reduced to only the neurologic prelude, without the attendant headache.

Neither the etiology nor the pathogenesis of migraine is fully understood. Most authorities contend that it is a hereditary disorder, since classic migraine occurs in several family members of the same and successive generations in 60 to 80 percent of cases. The figures for common migraine are less convincing. No one personality type has proved to be disproportionately vulnerable. In none of the so-called psychosomatic diseases or neuroses is the incidence of migraine higher than in the population at large. The worsening of migraine that occurs during periods of intense nervousness, anxiety, and depression is usually due to the superimposition of tension headache.

The conventional view of the pathogenesis of classic migraine, dating from the early observations of Wolff and colleagues, has been that vascular spasm accounts for the neurologic symptoms and vasodilatation for the headache and tenderness. The pulsatile character of the headache and its relief by carotid compression, the occasional occurrence of ischemic infarction, and the reduced blood flow (only in classic migraine, not in common migraine) all incriminate a vascular factor. More recent hypotheses place greater emphasis on the role of sensitized nerve endings in the blood vessels, which release substance P and other peptides. Presumably, a spreading cortical suppression (of the type described by Leão), associated with the aura, depolarizes the nerve endings and dilates the vessels, culminating in a throbbing, unilateral headache that causes vasoconstriction and regional reduction in blood flow. Yet another hypothesis favors an initial disturbance in the hypothalamus and limbic cortex. None of these hypotheses explains the periodicity of migraine.

Treatment   The control of an attack of *migraine* is most effective if the drug to be used is given at the very onset of an episode. If the attack is mild, 650 mg of aspirin (two tablets) or an equivalent amount of other nonnarcotic analgesic or anti-inflammatory agent, repeated as necessary, may be sufficient. Metoclopramide (10 to 20 mg), taken concomitantly, may have an independent beneficial effect on the headache; it also promotes gastric absorption and reduces nausea. For severe attacks, ergotamine tartrate and the "triptan"-based drugs (sumatriptan, zolmitriptan, etc.) are the most effective medications. These can be taken sublingually, by subcutaneous injection, orally, by suppository, or by inhalation. Each of these ergot preparations may be repeated after 30 to 60 min, but only once or twice.

Dihydroergotamine (DHE), 1 mg intramuscularly, intravenously, or subcutaneously, has fewer side effects (nausea, aching in the legs) than ergotamine tartrate. Also, DHE is more effective in terminating an established headache and status migrainosus. Metoclopramide is given beforehand.

For the *prevention of migraine*, oral propranolol (Inderal, 20 to 80 mg tid) is often effective, reducing the frequency and severity of headache in about 75 percent of patients. Clonidine (0.05 mg tid), indomethacin (150 to 200 mg/day) or another nonsteroidal anti-inflammatory drug, cyproheptadine (Periactin, 4 to 16 mg/day), or a course of methyscrgide (Sansert, 2 to 6 mg/day), amitriptyline (25 mg tid), phenelzine (Nardil, 30 to 60 mg/day), and phenytoin or valproic acid have been helpful in individual cases. Prednisone (45 mg/day for 3 to 4 weeks) or a calcium channel blocker (verapamil, nifedipine) can be tried in refractory cases. Each of these drugs has significant side effects, and one resorts to them only if the headaches are severe and disabling and cannot be controlled by the early use of ergotamine tartrate, one of the triptans, or DHE. Narcotics and barbiturates should be used sparingly if at all in order to avoid dependence and "rebound" headaches.

Tension Headache

This is the most frequent type of chronic headache encountered in general practice, constituting about two-thirds of all headache cases and affecting, at one time or another, about 25 percent of the general population. The main features are outlined in Table 10-1. The headache, though bilateral and usually diffuse, may predominate in any part of the cranium. Aching, fullness,

TABLE 10-2 Types of Facial Pain

Type	Site	Clinical characteristics	Aggravating-relieving factors	Associated diseases	Treatment
Trigeminal neuralgia (tic douloureux) (see p. xx)	Second and third divisions of trigeminal nerve, unilateral	Men/women 1:3; over 50 years; paroxysms (10–30 s) of stabbing, burning pain; persistent for weeks or longer; trigger points; no sensory or motor paralysis	Touching trigger points, chewing, smiling, talking, blowing nose, yawning	Idiopathic; in young adults, multiple sclerosis; vascular anomaly; tumor of fifth cranial nerve	Carbamazepine; phenytoin; glycerol injection; RF coagulation or surgical (vascular) decompression of nerve
Atypical facial neuralgia	Unilateral or bilateral; cheek or angle of cheek and nose; deep in nose	Predominantly female 30–50 years; continuous intolerable pain; mainly maxillary areas	None	Depressive and anxiety states; hysteria; idiopathic	Antidepressant and antianxiety medication
Postzoster neuralgia	Unilateral; usually ophthalmic division of fifth nerve	History of zoster; aching, burning pain; jabs of pain; paresthesias, slight sensory loss; dermal scars	Contact, movement	Herpes zoster	Carbamazepine or gabapentin, combined with antidepressants (amitriptyline, fluoxetine)

	Location	Clinical features	Precipitating factors	Cause	Treatment
Temporo-mandibular joint (Costen) syndrome	Unilateral, behind or front of ear, temple, face	Aching pain, intensified by chewing; tenderness over temporo-mandibular joints; malocclusion, missing molars	Chewing, pressure over temporo-mandibular joints	Loss of teeth; rheumatoid arthritis	Correction of bite
Tolosa-Hunt syndrome (see Chap. 47)	Unilateral, mainly retro-orbital	Intense sharp, aching pain, associated with ophthalmoplegias and sensory loss over forehead; pupil usually spared	None	Idiopathic or granulomatous lesion of cavernous sinus or superior orbital fissure	Corticosteroids
Raeder paratrigeminal syndrome	Unilateral, frontotemporal and maxillary	Intense sharp or aching pain, ptosis, miosis, preserved sweating	None	Tumors, granulomatous lesions, injuries in parasellar region	Depends on type of lesion
Carotidynia, "lower half" headache, sphenopalatine neuralgia, etc.	Unilateral; face, ear, jaws, teeth, upper neck	Both sexes, constant dull ache 2-4 h	Compression of common carotid at or below bifurcation reproduces pain in some	Occasionally with cranial arteritis, carotid tumor, dissection, migraine and cluster headache	Ergotamine acutely; methysergide for prevention

tightness, or pressure are the common descriptive terms. Persistence of the headache, with only mild fluctuations, for weeks, months, or even years is characteristic. Sleep is rarely disturbed, however. Accompanying symptoms are anxiety and depression, although in some patients these features are not prominent. In these respects, the headaches of the posttraumatic instability syndrome are similar (Chap. 35). Tension headache may be combined with typical attacks of migraine. Sustained, excessive muscle contraction was at one time the postulated mechanism of the pain, but it probably explains only a small proportion of the cases.

Antidepressive and anxiolytic medication—amitriptyline, imipramine, paroxetine, or one of the MAO inhibitors—or benzodiazepines are the usual treatment for severe and chronic tension headaches with symptoms of anxiety and depression. Patients in whom sustained excessive muscle contraction is prominent may benefit from massage and lidocaine or botulinum toxin injection of tender points in the temporal or neck muscles. For mild cases, nonsteroidal anti-inflammatory medications are effective.

Cluster Headache (Migrainous Neuralgia)

This type occurs nightly, less often daily, for many weeks to months (a cluster) and then disappears as mysteriously as it came. It occurs predominantly in young men (male-female ratio of 5:1). The pain is intense and nonpulsatile in and around one eye and is accompanied by one or more of the following features: tearing, conjunctival congestion, rhinorrhea, mild ptosis, and sweating and flushing of the forehead and cheek. It usually lasts for 20 to 30 min and subsides rapidly. The common pattern is abrupt onset within an hour or two after falling asleep; it is of such intensity as to awaken the patient and set him to pacing. At the peak of severity, it may occur several times a day. The entire cluster may recur several times, usually on the same side. In some patients, a cluster is provoked by consumption of alcohol. A chronic form, recurring daily for many years without respite, is known.

Cluster headaches can by treated with single doses of ergotamine at bedtime (for nocturnal attacks) or once or twice during the day, in anticipation of a headache. Sumatriptan and inhalation of 100% oxygen at the very onset of pain aborts most attacks. Once the diagnosis has been established, some physicians turn directly to a course of prednisone, beginning with 60 to 75 mg daily and reducing the dose at 3-day intervals unless the headaches reappear. In chronic cases, lithium carbonate (600 to 900 mg daily, with blood levels of 0.7 to 1.2 meq/L) or indomethacin may be effective.

Other Varieties of Headache

Postlumbar puncture headache and other headaches with low CSF pressure Characteristic of this type is the occurrence of headache and pain in the neck and upper back within a minute or less after sitting up or standing and relief on lying down. A persistent rent in the spinal arachnoid dura permits CSF to seep into the epidural tissues for hours or days after the lumbar puncture. The low CSF pressure, which is further reduced in the upright position, leads to caudal displacement of the brain and traction on dural attachments and sinuses. Once the leakage stops and the pressure is restored, the postural headache ceases. "Spontaneous," low-pressure headaches lasting several days may follow a sneeze or strain that has caused rupture of the arachnoid surrounding a nerve root. Either type of headache accompanied by low CSF pressure, if persistent for days, is treated by the epidural instillation at the lumbar level of 5 to 10 mL of autologous blood ("blood patch"). Caffeine seems to help some patients.

Headache of brain tumor   Headache is a significant symptom in approximately two-thirds of patients with intracranial tumor. With supratentorial tumors, the pain is usually anterior to the interauricular circumference of the skull; with posterior fossa tumors, it is postauricular or supraorbital. Early on, the location of the headache correlates more or less with the site of the tumor. Usually, the headache is deep-seated and nonthrobbing and lasts a few minutes to hours. Nocturnal and early-morning occurrences of the headache are characteristic features but are not specific. The headaches increase in frequency and severity as the tumor grows. As with all causes of elevated intracranial pressure, the headache tends eventually to be bilateral and fronto-occipital. Unanticipated vomiting may accompany tumor headaches. Colloid cysts of the third ventricle can produce severe constant or intermittent headache of several types.

Temporal (cranial or giant-cell) arteritis   This is an inflammatory disease of extracranial arteries, sometimes occurring in conjunction with polymyalgia rheumatica (p. 319). The patient is nearly always elderly and has some systemic symptoms, an elevated sedimentation rate, and palpably thickened, tender temporal arteries on one side of the head (however, other nonpalpable arteries may be affected). Diagnosis is confirmed by biopsy of a scalp artery; ultrasound insonation of tender vessels is being examined as an alternative. If untreated, the disease lasts for many months to a year or longer, the great dangers being an abrupt occurrence of visual loss (often permanent), ophthalmoplegia, and, rarely, cerebral infarction. Treatment is with corticosteroids.

Exertional headaches   Headaches, often severe and abrupt, related to *cough, weight lifting* and other *physical exertion*, and *sexual activity* are not uncommon but present no special difficulties in diagnosis or management (see *Adams and Victor's Principles of Neurology*, 7th ed., for details).

OTHER CRANIOFACIAL PAINS

There are many types, for the most part rare. Only trigeminal neuralgia occurs with any degree of frequency, and it is discussed with disorders of the cranial nerves (Chap. 47) The other types deriving from facial pain are summarized in Table 10-2.

For a more detailed discussion of this topic, see Victor and Ropper: *Adams and Victor's Principles of Neurology*, 7th ed, pp 175–203.

ADDITIONAL READING

Broderick JP, Swanson JW: Migraine-related strokes. *Arch Neurol* 44:868, 1987.
Dalessio DJ (ed): *Wolff's Headache and Other Head Pain*, 6th ed. New York, Oxford University Press, 1993.

Diamond S: Migraine headaches. *Med Clin North Am* 75:545, 1991.

Fields HL: Treatment of trigeminal neuralgia. *N Engl J Med* 334:1125, 1996.

Fisher CM: Late-life migraine accompaniments—Further experience. *Stroke* 17:1033, 1986.

Kittrelle JP, Grouse DS, Seybold ME: Cluster headache. *Arch Neurol* 42:496, 1985.

Lance JW: *The Mechanism and Management of Headache*, 5th ed. London, Butterworth, 1993.

Moskowitz MA: The neurobiology of vascular head pain. *Ann Neurol* 16:157, 1984.

Oleson J: The ischemic hypothesis of migraine. *Arch Neurol* 44:321, 1987.

Raskin NH: *Headache*, 2nd ed. New York, Churchill Livingstone, 1988.

Schulman EA, Silberstein SD: Symptomatic and prophylactic treatment of migraine and tension-type headache. *Neurology* 42(suppl 2):16, 1992.

11 | Pain in the Back, Neck, and Extremities

In the study of painful disorders of these parts, mainly a problem of ortho-pedics, the principal role of the neurologist is to help decide whether a dis-ease of the spine has implicated the spinal cord and the spinal roots and nerves. (The neurology of spinal cord and root compression is discussed in Chap. 44.) But the task of searching for the underlying disease and deter-mining the mechanism of the pain often falls to the neurologist, and this requires knowledge of many diseases outside the field of neurology.

PAIN IN THE LOWER BACK AND LEGS

The periosteum of the lumbosacral vertebrae, the ligaments that bind them together, their articulations (facet joints), and the muscles that provide spinal motility and postural support all contain pain receptors. Pain can be pro-duced by direct injury to these structures or may result from secondary (pro-tective) muscular spasm. Or pain can be referred to the low back from extravertebral sources (lower abdominal and genitourinary organs). Certain spinal diseases—particularly herniated ("prolapsed") intervertebral discs, spondylotic stenosis, and spondylolisthesis—as well as spinal trauma and tumors may implicate spinal roots and nerves. Pain from disease of the spine and that from involvement of sensory roots may then be combined. Seg-mental truncal pain from protective paravertebral muscle spasm and pain referred to parts remote from the lesion add to the difficulties of localization and diagnosis.

Types of Low Back Pain

1. *Pain due to involvement of lumbosacral spinal structures* is steady, aching (at times sharp), and poorly localized but is felt in the general vicinity of the affected part. If severe, it is accompanied by involuntary spasm (nocifensive reflex) of the corresponding paravertebral muscles. Certain movements are painful and the assumption of certain postures is thereby prevented. Pressure and percussion over the involved segment(s) may elicit tenderness.
2. *Pain of reflex muscle spasm* is a pressing, aching pain in palpably taut muscles. Tender points, small knots of contracted muscles, may be pal-pable.
3. *Referred pain* is of two types: One is projected from the spine to extravertebral structures (e.g., buttock, groin, and hamstring muscles) and the other from viscera (ovary, uterus, pancreas, prostate, kidney, colon) to the low back. Referred pain is usually diffuse and aching but at times is more sharp and superficial. The intensity of the referred pain cor-responds roughly to that of the local pain but is not affected by movement of the spine.

91

4. *Radicular, or root, pain* is more intense than referred pain and is characterized by a proximal-distal radiation in the territory of the root. It is sharp, knife-like, and intensified by movement, cough, or strain and is usually superimposed on a background of aching pain.

Examination of the Back

Much information can be obtained from simple *inspection* of the back, buttocks, and lower extremities as the patient assumes various positions. When the patient is standing, the presence of an excessive curvature (of the normal dorsal kyphosis or lumbar lordosis), a gibbus (from vertebral fracture), a step deformity (from lumbar spondylolisthesis), a pelvic tilt (from a lateral prolapsed disc), and a sagging gluteal fold (from an S1 root lesion) are all helpful diagnostic signs.

The patient is then observed walking, sitting, and lying down. All the natural motions may be impeded. Forward bending with knees extended may be limited by pain and spasm, the lumbar spine may be straight and immobile, and tautness of the sacrospinalis muscles may be visible. With degenerative spine disease, straightening up from a flexed position is characteristically slow, stiff, and variably uncomfortable. In unilateral sciatica, there is often a list to the painful side (sometimes to the opposite side), and the affected leg may be held slightly flexed at the hip and knee. However, hyperextension of the lumbar spine is usually not restricted or painful, either with the usual types of prolapsed disc (L4–5, L5–S1) or with lumbosacral strain. It is restricted with vertebral fracture or inflammatory disease of the articular facets or other structures. One also looks for muscle atrophy on the side of the pain.

Of the tests performed by the examiner, straight-leg raising is the most useful. In cases of prolapsed disc, with the patient supine, lifting the leg with the knee fully extended is limited by pain and hamstring muscle spasm (Lasègue sign). Straight-leg raising on the opposite side may also be limited and may evoke pain in the affected limb. Abduction and rotation of the hip are painful in diseases of the hip joint. A search for tender areas is the next step. The finding of such areas, as indicated in Fig. 11-1, suggests disease in the designated structures. Finally, the knee and ankle reflexes and sensation should be tested.

Ancillary Procedures

The selection of laboratory tests depends on the nature of the back problem and the degree of one's suspicion of the presence of disease. Helpful measurements include complete blood count, sedimentation rate, serum immunoelectrophoresis, calcium, potassium, acid and alkaline phosphatase, prostate-specific antigen (if metastatic carcinoma of the prostate is a diagnostic possibility), and rheumatoid factor. Tuberculin skin test and, in endemic areas, *Brucella* antibody test should be carried out if there is a suspicion of chronic infectious disease. Plain films of the spine, bone scans, computed tomography (CT) scans with or without enhancement or myelography, magnetic resonance imaging (MRI), and, in cases of discogenic disease, electromyography (EMG), nerve conduction studies, and sensory evoked potentials are important ancillary procedures. Myelography is customarily reserved for patients in whom there is a strong suspicion of rup-

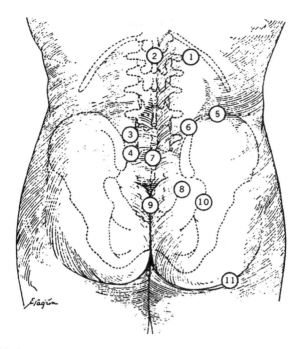

FIG. 11-1   (1) Costovertebral angle (renal pain). (2) Spinous process and interspinous ligament. (3) Region of L5–S1 articular facet (facet joint pain). (4) Dorsum of sacrum. (5) Region of iliac crest. (6) Iliolumbar angle. (7) Spinous processes of fifth lumbar to first sacral vertebrae (tenderness = metastasis, faulty posture, or occasionally spina bifida occulta). (8) Region between posterior superior and posterior inferior spines. Sacroiliac ligaments (tenderness = sacroiliac sprain, often tender with fifth lumbar to first sacral disc). (9) Sacrococcygeal junction (tenderness = sacrococcygeal injury, i.e., sprain or fracture). (10) Region of sacrosciatic notch (tenderness = fourth to fifth lumbar disc rupture and sacroiliac sprain). (11) Sciatic nerve trunk–sciatic notch (tenderness = ruptured lumbar disc or sciatic nerve lesion).

tured disc, tumor, or spinal stenosis not completely revealed by MRI and when there is a likely need of surgery.

Common Conditions Causing Low Back Pain

The age of the patient makes certain diagnostic possibilities more or less likely. Sprains, postural abnormalities (scoliosis, kyphosis), congenital malformations (e.g., spondylolisthesis and spondylolysis), and osteochondritis (Scheuermann disease) are the most frequent causes of chronic back pain in childhood and adolescence. Lumbosacral sprains, discogenic disease, rheumatoid spondylitis, ankylosing spondylitis, and trauma are the predominant sources of back pain in the early and middle adult years. Degenerative arthropathy ("arthritis"), stenosing spondylosis, osteoporosis with vertebral collapse, and metastatic tumor tend to occur in older people.

Lumbosacral strain or sprain At any age, but mostly in physically vigorous individuals, this disorder may cause intense low back pain and muscle spasm. Plain films of the lumbosacral region are usually unrevealing. Unless there are paresthesias, weakness unrelated to pain, or reflex changes, there is no way of deciding whether this condition is due to a prolapsed disc or to a ligamentous or muscular lesion (low back strain). Bed rest, the application of cold and heat, and sufficient analgesic medication relieve the pain in a few days. Hospitalization is only a matter of convenience. A history of one or several such episodes is often elicited in patients who are later found to have disc disease.

Spondylolisthesis This disorder is one in which a vertebral body, along with its pedicles and articulatory processes, slips forward on the vertebra below (usually L5 on S1, less often L4 on L5). It reveals itself in childhood and adolescence and at first may cause little difficulty. Later, low back pain, limitation of motion, a palpable "step" of the spinous process forward from the one below, and an exaggerated lumbar lordosis are the usual manifestations. In severe cases, the lower lumbar roots may be compressed, with slight weakness or sensory changes in the legs, diminished ankle reflexes, and disturbances of bladder function. The symptoms, like those of lumbar stenosis (see below), are increased by standing and walking.

Spondylolisthesis arising in later life is usually due to trauma or degenerative spinal disease. It may be a major component of lumbar stenosis. Treatment is surgical in both the congenital and acquired forms.

Spondylolysis is the name given to a common genetic defect of the pars interarticularis (the segment at the junction of pedicle and lamina) of the lower lumbar vertebrae. The defect predisposes to fracture at this location. The defect is occasionally unilateral but far more often bilateral. In the latter form, the vertebral body, pedicles, and superior articular facets move anteriorly, in which case the disorder results in spondylolisthesis.

Herniated intervertebral discs Trauma (usually a flexion injury) or chronic fraying of the annulus fibrosus and posterior longitudinal ligaments allows the soft nucleus pulposus to extrude posterolaterally into the spinal canal and compress a spinal root. Because of underlying degenerative changes, the injury need not be severe; a sudden twist or lifting from a flexed position of the trunk may be sufficient. The sites of rupture are usually at L5–S1 and L4–L5 and rupture is progressively less frequent at the upper lumbar and lower thoracic levels. The other common sites are C6–C7, C5–C6, and C4–C5. Of importance is the fact that bulging of the disc in itself is not generally a cause of any significant pain or radicular symptoms.

Protrusion of the L4–L5 disc, by compressing the L5 root, causes sciatica with pain extending along the lateral surface of the thigh and calf and dorsal surface of the foot and first three toes. With an L5–S1 disc (compression of S1), the pain, sciatica, is in the posterior thigh and calf, lateral border of the foot, and fourth and fifth toes; the ankle jerk is reduced or absent. Straight-leg raising stretches L5 and S1 roots, hence the presence of a Lasègue sign. With an L3–L4 disc, the pain extends to the anterior thigh and anteromedial leg into the knee, and the knee jerk is diminished. A large central disc protrusion may cause bilateral symptoms, with severe weakness of the legs and paralysis of bladder and bowel (cauda equina syndrome). The configurations of root compressions by protruded discs are illustrated in Fig. 11-2.

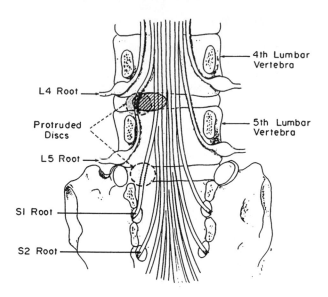

FIG. 11-2   Mechanisms of compression of the fifth lumbar and first sacral roots. A lateral disc protrusion at the L4–L5 level usually involves the fifth lumbar root and spares the fourth; a protrusion at L5–S1 involves the first sacral root and spares the fifth lumbar root. Note that a more medially placed disc protrusion at the L4–L5 level may involve the fifth lumbar root as well as the first (or second and third) sacral root.

Usually pain and paresthesias are more conspicuous than weakness, although weakness can be severe with anterior root compression. Despite overlapping effects, one finds S1 lesions to weaken plantar flexors; L5, extensors of ankle and big toe; L4, ankle evertors; L3, knee extensors; L2, thigh adductors; and L1, hip flexors.

Bed rest usually relieves the pain of lumbar root compression. If there is a large free fragment of nucleus pulposus (detached from the disc space), the patient may be most comfortable in the seated or standing position and bed rest may fail. An MRI or CT scan with or without myelography confirms the diagnosis and serves as a guide to hemilaminectomy and excision of disc tissue. If diagnostic procedures disclose a protruded disc, a protracted period of conservative therapy (rest for 2 weeks and analgesics) is usually tried before resorting to laminectomy. Recently the value of rest has been called into question, but clinical experience suggests that it is still helpful. Epidural injection of corticosteroids may give temporary relief. Unremitting sciatica with evidence of L5 or S1 root involvement responds to surgery 9 times out of 10. *A large central protrusion with signs of cauda equina compression demands immediate MRI or myelography and surgical removal.*

Only a small proportion of patients with low back pain have unmistakable signs of root compression that cannot be relieved by conservative measures and requires surgical decompression. Of those operated upon, as many as 10 percent in some series need further surgery, and as many as 25 percent are left with troublesome back pain ("failed back syndrome"; see *Adams and Victor's Principles of Neurology*, 7th ed., for details).

Degenerative arthropathy of lumbar spine (spondylosis) Wear and tear and repeated subclinical trauma are blamed for degenerative changes in the most mobile parts of the spine (low cervical and lumbar). This leads to osteophyte formation—both anteriorly and posteriorly into the spinal canal, infolding and thickening of the posterior longitudinal ligament and ligamentum flavum, bulging of discs, and osteophytic enlargement of facet joints, all leading to segmental pain, stiffness, and limitation of motion and, at times, to stenosis of the lumbar spinal canal (*lumbar spondylosis* and *lumbar stenosis*). Treatment follows conservative lines if no compression of roots is present. Superimposition of the osteoarthritic changes on a congenitally narrower-than-normal canal is particularly likely to cause compression of one or many of the lumbosacral roots.

Patients with lumbar stenosis may have pain in the low back with radiation into thighs and legs. Typically, the pain increases on standing and walking and may resemble the intermittent claudication associated with vascular disease. Weakness and numbness of the feet are added in some cases. Sitting, leaning forward, and flexing of the trunk reduce or abolish the symptoms. Weakness and reflex loss in the legs may be brought out by having the patient walk one or two blocks or sit in a chair and attempt to touch his toes with legs extended. The neurologic signs may be localized to the roots by EMG of paraspinal muscles and conduction studies of proximal nerves. CT, CT myelography, and MRI all show the narrowed canal, but the latter two examinations provide more detail and demonstrate the ligamentous contribution to compression of nerve roots.

Surgical decompression of the lumbar canal is necessary in severe cases with intractable pain or sphincteric dysfunction, but the results are not always satisfactory.

Other conditions that narrow the lumbar spinal canal will produce the same syndrome. The most frequent causes, after lumbar spondylosis, are central disc protrusion and spondylolisthesis.

Spinal cord and column, and other intraspinal tumors These important causes of back pain are considered in Chap. 44.

NECK AND SHOULDER-ARM PAIN

One must distinguish among diseases of the cervical spine (spondylosis, herniated disc), diseases of the brachial plexus (cervical rib, thoracic outlet syndrome, inflammation and neoplastic invasion), and diseases of the shoulder joint (bursitis, rotator cuff syndrome). Usually the symptoms indicate whether the pain originates in the neck or shoulder. If in the neck, the pain is felt in or near the spine; movements of the head are restricted in range and aggravate the pain. If in the shoulder, the pain is localized there and is worsened by lifting, abducting, or rotating the upper arm. More deceptive is the relatively rare thoracic outlet syndrome, in which the pain is mainly in the shoulder and upper arm or inner parts of the hand and forearm (see below), and brachial neuritis, which typically causes severe pain in the axilla, shoulder, or arm followed days later by weakness of restricted shoulder and arm muscles. On occasion, the pain of the carpal tunnel syndrome is referred to the region of the biceps muscle.

Cervical Disc Protrusion

This may result from injury, especially with hyperextension of the neck (as in diving, whiplash, and head injury), or it may develop without explanation. A lateral protrusion at C5–C6 compresses the C6 root. There is pain along the ridge of the trapezius and tip of the shoulder, with radiation to the anterior part of the upper arm, radial forearm, and often the thumb and index finger, and there are paresthesias and mild sensory impairment in the same regions. The biceps and supinator reflexes are diminished, and there may be slight weakness in flexion of the forearm and external rotation of the shoulder.

Protrusion of the disc between C6 and C7, compressing the C7 root, causes pain in the shoulder blade, with radiation into the pectoral region, axilla, posterolateral aspect of the upper arm, dorsal forearm, and index and middle fingers; paresthesias and sensory loss correspond to the distribution of the pain. There may be weakness in extension of the forearm and a diminished or absent triceps reflex.

Rupture of a disc may occur at other cervical levels, but that at C6–C7 accounts for 70 percent of cases and that at C5–C6 for 20 percent.

Treatment follows along the same lines as were indicated for lumbar disc disease. In the case of cervical root compression, immobilization of the neck with a soft collar or by traction with a halter is often helpful. Surgical discectomy is highly successful in cases of recalcitrant pain.

Degenerative Disease of the Cervical Spine

Osteoarthritis, the most common member of this group, affects men more often than women. Not well understood is its tendency to worsen abruptly and to induce symptoms of radicular disease. This suggests trauma or an inflammatory joint change, but evidence for either is usually lacking. The usual symptoms are cervical aching pain radiating into the occiput, shoulders, and upper arms and restriction of movement of the head. With advanced disease and the formation of bony ridges (ossification of protruded disc material), the spinal cord may be compressed (*cervical spondylosis*), resulting in spastic weakness and loss of position and vibratory sense in the legs. Osteophytic spur formation in and around the vertebral foramina may cause symptoms and signs of root compression that simulate the cervical disc protrusion syndromes outlined above. In patients with congenital narrowing of the cervical spinal canal (less than 10 to 11 mm in anteroposterior diameter), relatively mild trauma or osteoarthritic changes may result in cord and root compression. Temporizing, using analgesic medications, and particularly immobilization of the neck (soft collar, traction) frequently relieves the symptoms. Failure of conservative therapy may require surgical measures (see discussion of cervical spondylosis, Chap. 44).

Rheumatoid arthritis and *ankylosing spondylitis* of the cervical spine, in their advanced forms, may give rise to a number of acute and chronic spinal cord syndromes. The most serious is acute spinal cord compression due to vertebral subluxation, particularly atlantoaxial subluxation with odontoid displacement.

Thoracic outlet syndrome (cervical rib syndrome, anterior scalene syndrome) is a relatively infrequent condition seen often in women with drooping shoulders and poor muscle tone. The lower trunk of the brachial plexus, the subclavian vein, and the subclavian artery, together or in various combinations, are compressed in the lateral cervical region by a cervical rib, fascial bands, or possibly the anterior and medial scalene muscles. Shoulder and usually medial arm pain, slight weakness and atrophy of muscles in an ulnar distribution, dusky discoloration of the hand and forearm, venous distention, and ischemic changes in the hand and arm are the usual clinical manifestations. Definitive diagnosis depends on EMG findings (see *Adams and Victor's Principles of Neurology*, 7th ed., for details and treatment).

PAIN DUE TO DISEASES OF EXTREMITIES

Here one must distinguish pain due to rheumatoid and hypertrophic arthritis, atherosclerosis of iliac and femoral arteries, polymyalgia rheumatica, and reflex sympathetic dystrophy. The last named is of special neurologic interest (see below). Causalgia, one component of reflex sympathetic dystrophy, is described below and also with diseases of the peripheral nervous system (Chap. 46).

Reflex Sympathetic Dystrophy (RSD)

This is the name applied to a group of painful states that commonly affect the arm and hand; the leg and foot are less frequently involved. The syndrome occurs in a number of clinical settings so varied as to suggest more than one mechanism. These include shoulder injury, stroke, myocardial infarction (all of which result in immobilization of the arm), and partial traumatic interruption of peripheral nerves. Pain in the shoulder, arm, and hand, often causalgic (intense burning pain with allodynia), is accompanied by dystrophic and autonomic disturbances that may exceed sensory loss. When osteoporosis develops in the forearm and hand, the condition is called Sudeck's atrophy. Causalgic-type pain, the most dramatic aspect of RSD, has been considered in Chap. 8, on pain. The pathogenesis is not fully understood. Since sympathetic block abolishes the pain in some cases, ephaptic excitation of pain fibers by postganglionic sympathetic fibers is one of the postulated mechanisms. Another hypothesis attributes the pain to impaired function (hypersensitivity) of C fiber receptors.

For a more detailed discussion of this topic, see Victor and Ropper: *Adams and Victor's Principles of Neurology*, 7th ed, pp 204–233.

ADDITIONAL READING

Alexander E Jr, Kelly DL, Davis CH Jr, et al: Intact arch spondylolisthesis: A review of 50 cases and description of surgical treatment. *J Neurosurg* 63:840, 1985.

Borenstein DG, Wiesel SW: *Low Back Pain: Medical Diagnosis and Comprehensive Management*. Philadelphia, Saunders, 1989.

Cherkin DC, Devo RA, Battié M: A comparison of physical therapy, chiropractic manipulation, and provision of an educational booklet for the treatment of patients with low back pain. *N Engl J Med* 339:1021, 1998.

Devo RA, Weinstein JN: Low back pain. *N Engl J Med* 344:363, 2001.

Epstein NE, Epstein JA, Carras R, Hyman RA: Far lateral lumbar disc herniations and associated structural abnormalities: An evaluation in 60 patients of the comparative value of CT, MRI and myelo-CT in diagnosis and management. *Spine* 15:534, 1990.

Long DM: Low back pain, in Johnson RT, Griffin JW (eds): *Current Therapy in Neurologic Disease*, 5th ed. St. Louis, Mosby, 1997, pp 71–76.

Schwartzman RJ, McLellan TL: Reflex sympathetic dystrophy: A review. *Arch Neurol* 44:555, 1987.

Shannon N, Paul EA. L4/5, L5/S1 disc protrusions: Analysis of 323 cases operated on over 12 years. *J Neurol Neurosurg Psychiatry* 42:804, 1979.

Vroomen P, deKrom M, Wilmink JT, et al: Lack of effectiveness of bed rest for sciatica. *N Engl J Med* 340:418, 1999.

Wilbourn AJ: The thoracic outlet syndrome is overdiagnosed. *Arch Neurol* 47:328, 1990.

12 | Disorders of Smell and Taste

The senses of smell and taste are unique in that they are responsive only to chemical stimuli. Clinically, these senses are subtly combined; many gustatory experiences are largely olfactory, and patients often think that they have lost their sense of taste when actually the loss is one of smell.

While often a source of pleasure—we delight in certain aromas and savor our food—the senses of smell and taste seldom contribute in a fundamental way to health and survival (an exception might be the capacity to smell smoke). Nevertheless, disorders of these senses may be sources of complaint, and they may point to the presence of intracranial or systemic disease.

OLFACTORY SENSE

Nerve fibers subserving the sense of smell originate in the mucous membrane of the upper and posterior parts of the nasal cavity. The olfactory cells are bipolar neurons with peripheral processes (olfactory rods) from which project 10 to 30 fine hairs (cilia)—the sites of olfactory receptors. The central processes of these cells, or *olfactory fila*, are fine unmyelinated fibers that pass through openings in the cribriform plate of the ethmoid bone into the olfactory bulb. Collectively, the central processes of the olfactory receptor cells constitute the *first cranial, or olfactory, nerve*. In the olfactory bulb, the receptor-cell axons synapse with granule cells and mitral cells (triangular, like a bishop's mitre), the dendrites of which form brush-like terminals or olfactory glomeruli. The axons of the mitral and tufted cells form the *olfactory tract*, which courses along the olfactory groove of the cribriform plate to the cerebrum. Posteriorly, the olfactory tract divides into medial and lateral olfactory striae, which project to the amygdala and to the *primary olfactory cortex*. In humans, this occupies a restricted area on the anterior end of the parahippocampal gyrus and uncus. Thus olfactory impulses reach the cerebral cortex without relay through the thalamus—unique among sensory systems.

To be perceived as an odor, an inhaled substance must be volatile and soluble in water. Molecules provoking the same odor seem to be related more by their shape than by chemical quality. Intensity of olfactory sensation is determined by the frequency of firing of afferent neurons, while the quality is thought to be provided by "cross fiber" activation, since the individual receptor cells are responsive to a wide variety of odorants and exhibit different types of responses to stimulants. Most significant is the fact that the olfactory receptor cells are constantly dying and being replaced by new ones, as a result of division of the basal cells of the olfactory epithelium.

Clinical Disorders of Smell

Anosmia   Loss of the sense of smell is a frequent occurrence, but only if bilateral is it appreciated by the patient. Olfaction is tested by blocking one nostril and then the other and asking the patient to sniff nonirritating substances, such as coffee, tobacco, vanilla, and perfume. If the subject can detect and describe (but not necessarily identify) these odors, the olfactory nerves are intact. Commercial scratch-and-sniff test kits are available.

Numerous conditions and nasal disorders may cause anosmia or hyposmia by damaging the ciliated receptor cells in the upper nasal mucosa. The most common are chronic rhinitis of infective or allergic type, heavy smoking, influenza, and atrophic rhinitis (leprosy, local radiation). Receptor cells may be congenitally absent, notably in albinos.

Concussive head injury and particularly fractures of the ethmoid bone cause anosmia by shearing the delicate central processes of the olfactory receptor cells as they pass through the cribriform plate to the olfactory bulbs. The anosmia may be unilateral or bilateral and is often permanent. Subarachnoid hemorrhage, chronic meningitis, and cranial surgery, in which the frontal lobes and olfactory bulbs are retracted from the ethmoid bone, may have the same effect.

The olfactory bulb and tract (second olfactory neurons) may be compressed by a meningioma of the olfactory groove, in which case the optic nerve is often implicated as well. The association of unilateral anosmia and optic atrophy with a contralateral papilledema is known as the Foster Kennedy syndrome. Rarely, a large aneurysm causes the same syndrome. Children with anterior meningoencephaloceles or hydrocephalus are usually anosmic, and some of them exhibit CSF rhinorrhea as well.

A considerable proportion of patients with multiple sclerosis and Parkinson disease are hyposmic or anosmic, and odor recognition may be reduced in patients with Huntington chorea and Alzheimer disease. An impaired capacity to discriminate between odors, the primary perceptual aspects of olfaction being intact, is a characteristic feature of the alcoholic form of Korsakoff psychosis. Presumably these disorders of olfaction are due to involvement of the higher-order olfactory systems in medial-temporal and diencephalic regions.

Parosmia and dysosmia   These terms refer to perversions of the sense of smell; they occur with partial injuries of the olfactory bulbs or local nasopharyngeal infections, such as ozena or empyema of the nasal sinuses. Parosmia of extreme degree, in which every article of food has an intolerably disagreeable odor (and taste), is sometimes a manifestation of a depressive or psychotic illness. Parosmia of minor degree is not necessarily abnormal, since protracted exposure to unpleasant odors can later be reawakened by other olfactory stimuli (phantosmia).

Olfactory hallucinations   These are always of central origin. They are observed most often as the aura—the brief initial manifestation (lasting only seconds)—of seizures that originate in the mesial-temporal cortex ("uncinate seizures"). Gustatory hallucinations are sometimes conjoined. Persistent olfactory hallucinations accompanied by delusions signify a psychiatric disease, most frequently endogenous depression or schizophrenia. Rarely, hallucinations that occur during the alcohol withdrawal period are olfactory; these hallucinations may also occur in patients with senile dementia, but in such cases one needs always to consider the presence of an associated late-life depression.

GUSTATORY SENSE

There are four primary taste sensations: salty, sweet, bitter, and sour. The receptors are exquisitely sensitive taste buds distributed mainly over the surface of the tongue and to a lesser extent over the palate, pharynx, and larynx. Each receptor is preferentially but not solely sensitive to one type of stimulus, which in the case of taste is a chemical substance in solution. From the anterior two-thirds of the tongue, taste fibers run first in the lingual nerve (a branch of the trigeminal nerve) and then in the chorda tympani, which is a branch of the facial nerve. From the posterior third of the tongue and soft palate, the taste fibers are part of the glossopharyngeal nerve, and from the pharynx and larynx, of the vagus nerve. All of the primary taste fibers converge on the gustatory subnucleus of the nucleus solitarius. The second sensory neuron for taste projects to the ventroposteromedial nucleus of the thalamus, probably bilaterally, and also to the hypothalamus and other basal forebrain limbic structures. The cortical receptive area for taste is probably in the tongue-face region of the postrolandic sensory cortex, since gustatory sensations have been produced by electrical stimulation of this region. However, brief gustatory hallucinations may introduce a temporal lobe seizure, indicating that taste sensibility is also probably represented in the parietal operculum and the adjacent parainsular cortex.

Taste is tested by withdrawing the tongue with a gauze sponge and placing a few crystals of salt or sugar on discrete parts. The tongue is then wiped clean and the subject reports what he has tasted. If the taste loss is bilateral, mouthwashes with dilute solutions of sugar, salt, citric acid, and caffeine are used. Special instruments are available for measuring the thresholds for taste and olfactory perception.

Clinical Disorders of Taste

The causes of taste impairment are remarkably diverse. Heavy smoking, particularly pipe smoking, is probably the most common cause. Since taste stimuli, like olfactory ones, are effective only in a fluid medium, disorders that cause extreme dryness of the tongue (Sjögren syndrome, pandysautonomia, radiation therapy) will lead to a loss or reduction in taste sensation (ageusia or hypogeusia).

The influenza-like illnesses that impair the sense of smell (see above) also damage the taste buds and diminish or pervert the sense of taste (dysgeusia). Other conditions that may have the same effects are scleroderma, hepatitis, viral encephalitis, myxedema, adrenal insufficiency, and a deficiency of cobalamin and vitamin A. A wide variety of drugs may cause persistent distortions of taste, the most common ones being penicillamine (used in Wilson disease and rheumatoid arthritis); the antineoplastic drugs cisplatin, carboplatin, procarbazine, and vincristine; griseofulvin; amitriptyline; antithyroid drugs; chlorambucil; and cholestyramine. Henkin and coworkers have described a special form of hypogeusia in which the taste and aroma of food is unpleasant to the point of being revolting. Patients with this disorder have reportedly responded to small oral doses of zinc sulfate.

Taste is frequently lost over the anterior one-half of the tongue in Bell's palsy (see Chap. 47). Invasion of the lingual nerve or chorda tympani by tumor will have a similar effect.

For a more detailed discussion of this topic, see Victor and Ropper: *Adams and Victor's Principles of Neurology*, 7th ed, pp 237–246.

ADDITIONAL READING

Brodal A: *Neurological Anatomy in Relation to Clinical Medicine*, 3rd ed. New York, Oxford University Press, 1981, pp 640–654.

Doty RL, Kimmelman CP, Lesser RP: Smell and taste and their disorders, in Asbury AK, McKhann GM, McDonald WI (eds): *Diseases of the Nervous System*, 2nd ed. Philadelphia, Saunders, 1992, pp 390–403.

Douek E: *The Sense of Smell and Its Abnormalities*. London, Churchill Livingstone, 1973.

Hauser-Hauw C, Bancaud J: Gustatory hallucinations in epileptic seizures. *Brain* 110:339, 1987.

Henkin RJ, Larson AL, Powell RD: Hypogeusia, dysgeusia, hyposmia, and dysosmia following influenza-like infection. *Ann Otol* 84:672, 1975.

Kimmelman CP: Clinical review of olfaction. *Am J Otolaryngol* 14:227, 1993.

Pryse-Phillips W: Disturbances in the sense of smell in psychiatric patients. *Proc R Soc Med* 68:26, 1975.

Schiffman SS: Taste and smell in disease. *N Engl J Med* 308:1275, 1337, 1983.

13 | Common Disturbances of Vision

The diverse composition of the eye, containing epithelial, vascular, connective, muscular, pigmentary, and nervous tissue elements, renders it vulnerable to a wide variety of diseases. For this reason, it concerns physicians in several medical specialities other than ophthalmology.

To the neurologist, the eyes are the most important of all sense organs. A large part of human motility and numerous reactions to the environment are under visual control. This accounts for the large part of the cerebral cortex committed to visual and visually related functions. It has even been suggested that the peculiar neural arrangement wherein one-half of the body is represented in the opposite half of the brain is due to the biconvex lens of the eye, which projects all visual input from the right half of our world to the left hemisphere.

Since the eye is the sole organ of vision, impairment of vision is the main symptom of eye disease. Positive phenomena such as phosphenes (luminous sensations occurring with ocular movements or compression) and visual illusions and hallucinations are relatively unimportant. Other eye symptoms are irritation, photophobia, pain, diplopia and strabismus, and drooping of the eyelids.

The eyes are examined with two objectives: one is to search the eye and its adnexa for changes that might clarify the diagnosis of some systemic disease; the other, to find the cause of reduced vision. In Table 13-1 are listed the more common nonneurologic abnormalities of the eye and the local and systemic diseases of which they are a part. Some of them also impair vision.

APPROACH TO THE PROBLEM OF VISUAL LOSS

Examination for Visual Loss

First one measures *visual acuity* by means of a Snellen chart or, at the bedside, by a "near card," on which the letters have been reduced proportionately, to be read at a distance of 14 in. If the patient reads only the top line of the Snellen chart at 20 ft rather than 200 ft, the acuity is stated as 20/200 or 6/60, in meters. Normal vision is 20/20, or 6/6. If the patient has a refractive error, glasses should be worn during the test.

If visual impairment cannot be corrected to 20/20 with lenses (for either myopia or hyperopia), or by viewing through a pinhole, there must be some reason other than an uncorrected refractive error for the impaired visual acuity. It may be due to interference with light transmission through the refractive media (cornea, lens, or vitreous). One can inspect each of these structures by depth focusing with an ophthalmoscope. If each of these structures and the retina appear to be normal, the fault must lie in the optic nerves, chiasm, tracts, lateral geniculate bodies, geniculocalcarine tracts, or occipital lobes (see *Adams and Victor's Principles of Neurology*, 7th ed., and Fig. 13-1 for detailed anatomy of these structures).

TABLE 13-1 Ocular (Nonretinal) Manifestations of Local
and Systemic Diseases

Ocular abnormality	Causes
Conjunctivitis and uveitis with ulceration and fibrosis of cornea	Herpes simplex and zoster and other viral and bacterial infections; immune syndromes (Stevens-Johnson, Reiter, Behçet), lymphoma, sarcoid
Vascularization of conjunctiva	Ataxia-telangiectasia, orbital-vascular malformations
Keratitis	Congenital syphilis, tuberculosis, ocular pemphigus, fulminant thyroid exophthalmos
Corneal depositions	
Calcium salts (band keratopathy)	Vitamin D intoxication, sarcoid, hyperparathyroidism, multiple myeloma, rheumatoid arthritis
Cystine crystals	Cystinosis
Chloroquine crystals	Treatment with chloroquine
Clouding with polysaccharides	Mucopolysaccharidoses
Cholesterol	Arcus senilis
Kaiser-Fleischer ring (copper)	Wilson disease
Cataract	Diabetes mellitus, galactosemia, myotonic dystrophy, prolonged corticosteroid therapy, radiation therapy, aging
Vitreous hemorrhage	Trauma, ruptured aneurysm or arteriovenous malformation, diabetic proliferative retinopathy
Vitreous deposits	
Calcium (asteroid hyalosis)	Aging
Amyloid	Systemic amyloidosis
"Floaters"	Usually benign; sometimes retinal detachment
Neoplastic	Lymphoma

Next one examines the *visual fields*. At the bedside, this is done by having the patient cover one eye and aligning the other with the corresponding eye of the examiner. When a target (a moving finger or a white disc mounted on a stick) is brought into the visual field, from the periphery toward the center and equidistant between patient and examiner, the patient's visual fields, including the blind spot (representing the optic disc) can be compared to those of the examiner. Computerized perimetry and tangent screen testing are more accurate. The patterns of visual field loss from lesions in different parts of the visual pathway are illustrated in Fig. 13-1, and the common causes of these visual field defects are summarized in Table 13-2.

The third step in the examination is a careful *ophthalmoscopic inspection of the retina*, preferably through a pupil dilated with a short-acting mydriatic (e.g., 2.5 to 10% phenylephrine or 0.5 to 1.0% tropicamide). Common shortcomings in the ophthalmoscopic examination are a failure to examine the macular area (which lies 3 to 4 mm lateral to the optic disc and accounts for 95 percent of visual acuity), to search the periphery of the retina, and to appreciate the variations in the appearance of the normal disc. Ophthalmoscopy permits identification of most of the diseases that involve the

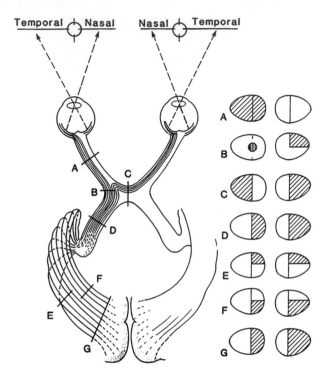

FIG. 13-1   Diagram showing the effects on the fields of vision produced by lesions at various points along the optic pathway (see Table 13-2): **A**, complete blindness in left eye; **B**, the usual effect is a left junctional scotoma in association with a right upper quadrantanopia. The latter results from interruption of right retinal nasal fibers that allegedly project into the base of the left optic nerve (Willebrand's knee). A left nasal hemianopia could occur from a lesion at this point but is rare; **C**, bitemporal hemianopia; **D**, right homonymous hemianopia; **E** and **F**, right upper- and lower-quadrant hemianopia; **G**, right homonymous hemianopia. See also Table 13-2.

retina, the retinal vessels, and the optic nerve head (see *Adams and Victor's Principles of Neurology*, 7th ed., for details).

Ancillary Examinations

A number of special tests are useful in the investigation of neuro-ophthalmic disorders. The *electroretinogram (ERG)* measures the electrical field generated by the retinal elements. The measurement is impaired in diseases affecting the retinal receptors but is normal with optic nerve lesions. This test is particularly helpful in the diagnosis of certain retinal degenerations that cause only minimal changes in the retina and pigment epithelium and are not easily detected by ophthalmoscopy. *Pattern shift visual evoked potentials* detect conduction delays caused by subtle and often asymptomatic lesions at various points in the visual pathways (Chap. 2). They are

TABLE 13-2 Lesions of the Conducting Visual Pathways (Retina to Calcarine Cortex): Effects on Visual Fields and Common Causes

Site of lesion	Field defect	Common causes
Optic nerve (A)*	Monocular scotoma or blindness	Multiple sclerosis; optic nerve glioma; ischemic optic neuropathy; sphenoid fracture, compression by tumor or sinus mucocele; Leber hereditary optic atrophy
Optic nerve and chiasm (B)	Heteronymous defect (scotomata or field defects that differ in the two eyes)	Craniopharyngioma and other suprasellar tumors
Optic chiasm (C)	Bitemporal hemianopia	Pituitary tumor; meningioma of tuberculum sellae; craniopharyngioma; aneurysm
Optic tract (D)	Homonymous hemianopia	Tumor; rarely demyelinative
Lateral geniculate	Homonymous hemianopia	Posterior cerebral artery occlusion; tumor
Geniculocalcarine pathway	Homonymous hemianopia	Infarction, mass lesion, demyelinative
Temporal loop of geniculocalcarine pathway (E)	Superior quadrantanopia	Temporal lobe infarction; mass lesion
Superior temporal lobe (F)	Inferior quadrantanopia or noncongruent homonymous hemianopia (with more posterior lesions)	Temporoparietal infarction; mass lesion
Occipital lobe and calcarine cortex (G)	Homonymous hemianopia, congruent; central homonymous hemianopic scotomata;	Posterior cerebral artery occlusion; infarction of one occipital pole
	homonymous altitudinal hemianopia (loss of vision in corresponding upper or lower visual fields);	Infarction above or below calcarine sulcus
	bilateral cortical blindness with retained pupillary reflexes	Bilateral infarction; central scotoma if only occipital poles are affected

*Letters in parentheses refer to structures in Fig. 13-1.

particularly useful in detecting nonsymptomatic optic neuritis as a manifestation of multiple sclerosis.

Other useful procedures are computed tomography (CT), magnetic resonance imaging (MRI), ultrasound examination of the orbit, and fluorescein retinography.

COMMON CAUSES OF VISUAL LOSS (Table 13-3)

Acute Retinal Lesions

Sudden painless loss of vision always suggests an ischemic lesion of the retina or optic nerve due to occlusive disease of the central retinal artery or vein or posterior ciliary arteries. Transient, painless monocular visual loss of one of several minutes duration (transient monocular blindness, or amaurosis fugax) is a common feature of stenosis or occlusion of the carotid artery on the same side; in these cases blindness or graying of vision may begin with an altitudinal "shade" effect. Macular and vitreous hemorrhages and retinal detachment are less common causes. Thrombotic or embolic occlusion of the central retinal artery renders the retina ischemic and causes a pale, bloodless appearance. Occlusion of the central retinal vein causes engorgement of the retinal veins and diffuse retinal hemorrhages. By contrast, in ischemic optic neuropathy, there may initially be few ophthalmoscopic changes or the nerve head may be swollen as a result of infarction (anterior ischemic optic neuropathy, AION); later the optic disc becomes pale. Usually these acute vascular accidents occur on a background of hypertensive atherosclerotic disease or diabetes; temporal arteritis is an important but less common cause in the elderly.

More chronic vascular changes, taking the form of straightening of the retinal arterioles, arteriolar-venular compression, and segmental narrowing of arterioles, are indicative of chronic hypertension. In malignant hypertension, there are also a number of extravascular lesions—papilledema, hemorrhages, and exudates. These retinal changes are referred to as hypertensive retinopathy, and the advanced changes are characteristically associated with hypertensive encephalopathy.

Syphilis, toxoplasmosis, cytomegalovirus, histoplasmosis, tuberculosis, and sarcoidosis may cause destructive inflammatory foci in the retina. Neoplastic foci are most often due to metastatic melanoma.

Degenerative Diseases of the Retina

Macular degeneration of late life and retinitis pigmentosa (RP) are the most common members of this group. RP is a hereditary disease in which the receptor layer of the retina degenerates, allowing melanin of the underlying pigment epithelium to collect in the thinned retina. The melanin deposits resemble bone corpuscles. The disease begins in adolescence and progresses slowly over years. The peripheral parts of the retina are first and more severely affected, constricting the visual fields and impairing twilight vision predominantly (nyctalopia). RP may occur alone or in conjunction with other hereditary metabolic and mitochondrial diseases of the nervous system—Kearns-Sayre syndrome (involving ocular muscles, corticospinal tracts, cerebellum, and myocardium), Refsum disease, Bassen-Kornzweig disease, Batten-Mayou lipid storage disease, endocrine-hypothalamic disease (Laurence-Moon-Biedl syndrome), and numerous others.

The finding of a "cherry-red spot" denotes one of the hereditary metabolic storage diseases (Tay-Sachs, Niemann-Pick). The entire retina is pale; only the macular area, which is not covered by ganglion cells, retains its color and appears red by contrast. An account of the aforementioned hereditary metabolic diseases, all of them rare, can be found in the monograph by Lyon and colleagues (see references).

PAPILLEDEMA ("CHOKED DISC")

This is a reflection of raised intracranial pressure. Here the disc margins are elevated and the retinal veins are congested and no longer pulsate. There may be peripapillary hemorrhages, but the macular and peripheral retina are normal. Cerebral tumors, abscesses, intracranial hemorrhage, chronic meningitis, pseudotumor cerebri, and tension hydrocephalus are the usual causes. Initially the visual acuity remains normal, but later the blind spots enlarge and the visual fields become constricted. With high pressure of long standing, rapid but transient visual failure may occur suddenly. Swelling of the optic nerve fibers and stasis of axoplasmic flow are thought to underlie the development of papilledema.

Other causes of disc swelling Inflammatory and demyelinative lesions, if located at the optic nerve head, may cause swelling of the disc ("*papillitis*")

TABLE 13-3 Common Clinical Types of Visual Loss

Clinical problem	Etiology
Acute (minutes to hours) blindness in one eye	Amaurosis fugax; vitreous hemorrhage; ischemic optic neuropathy; temporal arteritis; occlusion of central retinal artery or vein; glaucoma (usually painful); acute iridocyclitis; optic neuritis
Acute bilateral blindness	
Retinal lesions	Episode of hypotension; malignant hypertension; eclampsia; retinal burns (sunlight); methyl alcohol poisoning
Optic nerves	Retrobulbar neuritis; pituitary apoplexy
Chronic bilateral partial field defects	
Bilateral scotomata	Optic (retrobulbar) neuritis; nutritional amblyopia; ischemic optic neuropathy; hereditary optic atrophy
Heteronymous field defects	Lesions of chiasm and nerve(s): suprasellar tumors, arachnoiditis
Bitemporal hemianopia	Pituitary adenoma, meningioma, aneurysm, some craniopharyngiomas
Homonymous hemianopia; upper quadrantanopia (anterior and inferior temporal lobe); lower quadrantanopia (temporoparietal)	May be acute or chronic effects of infarction, tumor, abscess, or hemorrhage
Homonymous altitudinal hemianopia (above or below horizontal diameter)	Basilar or bilateral posterior cerebral artery occlusion

TABLE 13-4 Main Causes of Swelling of the Optic Disc

Ophthalmic abnormality	Underlying cause	Visual loss	Associated symptoms	Pupils
Papilledema	Increased intracranial pressure	None or transient blurring; constriction of visual fields and enlargement of blind spot; findings almost always binocular	Headache; signs of intracranial mass	Normal unless succeeded by optic atrophy
Anterior ischemic optic neuropathy (AION)	Infarction of disc and intraorbital optic nerve due to atherosclerosis or temporal arteritis	Acute visual loss, usually monocular; may be an altitudinal defect	Headache with temporal arteritis	Afferent pupillary defect
Optic neuritis[a] ("papillitis")	Inflammatory changes in disc and intraorbital part of optic nerve—usually due to MS, sometimes to ADEM	Rapidly progressive visual loss; usually monocular	Tender globe, pain on ocular movement	Afferent pupillary defect
Hyaline bodies[b] (drusen)	Congenital, familial	Usually none; may be slowly progressive enlargement of blind spot or arcuate inferior nasal defect	Usually none; rarely transient visual obscurations	Normal

Key: MS, multiple sclerosis; ADEM, acute disseminated encephalomyelopathy.
[a]Optic neuritis affecting the retrobulbar portion of the nerve shows no funduscopic changes.
[b]May be mistaken for papilledema (pseudopapilledema).

and even peripapillary hemorrhages, but there is always simultaneous impairment of visual acuity and pupillary reaction to light. With lesions located farther back in the optic nerve, the retina and optic disc may appear normal ("*retrobulbar neuritis*"), although later temporal or complete pallor of the disc becomes apparent as a result of atrophy of the optic nerve. These forms of optic neuropathy are nearly always due to a demyelinative process, mainly multiple sclerosis, and are discussed in Chap. 36. As mentioned earlier, infarction of the nerve head can also give the appearance of papilledema, but it too is associated with severe loss of visual acuity, sometimes with an altitudinal monocular visual loss. The main causes of swelling of the optic nerve head are described in Table 13-4.

For a more detailed discussion of this topic, see Victor and Ropper: *Adams and Victor's Principles of Neurology*, 7th ed, pp 247–270.

ADDITIONAL READING

Chester EM: *The Ocular Fundus in Systemic Disease*. Chicago, Year Book, 1973.

Glaser JS (ed.): *Neuro-ophthalmology*, 3rd ed. Philadelphia, Lippincott Williams & Wilkins, 1999.

Hayreh SS: Anterior ischemic optic neuropathy. *Arch Neurol* 38:675, 1981.

Lyon G, Adams RD, Kolodny EH: *Neurology of Hereditary Metabolic Diseases of Children*. New York, McGraw-Hill, 1996.

McDonald WI, Barnes D: Diseases of the optic nerve, in Asbury AK, McKhann GM, McDonald WI (eds): *Diseases of the Nervous System*, 2nd ed. Philadelphia, Saunders, 1992, pp 421–433.

Pearlman AL: Visual system, in Pearlman AL, Collins RC (eds): *Neurobiology of Disease*. New York, Oxford University Press, 1990, pp 124–149.

Tso MOM, Hayreh SS: Optic disc edema in raised intracranial pressure, III: A pathologic study of experimental papilledema. *Arch Ophthalmol* 95:1448, 1977.

14 | Disorders of Ocular Movement and Pupillary Function

The extraocular muscles, by their coordinated action, permit a visual stimulus to fall precisely on the two foveae and maintain foveal fixation when the stimulus or the subject is moving. For the latter functions, the labyrinths are essential. The precision with which the two eyes are coordinated in foveation is the most impressive sensory guidance mechanism in human neurophysiology. It makes possible two forms of ocular movement: one in which the eyes turn simultaneously in the same direction, called *conjugate* or *versional movements*, and the other in which the eyes move in opposite directions (convergence or divergence), called *disconjugate* or *vergence movements*.

The anatomic arrangements that underlie conjugate lateral eye movements are illustrated in Fig. 14-1. The signals for volitional horizontal gaze originate in the opposite frontal lobe (area 8 of Brodmann, p. 182). Descending fibers traverse the anterior limb of the internal capsule, decussate in the low midbrain, and terminate mainly in the paramedian pontine reticular formation (PPRF), which, in turn, projects to the ipsilateral sixth nerve nucleus and to the contralateral third nerve nucleus through fibers that run in the crossed medial longitudinal fasciculus (MLF). In this way, conjugate lateral gaze is accomplished by the simultaneous activation of the lateral rectus on one side and the medial rectus on the other. Medullary structures, including the medial vestibular nuclei, have important modulating influences on versional eye movements.

By contrast, *vertical eye movements* are under bilateral control of aggregates of neurons in the pretectal area of the midbrain tegmentum, in the region of the posterior commissure. The main structures in this region that govern vertical eye movements are the interstitial nucleus of Cajal (INC) and the rostral interstitial nucleus of the MLF (riMLF). The projections for upgaze cross beneath the superior colliculi; those for downgaze project directly and ipsilaterally to the superior rectus and inferior oblique subnuclei of the oculomotor complex. The pathways subserving vertical gaze are shown in Fig. 14-2.

Diseases of the nervous system result in four types of disordered ocular movements: (1) a misalignment of the eyes due to weakness or paralysis of individual ocular muscles, so that a stimulus no longer falls exactly alike on each fovea (there is then a diplopia and strabismus); (2) a failure of conjugate movement or gaze, in which the two eyes do not move synchronously in one direction, either up or down or to the right or left (in conjugate gaze palsies, there is no diplopia or strabismus); (3) a mixture of ocular muscle and gaze palsies; and (4) certain spontaneous eye movements that appear mainly in comatose patients. All of these disorders of movement must be

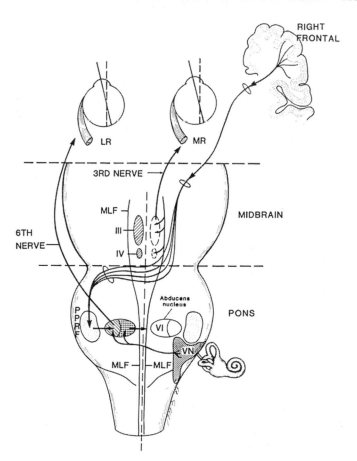

FIG. 14-1 The supranuclear pathway subserving *voluntary* conjugate horizontal gaze to the left. The pathway originates in the right frontal cortex, descends in the internal capsule, decussates at the level of the rostral pons, and descends to synapse in the left pontine paramedian reticular formation (PPRF). Further connections with the ipsilateral sixth nerve nucleus and contralateral medial longitudinal fasciculus are also indicated. Cranial nerve nuclei III and IV are labeled on left; nucleus of VI and vestibular nuclei (VN) are labeled on right. LR, lateral rectus; MR, medial rectus; MLF, medial longitudinal fasciculus.

separated from a congenital imbalance of ocular muscle tone, which misaligns the eyes at rest and in all directions of movement (nonparalytic strabismus, or phoria; see below).

THE TESTING OF EYE MOVEMENTS

To determine whether the axes of the two eyes are parallel, one observes the eyes as the patient looks straight ahead and fixates on a distant target. If one

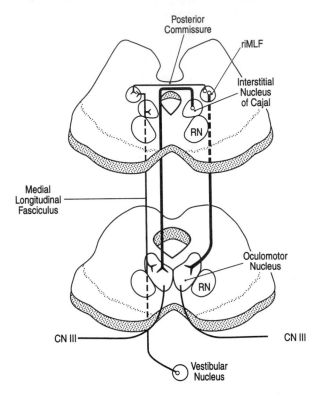

FIG. 14-2   Pathways for the control of vertical eye movements. The main structures are the interstitial nucleus of Cajal (INC), the rostral interstitial nucleus of the medial longitudinal fasciculus (riMLF), and the subnuclei of the third nerve, all located in the dorsal midbrain. Voluntary vertical movements are initiated by the simultaneous activity of both frontal cortical eye fields. The riMLF serves as the generator of vertical saccades and the INC acts tonically to hold eccentric vertical gaze. The INC and riMLF connect with their contralateral nuclei via the posterior commissure where fibers are subject to damage. Projections for upgaze cross through the commissure before descending to innervate the third nerve nucleus, while those for downgaze may travel directly to the third nerve, thus accounting for the frequency of selective upgaze palsies (see text). The MLF carries signals from the vestibular nuclei, mainly ipsilaterally, to stabilize the eyes in the vertical plane (VOR) and maintain tonic vertical position.

eye deviates inward (esotropia) or outward (exotropia) and covering the normal eye results in refixation of the deviant eye onto the target, there is an imbalance of ocular muscle tone (*congenital or nonparalytic strabismus*) rather than an ocular muscle palsy. Another way of detecting an ocular imbalance is for the patient to focus on a distant target; the examiner holds a light 1 meter away and observes the reflected image on the patient's pupils; in the eccentric eye, the light does not fall on the center of the pupil.

At the same time, one also observes the size of the pupils, the width of the two palpebral fissures, and relative prominence of the two eyes. Already one should have measured visual acuity and visual fields.

Next, one examines versional or conjugate movements, which are of two types. In one, the movements are initiated by will or by command ("look to the right" or to the left or up or down) or reflexly, as when a sudden visual or auditory stimulus causes a turning of the eyes (and usually the head) toward it. These movements are referred to as *saccadic* and are normally very accurate and rapid (about 200 ms) and hence do not in themselves interfere with vision. A single burst of ocular muscle contraction accomplishes the movement of both eyes. With certain diseases, such as Wilson disease and Huntington chorea, there may occur a marked slowness of saccadic movements. Failure to reach the target (*hypometria*), or overshoot of the target (*hypermetria*), followed by coarse corrective saccades is indicative of defective cerebellar control. Yet another abnormality is a failure to initiate voluntary saccades, which is characteristic of the late stages of progressive supranuclear palsy (see below) as well as so-called ocular apraxia of childhood (Cogan syndrome) and ataxia-telangiectasia.

A second type of versional, conjugate movement is referred to as "pursuit" or "smooth tracking." It is slower than saccadic movement and largely involuntary; it is tested by asking the patient to follow a moving target, first to one side and then the other and up and down. In addition, a slowly rotating striped drum or a striped cloth moved in front of the eyes can be used to evoke pursuit movements; the eyes follow the stripes and then make a quick corrective saccade to refocus centrally and to pursue the next stripe. These repeated rapid movements of refixation are called *optokinetic nystagmus*.

With parieto-occipital lesions, with or without hemianopia, the slow pursuit movements of the eyes *to the side of the lesion* are diminished or abolished. Cerebral control of visual pursuit movements, a function of the parietal cortex, is therefore ipsilateral. Pursuit movements, like the fast saccadic ones, may be slowed, fragmented, or dysmetric; these abnormalities are observed in progressive supranuclear palsy and other extrapyramidal diseases and as an adverse effect of sedative and anticonvulsant drugs. In a number of extrapyramidal disorders, particularly advanced Parkinson disease, the pursuit movements may be fragmented into a series of saccades.

When the patient fixates on a visual target and his head is passively turned, *vestibulo-ocular (oculocephalic) movements* are elicited. The ocular response normally is smooth and proportionate to the speed of head turning. The stimulated semicircular canals project information to the contralateral abducens nucleus, which simultaneously innervates the ipsilateral lateral rectus muscle and, via the medial longitudinal fasciculus, the opposite medial rectus muscle. Receptors in neck muscles are integrated with the vestibular end organs to produce these coordinated head and eye movements. So-called *caloric testing* utilizes the same mechanisms; stimulation of the semicircular canals by irrigation with cold water causes conjugate deviation of the eyes toward the cold stimulus. Warm water has the opposite effect. Awake patients make a series of corrective saccades in the direction opposite to the ocular deviation.

Other useful tests are observation of eye movements on forced flexion of the head (*doll's-head maneuver*) and on forced closure of the eyelids (*Bell phenomenon*). Retention of reflex upward ocular deviation in these maneuvers in the face of failure of voluntary elevation indicates that nuclear and peripheral mechanisms are intact and that the defect is supranuclear.

Vergence, or disconjugate eye movements, is tested by having the patient focus on a stimulus as it moves toward him. The eyes turn inward; concomitantly, the pupils constrict and the ciliary muscles relax to thicken the lens (near, or accommodative, triad). If convergence or divergence is inadequate, horizontal diplopia results on looking at near or distant objects, respectively. Paralysis of convergence implicates structures in the pretectal region of the midbrain; divergence paralysis is typically due to bilateral abducens weakness.

Finally, the size of the pupils and the pupillary reactions to light and dark and to near stimuli are recorded.

DISORDERS OF CONJUGATE MOVEMENT (GAZE)

Frontal lobe lesion, acute: Weakness or paralysis of contralateral gaze; eyes deviate to side of lesion temporarily (few days); retention of pursuit and vestibulo-ocular movements.

Bilateral frontal lesions: Loss of rapid voluntary (saccadic) movements to either side, with retention of visual pursuit and vestibulo-ocular movements.

Parieto-occipital lesion: Loss of pursuit movements to side of lesion; loss of the slow phase of optokinetic nystagmus to side of lesion and of the fast corrective phase contralaterally; retained voluntary, commanded, and vestibulo-ocular movements.

Midbrain periaqueductal lesion: Paralysis of vertical gaze, more often of upgaze than downgaze (Parinaud syndrome); loss of convergence; loss of horizontal gaze with large lesions; convergence and retraction nystagmus may occur on attempted upward gaze.

Pontine lesion: Ipsilateral palsy of horizontal gaze; eyes deviate away from a unilateral lesion; large lesions can cause bilateral horizontal gaze palsy.

Progressive supranuclear palsy: Loss of voluntary downward and upward and later horizontal eye movements initially sparing pursuit movements; lid retraction.

Parkinson disease: Saccadic eye movements are hypometric; pursuit movements are fragmented into a series of saccades.

Ocular "apraxia": With voluntary and commanded horizontal eye movements, the head and eyes move rapidly to one side and the eyes then move horizontally in a direction opposite to the head movement until fixation is obtained; horizontal movements are absent on pursuit; vertical movements intact; no optokinetic or vestibulo-ocular movements; seen as a congenital condition (Cogan syndrome) and in ataxia-telangiectasia.

NUCLEAR AND INFRANUCLEAR DISORDERS

A *complete oculomotor (third nerve) lesion* results in paralysis or weakness of superior, medial, and inferior rectus muscles, levator palpebrae, and usually of pupillary light and near reactions. Also, with complete lesions, there is ptosis of the eyelid, deviation of the eye outward and slightly downward (due to unopposed actions of abducens and superior oblique), and dilatation of the pupil. The pattern of diplopia on ocular movement conforms to that in Figs. 14-3 and 14-4. Compressive lesions of oculomotor nerve usually

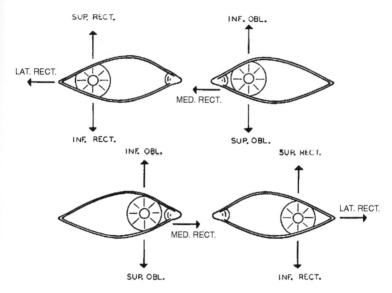

FIG. 14-3   Muscles chiefly responsible for vertical movements of the eyes in different positions of gaze. Right-gaze on top; left-gaze below.

dilate the pupil (aneurysm, tumor, herniation); ischemic lesions (e.g., diabetes), which involve the central portion of the nerve, usually do not.

A *lesion of the abducens (sixth nerve)* causes paralysis of the lateral rectus, with medial deviation of the eye, and results in uncrossed diplopia (image of abducting eye is projected lateral to image of adducting eye) on looking to the side of the lesion (Fig. 14-4). If the lesion is in the brainstem, it is often combined with a palsy of horizontal gaze or internuclear ophthalmoplegia (see below).

A *fourth (or trochlear nerve)* lesion causes paralysis of the superior oblique muscle and is manifest as extorsion and weakness of downward movement, most marked (diplopia) when the affected eye is looking downward and inward and corrected by tilting the head away from the side of the lesion.

The Analysis of Diplopia   Almost all instances of diplopia (i.e., seeing a single object as double) are the result of an acquired paresis or paralysis of one or more extraocular muscles, as described above. Usually, the faulty muscle or muscles are disclosed as the patient turns his eyes into the field of action of the paretic muscle. However, the muscle weakness may be so slight that no defect in ocular movement is obvious to the examiner. It is then necessary to determine (1) which of the cardinal positions of gaze causes the greatest separation of images and (2) which one of the pair of muscles that is active in that position is deficient; *this corresponds to the eye from which the image is displaced furthest from the neutral position.* To make these determinations, the clinician must have a working knowledge of the actions of the ocular muscles (Fig. 14-3). The eyes can be covered alternately to determine the one that produces the eccentrically displaced image. It is also helpful to become proficient in the use of the red-glass or Maddox rod test. These tests assist the patients in identifying the images derived from each eye. The essential strategy of these tests is to determine the position of gaze that produces the maximal diplopia and to identify the eye of origin, as depicted in Fig. 14-4 and elaborated in *Adams and Victor's Principles of Neurology*, 7th ed.

Causes of third, fourth, and sixth nerve palsies Common *central causes* are infarction (basilar artery and basilar branches), tumor (pontine glioma), hemorrhage, demyelinative disease, and Wernicke encephalopathy. *Peripheral causes* are infarction of nerve (particularly with hypertension and diabetes), basilar skull fractures, tumor (meningeal carcinomatosis), aneurysms or thrombosis of cavernous sinus (often with involvement of ophthalmic division of fifth nerve), saccular aneurysm (third nerve), giant compressive aneurysms, temporal arteritis, Tolosa-Hunt syndrome (painful, unilateral granulomatous infiltration of several nerves), Guillain-Barré syndrome, and increased intracranial pressure (bilateral abducens).

As a rule, pure ocular muscle weakness (without associated tract or segmental brainstem signs) indicates a peripheral nerve lesion or a disorder of muscle (thyroid ophthalmopathy, myotonic or oculopharyngeal dystrophy, certain congenital myopathies) or of neuromuscular transmission (myasthenia gravis, botulism). Muscular dystrophy and myasthenia cause ptosis of the eyelids and weakness of multiple extraocular muscles but spare pupillary function (intrinsic muscles). Botulism affects both extrinsic and intrinsic muscles of the eye.

MIXED GAZE AND OCULAR MUSCLE PARALYSIS

This is always an indication of an intrapontine or mesencephalic lesion, due usually to vascular, neoplastic, or demyelinative disease. The following are the most common of these mixed syndromes.

→

FIG. 14-4 Diplopia fields with individual muscle paralysis. The dark glass is in front of the right eye, and the fields are projected as the patient sees the images (i.e., the left side of each field diagram corresponds to the patient's right). *A.* Paralysis of right lateral rectus; right eye does not move to the right. Field: horizontal homonymous diplopia increased on looking to the right. *B.* Paralysis of right medial rectus; right eye does not move to the left. Field: horizontal crossed diplopia increased on looking to the left. *C.* Paralysis of right inferior rectus; right eye does not move downward when eyes are turned to the right. Field: vertical diplopia (image of right eye lowermost) increased on looking to the right and down. *D.* Paralysis of right superior rectus; right eye does not move upward when eyes are turned to the right. Field: vertical diplopia (image of right eye uppermost) increased on looking to the right and up. *E.* Paralysis of right superior oblique; right eye does not move downward when eyes are turned to the left. Field: vertical diplopia (image of right eye lowermost) increased on looking to the left and down. *F.* Paralysis of right inferior oblique; right eye does not move upward when eyes are turned to the left. Field: vertical diplopia (image of right eye uppermost) increased on looking to the left and up. (*Adapted, with permission, from DG Cogan, Neurology of the Ocular Muscles, 2nd ed, Springfield, IL, Charles C Thomas, 1956.*)

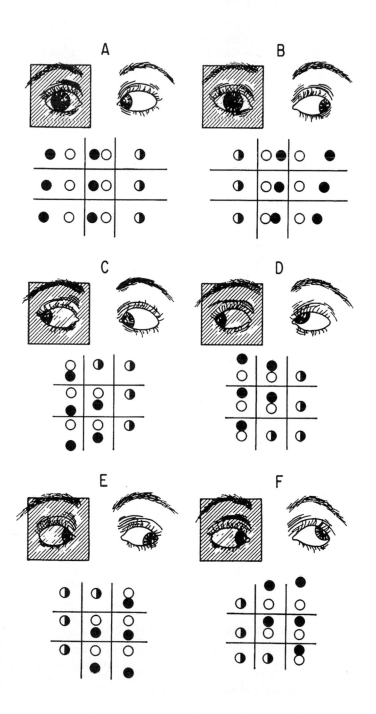

Internuclear ophthalmoplegia (see Fig. 14-1) As indicated earlier, the PPRF accomplishes horizontal gaze by the simultaneous innervation of the lateral rectus (via the ipsilateral abducens nucleus and nerve) and the contralateral medial rectus (via the MLF). Thus, with a lesion of the left MLF, the patient fails to adduct the left eye when attempting right lateral gaze, associated with nystagmus in the abducting right eye (left internuclear ophthalmoplegia). The medial rectus still functions normally in convergence, showing that it is not paralyzed. Bilateral internuclear ophthalmoplegia, affecting adduction bilaterally, is a common sign of multiple sclerosis. A unilateral lesion is usually due to a small infarction. With lesions *high in the MLF*, a loss of convergence may be added. With a lesion of the MLF near its origin in the pons, there may be involvement of the abducens nucleus, causing a homolateral paralysis of abduction combined with a failure of adduction on the opposite side (pontine gaze palsy).

The one-and-a-half syndrome (Fisher) With a lower pontine lesion, there may be involvement of the pontine gaze center and the ipsilateral MLF. One eye is paralyzed for all horizontal movements; the other eye can only abduct, with nystagmus in the direction of abduction. The abducting eye may be turned outward due to the gaze palsy (pontine paralytic exotropia).

Vertical gaze palsy with or without partial oculomotor paralysis This syndrome is due to a lesion of the midbrain tegmentum involving the pretectal centers for vertical gaze and one or both oculomotor nuclei. Dorsal midbrain lesions in the region of the superior colliculus interrupt the crossing fibers for upward gaze; often the pupils are dilated and convergence is impaired (Parinaud syndrome). Lesions of large lateral extent may interrupt horizontal gaze pathways as well (pseudoabducens palsy). The usual causes are pineal tumors, small infarctions of the midbrain, and hydrocephalus.

NYSTAGMUS

This refers to involuntary rhythmic movements of the eyes and is of two general types: (1) *jerk nystagmus*, in which the movements alternate between a slow phase in one direction and a rapid, corrective phase in the opposite direction (by custom, the nystagmus is named according to the direction of the fast phase), and (2) a less common *pendular nystagmus*, in which the oscillations are more or less equal in the two directions, although on lateral gaze two distinct phases may become evident, with the fast phase to the side of gaze. A very fine, rhythmic nystagmus, appearing at the end point of gaze, is physiologic and is abolished by allowing the eyes to move a few degrees toward the midline. Sedative and anticonvulsant drugs are the most common causes of coarse end gaze nystagmus.

The several types of pendular and jerk nystagmus, their identifying features, and their causes are summarized in Table 14-1.

OTHER DISORDERS OF OCULAR MOVEMENT

A number of abnormalities of conjugate movement are seen in comatose patients. In those with bilateral damage to a cerebral hemisphere, the eyes may rove conjugately from side to side. This is similar to—and accompanied by—oculocephalic induced movements.

TABLE 14-1 Types of Nystagmus

Type	Identifying features	Causes
Jerk nystagmus		
Optokinetic (induced by moving stripes)	Involuntary slow pursuit followed by fast corrective saccade (refixation)	Lost with parietal lesion and transiently with acute frontal lesion
Labyrinthine-vestibular	Mixed horizontal and torsional nystagmus associated with vertigo, nausea and vomiting, staggering, often tinnitus and deafness; greater amplitude to side away from lesion	Ménière disease; acute labyrinthitis; vestibular neuronitis; eighth nerve tumor; lateral medullary infarction
Fastigiovestibular (inferior cerebellum, lateral medulla)	Greatest amplitude toward side of lesion; may or may not have vertigo, nausea, or vomiting	Multiple sclerosis, brainstem infarction and tumor; hereditary ataxias
Pendular	Always binocular; oscillations in one plane	Albinism and other congenital diseases of retina and refractive media; congenital nystagmus with normal vision
Spasmus nutans	Occurs in infancy with head-nodding and wry neck	Cause unknown; prognosis good
Gaze paretic	Inability to sustain horizontal gaze with drifting of eyes to midline	Pontine reticular or cerebellar lesion
Drug-induced	Usually horizontal, may be vertical and asymmetrical	Intoxication with alcohol, phenytoin, barbiturates
Upbeat	Precise anatomy uncertain, probably pontine	Multiple sclerosis, infarction, tumors, Wernicke disease
Downbeat	Lesions in medullary-cervical region	Chiari malformation, syringobulbia, basilar invagination, Wernicke disease, Li intoxication
Special types		
Monocular in abducting eye	Incompletely developed internuclear ophthalmoplegia	Multiple sclerosis, vascular lesions, Wernicke disease
Retraction and convergence	Slow abduction, followed by quick adduction and retraction of both eyes, often with paralysis of upward gaze	Infarcts, tumors (pinealoma) of midbrain
Seesaw	Torsional-vertical oscillation; intorting eye moves up, extorting eye down, then reverse	Sellar or parasellar masses

Ocular bobbing consists of fast downward (or upward) movements of both eyes, followed by a slow return to the central position. These movements are usually observed in comatose patients, in whom horizontal movements are absent, and are associated most often with extensive pontine lesions. *Ocular dipping* is the name that has been given to a slow downward movement of the eyes, followed in a few seconds by a more rapid upward movement in the context of preserved horizontal movements. Anoxic encephalopathy is the most common cause.

Ocular myoclonus is a rapid, continuous, rhythmic pendular oscillation of the eyes, usually occurring in the vertical plane and in conjunction with movements of similar rhythm involving the palate, face, neck, or thoracic muscles (p. 47). The lesion (vascular or tumor) involves the central tegmental tracts between the red nuclei and the medulla.

Opsoclonus refers to rapid multidirectional conjugate oscillations of the eyes ("dancing eyes"). *Ocular flutter* is a closely related disorder in which bursts of very rapid horizontal oscillations occur around the point of fixation. These disorders are often part of a paraneoplastic syndrome in adults and may be associated with widespread myoclonus; neuroblastoma in children and viral encephalitis of childhood are other causes.

Sustained spasm of convergence may occur with lesions of the upper midbrain tegmentum. As an isolated phenomenon, it is usually a hysterical symptom.

ABNORMALITIES OF THE PUPILS

The size of the pupil is controlled by the degree of retinal illumination and depends on the integrity of a reflex pathway along the optic nerves and tracts, superior colliculi, oculomotor nuclei (Edinger-Westphal) and nerves, ciliary ganglia, and irides. In addition, a sympathetic hypothalamic-cervical cord pathway, with exit mainly at T2, sends preganglionic fibers to the superior cervical ganglion and postganglionic fibers along the internal carotid artery to pupillodilator muscles (see Chap. 26). The pathways concerned with the pupillary light reflex are illustrated in Fig. 14-5.

Parasympathetic stimulation constricts the pupil and sympathetic stimulation dilates it; i.e., parasympathetic and sympathetic paralyses have opposite effects. Usually, lesions that interrupt the parasympathetic innervation of the pupil also interfere with accommodation. This is true of botulinum and diphtheria infections, Guillain-Barré syndrome, and the periaqueductal (Parinaud) syndrome. But in certain diseases, mainly syphilis and diabetes, pupillary constriction to light is lost while that of convergence is retained (Argyll Robertson pupil). Lesions that involve the parasympathetic fibers within the third nerve usually also affect the levator palpebrae, causing ptosis, and affect ocular muscles (mainly medial rectus) to a variable degree. The main pupillary syndromes are summarized in Table 14-2.

The functional integrity of the sympathetic and parasympathetic innervation of the pupils can be determined pharmacologically. The small pupil that is due to sympathetic denervation (*Horner syndrome*) fails to dilate in the dark and in response to the conjunctival instillation of 4 to 10% cocaine. If the lesion is in the postganglionic neuron, the pupil still does not react to hydroxyamphetamine (1%); however, if the lesion is central or preganglionic, the pupil will dilate with the latter drug. A *tonic (Adie) pupil* constricts to a tiny size with 0.1% pilocarpine (denervation supersensitivity). A

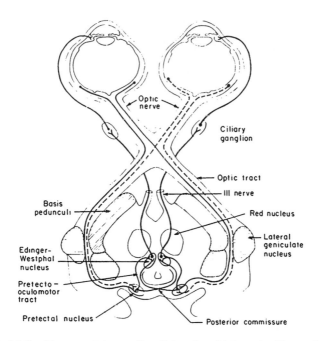

FIG. 14-5   Diagram of the pupillary light reflex. (*Adapted, with permission, from FB Walsh, WF Hoyt, Clinical Neuro-Ophthalmology, 3rd ed, Baltimore, Williams & Wilkins, 1969.*)

large pupil that is due to a mydriatic (anticholinergic) drug does not constrict, even to 1.0% pilocarpine.

With blindness due to interruption of the optic nerve, the reflex constriction to direct light is abolished (*afferent defect*) and there is also absence of the reflex constriction that normally occurs in the opposite eye (*consensual reflex*). However, the pupil of the blind eye is still capable of consensual constriction from a light stimulus to the opposite normal eye. Damage to the retina or optic nerve may weaken the direct light reflex and, after a brief constriction, the pupil dilates (Gunn pupil sign). Inequality of the pupils (*anisocoria*) of mild degree, unaccompanied by other pupillary abnormalities, is present in many normal persons. *Hippus* refers to small, arrhythmic fluctuations in pupillary size; it is seen mostly in metabolic encephalopathies.

DISORDERS OF THE EYELIDS AND BLINKING

The eyelids serve to protect the corneas. The width of the two palpebral fissures is usually equal, maintained by the constant action of the levator palpebrae muscle (innervated by the third nerve) and by Müller's muscle (sympathetically innervated). Closure is effected by the orbicularis oculi muscle, which is innervated by the facial nerve.

Ptosis, a drooping of the lid, may be a manifestation of levator weakness, signifying dysfunction of the third nerve, in which case it is often associated

TABLE 14-2 Major Pupillary Syndromes

Type	Main features	Causes
Horner syndrome	Ptosis upper eyelid (paresis of Müller's muscle), miosis, apparent enophthalmos (narrowed palpebral fissure); ipsilateral anhidrosis and warmth of face	Lesions involving sympathetic pathway in brainstem and cervical cord (no anhidrosis) or in upper thorax, neck, internal carotid, cavernous sinus, or orbit
Adie syndrome (pupillotonia)	Blurred vision, one enlarged pupil, anisocoria, more common in women, knee and ankle jerks often absent; pupil dilates only slowly to strong maximal stimulation, dilatation sustained, sensitive (constricts) to 0.1% pilocarpine	Idiopathic degeneration of ciliary ganglia and postganglionic parasympathetic fibers; occasionally diabetes
Argyll Robertson pupil	Pupils small, irregular, unequal; do not react to light, but near response is intact; no response to mydriatics; iris atrophy; vision intact	Neurosyphilis, especially tabes; occasionally diabetes
Other light–near dissociation syndromes	Pupils do not react to light; react on accommodation; pupils normal size; vision intact	Neurosyphilis; diabetes; high midbrain lesions (pinealoma, multiple sclerosis)
Dilated pupil	Unreactive to light and accommodation	Part of oculomotor palsy, always with some degree of ptosis and extraocular muscle weakness; if a solitary finding, usually due to a mydriatic drug

with pupillary enlargement and oculomotor weakness as mentioned above; or it may be due to loss of sympathetic tone that also affects the lower lid and causes miosis (Horner syndrome). Disorders of the facial nerve may cause an apparent ptosis on the opposite side by enlarging the affected palpebral fissure. Paralysis of eyelid closure is caused by Bell's palsy and other lesions of the facial nerve (see Chap. 47). Combined weakness of lid elevation and closure is usually myopathic (myasthenia gravis, ocular myopathy, etc.).

The normal frequency of blinking is 12 to 20 times per minute and is increased in frequency and forcefulness in *blepharospasm*, a condition often associated with other dyskinesias. Blinking is reduced in Parkinson disease and drug-induced parkinsonism.

Exophthalmos is a protrusion of the globe and overlying lid. Thyroid disease, which also enlarges the extraocular muscles, is a frequent cause of bilateral exophthalmos and rarely of unilateral exophthalmos. The latter may be due to a mass in the orbit or cavernous sinus thrombosis.

For a more detailed discussion of this topic, see Victor and Ropper: *Adams and Victor's Principles of Neurology*, 7th ed, pp 271–300.

ADDITIONAL READING

Caplan LR: "Top of the basilar" syndrome. *Neurology* 30:72, 1980.

Corbett JJ, Thompson HS: Pupillary function and dysfunction, in Asbury AK, McKhann GM, McDonald WI (eds): *Diseases of the Nervous System*, 2nd ed. Philadelphia, Saunders, 1992, pp 490–500.

Daroff RB: Ocular oscillations. *Ann Otol Rhinol Laryngol* 86:102, 1977.

Glaser JS (ed): *Neuro-ophthalmology*, 3rd ed. Philadelphia, Lippincott, 1999.

Keane JR: Acute bilateral ophthalmoplegia: 60 cases. *Neurology* 36:279, 1986.

Leigh RJ, Zee DS: *The Neurology of Eye Movements*, 2nd ed. Philadelphia, Davis, 1991.

Rush JA, Younge BR: Paralysis of cranial nerves III, IV, and VI: Cause and prognosis in 1000 cases. *Arch Ophthalmol* 99:76, 1981.

Spector RW, Troost BT: The ocular motor system. *Ann Neurol* 9:517, 1981.

Thompson HS, Pilley SFJ: Unequal pupils: A flow chart for sorting out the anisocorias. *Surv Ophthalmol* 21:45, 1976.

15 | Deafness, Dizziness, and Disorders of Equilibrium

The eighth cranial nerve contains fibers that subserve hearing and equilibrium. These two neurologic systems and the diseases that derange these functions are quite distinct; for that reason, they are considered separately.

DEAFNESS

There are three types of deafness: (1) *conductive* deafness, which is caused by a defect of the external or middle ear (i.e., the structures that amplify and conduct sound to the receptive elements in the cochlea); (2) *sensorineural* or *nerve* deafness, which is caused by disorders of the cochlea or auditory (eighth cranial) nerve; and (3) *central* deafness, which is due to abnormalities of the cochlear nuclei in the brainstem and their connections in the upper brainstem and with the primary receptive areas in the temporal lobes. The first of these types is mainly of interest to otologists and the second and third types, to neurologists, although specialists in both fields must be able to differentiate all types of deafness.

Tests of Hearing

The patient's report of hearing loss is usually reliable; the examiner can confirm this by testing the patient's ability to hear a whispered voice in each ear. A number of simple tuning fork tests are helpful in separating conductive from sensorineural deafness. When a tuning fork, vibrating at 512 Hz (middle C), is applied to the middle of the forehead, the sound is normally heard in both ears. In nerve deafness, the sound is localized in the normal ear; in conductive deafness, it is localized in the affected ear (*Weber test*). In the *Rinne test*, the vibrating fork is applied to the mastoid bone, and as soon as the sound ceases, the fork is held at the auditory meatus. Normally, air conduction (AC) is greater than bone conduction (BC). In middle ear deafness, BC > AC; in nerve deafness, the reverse is true (positive Rinne), although both AC and BC may be quantitatively reduced.

Sensorineural deafness, if partial, affects high tones more than low tones; the opposite occurs in conduction deafness. This is determined most accurately by the use of an audiometer and the construction of an audiogram, which is an essential procedure in any investigation of hearing loss.

Special Audiologic Procedures

Often it is difficult to distinguish between lesions that affect the organ of Corti (the cochlear receptor) and those of the auditory nerve (retrocochlear lesions). It is nonetheless important to make this distinction because retrocochlear lesions (one of the most common of which is an acoustic neuroma) are surgically treatable. In addition to the audiogram, a number of special laboratory tests are useful. These are Békésy audiometry, loudness recruitment and threshold "tone decay" (often the most helpful), speech discrimination, short-increment sensitivity index, and brainstem auditory evoked responses (see *Adams and Victor's Principles of Neurology*, 7th ed., for details). Magnetic resonance imaging (MRI) provides clear images of the brainstem and internal auditory meati and can identify tiny intracanalicular tumors of the eighth nerve.

Tinnitus

Tinnitus refers to sounds emanating from the ear: ringing, buzzing, humming, whistling, hissing, clicking, or pulse-like sensations. Tinnitus is of two general types: *tonal*, which can be heard only by the patient (subjective), and a far less frequent type, *nontonal*, which can sometimes be heard by the examiner as well as by the patient (hence, objective).

Tonal tinnitus, transient and of short duration, is experienced by most normal adults in very quiet surroundings (physiologic tinnitus); under ordinary conditions, it is masked by the ambient noise level. A persistent complaint of tinnitus usually signifies a disturbance of the tympanic membrane, ossicles, cochlea, or auditory nerve. As a generalization, ringing and high-pitched musical sounds are associated with impairment of neurosensory (cochlear) function. Tinnitus due to middle ear disease (e.g., otosclerosis) tends to be more constant, of variable intensity, and of lower pitch.

Nontonal tinnitus consists of noises that are conducted to the ear from various structures of the head and neck: clicks from the eustachian tube, temporomandibular joint, or tensor tympani muscle; a bruit transmitted from neck vessels or from an intracranial arteriovenous malformation or glomus tumor; or the rhythmic (1- to 2-per-second) beat of palatal myoclonus.

Table 15-1 lists the common causes of acquired deafness and tonal tinnitus. The numerous types of hereditary deafness are classified and tabulated in *Adams and Victor's Principles of Neurology*, 7th ed.

DIZZINESS AND VERTIGO

Dizziness is among the most common of all neurologic complaints, and an essential step in dealing with it is to determine how the patient is using the word. Most often it is found to refer to a feeling of light-headedness, giddiness, weakness, or faintness. The patient, given a choice of terms, usually likens it to a swaying sensation rather than a feeling of rotation or other illusion of movement characteristic of vertigo. If uncertainty exists, deep breathing will usually reproduce the feeling of light-headedness, precluding a labyrinthine disorder. In contrast, dizziness that is greatly worsened by head shaking is most often a type of vertigo.

Clinical settings in which one encounters pseudovertiginous symptoms are anxiety states, hyperventilation, severe anemia, chronic obstructive pulmonary disease, and orthostatic hypotension. Such symptoms may also be found in patients taking antihypertensive drugs or who have been recently bedfast, as well as in some elderly but otherwise asymptomatic persons. Rising quickly from a sitting or recumbent position may be followed by a swaying dizziness and "spots before the eyes"; the symptoms abate after several seconds, during which time the patient stands still and steadies himself.

TABLE 15-1 Common Causes of Deafness and Tonal Tinnitus

Type	Site of lesion	Treatment
Conduction		
Chronic otitis, mastoiditis	Middle ear, mastoid air cells	Control of infection
Otosclerosis	Ossicles	Surgery
Disorders of external ear or eustachian canal	—	Symptomatic
Cochlear		
Degenerative deafness (over 35 types, many of them hereditary and associated with other neurologic disorders)	End organ (cochlea) often with retinal, systemic, or neurologic abnormalities	See *Adams and Victor's Principles of Neurology,* 7th ed.
Infections	Cochlea, nerve (?)	For measles, mumps, herpes zoster, otitis media, etc.
Presbycusis	Cochlea and spiral ganglion	
Drugs (kanamycin, streptomycin, gentamicin, ethacrynic acid, furosemide)	Organ of Corti	Preventive
Explosions, intense noise	Organ of Corti	—
Ménière disease	Organ of Corti	See text, under vertigo
Auditory nerve		
Tumor, trauma, vascular loop Postmeningitis	Usually both portions of eighth nerve	Surgery in some cases
Central		
Unilateral	Cochlear nuclei	—
Bilateral	Temporal lobes (infarction, tumor)	Surgery in some cases of tumor

True vertigo usually comes in attacks, which, if severe, are accompanied by nausea and vomiting, sometimes with pallor and perspiration, difficulty in walking, and the need to sit or lie down. In its most common form, the patient reports a whirling or turning sensation, either of objects in the environment or of himself. Less frequently, other feelings of movement are described, such as tilting or leaning or being pulled to one side, or the environment may appear tilted. Nystagmus, horizontal and rotary, is usually present during an attack. Certain motions of the head or body, such as turning over in bed, may provoke brief episodes of vertigo. The site of disease is almost always in some part of the labyrinthine-vestibular apparatus—in the semicircular canals, vestibular nerve, or vestibular nuclei of the brainstem. Less commonly, vertigo arises from a lesion of the vestibulocerebellum (flocculonodular lobe) or, rarely, as part of a seizure arising in the temporal lobe.

Causes of Vertigo

The common causes of an acute attack of vertigo are benign positional vertigo, Ménière disease, and vestibular neuronitis. It may also follow head injury.

Benign positional vertigo This is the most frequent in clinical practice. It is characterized by brief (a minute or less) attacks of vertigo and nystagmus that occur immediately upon assuming certain positions of the head, such as lying down, turning over in bed, or tilting the head backward. Symptoms may recur periodically for several days or months. *Hearing is unaffected.* Diagnosis is confirmed by moving the patient from the sitting position to recumbency with the head tilted 30° over the end of the table and 30° to one side (Fig. 15-1A and B; Hallpike maneuver). This maneuver produces a brief attack of vertigo and nystagmus; return to the sitting position changes the direction of the vertigo and nystagmus. After about three successive trials, the attacks can no longer be elicited. As to pathogenesis, it is generally

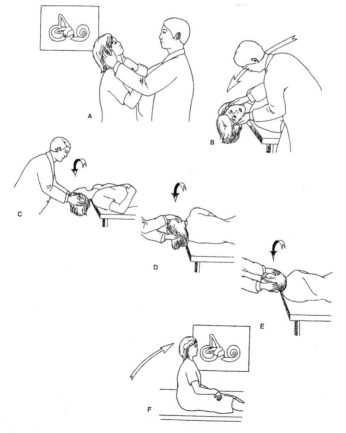

FIG. 15-1   Dix-Hallpike maneuver to elicit benign positional vertigo (*A* and *B*) and treatment with the canalith repositioning maneuver (*C* to *F*). See text for details. (*Adapted from Fife, with permission.*)

TABLE 15-2 Vertiginous Syndromes with Lesions of Different Parts of the Vestibular System

Site and type of lesion	Other neurologic findings	Disorders of equilibrium	Type of nystagmus*	Hearing	Laboratory exam
Labyrinthine, *unilateral* (trauma, Ménière disease, vestibular neuronitis, labyrinthitis, benign positional)	None	Ipsilateral past pointing and lateral propulsion to side of lesion	Horizontal to side opposite lesion, or rotary; paroxysmal, positionally induced	Normal, or conduction or neurosensory deafness with recruitment (normal in benign positional type)	Vestibular paresis by caloric testing
Labyrinthine, *bilateral* (aminoglycoside toxicity; idiopathic vestibulopathy)	None	Slightly wide base and tottering to both sides	Bilateral fine horizontal or rotary, or none	Normal, or sensorineural deafness	Vestibular paresis by caloric testing, bilateral
Vestibular nerve and ganglia (vestibular neuropathy, herpes zoster)	Auditory eighth, seventh, and sometimes other cranial nerve abnormalities	Ipsilateral past pointing and lateral propulsion to side of lesion	Horizontal to side opposite lesion, or rotary; positionally induced	Usually sensorineural deafness, without recruitment; speech discrimination diminished	MRI and CT may be normal or abnormal; vestibular paresis on caloric testing

Cerebellopontine angle (acoustic neuroma, glomus and other tumors)	Ipsilateral fifth, seventh, ninth, tenth cranial neuropathies; cerebellar ataxia; increased intracranial pressure (late)	Ataxia and falling ipsilaterally	Gaze-paretic, positionally induced, coarser to side of lesion	Sensorineural deafness without recruitment	CT and MRI abnormal; vestibular paresis on caloric testing; increased CSF protein
Brainstem and cerebellum (infarcts, tumors, viral infections)	Multiple cranial neuropathies, brainstem tract signs, cerebellar ataxia	Ataxia present with eyes open	Coarse horizontal and vertical; gaze-paretic	Usually normal	Hyperactive labyrinths or directional preponderance on caloric testing; CT and MRI abnormal in some cases
Higher (cerebral) connections	Aphasia, visual field, hemimotor, hemisensory, and other cerebral abnormalities, seizures	No change	Usually absent	Normal	No change in caloric responses; CT and EEG may be abnormal

*See Chap. 14 for description of types of nystagmus.

believed that otolithic debris comes loose from the utricular macula and, with changes in head position, gravitates into the posterior semicircular canal, where it induces push-and-pull forces on the cupula, triggering an attack of vertigo (Shuknecht).

Benign positional vertigo usually requires no special therapy. For patients with severe and frequent attacks, a *canalith repositioning maneuver* has been devised (see Fife; also Fig. 15-1*C* to *F*). The first part of the canalith repositioning maneuver (Fig. 15-1*A* and *B*) is identical to the diagnostic Hallpike maneuver, outlined above. With the patient in the head-hanging position that causes symptoms, the head is turned in a series of three steps, each separated by about 20 s (*C* to *F*): first the head is turned 45 to 60° toward the opposite ear; then turned onto his left side and the head turned an additional 45°, until the head is parallel to the ground; then the head is turned once more until it nearly faces the floor. After 20 s, the patient is returned to the upright position and must remain at least 45° upright for the next 24 h. Often a single sequence suffices to terminate an attack of positional vertigo. Antihistaminics are useful in patients with vestibular neuronitis (see below).

Ménière disease   In this disease the attacks of vertigo are characteristically abrupt, several minutes to an hour in duration, and of such severity that the patient must lie still, preferentially with the faulty ear uppermost. Nystagmus, induced by rotation or caloric stimulation, is impaired or lost on the affected side. Tinnitus, a sense of head or ear fullness, and deafness are usually associated and may worsen during an attack.

During an acute attack of Ménière disease, the patient recognizes the need to remain immobile in a position that minimizes the vertigo. Fortunately, the severe vertigo is usually of brief duration; if it is protracted, the administration of one of several antihistaminic drugs is helpful: dimenhydrinate (Dramamine), cyclizine (Marezine), meclizine (Bonine, Antivert), or promethazine (Phenergan) in doses of 25 to 50 mg every 4 h. Trimethobenzamine (Tigan) in 200-mg suppositories every 6 h is useful in controlling the nausea and vomiting. If the attacks are frequent and disabling, permanent relief can be obtained by surgical destruction of the labyrinth—undertaken only if the disease is strictly unilateral and hearing loss is nearly complete. Or the vestibular portion of the eighth nerve can be sectioned.

Vestibular neuronitis   This process is distinguished by the occurrence of a single protracted attack of vertigo, which persists in severe form for several days and, to a lesser degree, for several weeks. There is a reduced response to caloric stimulation on one side, and *tinnitus and deafness are absent*. Rare recurrent and epidemic forms have been noted. The cause of this disorder and exact site of the lesion have not been firmly established; an inflammatory lesion of the vestibular portion of the eighth nerve, presumably of viral origin, has been postulated.

Vertigo, usually fluctuating in severity but not occurring in attacks and accompanied by neural deafness and other cranial nerve signs, is a rare but characteristic symptom of acoustic neuroma. Some cases of intractable vertigo, previously thought to be idiopathic, have been relieved by the repositioning of a tortuous branch of the basilar artery, a loop of which has come into contact with the eighth nerve (Janetta and colleagues). These and other common vertiginous syndromes and their main clinical features are summarized in Table 15-2.

For a more detailed discussion of this topic, see Victor and Ropper: *Adams and Victor's Principles of Neurology*, 7th ed, pp 301–328.

ADDITIONAL READING

Baloh RW: *Dizziness, Hearing Loss, and Tinnitus: The Essentials of Neurotology.* Philadelphia, Davis, 1984.

Baloh RW, Honrubia V, Jacobson K: Benign positional vertigo: Clinical and oculographic features in 240 cases. *Neurology* 37:371, 1987.

Baloh RW, Jacobson K, Honrubia V: Idiopathic bilateral vestibulopathy. *Neurology* 39:272, 1989.

Brandt T, Steddin S, Daroff RB: Therapy for benign paroxysmal positional vertigo, revisited. *Neurology* 44:796, 1994.

Fife TD: Bedside cure for benign positional vertigo. *Barrows Neurol Inst Q* 10:2, 1994.

Janetta PJ, Moller MB, Moller AR: Disabling positional vertigo. *N Engl J Med* 310:1700, 1984.

Konigsmark BW: Hereditary progressive cochleovestibular atrophies, in Vinken PJ, Bruyn GW (eds): *Handbook of Clinical Neurology*, vol 22. Amsterdam, North-Holland, 1975, pp 481–497.

Konigsmark BW: Hereditary diseases of the nervous system with hearing loss, in Vinken PJ, Bruyn GW (eds): *Handbook of Clinical Neurology*, vol 22. Amsterdam, North-Holland, 1975, pp 499–526.

Nadol JB Jr: Hearing loss. *N Engl J Med* 329:1092, 1993.

Shuknecht HF: Cuprolithiasis. *Arch Otolaryngol* 90:765, 1965.

Shuknecht HF, Kitamura K: Vestibular neuronitis. *Ann Otol Rhinol Laryngol* 90:1, 1981.

16 | Epilepsy and Other Seizure Disorders

Epilepsy is one of the most frequent and dramatic of all neurologic disorders. Often it is the only manifestation of a disease state that is otherwise inapparent but persists for a lifetime and requires regular medical care. In many other cases, seizures complicate intercurrent medical and neurologic illnesses or brain injuries.

The term *epilepsy* refers to recurrent seizures that were recognized by Hughlings Jackson more than a century ago as being due to the intermittent, sudden, excessive discharge of cerebral cortical neurons. The term *convulsion* applies to a seizure in which motor manifestations predominate. *Seizure* is the more appropriate term, since many attacks are purely sensory or akinetic and also because the term can be qualified (e.g., psychic seizure and convulsive seizure).

Seizures take many forms, varying according to cause, location of the lesion, electroencephalographic (EEG) correlates, and the level of maturity of the nervous system at the time of their occurrence. Many classifications have been elaborated on the basis of these and other features. For all practical purposes, however, only two major categories need be recognized:

1. *Primary, generalized seizures:* bilaterally symmetrical, without local onset. These are of two main types: one first called by the French and now known to everyone as *grand mal* and the other, consisting of a brief lapse of consciousness, referred to originally as *petit mal* and now as *absence* seizures.
2. *Partial seizures:* seizures beginning locally. These are also of two main types: *simple*, in which consciousness is not impaired, and *complex*, with impairment or alteration of consciousness. These seizures vary with the site of the discharging focus and often become generalized. Partial seizures are also called *focal* or *secondary seizures*, emphasizing the facts that they usually have an identifiable structural cause and that there is a need to ascertain the localization and nature of the epileptogenic lesion.

In all forms of epilepsy, the EEG is the most effective way of identifying a seizure discharge, and magnetic resonance imaging (MRI) and computed tomography (CT) scanning provide the best means of demonstrating an epileptogenic lesion.

GENERALIZED SEIZURES

Grand Mal

Sometimes without warning or only after a brief (seconds) unnatural visceral sensation, the patient abruptly loses consciousness and emits a cry as the entire musculature becomes engaged in a violent contraction. The patient falls to the ground and the jaws snap shut, often biting the tongue; breathing is arrested, and if the bladder is full, it empties. The tonic contraction is sustained for about 20 s, and the patient becomes cyanotic; then the tonic contraction breaks into a series of clonic contractions, which last for a minute or less as a rule (tonic-clonic seizure). Less often the sequence differs; for example, a brief clonic phase precedes the tonic phase (clonic-tonic-clonic seizure). At the end of the final clonic phase, breathing resumes and the patient lies comatose, flaccid, and breathing quietly. After a few minutes, consciousness is regained, but the patient is confused and drowsy and has no recollection of the event. Later there may be headache, a sore, bitten tongue, aching of overexercised muscles, and the aftereffects of a hurtful fall. Vertebrae may be crushed and serious craniocerebral injury incurred. Almost always, the serum CK is elevated for several hours, a useful way to corroborate the occurrence of a convulsion that has not been witnessed. During a seizure the EEG shows a continuous train of rhythmic spikes or sharp waves and a suppression of normal background rhythms. In the immediate postictal period, there is slowing of the EEG, which may still display sharp waves or brief seizure discharges.

If one grand mal seizure after another occurs before full recovery from the preceding one, and more particularly before consciousness is regained, the condition is known as *grand mal*, or *tonic-clonic status epilepticus*.

Petit Mal (Absence)

The absence seizure consists of a brief lapse of consciousness, which comes without warning, lasts for 2 to 10 s, and is followed by immediate and full resumption of consciousness. Often there is blinking of the eyelids or rhythmic (3-per-second) movement of the arms or fingers. The patient remains sitting or standing and afterward may be unaware that anything has happened. Hyperventilation may induce an attack.

This form of petit mal is a disease of childhood, with onset between 4 and 12 years of age. The attacks tend to become less frequent (but rarely disappear) in adolescence, when a major seizure may appear for the first time. During an attack, the *EEG shows a characteristic generalized, highly rhythmic, 3-per-second spike-and-wave abnormality.*

Petit Mal Variants

A number of unusual epilepsies, seen mostly in infancy and childhood, are not easily classified but bear some resemblance to petit mal. In these varieties, loss of consciousness is less complete and myoclonus more prominent than in typical absence. The spike-and-wave EEG discharge may occur at a frequency of 2 to 2.5 per second, or there may be 2- to 6-Hz multiwave and spike complexes.

One particular variant, called the *Lennox-Gastaut syndrome*, consists of atonic (astatic) postural lapses succeeded by various combinations of minor tonic-clonic seizures and tonic spasms, intellectual impairment (not part of typical absence), and a distinctive slow (1- to 2.5-per-second) spike-and-wave EEG pattern. Often this syndrome occurs in a patient who in previous years had infantile spasms, an EEG with continuous multifocal spikes and delta waves of large amplitude ("hypsarrhythmia"), and retardation in mental development—a triad known as the West syndrome. The seizures of Lennox-Gastaut syndrome are frequently associated with extensive lesions of the brain. These seizures may persist into adult life. They take various forms and are often recalcitrant to many combinations of anticonvulsant therapy.

Pathogenesis The pathologic basis and cause of the primary seizure states described above has not been established, hence the term *idiopathic*. In various series, 3 to 6 percent have a family history of seizures. In identical twins, there is concordance in more than half. Several special disorders, notably juvenile myoclonic epilepsy, appear to have a genetic basis, but the mechanism of generation of seizures is still unknown. Increasingly, a subtle loss of tissue and a change in magnetic resonance (MR) signal intensity are being found in the inferomedial temporal gyri. This presumably represents perinatal injury (medial temporal, or hippocampal sclerosis).

PARTIAL, OR FOCAL, SEIZURES

Seizures that make up this category, in distinction to primary generalized ones, usually have readily identifiable structural causes. Recognition of the focal symptoms of the seizure, particularly at its outset, is of prime importance, because it enables one to localize the discharging lesion. These localizing clinical correlates are listed in Table 16-1.

Both simple and complex patterns occur. *Simple*, or *elementary*, *partial seizures* are unaccompanied by a loss of consciousness if the motor, sensory, or psychic symptoms remain confined to one region or one side of the brain. Focal motor seizures attributable to a lesion of the opposite frontal lobe are characterized by forceful turning of the eyes and head to the side opposite the discharging focus, often with tonic contraction and then clonic movements of the limbs on that side. The *jacksonian motor seizure*, in which there is, within seconds, an orderly spread ("march") of clonic movements from the muscles first affected to other muscles on the same side, although quite uncommon, has the same localizing significance as a focal motor seizure of the more common type.

Rolandic epilepsy (sylvian epilepsy; epilepsy with central-temporal spikes) is a relatively common and benign type of focal motor epilepsy with a strong heritable predisposition. It begins between 5 and 9 years of age and takes the form of clonic contractions of one side of the face and body, with high-voltage spikes in the opposite lower rolandic area. The spike activity is accentuated during slow-wave sleep. The seizures tend to disappear during adolescence. Similar benign types of epilepsy are designated by the predominant focus of spike activity (occipital, parietal, frontal).

Epilepsia partialis continua is a special form of focal motor seizure characterized by clonic movements of one group of muscles, most often of the face, hand, or foot. The movements are repeated at regular intervals of a few seconds and may continue without interruption for days or months on end without spreading to other parts. This form of epilepsy is related to a

TABLE 16-1 Common Seizure Patterns

Clinical type	Localization
Somatic motor	
Jacksonian (local motor)	Prerolandic gyrus
Masticatory	Amygdaloid nuclei
Simple contraversive	Frontal
Head and eye turning	Supplementary motor cortex
associated with arm posturing	
Somatic and special sensory (auras)	
Somatosensory	Contralateral postrolandic
Unformed visual images, lights,	
patterns	Occipital
Auditory	Heschl gyri (temporal lobe)
Vertiginous	Superior temporal
Olfactory	Mesial temporal
Gustatory	Parietal and/or rolandic operculum
Visceral: autonomic	Insular-orbital-frontal cortex
Complex partial	
Formed hallucinations	Temporal neocortex or amygdaloid-hippocampal complex
Illusions	—
Dyscognitive experiences	Temporal
(déjà vu, dreamy states, depersonalization)	
Affective states (fear,	Temporal
depression, or elation)	
Automatism (ictal and postictal)	Temporal and frontal
Absence	Frontal cortex, amygdaloid-hippocampal complex, reticulocortical system
Bilateral epileptic myoclonus	Reticulocortical

Source: Modified from Penfield and Jasper.

cortical-subcortical lesion of the opposite side and usually does not respond favorably to anticonvulsant medication.

Somatosensory seizures, either focal or "marching," point to a lesion in or near the opposite postcentral gyrus. Other focal sensory seizures—visual, auditory, olfactory, vertiginous—also have discrete localizing value, but all of these types are infrequent (Table 16-1).

Seizure discharges arising in the temporal lobe (temporal lobe epilepsy) are unique in that *the initial event in the seizure* (i.e., *the aura*) is often a hallucination or perceptual illusion, such as a feeling of familiarity, strangeness, fear, visceral sensation, and so forth. If these subjective experiences constitute the entire attack, it is classified as a *simple partial seizure.* If the aura is followed by a period of unresponsiveness and altered behavior (lip smacking, chewing or swallowing movements, and walking in a daze, so-called *automatisms*), the seizures are classified as *complex partial* or *psychomotor seizures.*

Brain lesions of many types are regularly found in patients with simple and complex partial seizures. They give rise to epileptogenic foci in the surrounding tissue and are sometimes amenable to excision.

Myoclonus as a neurologic phenomenon and some of its relationships to epilepsy have been discussed in Chap. 6. The small rhythmic myoclonic jerks that occur as part of absence seizures, the isolated myoclonic jerks that portend clonic-tonic-clonic seizures, and the massive myoclonic spasms that characterize West syndrome have all been alluded to earlier in this chapter. Myoclonus, focal or diffuse, is often the main feature of *juvenile myoclonic epilepsy*—a common and relatively benign form of epilepsy that begins in adolescence and responds well to valproic acid. Widespread stimulus-sensitive myoclonus is a feature of certain grave disorders of childhood, such as Lafora body disease and hereditary neuronal storage disease, which lead to progressive dementia and death.

Finally, it should be emphasized that any focal seizure may evolve into a generalized convulsion. If this happens rapidly or if the initial focal symptom is not recognized, the seizure is indistinguishable from grand mal.

Common Clinical Problems

Medical care will be sought in the clinical circumstances listed below. Although each type of seizure problem requires a somewhat different approach, a number of clinical principles are applicable to all of them. Initially, one must always ask whether the patient has indeed had a cerebral cortical seizure and not some other neurologic disorder—syncope, migraine, transient ischemic attack, episodic disturbances of behavior, episodic ataxia or dystonia, or confusion and stupor of various toxic or metabolic types. If the disorder fulfills the diagnostic criteria for a seizure, one must ascertain the clinical setting in which it occurred: in a patient with a known seizure disorder, brain tumor or cerebral trauma, drug overdose, systemic disease, or withdrawal state. Finally, the type of seizure needs to be identified, since this feature more than any other permits one to localize the discharging lesion (Table 16-1) and determine the proper therapy (Table 16-2).

A useful approach to the common clinical seizure types is one that relates to the age of onset of seizures (Table 16-3).

1. For the pediatrician, *neonatal seizures* are a special problem. Because of the immature state of cerebral development, the seizures are brief and fragmentary—a forced deviation of the head and eyes, an apneic episode, a stiffening of a limb, or a clonic twitching of several limbs and trunk. A skilled interpreter of neonatal EEGs can often settle the issue. Seizures in these circumstances are usually of dire significance, often being due to birth injury or metabolic disease. There is, however, a benign form of neonatal myoclonus that disappears in days or weeks. Blood gases, glucose, and calcium (Ca) should be measured. Phenobarbital is the most useful anticonvulsant in this age group.

2. *In an infant or young child*, there may be episodes of a few seconds' duration of massive flexion myoclonus ("salaam" or jacknife seizures). These may follow neonatal seizures. A variety of pathologic changes underlie the massive myoclonus (tuberous sclerosis, phenylketonuria, etc.), but many are idiopathic. If the unique EEG abnormality hypsarrhythmia (see above) is present, a trial of ACTH or an anticonvulsant is mandated. The massive myoclonic seizures tend to subside by 5 or 6 years of age, but they may be replaced by other types of seizure activity, and in many instances the child remains mentally retarded.

TABLE 16-2 Common Antiepileptic Drugs

Generic name	Trade name	Usual daily dosage		Principal therapeutic indications	Serum half-life, h	Effective blood level, μ/mL*
		Children	Adults, mg			
Phenobarbital	Luminal	3–5 mg/kg (8 mg/kg infants)	60–200	Tonic-clonic seizures; simple and complex partial seizures; absence partial seizures	96 ± 12	10–40
Phenytoin	Dilantin	4–7 mg/kg	300–400	Tonic-clonic seizures; simple and complex partial seizures	24 ± 12	10–20
Carbamazepine	Tegretol	20–30 mg/kg	600–1200	Tonic-clonic seizures; complex partial seizures	12 ± 3	4–10
Valproic acid	Depakene, Depakote	30–60 mg/kg	1000–3000	Absence and myoclonic seizures; as a primary or adjunctive drug in tonic-clonic and complex partial seizures	8 ± 2	50–100
Primidone	Mysoline	10–25 mg/kg	750–1500	Tonic-clonic seizures; simple and complex partial seizures	12 ± 6	5–15
Ethosuximide	Zarontin	20–40 mg/kg	750–2000	Absence	40 ± 6	50–100
Diazepam	Valium	0.15–2 mg/kg (IV)	10–150	Status epilepticus		
Lorazepam	Ativan	0.1 mg/kg (IV)	0.03–0.1 mg/kg (IV)	Status epilepticus		
Clonazepam	Klonopin	0.01–0.2 mg/kg	1.5–5	Absence; myoclonus	18–50	0.01–0.07
Gabapentin	Neurontin	—	1200	Adjunctive therapy	6	—
Lamotrigine	Lamictal	—	400	Adjunctive	14	—
Topiramate	Topamax	—	200–600	Adjunctive in adult partial seizures; Lennox-Gastaut syndrome	21	—
Levetiracetam	Keppra	—	1500–3000	Partial seizures	7	—
Tiagabine	Gabitril	—	16–32	Partial seizures	—	—

*Common trough levels.

139

TABLE 16-3 Causes of Recurrent Seizures in Different Age Groups

Age of onset	Probable cause
Neonatal	Congenital maldevelopment, birth injury, anoxia, metabolic disorders (hypocalcemia, hypoglycemia, vitamin B_6 deficiency, phenylketonuria, and others)
Infancy (1–6 months)	As above; infantile spasms
Early childhood (6 months–3 years)	Infantile spasms, febrile convulsions, birth injury and anoxia, infections, trauma, accidental drug poisoning
Childhood (3–10 years)	Perinatal anoxia, injury at birth or later, infections, thrombosis of cerebral arteries or veins, or "idiopathic" probably inherited epilepsy (rolandic epilepsy and its variants)
Adolescence (10–18 years)	Idiopathic epilepsy, including genetically transmitted types (juvenile myoclonic epilepsy), trauma
Early adulthood (18–25 years)	Idiopathic epilepsy, trauma, neoplasm, withdrawal from alcohol or other sedative-hypnotic drugs, eclampsia
Middle age (35–60 years)	Trauma, neoplasm, vascular disease, alcohol or other drug withdrawal
Late life (over 60 years)	Vascular disease, tumor, abscess, degenerative disease, trauma

Note: Meningitis and its complications may be a cause of seizures at any age. In tropical and subtropical countries, parasitic infections of the brain are frequent causes.

3. *Febrile states* are accompanied by one or more generalized seizures in one of every 20 young children. This tendency disappears after 5 to 6 years. Often there is a family history of such an occurrence. Quick recovery and a normal neurologic examination and EEG are the general rule. Treatment of the fever and infection and a brief period of administration of barbiturates usually suffice. Some of the patients will prove later to have focal or unilateral seizures unassociated with fever. These attacks are then examples of focal or secondary epilepsy, which is likely to continue thoughout life, often changing to the temporal lobe type and requiring the use of carbamazepine, phenytoin, or other medications.

4. A child or adolescent may present in *status epilepticus*. It is often the first manifestation of idiopathic epilepsy but may be caused by meningitis, encephalitis, or brain tumor and less often by an acquired metabolic disorder such as hyper- or hypoglycemia or hyponatremia. Appropriate diagnostic steps are undertaken after a therapeutic regimen for status epilepticus has been instituted (see #10, below).

5. A common problem is that of a *child or adolescent who has had his first major generalized seizure* and has a normal neurologic examination. An EEG and computed tomography (CT) scan or MRI should be obtained. If they are normal, the problem is whether to wait and observe the patient or administer anticonvulsant medication. The latter course is more clearly indicated if the EEG shows a paroxysmal abnormality. A substantial proportion of these patients will be found to have medial temporal sclerosis by careful MRI examination.

6. A *child or adult known to be epileptic* may still be having seizures despite medication. One must check the patient's compliance and the dosage and blood levels of the drug. The EEG as well as serum electrolytes, glucose, blood urea nitrogen (BUN), and Ca should also be checked. If the blood level of anticonvulsant is low, the dosage is adjusted; if the level is normal or high, the medication is changed in accordance with the type of seizure or a second medication is added (see Table 16-2). In the latter case, interactions between anticonvulsants must be considered.

7. The first appearance of a *focal or partial seizure* disorder in an adult requires a neurologic investigation with EEG, CT scan, or MRI and, usually, lumbar puncture (LP). Almost always, a focal brain lesion will be found—infarction, healed contusion, tumor, subdural hematoma, abscess, etc. Treatment is directed at both the primary lesion and the seizures.

8. A burst of *generalized or multifocal seizures* occurring for the first time in the patient's life raises a number of diagnostic possibilities, again depending on the age at which they occur (Table 16-3): withdrawal from alcohol, barbiturate, or other sedative drug; abuse of cocaine or other stimulant drugs; recovery phase from hypoxic-ischemic encephalopathy with coma; hypo- or hyperglycemia, hypocalcemia, hypomagnesemia; hyponatremia; uremia; hypertensive encephalopathy and eclampsia; encephalitis; abscess; chronic meningitis; tumor; rarely, porphyria or an aminoaciduria. Cerebral infarction and healed traumatic cortical lesions are common causes of seizures that arise for the first time in late adult life. Usually the seizures occur several months or years after the infarction or contusion, either of which may have been clinically inevident. Seldom, however, is a convulsive seizure the presenting feature of a stroke.

9. A patient who continues to have *frequent complex partial and generalized seizures* despite protracted trials of all known medications should be referred to an epilepsy center, where a search for cortical epileptogenic lesions is made by special techniques. If such lesions are found, surgical excision or other procedures may be considered.

10. The most serious seizure problem is the recurrence of generalized convulsions at a frequency that does not allow consciousness to be regained in the interval between seizures—*grand mal status epilepticus. Treatment must be undertaken at once*, because persistent status epilepticus has a mortality of about 10 percent, and many survivors are left with brain damage. An IV line is established with normal saline, and blood is drawn for serum chemistries and antiepileptic drug concentrations. The first drug to be administered should be a benzodiazepine, for example, *lorazepam*, 0.1 mg/kg by IV push ($<$2 mg/min). Immediately afterward, phenytoin or its prodrug *fosphenytoin* is given, 18 mL/kg IV ($<$50 mg/min for phenytoin, $<$150 mg/min for fosphenytoin), blood pressure and ECG being closely monitored during the infusion. Additional doses of 5 mg/kg are given if necessary to a maximum of 30 mg/kg. If status persists, the patient should be intubated and a second drug such as phenobarbital administered, 20 mg/kg by IV push ($<$100 mg/min), but we favor anesthetic doses of midazolam, 5 to 10 mg initially, then 6 to 20 mg/h or propofol in an infusion of 2 to 8 mg/h. The rate of infusion is slowed every few hours to determine whether seizure activity (on the EEG tracing) has stopped.

HYSTERICAL SEIZURES

These are sham seizures (also referred to as "psychogenic" or "pseudo-seizures"); they are nonepileptic. They are observed in female hysterics and in malingering males and females (compensation neurosis). It should be pointed out, however, that some patients with genuine epilepsy may have sham seizures as well, adding to the difficulty in diagnosis. Completely asynchronous thrashing of the limbs; repeated side-to-side movements of the head; hand-biting, kicking, and trembling; pelvic thrusting and opisthotonic arching postures; and screaming and talking during the attack all point to the seizure as hysterical, although no single feature is specific. The serum CK is usually normal after a hysterical seizure. A combined video and EEG recording of an attack usually settles the issue.

TREATMENT

For most patients with seizures, medical therapy is the mainstay. It consists of eliminating causative factors, instituting sound physical and mental routines, and administering drugs of appropriate type and in adequate amounts. Table 16-2 lists the most commonly used drugs along with their dosages, principal therapeutic indications, effective blood levels, and serum half-life. The artful management of anticonvulsants, their side effects, and their interactions is a major part of the overall treatment of the epileptic patient.

The principal drugs for the treatment of grand mal and partial complex seizures are phenytoin, carbamazepine, valproic acid, and phenobarbital; for absence seizures, ethosuximide and many of the newer drugs listed in the latter part of Table 16-2 are effective. The physician should make an effort to control seizures with one drug alone. Only if sustained use has failed should a second drug be added, with the dosage gradually increased to optimum levels while the dosage of the old drug is slowly reduced. If seizures are still not controlled, another primary anticonvulsant can be added. Second-line anticonvulsants that have an auxiliary use in recalcitrant cases include gabapentin, lamotrigine, topiramate, levetiracetam, tiagabine, and clonazepam, some of which are also apparently effective as first-line anticonvulsants. Rarely if ever are more than two drugs necessary. Most anticonvulsants have noticeable interactions with other drugs, especially those that are highly protein-bound or are metabolized by the liver, including other anticonvulsants. Drug management in pregnant women and those of childbearing age is also complex, in part because of the slight teratogenic effect of most of the anticonvulsants (see *Adams and Victor's Principles of Neurology*, 7th ed., for details).

Increasingly in patients with an isolated seizure focus defined by EEG, MRI, and positron emission tomography (PET), and unresponsive or poorly responsive to drug therapy, surgical excision of the epileptogenic cortex is being successfully accomplished.

For a more detailed discussion of this topic, see Victor and Ropper: *Adams and Victor's Principles of Neurology*, 7th ed, pp 331–365.

ADDITIONAL READING

Annegers JF, Hauser WA, Shirts SB, Kurland LT: Factors prognostic of unprovoked seizures after febrile convulsions. *N Engl J Med* 316:493, 1987.

Browne TR, Holmes GL: Epilepsy. *N Engl J Med* 344:1145, 2001.

Engel J, Pedley TA: *Epilepsy: A Comprehensive Textbook*. Philadelphia, Davis, 1998.

Kumar A, Bleck TP: Intravenous midazolam for the treatment of status epilepticus. *Crit Care Med* 20:438, 1992.

Lowenstein DH, Aldredge BK: Status epilepticus. *N Engl J Med* 338:970, 1998.

Mattson RH: Current challenges in the treatment of epilepsy. *Neurology* 44(Suppl 5), S4–S9, 1994.

Niedermeyer E: *The Epilepsies: Diagnosis and Management*. Baltimore, Urban and Schwarzenberg, 1990.

Penfield W, Jasper HH: *Epilepsy and Functional Anatomy of the Human Brain*. Boston, Little, Brown, 1954.

Porter RJ: *Epilepsy: 100 Elementary Principles*, 2nd ed. Philadelphia, Saunders, 1989.

Scheuer ML, Pedley TA: The evaluation and treatment of seizures. *N Engl J Med* 323:1468, 1990.

Thomas JE, Regan TJ, Klass DW: Epilepsia partialis continua: A review of 32 cases. *Arch Neurol* 34:266, 1977.

Treiman DM, Meyers PD, Walton NY, et al: A comparison of four treatments for generalized status epilepticus. *N Engl J Med* 339:792, 1998.

17 | Coma and Related Disorders of Consciousness

Coma and lesser degrees of impaired consciousness are alarming neurologic emergencies. If persistent, the conditions that cause them often end fatally or leave the patient irreparably damaged, mentally and physically.

Coma is the equivalent of loss of consciousness, which in practical terms means a loss of awareness of self and environment and an inability to respond to external stimuli or inner needs. Coma differs from natural sleep in that the patient is unarousable; syncope differs by virtue of its brevity and natural resolution (see Chaps. 18 and 19).

One can identify different degrees of coma. In profound coma, all stimuli, even the most severely painful ones, have no effect. A somewhat lighter state of coma ("semicoma") is manifest by groaning, stirring, quickening of respiration, or a brief opening of the eyes when the patient is pinched or shaken. Still lesser degrees of impaired consciousness, through which the patient may pass as he sinks into or emerges from coma, are designated as stupor and drowsiness. A stuporous patient will open his eyes and make some simple response to loud voice or manipulation of his body and may even mumble but does not speak. A drowsy and confused patient reveals in conversation an inability to respond properly and to think with customary speed and clarity as well as a tendency to fall into an inattentive, stupefied state if left unstimulated.

Notable is the fact that the foregoing states of impaired consciousness include *both* a reduced receptivity to stimulation and a reduced responsivity. When only the latter defect exists, the patient being paralyzed but alert and aware of his surroundings, the condition is referred to as the "*locked in*" syndrome (also as "de-efferented state"). It is due most often to a lesion of the basis pontis, which interrupts the descending motor pathways but spares the ascending sensory pathways—both the somatosensory ones and the diencephalic-cortical mechanisms responsible for arousal, wakefulness, and continuity of self-awareness. If the patient lacks the impulse to move, though not paralyzed, the condition is one of *catatonia* or *abulia* (also spoken of, in its most severe form, as "*akinetic mutism*"); its specific anatomic basis is uncertain, but it is often observed with bilateral medial-orbital frontal or bilateral medial thalamic lesions. *A persistent vegetative state* is observed in patients who have barely emerged from coma or have progressed into a state of profound dementia. The patient is awake, blinks to threat, and is capable of a few primitive postural and reflex movements but is otherwise without awareness, responsiveness, or any recognizable cognitive function. Vegetative (autonomic) functions are maintained.

Profound coma, with total unreceptivity of all forms of stimulation and total unresponsivity, is often accompanied by loss of all brainstem and spinal reflexes. The pupils are dilated or midsized and unreactive to light. Spontaneous breathing and blink as well as vestibulo-ocular and oropharyngeal reflexes are abolished. Provided that there is no hypothermia or the effects of depressant medication and in the absence of all EEG activity, the condition is indicative of *brain death*, as defined below. Such patients rarely survive for more than a few days, even with respiratory support. The criteria for the diagnosis of brain death are (1) deep unresponsive coma; (2) absence of brainstem activity as demonstrated by large or midsized unreactive pupils, absence of corneal response, absence of eye movements with caloric stimulation of the labyrinths, and apnea despite adequate CO_2 stimulation ($P_{CO_2} > 50$ mmHg); and (3) exclusion of drug overdose and profound hypothermia.

MECHANISMS WHEREBY CONSCIOUSNESS IS DISTURBED BY DISEASE

Consciousness depends on the continuity of normal functioning of the reticular formations of the midbrain and thalamus and their connections with all parts of the cerebral cortex, to which they send and from which they receive fibers. Therefore, any process that affects the cortex diffusely renders a person comatose. The smallest lesions that produce coma are always to be found in the upper brainstem and thalamic reticular formations; damage in these deep central regions deactivates the cerebral cortex. Lesser degrees of impairment of these structures cause drowsiness, inattentiveness, and an inability to sustain mental activity.

The following are the main mechanisms by which the reticular activation of the cerebral cortex can be impaired:

1. *A generalized seizure*, in which the sudden excessive neuronal discharge originates in or spreads to and temporarily paralyzes deep central neuronal structures.
2. *Cerebral concussion*, in which a swirling motion of the brain and torque of the upper brainstem temporarily impair neuronal function in the diencephalic-midbrain regions.
3. *Drugs*, particularly anesthetics, alcohol, barbiturates, and other sedatives, each of which, by its own physiologic effect, paralyzes the cells of the reticular activating system.
4. *Metabolic derangements*, as in uremia, diabetic or other acidoses, hepatic failure, hypoglycemia, hypercalcemia, hypo- and hypernatremia, hypoxia, and hypercapnia, which affect the function of upper reticular and cortical neurons.
5. *Destructive lesions*—tumor, infarction (basilar artery occlusion), and hemorrhage—directly involving the upper brainstem tegmental and thalamic reticular formations. The effect may be permanent.
6. *Massive lesion of one cerebral hemisphere*—tumor, hemorrhage, contusion, or a subdural or epidural hematoma—secondarily displacing and compressing the high midbrain and diencephalic reticular formations. The degree of horizontal displacement of midline structures corresponds to the level of unresponsiveness (drowsiness, 3 to 5 mm; stupor, 6 to 8 mm; coma, greater than 9 mm; displacement of the pineal body from the midline).

7. Critical *decline in blood pressure* (below 60 mm systolic) in normotensive subjects—e.g., diffuse effects of sepsis, blood loss, and cardiac arrest.

Most frequent causes of coma   In the New York Hospital series of Plum and Posner, approximately one-third of the patients admitted in coma proved to be suffering from drug overdose, one-third from metabolic disease, and one-third from cerebrovascular disease (see Table 17-1). These were patients in whom the initial diagnosis was uncertain, so that obvious poisonings were underrepresented. Also, cases of traumatic coma were not included, since the cause was usually apparent and those patients were admitted to the neurosurgical service. Overall, global brain ischemia and

TABLE 17-1 Final Diagnosis in 500 Patients Admitted
to the Hospital with "Coma of Unknown Etiology"

Supratentorial mass lesions	101
Intracerebral hematoma	44
Subdural hematoma	26
Epidural hematoma	4
Cerebral infarct	9
Thalamic infarct	2
Brain tumor	7
Pituitary apoplexy	2
Brain abscess	6
Closed-head injury	1
Subtentorial lesions	65
Brainstem infarct	40
Pontine hemorrhage	11
Brainstem demyelination	1
Cerebellar hemorrhage	5
Cerebellar tumor	3
Cerebellar infarct	2
Cerebellar abscess	1
Posterior fossa subdural hemorrhage	1
Basilar migraine	1
Metabolic and other diffuse disorders	326
Anoxia or ischemia	87
Hepatic encephalopathy	17
Uremic encephalopathy	8
Pulmonary disease	3
Endocrine disorders (including diabetes)	12
Acid-base disorders	12
Temperature regulation	9
Nutritional	1
Nonspecific metabolic coma	1
Encephalomyelitis and encephalitis	14
Subarachnoid hemorrhage	13
Drug poisoning	149
Psychiatric disorders	8

Note: Listed here are only the patients in whom the initial diagnosis was uncertain and a final diagnosis was established. Thus, obvious poisonings and closed-head injuries are underrepresented.
(From Plum and Posner, with permission.)

overdose were the commonest cause; encephalitis and brain abscess were infrequent, being found in only 22 of 500 cases.

CLINICAL APPROACH TO THE COMATOSE PATIENT

When the patient is first seen, it is essential to obtain information about the events that led up to the coma. But one must first make certain that the patient's airway is clear, that he is able to sustain respiration, and that his blood pressure is adequate. If not, cardiorespiratory resuscitative measures should be undertaken. As indicated below, if shock, bleeding, or airway obstruction has supervened, the immediate institution of certain therapeutic measures—insertion of an endotracheal tube, administration of O_2, pressor agents, blood, or glucose—takes precedence. There follows a complete medical and neurologic examination, including a computed tomography (CT) scan or magnetic resonance imaging (MRI) in appropriate circumstances and examination of the cerebrospinal fluid (CSF) if there is any suspicion of meningitis. The demonstration of focal brain disease or meningeal inflammation with pleocytosis permits the categorization of coma-producing diseases into one of three groups, a practice that is particularly helpful in differential diagnosis. The diseases that constitute each of these groups and their main clinical and laboratory features are summarized in Table 17-2.

MANAGEMENT OF THE COMATOSE PATIENT

This requires the services of a well-coordinated team of nurses under the constant guidance of a physician. Treatment must start at once, even before the necessary diagnostic steps are completed. The principles of management are listed below; details of management of shock, fluid and electrolyte imbalance, and other complications to which the insensate patient is subject (e.g., pneumonia, urinary tract infections, phlebothrombosis) can be found in *Harrison's Principles of Internal Medicine*.

1. The management of shock, if present, takes precedence over all other diagnostic and therapeutic measures.
2. Shallow and irregular respirations, stertorous breathing (indicating partial obstruction to inspiration), and cyanosis require the establishment of a clear airway and delivery of oxygen. If the cerebral disease is not complicated by a fracture-dislocation of the cervical spine, the patient should initially be placed in a lateral position so that secretions and vomitus do not enter the tracheobronchial tree. Usually the pharyngeal reflexes are suppressed; therefore an endotracheal tube can be inserted without difficulty. Secretions should be removed by suctioning as soon as they accumulate; otherwise they will lead to atelectasis and bronchopneumonia. Oxygen can be administered by mask or endotracheal tube, guided by the arterial oxygen saturation and other arterial blood gas measurements. Respiratory insufficiency and intracranial hypertension dictate the use of endotracheal intubation and a positive pressure respirator.
3. Concomitantly, an IV line is established, an electrocardiogram (ECG) is obtained, and blood samples are drawn for measurement of glucose, drug levels, and electrolytes and for tests of liver and kidney function. Dextrose 50% and thiamine 100 mg should be administered in cases of

TABLE 17-2 Important Points in the Differential Diagnosis of the Common Causes of Coma

General group	Specific disorder	Main clinical findings	Main laboratory findings	Remarks
Coma *with* focal or lateralizing signs	Cerebral hemorrhage	Hemiplegia, hypertension, cyclic breathing, specific ocular signs (see Chaps. 14 and 34)	CT scan +	Sudden onset, with headache, vomiting; history of chronic hypertension or coagulopathy; late pupillary enlargement
	Basilar artery occlusion (thrombotic or embolic)	Extensor posturing and bilateral Babinski signs; loss of oculocephalic responses; ocular bobbing (Chap. 34)	Normal early CT; MRI shows cerebellar and brainstem or thalamic infarction, normal CSF	Onset subacute (thrombosis), or sudden (rostral basilar embolism)
	Massive infarction and edema in carotid territory	Hemiplegia, unilateral unresponsive or enlarged pupil	CT and MRI show massive edema of hemisphere	Coma preceded by drowsiness for several days after stroke
	Subdural hematoma	Slow or cyclic respiration, rising blood pressure, hemiparesis, unilateral enlarged pupil	CT scan +; CSF xanthochromic with relatively low protein	Signs or history of trauma, headache, confusion, progressive drowsiness

Trauma	Signs of cranial and facial injury	CT and MRI show brain contusions and other injuries (see Chap. 35)	Unstable blood pressure, associated systemic injuries
Brain abscess	Neurologic signs depending on location	CT scan and MRI +	Systemic infection or neurosurgical procedure, inconsistent fever
Hypertensive encephalopathy; eclampsia	Blood pressure > 210/110 (lower in eclampsia and in children), headache, seizures, hypertensive retinal changes	CT ±; MRI posterior white matter edema; CSF pressure elevated	Acute or subacute evolution, use of aminophylline or catecholamine medications
Meningitis and encephalitis	Stiff neck, Kernig sign, fever, headache	CT scan ±; pleocytosis, increased protein, low glucose in CSF	Subacute or acute onset
Subarachnoid hemorrhage	Stertorous breathing, hypertension, stiff neck, Kernig sign	CT scan may show blood and aneurysm; bloody or xanthochromic CSF under increased pressure	Very sudden onset with severe headache

Coma *without* focal or lateralizing signs, but *with* signs of meningeal irritation

(continued)

TABLE 17-2 (continued) Important Points in the Differential Diagnosis of the Common Causes of Coma

General group	Specific disorder	Main clinical findings	Main laboratory findings	Remarks
Coma *without* focal neurologic signs or meningeal irritation; CT scan and CSF normal	Alcohol intoxication	Hypothermia, hypotension, flushed skin, alcohol breath	Elevated blood alcohol	May be combined with head injury, infection, or hepatic failure
	Sedative intoxication	Hypothermia, hypotension	Drug in urine and blood; EEG often shows fast activity	History of intake of drug; suicide attempt
	Opioid intoxication	Slow respiration, cyanosis, constricted pupils		Administration of naloxone causes awakening and withdrawal signs
	Carbon monoxide intoxication	Cherry-red skin	Carboxyhemoglobin	Faulty ventilation or furnace, suicide attempt
	Anoxia	Rigidity, decerebrate postures, fever, seizures, myoclonus	CSF normal; EEG may be isoelectric or show high-voltage delta	Abrupt onset following cardiopulmonary arrest; damage permanent if anoxia exceeds 3–5 min
	Hypoglycemia	Same as in anoxia	Low blood and CSF glucose	Diabetes medications, slow evolution through stages of nervousness, hunger, sweating, shallow respirations and seizures

Diabetic coma	Signs of extracellular fluid deficit, hyperventilation with Kussmaul respiration, "fruity" breath	Glycosuria, hyperglycemia, acidosis; reduced serum bicarbonate; ketonemia and ketonuria, or hyperosmolarity	History of polyuria, polydipsia, weight loss, or diabetes
Uremia	Hypertension; sallow, dry skin, uriniferous breath, twitch-convulsive syndrome	Protein and casts in urine; elevated BUN and serum creatinine; anemia, acidosis, hypocalcemia	Progressive apathy, confusion, and asterixis precede coma
Hepatic coma	Jaundice, ascites, and other signs of portal hypertension; asterixis	Elevated blood NH_3 levels; CSF yellow (bilirubin) with normal or slightly elevated protein	Onset over a few days or after paracentesis or hemorrhage from varices; confusion, stupor, asterixis, and characteristic EEG changes precede coma
Hypercapnia	Papilledema, diffuse myoclonus, asterixis	Increased CSF pressure; P_{CO_2} may exceed 75 mmHg; EEG theta and delta activity	Advanced pulmonary disease; profound coma and brain damage uncommon
Severe infections (septic shock); heat stroke	Extreme hyperthermia, rapid respiration	Vary according to cause	Evidence of a specific infection or exposure to extreme heat
Seizures	Episodic disturbance of behavior or convulsive movements	Characteristic EEG changes	History of previous attacks

unclear etiology or if hypoglycemia is a diagnostic possibility. Naloxone, 0.5 to 2 mg IV, should be given cautiously if a narcotic overdose is a diagnostic possibility. In the heroin addict, arrhythmias and seizures may result. Flumazenil is useful in cases of overdose with diazepines.

4. If a mass lesion is strongly suspected on the basis of coma, a dilated pupil, and contralateral hemiplegia, or if one is evident on the CT scan, the control of raised intracranial pressure becomes paramount. Mannitol, 50 g in a 20% solution, should be given IV over 10 to 20 min. Repeated CT scans allow the physician to follow the size of the lesion and degree of localized edema and to detect displacements of cerebral tissue.

5. A lumbar puncture (LP) should be performed if meningitis (fever, leukocytosis, stiff neck) or subarachnoid hemorrhage (sudden coma preceded by headache) is suspected, although one must keep in mind the risks of this procedure and the means of dealing with them (Chap. 2). If time permits, brain imaging is advisable before an LP. A CT scan may have disclosed a subarachnoid hemorrhage, in which case LP is not necessary.

6. Convulsions should be controlled by measures outlined in Chap. 16.

7. Gastric aspiration and lavage with normal saline may be useful in some instances of coma due to drug ingestion. Salicylates, opiates, and anticholineric drugs (tricyclic antidepressants, phenothiazines, scopolamine), all of which induce gastric atony, may be recovered many hours after ingestion. Patients in whom the ingested drug is unidentified are treated with activated charcoal, 50 to 100 g by nasogastric tube, after the airway has been secured. Induction of emesis by ipecac or apomorphine should be reserved for alert patients.

8. The temperature-regulating mechanisms may be disturbed, and extreme hypothermia, hyperthermia, or poikilothermia may occur. In hyperthermia, the use of evaporative cooling with sprayed water and a fan is the most efficient. A cooling mattress may be used as well.

9. The bladder should not be permitted to become distended; if the patient does not void, a catheter should be inserted. The patient should not be permitted to lie in a wet or soiled bed.

10. Diseases of the central nervous system may upset the control of water, glucose, and sodium. The unconscious patient can no longer adjust the intake of food and fluids by hunger and thirst. Both salt-losing and salt-retaining syndromes have been seen with brain disease. Water intoxication and severe hyponatremia may of themselves prove fatal. If coma is prolonged, the insertion of a gastric tube will ease the problems of feeding the patient and maintaining fluid and electrolyte balance.

11. Aspiration pneumonia is avoided by intubation, prevention of vomiting (gastric tube), proper positioning of the patient, and restriction of oral fluids. The legs should be examined regularly for signs of venous thrombosis; if that is found, it should be treated with anticoagulants or surgical measures. Deep vein thrombosis, which is a common occurrence in comatose and hemiplegic patients, often does not manifest itself by clinical signs. If the bedridden state is prolonged, the legs should be fitted with intermittent pneumatic compression boots. Thrombosis can also be prevented by the administration of subcutaneous heparin, 5000 units q 12 h, or other anticoagulant drug.

TABLE 17-3 Glasgow Coma Scale Score (Sum of Three Categories)

Eye opening	
Never	1
To pain	2
To verbal stimuli	3
Spontaneously	4

Best verbal response	
No response	1
Incomprehensible sounds	2
Inappropriate words	3
Disoriented and converses	4
Oriented and converses	5

Best motor response	
No response	1
Extension (decerebrate rigidity)	2
Flexion abnormal (decorticate rigidity)	3
Flexion withdrawal	4
Localizes pain	5
Obeys	6
	3–15

12. If the patient is restless, suitable restraints should be used to prevent falling out of bed. Sedation for this purpose should be avoided.

Prognosis

The outcome of metabolic and drug-induced coma is generally favorable and that from trauma, cerebral hemorrhage, and infarction of the brainstem is usually poorer; brain anoxia-ischemia after cardiac arrest occupies an intermediate position. Deep coma that lasts for 48 to 72 h carries a grave prognosis; many such patients fall into the category of brain death, usually with fatal outcome in a few days. A small number emerge into the category of vegetative state, for which the prognosis is equally grave. A few patients survive in a persistent vegetative state for years, but in most cases survival is measured in weeks or months. In a number of others, the vegetative state is a transitional stage between deep coma and recovery of some degree of neurologic functioning. The absence of pupillary and corneal reflexes and ocular movements after 1 to 3 days of coma is predictive to a high degree of a fatal outcome or a vegetative state. Low scores on the Glasgow Coma Scale (Table 17-3) may be of help in predicting the outcome, particularly in cases due to cerebral trauma. Few patients with scores below 8 emerge from traumatic coma and regain meaningful function.

For a more detailed discussion of this topic, see Victor and Ropper: *Adams and Victor's Principles of Neurology*, 7th ed, pp 366–389.

ADDITIONAL READING

Beecher HK, Adams RD, Sweet WH: A definition of irreversible coma. Report of the Committee of Harvard Medical School to examine the definition of brain death. *JAMA* 205:85, 1968.

Fisher CM: The neurological examination of the comatose patient. *Acta Neurol Scand Suppl* 45 (Suppl 36):1, 1969.

Jennett B, Plum F: Persistent vegetative state after brain damage. *Lancet* 1:734, 1972.

Kennard C, Illingworth R: Persistent vegetative state. *J Neurol Neurosurg Psychiatry* 59:347, 1995.

Levy DE, Caronna JJ, Singer BH, et al: Predicting outcome from hypoxic-ischemic coma. *JAMA* 253:1420, 1985.

Plum F, Posner JB: *Diagnosis of Stupor and Coma*, 3rd ed. Philadelphia, Davis, 1980.

Ropper AH: Lateral displacement of the brain and level of consciousness in patients with an acute hemispheral mass. *N Engl J Med* 314:953, 1986.

Ropper AH (ed): *Neurological and Neurosurgical Intensive Care*, 3rd ed. New York, Raven Press, 1993.

Young GB, Ropper AH, Bolton CF: *Coma and Impaired Consciousness*. New York, McGraw-Hill, 1998.

18 | Faintness and Syncope

Syncope is synonymous with the common faint. In most cases, it is a transitory, spontaneously reversible state. A lesser form, a feeling as though one were about to faint, is referred to as *faintness*, or *presyncope*. Most otherwise healthy persons have experienced the latter, and many have at some time fainted.

CLINICAL FEATURES

In the common (vasovagal) type of faint, the person is assailed by a sense of weakness, as though all energy had been drained from the body. He feels uneasy and queasy and has a sense of giddiness and swaying. Headache, dimness of vision, and ringing in the ears are common accompaniments, and the subject may have difficulty in thinking clearly. The face blanches; a cold sweat breaks out. Pallor of the face coincides with pallor of the brain, which is the mechanism common to all types of faint. Signs of autonomic overactivity—salivation, nausea, and sometimes vomiting and sweating—are variably prominent and represent the body's attempts to counteract the fall in blood pressure.

The victim, who is usually standing or sitting, looks for a place to lie down. If unable to lie down promptly, he loses consciousness and falls to the ground. Breathing and pulse are imperceptible or almost so. For a brief period, the appearance is one of death. Once horizontal for a few seconds or a minute or two, the patient stirs, opens his eyes, and quickly takes in the situation. Strength and color soon return as well. Bystanders are relieved by the rapid recovery.

The pulse is often slowed during recovery, suggesting vagal overactivity (hence the name *vasovagal*). But the loss of vasoconstrictive tone is a more important factor than bradycardia in the genesis of the faint (vasodepressor effect).

Such an episode has at some time been witnessed or experienced by most people, but there are variations that may cause uncertainty. If unconsciousness persists for 15 to 20 s or the patient, for some reason, is maintained upright as the faint comes on, the limbs and trunk may jerk several times or stiffen, as in a convulsive seizure. Or the patient may not lose consciousness completely; he can hear voices of those around him but his responses betray confusion ("grayout"). Syncope of cardiac origin may be so abrupt that the fall results in injury, even a concussion. In general, however, the loss of strength and consciousness, though of sudden onset, provides sufficient warning for a hurtful fall to be averted. Sphincteric incontinence is also exceptional.

With these characteristics in mind, the distinction between a faint and a seizure should rarely occasion difficulty. Only the akinetic (astatic) seizure resembles a faint, but usually it comes without warning or facial pallor. The seizure-like clonic jerking or tonic spasm of limbs and trunk that sometimes complicates a protracted faint is usually attended by the other manifestations of hypotension. Unless there has been severe muscle trauma, serum CK is not elevated after syncope, as it is following a convulsive seizure.

CAUSES OF SYNCOPE AND FAINTNESS

In Table 18-1 are listed the many types of syncope and faintness on the basis of their established or presumed physiologic mechanisms. In practice, only a small proportion of the conditions listed in the table are encountered with any degree of frequency. Moreover, the fundamental mechanism in all of them is the same—an inadequacy of blood flow to the brain, which in turn may be due to (1) an active, centrally mediated withdrawal of peripheral vascular tone (e.g., vasodepressor fainting due to strong emotion, painful injury, sight of blood, etc.); (2) an inability to maintain peripheral vascular resistance upon standing (orthostatic hypotension due to peripheral neuropathy, antihypertensive medication, prolonged bed rest, central autonomic failure); or (3) inadequate delivery of oxygen and glucose (failure of cardiac output from arrhythmia or myocardial pump failure, aortic stenosis, blood loss, dehydration).

Details of the clinical features and mechanisms of the various types of syncope will be found in *Adams and Victor's Principles of Neurology*, 7th ed.

CLINICAL APPROACH TO SYNCOPE

If on the scene of a common vasovagal faint, one need only ensure that the patient remains recumbent until the vasodepressor inadequacy has corrected itself. For the patient who reports one or more faints and is normal when seen, one must ascertain, from the descriptions of the episode, that it was a faint and not a seizure or an attack of anxiety, transient ischemia, or hypoglycemia. Having satisfied oneself on this point, the mechanism of the faint and the likelihood of its recurrence should be determined. Some types of syncope, such as those of cardiac and orthostatic origin, must be taken seriously; others are obviously benign. An otherwise healthy adolescent or young adult who faints at the scene of an accident or when sitting or standing still in an overheated atmosphere needs no further study—only an explanation of the nature of vasovagal syncope and the admonition to avoid situations that are known to induce fainting. In fainting of orthostatic type, one must not fail to consider the possible hypotension-producing effects of certain drugs—the common ones being antihypertensive agents, diuretics, phenothiazines, benzodiazepines, tricyclic antidepressants, L-dopa, and centrally acting dopamine agonists, the last two being used for the treatment of Parkinson disease.

A person *convalescing from illness* or one with an *inadequate peripheral vasoconstrictor mechanism* (e.g., diabetic neuropathy, Parkinson disease, striatonigral degeneration, and Shy-Drager syndrome) requires investigation of the underlying disease and the institution of certain corrective measures to help avoid future attacks. Such measures include sleeping with the head of the bed elevated by 8 to 12 in., arising slowly from a recumbent position, the use of a snug elastic abdominal binder and stockings, increasing salt intake to expand blood volume, and the administration of fludrocortisone acetate (Florinef), 0.01 to 0.02 mg/day in divided doses or the α-1 sympathetic agonist Midodrine given in doses of 10 mg every 4 h, with care taken to monitor supine blood pressure for an excessive rise.

TABLE 18-1 Types of Syncope and Faintness

I. Neurogenic vasodepressor and vasovagal reactions
   A. Elicited by *extrinsic signals* to the medulla from baroreceptors
       1. Vasodepressor (vasovagal)
       2. Neurocardiogenic (receptors in cardiac wall)
       3. Carotid sinus hypersensitivity
       4. Vagoglossopharyngeal and glossopharyngeal neuralgia
   B. Coupled with diminished venous return to the heart
       1. Micturitional
       2. Tussive
       3. Valsalva, straining, weightlifting
       4. Postprandial
   C. Intrinsic psychic stimuli
       1. Fear, anxiety, pain (presyncope more common)
       2. Sight of blood
       3. Hysterical fainting

II. Sympathetic nervous system failure (postural-orthostatic hypotension)
   A. Autonomic neuropathy
       1. Diabetes
       2. Pandysautonomia
       3. Guillain-Barré syndrome
       4. Amyloidosis
       5. Surgical sympathectomy
       6. Antihypertensive medications and other blockers of vascular innervation
   B. Central autonomic failure
       1. Primary autonomic failure
       2. Parkinsonian syndromes (Shy-Drager, multiple system atrophy,
           Parkinson disease)
       3. Tabes dorsalis
       4. Syringomyelia
       5. Spinal cord transection
       6. Centrally acting antihypertensive medications

III. Reduced cardiac output or inadequate intravascular volume (hypovolemia)
   A. Reduced cardiac output
       1. Obstruction to left ventricular outflow: aortic stenosis; hypertrophic
           subaortic stenosis
       2. Obstruction to pulmonary flow: pulmonic stenosis, tetralogy of Fallot,
           primary pulmonary hypertension, pulmonary embolism
       3. Myocardial: infarction or severe congestive heart failure
       4. Pericardial tamponade
       5. Cardiac arrhythmias (with reduced cranial circulation)
           Bradyarrhythmias
           a. AV block (second and third degrees) with Stokes-Adams attacks
           b. Ventricular asystole
           c. Sinus bradycardia, sinoatrial block, sinus arrest, sick-sinus syndrome
           Tachyarrhythmias
           a. Episodic ventricular fibrillation
           b. Ventricular tachycardia
           c. Supraventricular tachycardia without AV block (infrequently
               causes syncope)
   B. Inadequate intravascular volume (dehydration, blood loss)

IV. Other causes of episodic faintness and syncope
   A. Hypoxia
   B. Anemia
   C. Diminished CO_2 due to hyperventilation (faintness common, syncope rare)
   D. Hypoglycemia (faintness frequent, syncope rare)

In patients with *cardiac syncope*, it may be necessary to monitor cardiac rhythm for several days or weeks or even longer. The drug treatment of the various arrhythmias that induce syncope and the need for a pacemaker require consultation with a cardiologist. The treatment of *carotid sinus syncope* can be difficult. Atropine or ephedrine should be tried in patients whose attacks are associated with bradycardia or hypotension, respectively. If these medications fail and the attacks are incapacitating, surgical denervation of the carotid sinus or the placement of a demand pacemaker needs to be considered.

Tussive syncope, micturition syncope, and *"weight-lifter's syncope"* simply require the use of antitussive medicines and treatment of tracheobronchitis, instruction to urinate while sitting, and interdiction of straining and heavy lifting, as the case may be. In patients who faint because of hypovolemia or the effects of antihypertensive drugs, it may suffice to restore the blood volume or discontinue or adjust the dosage of the offending drug(s).

A number of simple maneuvers may help to clarify the medical problem of syncope. Measurement of blood pressure while the patient is lying down and after standing relaxed for 2 to 3 min may disclose a fall of 20 to 30 mmHg or more, supporting the hypothesis of faulty vasoconstriction. Orthostatic hypotension that becomes evident only after even more prolonged standing suggests a vasodepressor response that is triggered by afferent impulses from the cardiac chambers as their filling volume is diminished (*"neurocardiogenic" syncope*). Syncope during exercise in young athletes is often imputed to this mechanism. An even better method of studying neurocardiogenic syncope is to subject the patient to an 80° head-up tilt on a special table for 10 min. The upright posture, by emptying the cardiac chambers of blood, produces, in susceptible individuals, vigorous contractions that stimulate receptors in the cardiac wall; the afferent signal from these receptors elicits a vasodepressor response. Combining an isoproterenol infusion with the upright-tilt test may be a useful method of reproducing neurocardiogenic syncope.

Purely *orthostatic fainting* characterizes a number of processes, including peripheral neuropathy (distal sensory loss and absent ankle jerks), isolated central autonomic insufficiency (loss of sweating, slowed pupillary reactions, sphincteric difficulties, dry mouth), or central autonomic failure as a component of an extrapyramidal or cerebellar degeneration—a condition that goes by several names, commonly, multiple system atrophy.

Gentle massage of first one and then the other carotid sinus, while recording pulse and blood pressure, may reproduce *carotid sinus syncope*. Hyperventilation for 3 min often induces part of an anxiety attack and absence seizures. Hysterical fainting can be recognized by the normality of pulse and blood pressure during the attack, and the presence of other features of hysteria (see Chap. 56). Continuous portable ECG and EEG recordings are helpful if repeated spells defy explanation.

In some cases, even after all these tests, one may not be sure of having discovered the basis of the patient's syncopal attacks. The plan then is to have the patient avoid situations that induce postural hypotension and to make further observations of the circumstances surrounding future attacks.

For a more detailed discussion of this topic, see Victor and Ropper: *Adams and Victor's Principles of Neurology,* 7th ed, pp 390–403.

ADDITIONAL READING

Almquist A, Goldenberg IF, Milstein S, et al: Provocation of bradycardia and hypotension by isoproterenol and upright posture in patients with unexplained syncope. *N Engl J Med* 320:346, 1989

Kapoor WN: Evaluation and management of the patient with syncope. *N Engl J Med* 328:1117, 1993.

Kapoor WN: Syncope. *N Engl J Med* 343:1856, 2000.

Lipsitz LA: Orthostatic hypotension in the elderly. *N Engl J Med* 321:952, 1989.

Manolis AS, Linzer M, Salem D, Estes NAM: Syncope: Current diagnostic evaluation and management. *Ann Intern Med* 112:850, 1990.

Mathias CJ, Keguchi K, Bleasdale-Barr K, Kimber JR: Frequency of family history in vasovagal syncope. *Lancet* 352:33, 1998.

Mathias CJ, Kimber JR: Treatment of postural hypotension. *J Neurol Neurosurg Psychiatry* 65:285, 1998.

Meissner L, Wiebers DO, Swanson JW, O'Fallon WM: The natural history of drop attacks. *Neurology* 36:1029, 1986.

Ross RT: *Syncope.* Philadelphia, Saunders, 1988.

19 | Sleep and Its Abnormalities

Sleep laboratories, which are now found in practically all medical centers, have greatly advanced our knowledge of the physiology of sleep and have given physicians new insights into the nature of many common sleep abnormalities.

Normal sleep obeys an elemental 24-h (circadian) rhythm, the neural control of which lies mainly in the anterior hypothalamus. Nocturnal sleep is of two types: *rapid eye movement (REM) sleep*, which is linked to dreaming, and *non–rapid eye movement (NREM) sleep*, which constitutes about 80 percent of the sleep cycle. The latter is divided into four stages on the basis of the depth of sleep and accompanying physiologic, endocrine, and electroencephalographic (EEG) changes. REM sleep occurs as a single phase and normally follows NREM sleep. Together they form a predictable sequence or cycle that lasts 70 to 100 min and repeats itself four to six times per night. The number of cycles and the proportions of NREM sleep and REM sleep vary with age. The total hours of sleep also are age-linked—16 to 20 h in the newborn, 10 to 12 h in the child, 7 to 8 h in the adolescent, and progressively less in the elderly—but there are wide individual variations.

As one falls asleep, there is a progression from an alert to a drowsy state and then into stage 1 NREM sleep, wherein muscles are relaxed, breathing is slowed, and eyelids are closed; low-voltage, mixed-frequency waves replace the alpha rhythm in the EEG. In stage 2, sleep spindles (12 to 14 Hz), vertex sharp waves, and high-amplitude, sharp slow-wave (K) complexes appear in the EEG. Stages 3 and 4 are characterized by deep sleep and high-amplitude delta waves (1 to 2 Hz) in the EEG. After 80 to 90 min, REM sleep interrupts the cycle, with bursts of rapid eye movements, stirring of the limbs, changes in blood pressure and respiration, and low-voltage, fast-frequency waves in the EEG; if the subject is awakened at this time, he often reports dreams, although dreaming also occurs during NREM sleep. After a period of 5 to 10 min of REM sleep, NREM sleep recurs. With succeeding cycles, however, the four discrete stages of NREM sleep can no longer be recognized; in the later portion of a night's sleep, the cycles consist essentially of two alternating stages—REM sleep and stage 2 (spindle–vertex wave–K complex) sleep (Fig. 19-1).

Experimental physiologists have proposed that the alternations of sleep and wakefulness depend on the reciprocal interaction of excitatory (cholinergic) and inhibitory (aminergic) neurotransmitters produced by two interconnected neuronal populations in the pontine reticular formation. Details of this theoretical concept should be sought in the references listed at the end of the chapter.

SLEEP DISORDERS

Insomnia

Strictly defined, insomnia is a chronic (lasting more than 3 weeks) inability to sleep at times when sleep normally occurs, but the term is commonly used

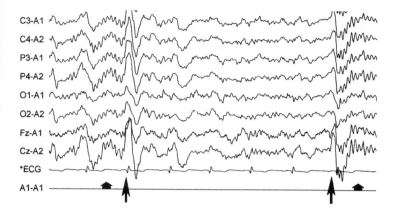

FIG. 19-1   Conventional EEG (30 mm/s) of a young healthy woman in stage 2 sleep showing vertex waves (*large arrows*) and sleep spindles (*small arrow*) of highest amplitude in the central regions.

to designate any short- or long-term disturbance in the depth, duration, or restorative powers of sleep. There may be delay in falling asleep, frequent or easy awakening during the night, or early-morning awakening. Apart from *pseudoinsomnia*, in which an individual expresses dissatisfaction with his sleep despite its normal depth and duration, there are two major types of insomnia, primary and secondary.

In *primary insomnia*, there is a chronic derangement of the sleep mechanism, affecting the quantity and quality of sleep in the absence of any medical or psychiatric illness. It may be a lifelong condition. Unlike the rare individual who functions adequately on 4 to 5 h of sleep, the primary insomniac complains of the effects of sleep deprivation. Moreover, sleep-laboratory recordings can verify the inadequacy of his sleep, with failure to progress to deeper stages of sleep, limited REM sleep, or frequent arousals (often due to sleep apnea, as discussed below).

Secondary (situational) insomnia is most often related to worry and anxiety (difficulty in falling asleep), depression (early-morning awakening), and the abuse of alcohol or drugs. Also, breathing difficulty (chronic pulmonary or cardiac disease) and painful medical or surgical conditions (e.g., pain in the spine, abdominal pain from peptic ulcer or carcinoma) are conducive to excessive wakefulness.

In addition, there are a number of special conditions in which a disturbance of sleep is the main abnormality and a source of distress to the patient, often delaying the onset of sleep. These are as follows: (1) The "*restless legs*" syndrome (anxietas tibiarum), which consists of unpleasant aching, drawing, and crawling sensations in the calves and thighs that are temporarily relieved by movement of the limbs. (2) *Periodic leg movements*, which are repetitive, rapid contractions of the tibialis anterior with extension of the big toe, followed sometimes by flexion of the hip, knee, and ankle; these movements occur every 20 to 40 s for long periods during sleep and cause partial or full arousals. (3) *Acroparesthesias of the hands*, usually due to carpal tunnel syndrome. (4) *Cluster headaches*, described in Chap. 10.

(5) *Nightmares and night terrors* (pavor nocturnus), which usually occur in children who are also sleepwalkers and sometimes persist into adult life.

Of the more strictly neurologic diseases, acute confusional states and deliria are known to derange sleep. In their most severe form (e.g., delirium tremens), the patient may be sleepless for days on end. During the inexhaustible activity of mania and hypomania, the patient seems to require little sleep to restore energy. Pontine infarction may reduce the amount and pattern of sleep (little or no REM sleep and reduced NREM sleep). This may also be observed in some cases of Huntington chorea, certain cerebellar degenerations, striatonigral degeneration, and progressive supranuclear palsy. Fatal familial insomnia is a rare inheritable disease characterized by intractable insomnia and related to the prion diseases (Chap. 32).

Treatment If the insomnia is of secondary type, it stands to reason that treatment needs to be directed to the underlying disease (antianxiety or antidepressant drugs or analgesics). In the patient with "restless legs," a benzodiazepine (diazepam, clonazepam) taken at bedtime may be helpful. Several medications are effective in the treatment of both "restless legs" and periodic nocturnal leg movements: L-dopa, bromocriptine, propoxyphene, baclofen, clonazepam, and others.

The management of primary insomnia is more difficult. In general, the long-term use of sedative-hypnotic drugs is not the answer. Barbiturates, short- or long-acting, should not be used because of the danger of addiction and of rebound insomnia (i.e., an intense worsening of the sleep disorder following withdrawal of the drug). The danger is less but still exists with drugs such as diazepam and chloral hydrate; their nightly use has a cumulative effect, causing daytime drowsiness. Drugs with the least tendency to the development of tolerance and dependence include diphenhydramine (Benadryl) 25 to 50 mg, the benzodiazepines flurazepam (Dalmane) in doses of 15 to 30 mg and triazolam (Halcion) in doses of 0.25 to 0.5 mg, and the unrelated drug zolpidem (Ambien), 10 mg. In each case, the lesser dose should be used if possible. In general, sleeping medication should not be used on consecutive nights for more than a week or two.

Hypersomnic States

Of the hypersomnic states, two are of particular importance because of their frequency and disturbing effects on the life of the patient: the narcolepsy-cataplexy syndrome and sleep apnea with daytime hypersomnolence. Some depressed and asthenic patients sleep excessively, as do patients with severe hypothyroidism and hypercapnia.

Narcolepsy-cataplexy syndrome This is a disease of obscure cause and pathology characterized by frequently recurring (two to six per day) attacks of sleepiness. The unique features of narcoleptic attacks are their irresistibility, their occurrence in unusual circumstances (while standing, eating, or conversing, for example), and their electroencephalographic (EEG) findings, which show the attacks to coincide with episodes of REM sleep that arise suddenly from a background of wakefulness. Most narcoleptic individuals also have occasional attacks of *cataplexy*, a sudden loss of muscle tone, which is provoked by hearty laughter or other strong emotion. The cataplexy is momentary and may affect only certain muscles, such as those of the jaw or arms, or it may be complete, with a fall to the ground but with retention of consciousness and immediate recovery. Less often, patients experience *sleep paralysis*—a brief powerlessness of muscles occurring during the period of falling asleep or awakening—and *vivid hallucinations* occurring soon after the onset of sleep and termed "hypnagogic," which complete the tetrad that constitutes the narcolepsy syndrome.

Narcolepsy usually begins in adolescence or early adult years and, once begun, is lifelong. The prevalence in the general population is approximately 40 per 100,000 and males are more often affected than females. A genetic cause has been postulated, but the pattern of inheritance is not established. However, the presence of HLA-DR2 or -Dqw1 is nearly universal. As to causation, two previously unknown hypothalamic peptides, each derived from the same gene, have been implicated. These are referred to as hypocretin 1 and 2, or as orexin A and B. In patients with narcolepsy, a severe loss of hypocretin-containing neurons has been demonstrated in the tuberolateral region of the hypothalamus.

The *treatment* of narcolepsy consists of having the patient take strategically spaced naps during the day and analeptic drugs—modafinil (Provigil), 200 mg; dextroamphetamine (Dexedrine), 5 to 20 mg/day; or methylphenidate (Ritalin), 10 to 30 mg/day. Imipramine (Tofranil), 25 mg tid or similar drug is prescribed for cataplexy. These drugs act by inhibiting REM sleep. Cataplexy, which is neither as frequent nor as troublesome as sleep attacks, can be avoided by the wary patient.

Sleep apnea and daytime hypersomnolence In certain individuals, notably those with upper airway obstruction or decreased respiratory drive, sleep may induce repeated episodes of prolonged ($>$ 10 s) apnea. The common *obstructive type* of apnea, seen especially in males, is often associated with obesity and adenotonsillar hypertrophy and less often with micrognathia, neuromuscular diseases of many types, acromegaly, and hypothyroidism. Loud snoring is indicative of the upper airway obstruction. The anatomy and physiology of the rare *central*, or *primary*, *type* are poorly understood, but a severe form of this disorder has been identified as *idiopathic central hypoventilation* (Ondine's curse). The central form is also observed in patients with medullary lesions (e.g., lateral medullary infarction, syringobulbia, bulbar poliomyelitis, olivopontocerebellar degeneration). Most cases of sleep apnea appear to have both central and obstructive components, but the latter, due to pharyngeal hypotonia, appears to be the more important.

Periods of obstructive apnea usually occur during REM sleep. As a result of the repeated interruptions of nocturnal sleep, there is increased drowsiness throughout the day. In fact, the occurrence of persistent daytime drowsiness should always raise the suspicion of obstructive sleep apnea, especially in heavy-set men.

The treatment of obstructive sleep apnea consists of weight reduction, the placement of pillows in such a way as to force the patient to sleep on one side, and surgical measures that relieve nasopharyngeal obstruction. If these fail to improve daytime alertness, the upper airway can be kept open and breathing stimulated by nasally administered biphasic positive airway pressure (BIPAP) during sleep. In central sleep apnea, administration of medroxyprogesterone and protriptyline is thought to be beneficial.

Other hypersomnic states Midbrain-diencephalic encephalitis, known during the decade that followed World War I as "encephalitis lethargica," produced hypersomnolence that could last for months on end. In central Africa, trypanosomiasis is the cause of a similar disorder ("sleeping sickness"). Patients with severe hypothyroidism may sleep for 15 to 20 h a day. Periodic hypersomnia is part of the rare and obscure Kleine-Levin syndrome, in which adolescent boys, and infrequently girls, lapse into a state of somnosis for days or weeks, associated with episodes of greatly increased appetite (bulimia), negativism, and social withdrawal. Its cause is unknown. Hypothalamic tumors are a rare cause of hypersomnolence, and usually other hypothalamic, pituitary, and visual symptoms are present.

Other Sleep Disorders

Benign parasomnic phenomena Numbered among these disorders are *somnolescent starts*—sudden, massive jerks of the legs or trunk at the moment of falling asleep; *sensory paroxysms*—a flash of light, clanging sound, or explosive sensation in the head ("exploding head syndrome"), also occurring as the individual dozes off and often associated with a somnolescent start; and *postdormital paralysis*—a brief state of paralysis on "too soon" awakening.

Somnambulism and sleep automatism This is a condition in which a child, less often an adult, sleepwalks. In children it may be associated with *enuresis* and *night terrors*. Somnambulism occurs almost exclusively during stages 3 and 4 of NREM sleep. Children usually outgrow this disorder. Somnambulism in the adult can be a relatively benign event, as it usually is in children, but more often it is associated with awake-appearing, undirected violent behavior, fear, tachycardia, and self-injury (night terror) for which the patient is amnesic. These attacks can be suppressed by the administration of clonazepam (0.5 to 1.0 mg) at bedtime or by awakening the individual for several consecutive nights, just before the usual time of the attack.

Nocturnal epilepsy This is a well-established entity and is easily recognized if the seizure is generalized. If the seizure is of psychomotor (temporal lobe) type, it must be distinguished from night terrors, nightmares, somnambulism, and nocturnal paroxysmal dystonia or certain sleep automatisms.

Nocturnal enuresis (bedwetting) Approximately 10 percent of children 4 to 14 years of age are afflicted with this disorder. It is more frequent in boys than in girls. The child is not awakened by relatively high intravesicular pressures, which usually occur during the first part of the night; an enuretic episode is most likely to occur about 4 h after the onset of sleep. Imipramine (Tofranil), 25 mg at bedtime, has proved to be effective, as have several behavioral modifications; almost all cases are self-limited by early adolescence. Diseases of the bladder or its innervation, diabetes mellitus, diabetes insipidus, epilepsy, and sickle cell anemia must be excluded but are seldom found.

REM sleep behavior disorder This disorder occurs primarily in older men *without* a history of childhood sleepwalking. The attacks occur exclusively during REM sleep and are characterized by shouting and violent motor activity; typically the patient recalls a nightmare of being attacked and fighting back or attempting to flee. This disorder can also be effectively suppressed by the bedtime administration of clonazepam (0.5 to 1.0 mg).

For a more detailed discussion of this topic, see Victor and Ropper: *Adams and Victor's Principles of Neurology*, 7th ed, pp 404–427.

ADDITIONAL READING

Aldrich MS: Diagnostic aspects of narcolepsy. *Neurology* 50(suppl):S2, 1998.

Bassetti C, Aldrich MS: Idiopathic hypersomnia: A series of 42 patients. *Brain* 120:1423, 1997.

Culebras A (ed): The neurology of sleep. *Neurology* 42 (Suppl 6), 1992.

Gillin JC, Byerley WF: The diagnosis and management of insomnia. *N Engl J Med* 322:239, 1990.

Guilleminault C, Dement WC: 235 cases of excessive daytime sleepiness: Diagnosis and tentative classification. *J Neurol Sci* 31:13, 1977.

Krueger BR: Restless legs syndrome and periodic movements of sleep. *Mayo Clin Proc* 65:999, 1990.

Kryger MH, Roth T, Dement WC (eds): *Principles and Practice of Sleep Medicine*, 2nd ed. Philadelphia, Saunders, 1994.

Kupfer DL, Reynolds CF: Management of insomnia. *N Engl J Med* 336:341, 1998.

Thannickal TC, Moore RY, Nienhuis R, et al: Reduced number of hypocretin neurons in human narcolepsy. *Neuron* 27:469, 2000.

20 | Delirium and Other Confusional States

In this chapter and the ones that follow we use the term *confusion* in a general sense, to embrace all states in which a patient is unable to think with his customary speed, clarity, and coherence. Disorientation, impaired attentiveness and concentration, impaired registration of immediate events and information, and a quantitative reduction in all mental activity are its most prominent features; reduced perceptiveness, sometimes with visual and auditory illusions and even hallucinations, is another but more variable feature.

By contrast, we use the term *delirium* to denote a special type of confusional state, the predominant features of which are agitation, a disorder of perception or "clouding of the sensorium" (misinterpretations and misidentifications), vivid and terrifying hallucinations and dreams, a kaleidoscopic array of strange and absurd fantasies and delusions, intense emotional experiences, insomnia, and a tendency to convulse. Delirium is also distinguished by a state of heightened alertness (i.e., an increased readiness to respond to stimuli) and by overactivity of psychomotor and autonomic nervous system functions.

Some authors, particularly psychiatrists, use the word *delirium* to designate all forms of confusion resulting from acute and even chronic cerebral disease; they make no distinction between delirium and any other confusional state. In our view, however, the clinical context in which delirium occurs, its symptomatology, and its pathogenesis are sufficiently distinctive to warrant its separation from other confusional states, as discussed further on.

Acute Confusional States Associated with Reduced Alertness and Psychomotor Activity

Some features of this syndrome have already been described in Chap. 17, under "Coma." In the most typical of these states—due to drug intoxications and metabolic disorders—all mental functions are reduced to some degree, but alertness and the ability to grasp all elements of the immediate situation, to maintain a coherent stream of thought, to keep in mind recent happenings, and to react quickly and decisively are affected most of all. The patient is inattentive and easily distracted; he cannot converse for long on any single topic. Illusory phenomena and hallucinations may be present but are variable. There is a tendency to doze. As the confusion deepens, alertness and responsivity diminish until stupor supervenes.

The main causes of this acute confusional state are listed in Table 20-1. As to the pathology and pathophysiology, all that has been said on the subject in Chap. 17 is applicable to at least one large subgroup of the confusional states. In most cases no consistent pathology is found, and in many the cause is uncertain. The electroencephalogram (EEG) is almost invariably abnormal, the degree of disturbance in background rhythms reflecting the severity of the encephalopathy; high-voltage slow waves in the theta or delta range are the usual findings in severe forms of this syndrome.

Delirium

This syndrome is exemplified most completely in the chronic alcoholic patient with delirium tremens. Upon cessation of drinking, after a sustained period of inebriation, the patient becomes restless, apprehensive, and tremulous (fast-frequency kinetic tremor); sleep is disturbed and he may experience visual and auditory illusions and hallucinations. One or several generalized convulsions precede or initiate the delirium in about one-quarter of the patients. These symptoms rapidly give way to the full-blown syndrome of delirium—the patient is grossly tremulous, profoundly disoriented, distractible, and preoccupied with his hallucinations. He talks incessantly and incoherently. Sleep is impossible. His temperature may be elevated. With concomitant illnesses—such as pneumonia, meningitis, liver failure, or cranial trauma—psychomotor activity is depressed, in which case the line that separates delirium from other confusional states becomes indistinct. In most instances, recovery from delirium tremens is complete in a matter of several days.

In the most typical cases, the EEG, if one can be obtained in such restless patients, may show either fast activity or nonfocal 5- to 7-per-second theta activity, but not the diffuse slowing that is characteristic of most other confusional states. No consistent cellular pathology has been observed in fatal cases—which is not surprising, for recovery is complete with resolution of the delirium.

Other types of delirium, listed in Table 20-1, differ in minor ways from delirium tremens.

Beclouded Dementia

We use this term to denote the acute confusional states of elderly persons in whom a preexisting brain disease, most often Alzheimer disease, is complicated by some medical or surgical illness or drug intoxication. *It is the most common mental disorder seen on the wards of a general hospital.*

In such a person, almost any complicating illness may precipitate the confusional state, but certain ones stand out: therapeutic use or intoxication with one or more drugs, electrolyte imbalance, and alcoholism; concussive brain injuries; infections (particularly of lungs and bladder); major surgical operations; congestive heart failure and chronic pulmonary disease; and severe anemia, notably pernicious anemia. Frequently, more than one of these factors is operative. Sometimes, the coming of nighttime alone arouses an agitated confusional state ("sundowning").

TABLE 20-1 Classification of Delirium and Acute Confusional States

I. *Acute confusional states associated with psychomotor underactivity*
  A. Associated with a medical or surgical disease (no focal or lateralizing neurologic signs; CSF clear)
      1. Metabolic disorders; hepatic stupor, uremia, hypoxia, hypercapnia, hypoglycemia, porphyria, hyponatremia, hypercalcemia, etc.
      2. Sepsis
      3. Congestive heart failure
      4. Postoperative and posttraumatic states
  B. Associated with drug intoxication (no focal or lateralizing signs; CSF clear): opiates, barbiturates and other sedatives, trihexyphenidyl, etc.
  C. Associated with diseases of the nervous system (with focal or lateralizing neurologic signs or CSF changes)
      1. Cerebral vascular disease, tumor, abscess, contusion (especially of the right parietal, inferofrontal, and temporal lobes)
      2. Subdural hematoma
      3. Meningitis and encephalitis
      4. Nonconvulsive seizures and postictal state
II. *Delirium*
  A. In a medical or surgical illness (no focal or lateralizing neurologic signs; CSF usually clear)
      1. Pneumonia and other infections
      2. Postoperative and postconcussive states
      3. Thyrotoxicosis and ACTH intoxication (rare)
  B. In neurologic disease that causes focal or lateralizing signs or changes in the CSF
      1. Vascular, neoplastic, or other diseases, particularly those involving the right temporal lobe and upper brainstem
      2. Cerebral concussion and contusion (traumatic delirium)
      3. Acute meningitis (Chap. 32)
      4. Encephalitis due to viral causes (e.g., herpes simplex, infectious mononucleosis) and to unknown causes (Chap. 33)
  C. The abstinence states, exogenous intoxications, and postseizure states; signs of other medical, surgical, and neurologic illnesses absent or coincidental
      1. Withdrawal of alcohol (delirium tremens), barbiturates, and nonbarbiturate sedative drugs, following chronic intoxication (Chaps. 42 and 43)
      2. Drug intoxications: atropine, amphetamine, cocaine, PCP
      3. Postconvulsive delirium
III. *Beclouded dementia*—i.e., senile or other brain disease in combination with infective fevers, drug effects, heart failure, or other medical or surgical diseases

Quite often the occurrence of this type of confusional state first draws attention to a preexisting mental impairment that may have passed unnoticed or may have been attributed by the patient's family to the benign effects of aging. Upon the patient's recovery from the medical illness and return to the premorbid mental state, the family may become more aware of the patient's deficiencies.

DIAGNOSIS AND MANAGEMENT OF THE CONFUSED OR DELIRIOUS PATIENT

This should be carried out in a general hospital rather than a psychiatric one, because the confusional and delirious states are reversible, as a rule, and the primary need is the diagnosis and treatment of the underlying medical disorder.

The patient should be placed in relative isolation, so as not to disturb the rest of the ward. A well-lighted, quiet room and constant reassurance and explanation of all procedures are helpful. A family member or nurse should be in constant or near-constant attendance if possible, or the patient must be restrained to prevent self-injury. All drugs that could possibly be causative should be discontinued, and any infection should be identified and treated with appropriate antibiotics.

Blood count, electrolytes, BUN, calcium, and ammonia levels should be evaluated and other blood tests obtained in appropriate clinical circumstances. The EEG may also be helpful in disclosing diffuse slowing, nonconvulsive seizures, or unsuspected focal abnormalities. The slightest suspicion of meningitis requires a cerebrospinal fluid (CSF) examination. Fluid intake and output should be carefully recorded and fluid and electrolyte abnormalities corrected. Adequate nutrition and B vitamins should be administered. When mild restlessness and agitation of delirium require sedation, chlordiazepoxide and lorazepam are the favored drugs. In the case of more severe agitation, the antipsychotics haloperidol, olanzapine, and risperidone are useful. Beta-blocking agents and clonidine can be used to mute the autonomic hyperactivity. The purpose of sedation in these circumstances is not to suppress the agitation completely but only to moderate it to the point where nursing care is facilitated. In elderly patients, frequent reorientation, mentally stimulating activities, ambulation, attention to hearing, and visual aids reduce the frequency of beclouded dementia.

For a more detailed discussion of this topic, see Victor and Ropper: *Adams and Victor's Principles of Neurology*, 7th ed, pp 431–443.

ADDITIONAL READING

Inouye SK, Bogardus ST, Charpentier PA, et al: A multicomponent intervention to prevent delirium in hospitalized older patients. *N Engl J Med* 340:669, 1999.

Mesulam M-M: Attentional networks, confusional states, and neglect syndromes, in Mesulam M-M (ed): *Principles of Behavioral and Cognitive Neurology*. Oxford, Oxford University Press, 2000, pp 174–256.

Moller JT, Cluitmans P, Rasmussen LS: Long-term postoperative cognitive dysfunction in the elderly: ISPOCD1 study. *Lancet* 351:857, 1998.

Mori E, Yamadori A: Acute confusional state and acute agitated delirium. *Arch Neurol* 44:1139, 1987.

21 | Dementia and the Amnesic (Korsakoff) Syndrome

In medical practice, the term *dementia* is used conventionally to denote a chronic deterioration of intellectual or cognitive functions, particularly learning and remembering but also verbal facility, numerical skill, visual-spatial perception, and the capacity to make proper deductions from given premises and to analyze and solve problems. Because these functions are clinically separable and may occur in varying degrees and in several combinations, it is evident that dementia may assume a variety of forms. Moreover, the anatomic substrates of the many diseases causing intellectual decline involve different parts of the cerebral cortex and their related thalamic nuclei and often the basal ganglia as well. It is not surprising, therefore, that the dementing diseases may also cause a number of noncognitive disturbances, such as loss of emotional control, changes in behavior and personality, and even disturbances of posture, movement, and coordination.

The very existence of several dementia syndromes signifies that in humans all parts of the cerebrum are not equivalent. For example, the hippocampi and medial thalamic nuclei and the basal frontal nuclei play a special role in learning and retentive memory. Yet it is a mistake to assume an absolutely strict localization of these functions, since lesions in each of these regions also have subtle and more general effects on widely distributed neuronal systems. For these reasons, it is not entirely correct to use the all-inclusive term *dementia*; it is preferable to speak of the *dementia syndromes* or the *dementing diseases*, each of which may reflect a disproportionate affection of a certain function or part of the brain.

It is therefore necessary to become skilled in the bedside examination of patients with mental disorders of all types. (A simplified mental status examination can be found at the end of this chapter.) The student or physician who has more than a passing interest in these aspects of cerebral neurology would do well to review the discussions of perception, thinking, emotion, mood, impulse, and insight in *Adams and Victor's Principles of Neurology*, 7th ed., or some other textbook of neurology and psychiatry.

NEUROLOGY OF THE DEMENTIAS

Table 21-1 lists the dementing diseases, which are subdivided into three categories on the basis of their associated neurologic signs and the clinical and laboratory evidence of medical disease.

The special clinical and pathologic features of the dementing diseases are discussed in subsequent chapters, but several general points should be made here. An inspection of Table 21-1 discloses that some dementing diseases are treatable, a fact that places a premium on accurate diagnosis. Most importantly, the cognitive slowing of a late-life depression, a treatable

TABLE 21-1 Bedside Classification of the Dementias

I.   Diseases in which dementia is usually the only evidence of neurologic or medical diseases
    A. Alzheimer disease
    B. Pick disease
    C. Some cases of AIDS
    D. Progressive aphasia syndromes
    E. Frontotemporal and "frontal lobe" dementias associated with tau deposition, Alzheimer change, or with no specific pathologic alteration
    F. Degenerative disease of unspecified type

II. Diseases in which dementia is associated with clinical and laboratory signs of other medical diseases
    A. AIDS
    B. Endocrine disorders: hypothyroidism, Cushing syndrome, rarely hypopituitarism
    C. Nutritional deficiency states: Wernicke-Korsakoff syndrome, subacute combined degeneration (vitamin B_{12} deficiency), pellagra
    D. Chronic meningoencephalitis: general paresis, meningovascular syphilis, cryptococcosis
    E. Hepatolenticular degeneration—familial (Wilson disease) and acquired
    F. Chronic drug intoxications (including CO poisoning)
    G. Prolonged hypoglycemia or hypoxia
    H. Paraneoplastic "limbic" encephalitis
    I. Heavy metal exposure: arsenic, bismuth, gold, manganese, mercury
    J. Dialysis dementia (now rare)

III. Diseases in which dementia is associated with other neurologic signs but not with other obvious medical diseases
    A. Invariably associated with other neurologic signs
       1. Huntington chorea (choreoathetosis)
       2. Multiple sclerosis, Schilder disease, adrenal leukodystrophy, and related demyelinative diseases (spastic weakness, pseudobulbar palsy, blindness)
       3. Lipid-storage diseases (myoclonic seizures, blindness, spasticity, cerebellar ataxia)
       4. Myoclonic epilepsy (diffuse myoclonus, generalized seizures, cerebellar ataxia)
       5. Subacute spongiform encephalopathy; Creutzfeldt-Jakob disease; Gerstmann-Strausler-Scheinker (prion, myoclonic dementias)
       6. Cerebrocerebellar degeneration (cerebellar ataxia)
       7. Cerebral-basal ganglionic degenerations (apraxia-rigidity)
       8. Dementia with spastic paraplegia
       9. Progressive supranuclear palsy
      10. Parkinson disease
      11. Amyotrophic lateral sclerosis (ALS) and ALS-Parkinson-dementia complex
      12. Other rare hereditary metabolic diseases
    B. Often associated with other neurologic signs
       1. Lewy-body disease (parkinsonian features)
       2. Communicating, normal-pressure, or obstructive hydrocephalus (usually with ataxia of gait)
       3. Multiple thrombotic or embolic cerebral infarctions and Binswanger disease
       4. Brain tumor (primary or metastatic) or abscess
       5. Brain trauma, such as cerebral contusions, midbrain hemorrhages, chronic subdural hematoma
       6. Progressive multifocal leukoencephalitis
       7. Marchiafava-Bignami disease (often with apraxia and other frontal lobe signs)
       8. Granulomatous and other vasculitides of the brain
       9. Viral encephalitis (herpes simplex)

Note: The special clinical features and pathologic anatomy of these many dementing diseases are discussed in appropriate chapters throughout this book, particularly Chap. 39 on degenerative disorders, Chaps. 37 and 41 on metabolic and nutritional disturbances, and Chap. 33 on chronic infections.

entity, can closely simulate dementia. The other treatable forms of dementia are those due to neurosyphilis and other chronic meningitides, chronic subdural hematoma, brain tumor, chronic drug intoxication, normal-pressure hydrocephalus, pellagra, vitamin B_{12} deficiency and other deficiency states, cerebral vasculitides, hypothyroidism, and other metabolic and electrolyte disorders. To the extent that infection with HIV is becoming a partially treatable disease, it should be numbered among this important type of dementia. Obviously, the correct diagnosis of these diseases is of greater practical importance than the diagnosis of the untreatable ones. Unfortunately, most dementias are due to untreatable degenerative diseases of the brain, mainly Alzheimer disease.

Dementia due to Degenerative Diseases

It is in this category of disease that a generic syndrome of dementia can most readily be discerned. The earliest signs are often subtle and easily overlooked. The old-age tendency to forget proper names becomes perceptibly worse. An employer or observant family member may remark on a reduction in the level of mental and physical activity, a certain lack of initiative and interest, a disinclination to converse, a neglect of routine tasks, and an abandonment of pleasurable activities. There follows a more obvious forgetfulness not only of proper names but also of the date, appointments, and assigned tasks. The patient asks the same question repeatedly, the answer being quickly forgotten. He becomes increasingly distracted by passing incidents or unreasonably preoccupied with some unimportant event. Complex activities can no longer be accomplished. Difficulties in calculation make it impossible to balance the checkbook, and household finances need to be removed from the patient's responsibility. A febrile illness, infection, seemingly mild craniocerebral injury, or excess of medication may provoke a state of more severe confusion, a "beclouded dementia," as discussed in Chap. 20.

Emotions may become labile, often with outbursts of tearfulness, irritability and unreasonable anger. Those who are by nature suspicious may become frankly paranoid. Judgment is increasingly impaired. Loss of social graces usually comes late in the illness. All this happens with the patient usually making little or no complaint and seemingly unaware of the changes (i.e., lack of insight). Some complain of mental "fuzziness," dizziness, or vague physical symptoms.

As the condition progresses, all intellectual faculties gradually fail, memory most of all. Language functions deteriorate sooner or later, and vocabulary becomes restricted. There is groping not only for proper names but also for common nouns. Even simple ideas can no longer be conveyed in properly constructed phrases or sentences, and the patient resorts to clichés and stereotyped phrases. Writing shows similar faults, and there is an increasing inability to comprehend complex spoken or written requests. As language function deteriorates, palilalia and echolalia may appear. Agnosias and apraxias become increasingly prominent, and eventually the patient requires help in all activities, even the most personal ones.

Late in the illness, there is also a change in the patient's physical and facial appearance, seemingly in parallel with his cognitive deterioration. Food intake is sometimes increased, but then it diminishes gradually with loss of weight. Walking becomes more difficult and the patient sits in idleness much of the time. Later, bed is preferred. Grasp and suck reflexes become easy to evoke. Even in this progressive vegetative state, somatic sensation, vision, hearing, and capacity for movement are retained until near the end. The final stage is one of cerebral paraplegia in flexion, in which the patient lies curled up, immobile and mute, until pneumonia or some other intercurrent infection mercifully terminates his life. In most cases, the duration of the entire illness is 5 to 10 years.

Problems in diagnosis In an elderly person, one of the problems is to distinguish Alzheimer disease from the natural forgetfulness and dysnomia of the aging process. The difference becomes clear by listening to the family's report of the patient's performance and behavior and by observing the patient over time and noting the lack of progression of symptoms, in contrast to the slow, steady decline in Alzheimer disease. In the latter illness, the memory loss begins to interfere seriously in the patient's daily life: e.g., his ability to keep appointments, drive, and maintain interpersonal relationships is disturbed.

Many of the diseases listed in Table 21-1 are identifiable by a slightly differing configuration of the dementing syndrome described above and also its temporal profile. *Lewy body dementia* may be identified by periods of psychosis lasting days or by prominent parkinsonian features. In *Huntington chorea*, an altered mood, particularly depression, or changes in personality and character (heightened irritability, suspiciousness, impulsive behavior, and other emotional disturbances) commonly precede the cognitive impairment. In *multi-infarct dementia*, the effects of one or more strokes may be added—hemiparesis, hemisensory loss, pseudobulbar palsy, homonymous hemianopia, or an early aphasia. As noted in Table 21-1, many of the dementing diseases have other identifying neurologic characteristics. An important example is *normal-pressure hydrocephalus*, in which a gait disorder is early and prominent, coming on before or with only slight mental change, and long before incontinence. As already noted, an *endogenous late-life depression* may simulate a type of progressive dementia. The patient's lack of interest and unwillingness to participate in tests of mental status make clinical evaluation difficult. Complaints by the patient of loss of memory, the presence of a sad facial expression, crying, talk of dying, discrepancies in memory tests coupled with intactness of language function and capacity for calculation, and a history of previous depression in the patient or in family members are helpful in differential diagnosis.

More than one factor may contribute to the dementia syndrome. Many patients with the Alzheimer–senile dementia complex may have one or more strokes. A considerable proportion of older patients with Parkinson disease develop senile dementia; conversely, the patient with advanced Alzheimer disease—with his impassive facies, stiff movements, and small steps—may simulate Parkinson disease. The special features of the dementias that complicate the cerebral degenerative diseases are described further in Chap. 39.

The Amnesic Syndrome (Korsakoff Psychosis, Amnestic-Confabulatory Syndrome)

These terms, which are used interchangeably, denote a special form of cognitive impairment in which learning and memory are deranged out of proportion to all other intellectual functions. Two features distinguish this category of disease: (1) an inability to recall events and other information that had been well established for months or years before the onset of the illness (*retrograde amnesia*) and (2) an inability to learn and retain new information, such as verbal, topographic, and complex motor skills (*anterograde amnesia*). The level of general intelligence may be affected very little, and language function, ability to calculate, and previously learned skills are retained (there is no aphasia, apraxia, or agnosia). While a global amnesia is the main disorder, there are usually relatively minor abnormalities in cognitive function as well. Psychometric tests disclose an impairment in concentration and visual and verbal abstraction and difficulty in changing from one task to another. Most patients with the amnesic syndrome are apathetic, indifferent to their surroundings, and lacking in initiative, spontaneity, and insight. Confabulation (fabrication of past events) is variably present and is not a requisite for the diagnosis.

The common diseases causing an amnesic syndrome are listed in Table 21-2 and classified according to their mode of onset and clinical course, associated neurologic signs, and ancillary findings. It will be recognized that the structures commonly damaged by these diseases are the diencephalon (more specifically the medial and anterior thalamic or basal forebrain nuclei) and the hippocampal formations. This is not to say that these structures necessarily constitute "memory centers" or that large hemispheric lesions do not impair memory, but that only in diencephalic-hippocampal structures do small, strategically placed lesions have a devastating effect on all learning and memory functions.

The diseases that cause an amnesic syndrome are discussed in the appropriate chapters. Also, special types of amnesia—e.g., for words (verbal or semantic) or for faces (prosopagnosia), each with its own anatomy—are discussed with the aphasias, and acalculia with parietal-occipital lesions in Chaps. 22 and 23. A unique amnesic syndrome, *transient global amnesia*, cannot with assurance be included with the epilepsies or with the cerebrovascular diseases and therefore is described below.

Transient Global Amnesia

This is the term given by Fisher and Adams to an acute syndrome in elderly patients who suddenly lose their temporal and spatial orientation for several hours. The affected patient characteristically repeats a question moments after being satisfied by a response to the same question ("Why are we here?" "How did we get to this place?") Other notable characteristics are a retrograde amnesia for events that had occurred in the hours or days before the episode began and a retained capacity, during the attack, to calculate, perform complex tasks, and recognize old friends and family. In this respect, the condition differs from the transient disorder of consciousness and the apparent amnesia (actually a failure of registration) that attends temporal lobe seizures, concussion, hypoxia, and other confusional states. The electroencephalogram (EEG) may show a slight slowing in temporal leads during the attack, but otherwise all studies are normal.

The mechanism is unclear. Transient ischemia and seizure have both been postulated, but proof of either is lacking. When followed for years, the patient is no more liable to stroke than his age-matched peers and is not disposed to seizures. As a rule, no treatment is needed and the disorder abates, leaving a permanent gap in the patient's memory for the acute event. The condition can recur up to five or more times over the years, but this happens

TABLE 21-2 Classification of Diseases Characterized
by an Amnesic Syndrome

I. *Amnesic syndrome of sudden onset*—usually with gradual but
    incomplete recovery
    A. Bilateral or left hippocampal infarction due to atherosclerotic-
        thrombotic or embolic occlusion of the posterior cerebral arteries or
        their inferior temporal branches
    B. Infarction of the basal forebrain due to occlusion of anterior
        cerebral-anterior communicating arteries
    C. Trauma to the diencephalic, inferomedial temporal, or orbitofrontal
        regions
    D. Rupture of anterior communicating artery aneurysm
    E. Carbon monoxide poisoning and other hypoxic states (rare)
II. *Amnesia of sudden onset and short duration*
    A. Temporal lobe seizures
    B. Postconcussive states
    C. Transient global amnesia
III. *Amnesic syndrome of subacute onset* with varying degrees of
     recovery, usually leaving permanent residue
     A. Wernicke-Korsakoff syndrome
     B. Herpes simplex encephalitis
     C. Tuberculous and other forms of meningitis characterized by a
         granulomatous exudate at the base of the brain
     D. Paraneoplastic "limbic" encephalitis
IV. *Slowly progressive amnesic states*
    A. Tumors involving the floor and walls of the third ventricle and limbic
        cortical structures
    B. Alzheimer disease (early stage) and other degenerative disorders
        with disproportionate affection of the temporal lobes

---

in only a small proportion of cases. A late-life migraine equivalent has been
postulated because some amnesic episodes are followed by a supraorbital
headache and others, accompanied by positive visual phenomena, have been
induced by vertebrobasilar angiography. Also, there appears to be an
increased history of migraine in this group of patients.

As remarked above, there are, apart from global memory loss for facts
and events, restricted impairments of memory. There may be an amnesia for
certain classes of spoken and written words (verbal memory loss) or for
visualized objects, while immediate memory (for repeated numbers) is
retained. In actuality, these special forms of memory loss overlap the conventional categories of apraxia; visual, auditory verbal, and object agnosias;
and aphasia, which are considered in Chaps. 22 and 23.

Management of the Demented Patient

Ideally, the demented patient should be admitted to the hospital for the purpose of fully assessing the clinical state and determining the presence or
absence of the treatable causes enumerated above, although this is often not
feasible. In addition to the history (which should always include information
from a person other than the patient) and the neurologic and mental status
examinations (see below), a number of ancillary examinations can be carried out as guided by clinical circumstances. These include blood counts,
vitamin B_{12} and drug levels, tests for thyroid function, evaluation of
endocrine and liver functions, serologic tests for HIV and syphilis,

sedimentation rate, cerebrospinal fluid (CSF) examination, and special tests of central nervous system (CNS) function—electroencephalography (EEG), computed tomography (CT), and, increasingly, magnetic resonance imaging (MRI). Neuropsychologic testing may be valuable in assessing the degree and nature of cognitive loss and following its progress.

Once it is established that the patient has an untreatable dementing disease, the cooperation of a responsible family member who is apprised of the situation is essential, for this person must assist in deciding upon time of retirement, guardianship, the assumption of legal and financial responsibility, the need for an attendant, placement in a nursing home, etc. This can be accomplished in a series of unobtrusive steps, since most of the underlying diseases are slowly progressive and incurable. In the very early stages of disease, the patient himself may have the wherewithal to guide some of these decisions. Adjustments to work, home life, and driving a car depend largely on the patient's circumstances, the degree of disability, and treatability of associated disease(s).

At times, medical treatment is indicated. Antidepressant medication helps alleviate mood change and insomnia. Severe paranoia may be controlled with olanzapine, quietapine, risperidone, or haloperidol. Nocturnal wandering can be controlled with diazepam or other sedative drugs. A sudden worsening in the mental state should always raise suspicion of an infection or electrolyte imbalance, a cardiac or cerebrovascular event, a pulmonary embolism, or the injudicious use of one or another drug.

THE MENTAL STATUS EXAMINATION

This must be systematic and should include most of the following categories of mental function (examples are given); of course, the patient must be fully awake and not aphasic in order to understand and respond to these questions.

1. *Insight* (patient's replies to questions about the chief symptoms): What is your difficulty? Are you ill? When did your illness begin?
2. *Orientation. Personal identity and present situation:* What is your name, your address, current location (building, city, state)? What is your occupation? Are you married?
   Place: What is the name of the place where you are now (name of hospital, city, state)? How did you get here? On what floor is it? Where is the bathroom?
   Time: What is the date today (year, month, day of the week)? What time of the day is it? What meals have you had? When was the last holiday?
3. *Memory*
   Remote: Tell me the names of your children and their birth dates. When were you married? What was your mother's maiden name? What was the name of your first schoolteacher? What jobs have you held? Identification of cultural icons appropriate to the patient's age (e.g., who was Fala, Groucho, Johnny Weismuller, O. J., John Lennon, etc.).
   Recent past: Tell me about your recent illness (compare with previous statements). What did you have for breakfast today? What is my name (or the nurse's name)? When did you see me for the first time? What tests have you had? What were the headlines in the newspaper today?
   Attention and immediate recall ("short-term memory"): Repeat these numbers after me (give a series of 4, 5, 6, 7, digits at a speed of one per

second). Now when I give a series of numbers, repeat them in reverse order. No fewer than 7 digits forward and 4 digits backward is acceptable. Spell the world *world* forward and backward.

Memorization (learning): The patient is given three simple data (e.g., examiner's name, date, time of day, and an article of clothing) and asked to repeat them until he can do so without prompting. Give the patient a simple story, oral or written, and ask him to retell it after 3 to 5 min. The capacity to reproduce these items at intervals after committing them to memory is a test of *retentive memory span.*

Visual span: The patient is shown a picture of several objects and then asked to name the objects; any inaccuracies are noted.

Names: The patient is asked to name as many items in a category as possible (e.g., cars, farm animals, words beginning with the letter *p*). Most normal adults can list 12 to 15 items in less than 1 min.

4. *General information:* Ask the names of the current president, the first president, and recent presidents, well-known historic dates, the names of large rivers and cities, the number of weeks in a year, and the definition of an island.

5. *Capacity for sustained mental activity:* Crossing out all the *a*'s on a printed page; counting forward and backward; saying the months of the year forward and backward.

Calculation: Test ability to add, subtract, multiply, and divide. Subtraction of serial 7's from 100 is a good test of calculation as well as of concentration.

Construction: Ask the patient to draw a clock and place the hands at 7:45, to draw a map of the United States or a floor plan of his house, to copy a cube.

Abstract thinking: Test the patient's ability to detect similarities and differences between classes of objects (orange and apple, horse and dog, desk and bookcase) or to explain a proverb or a fable.

6. *General behavior:* Note the patient's attitudes, general bearing, stream of thought, attentiveness, delay in responding, mood, manner of dress.

7. *Special tests of localized cerebral functions:* Grasp and suck reflexes, aphasia battery, praxis with both hands, and cortical sensory function.

The many available formal psychologic tests for dementia yield useful quantitative data of comparative value but in themselves cannot be used for the diagnosis of the underlying cerebral disease. However, comparison of the Wechsler Adult Intelligence Scales (WAIS) and the Wechsler Memory Scale is useful in distinguishing the amnesic state from a more general dementia (a discrepancy of 20 or more points between the two tests). The Raven matrix test is a standardized measure of nonverbal intelligence. The Hamilton and Beck scales for depression can be useful in excluding depressive pseudodementia.

"Mini-Mental State"

This is a simplified mental status examination, which includes 11 questions (maximum score, 30) and requires only 5 to 10 min to administer (Folstein et al). It is a widely used method of scoring cognitive impairment and following its progress, particularly in elderly patients who can cooperate for only short periods. This test is reproduced below (Table 21-3).

TABLE 21-3 The Mini-Mental State Examination*

Maximum score	Score		
		ORIENTATION	
5	( )	What is the (year) (season) (date) (day) (month)?	
5	( )	Where are we?: (state) (county) (town) (hospital) (floor).	
		REGISTRATION	
3	( )	Name 3 objects: 1 s to say each. Then ask the patient to repeat all 3 after you have said them. Give 1 point for each correct answer. Then repeat them until he learns all 3. Count trials and record. Trials _____	
		ATTENTION AND CALCULATION	
5	( )	Serial 7's. 1 point for each correct. Stop after 5 answers. Alternatively, spell "world" backward.	
		RECALL	
3	( )	Ask for the 3 objects repeated above. Give 1 point for each correct.	
		LANGUAGE	
9	( )	Name a pencil and a watch (2 points) Repeat the following: "No ifs, ands, or buts" (1 point) Follow a 3-stage command: "Take a paper in your right hand, fold it in half, and put it on the floor" (3 points) Read and obey the following: Close your eyes (1 point) Write a sentence (1 point) Copy design (1 point)	
_____		Total score	
		Assess level of consciousness along a continuum	

Alert	Drowsy	Stupor	Coma

A score of <20 is indicative of a dementia. Patients with the benign forgetfulness of senility generally score >25.
*From Folstein et al.

For a more detailed discussion of this topic, see Victor and Ropper: *Adams and Victor's Principles of Neurology*, 7th ed, pp 431–443.

ADDITIONAL READING

Deutsch JA (ed): *The Physiological Basis of Memory*, 2nd ed. New York, Academic Press, 1983, pp 199–268.
Esiri MM: The basis for behavioral disturbances in dementia. *J Neurol Neurosurg Psychiatry* 61:127, 1996.

Fisher CM, Adams RD: Transient global amnesia. *Acta Neurol Scand* 40 (Suppl 9):1, 1964.

Folstein M, Folstein S, McHugh PR: "Mini-mental state": A practical method for grading the cognitive state of patients for the clinician. *J Psychiatr Res* 12:189, 1975.

Growdon JH, Rossor MN: *The Dementias*. Boston, Butterworth-Heinemann, 1998.

Neary D, Snowden JS, Gustafson L, et al: Frontotemporal lobar degeneration: A consensus on clinical diagnostic criteria. *Neurology* 51:1546, 1998.

Victor M, Adams RD, Collins GH: *The Wernicke-Korsakoff Syndrome*, 2nd ed. Philadelphia, Davis, 1989.

Victor M, Agamanolis D: Amnesia due to lesions confined to the hippocampus: A clinical-pathologic study. *J Cog Neurosci* 2:246, 1990.

Wade JPH, Mirsen TR, Hachinski VC, et al: The clinical diagnosis of Alzheimer's disease. *Arch Neurol* 44:24, 1987.

Warrington EK, McCarthy RA: Disorder of memory, in Asbury AK, McKhann GM, McDonald WI (eds): *Diseases of the Nervous System*, 2nd ed. Philadelphia, Saunders, 1992, pp 718–728.

22 | Neurologic Syndromes Caused by Lesions in Particular Parts of the Cerebrum

In contrast to the dementing diseases discussed in Chap. 21, the lesions of which are diffuse or multifocal, the syndromes to be discussed here relate to lesions that are restricted to particular parts of the cerebral cortex and subcortical white matter. These focal syndromes are described in terms of the conventional lobar divisions of the cerebrum. However, it is obvious that most disease processes do not respect these boundaries. Hence the syndromes by which these diseases express themselves may reflect the involvement of more than one lobe or closely related systems.

It also needs to be remembered that all parts of the cerebral cortex are widely connected with other parts via tracts in the central white matter and with the thalamic nuclei via corticothalamic and thalamocortical pathways. For this reason, even though localized lesions may give rise to certain syndromes manifesting themselves as disorders of thinking, speaking, and behavior, one must guard against the presumption of a too discrete localization of function in the cerebral cortex. Evidence from blood flow studies attests to the wide extent of cerebral activation in all mental processes; the simple act of seeing, reading, and speaking a word successively activates the occipital, left temporal, and left frontal lobes. Surprising also is the magnitude of many cerebral lesions that result in no cerebral symptoms or signs whatsoever. However, in general, the degree of intellectual deficit correlates with the amount of brain destroyed by a lesion.

The lobar division of the cerebrum, as well as the gyral and sulcal pattern of its (left) lateral surface, are illustrated in Fig. 22-1. Figure 22-2 is a map of the surfaces of the cerebral cortex, numbered according to the different cytoarchitectonic areas recognized by Brodmann. The cortical surface can also be subdivided into broad functional zones, as depicted in Fig. 22-3. These schemes are the ones that are conventionally used in discussions of the functional anatomy of the human brain.

SYNDROMES CAUSED BY LESIONS OF THE FRONTAL LOBES

The frontal lobes are often conceived to be the human being's supreme evolutionary attainment. They lie anterior to the central (rolandic) sulcus and superior to the sylvian fissure and consist of several functionally different parts, as indicated in Figs. 22-1, 22-2, and 22-3.

The posterior parts of the frontal lobes are specifically related to motor function. Movements of the face, arm, and hand originate in the motor cortex of the convexity, and movements of the leg and foot, in the medial frontal

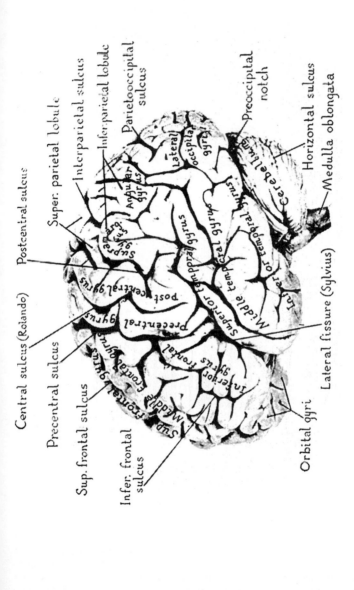

Central sulcus (Rolando)

Precentral sulcus

Sup. frontal sulcus

Infer. frontal sulcus

Postcentral sulcus

Super. parietal lobule

Interparietal sulcus

Interparietal lobule

Parietooccipital sulcus

Preoccipital notch

Horizontal sulcus

Medulla oblongata

Lateral fissure (Sylvius)

Orbital gyri

Sup. frontal gyrus

Middle frontal gyrus

Inferior frontal gyrus

Precentral gyrus

Postcentral gyrus

Supramarginal gyrus

Angular gyrus

Superior temporal gyrus

Middle temporal gyrus

Inferior temporal gyrus

Lateral occipital gyri

Cerebellum

FIG. 22-1 Photograph of the lateral surface of the human brain. (*From MB Carpenter and J Sutin, Human Neuroanatomy, 8th ed, Baltimore, Williams & Wilkins, 1982, with permission.*)

181

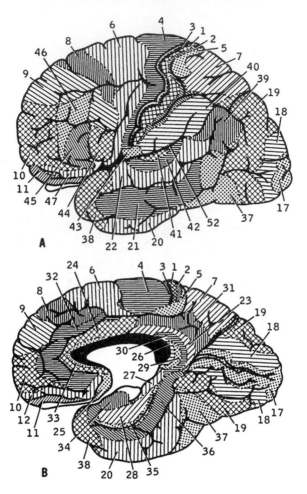

FIG. 22-2   Zones of the human cerebral cortex according to the scheme of Brodmann. *A*. Lateral surface. *B*. Medial surface.

cortex. Voluntary movement depends on the integrity of the motor and premotor areas (areas 4 and 6), and lesions that involve both these parts produce spastic paralysis of the contralateral face, arm, and leg. There is also a supplementary motor area in the posterior part of the superior frontal convolution. A lesion of this area and the premotor area is accompanied by a contralateral grasp reflex; bilateral lesions of this area are associated with a suck reflex. A lesion in area 8 interferes with turning the head and eyes contralaterally and with coordination of the two hands. A lesion in areas 44 and 45 (Broca area) of the dominant hemisphere results in loss of verbal expression and in dysarthric and effortful dysmelodic speech (p. 193). There is also a motor apraxia of the tongue and lips and, at times, the left hand. The

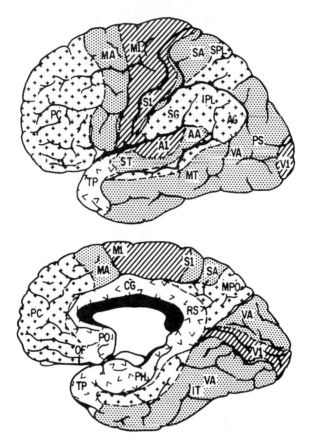

FIG. 22-3   Approximate distribution of functional zones on lateral (above) and medial (below) aspects of the cerebral cortex. Abbreviations: AA, auditory association cortex; AG, angular gyrus; A1, primary auditory cortex; CG, cingulate cortex; IPL, inferior parietal lobule; IT, inferior temporal gyrus; MA, motor association cortex; MPO, medial parieto-occipital area; MT, middle temporal gyrus; M1, primary motor area; OF, orbitofrontal region; PC, prefrontal cortex; PH, parahippocampal region; PO, parolfactory area; PS, peristriate cortex; RS, retrosplenial area; SA, somatosensory association cortex; SG, supramarginal gyrus; SPL, superior parietal lobule; ST, superior temporal gyrus; S1, primary somatosensory area; TP, temporopolar cortex; VA, visual association cortex; V1, primary visual cortex. (*Redrawn, with permission, from M-M Mesulam.*)

remaining parts of the frontal lobes (areas 9 through 12 of Brodmann), sometimes called the prefrontal areas, have less specific and measurable functions. They contribute to the planning of motor activity and, more importantly, to the control of behavior. If the lesions are large, they cause changes in drive and motivation (conation), emotional control, and personality—changes that in mild form may be more clearly realized by the family than by the physician from his survey of the mental status. Impulsivity, irritability, lack of initiative, apathy and slowness of response (abulia), and idleness are the observable changes in personality and behavior. Other frontal lobe disturbances of thinking and adaptive behavior are more subtle and difficult to detect even with sophisticated psychologic tests. With prefrontal lesions there may also be mental inflexibility, poor abstract reasoning, deficient sequencing (temporal ordering) of information, difficulty in shifting from one problem or paradigm to another, paucity of inner thoughts, and perseveration (or impersistence with right-sided lesions). A small unilateral anterior lesion may produce no detectable changes.

The *effects of frontal lobe lesions*, unilateral and bilateral, may be summarized as follows:

   I. Effects of unilateral frontal disease, either left or right
      A. Contralateral spastic hemiparesis or hemiplegia
      B. Slight elevation of mood, increased talkativeness, tendency to joke, lack of tact, difficulty in adaptation, loss of initiative
      C. If entirely prefrontal, no hemiplegia; a contralateral grasp reflex may be released
      D. Anosmia with involvement of medial-orbital parts
  II. Effects of right frontal disease
      A. Left hemiplegia
      B. Changes as in 1B, C, and D
      C. Confusional states with acute lesions
 III. Effects of left frontal disease
      A. Right hemiplegia
      B. Motor speech disorder with agraphia (Broca type), loss of verbal fluency with or without apraxia of the lips and tongue (see Chap. 23)
      C. Sympathetic apraxia of left hand
      D. Changes as in 1B, C, and D
 IV. Effects of bifrontal disease
      A. Bilateral hemiplegia
      B. Spastic bulbar (pseudobulbar) palsy
      C. If prefrontal, abulia (slowness of response and ideation) or, in its most severe form, akinetic mutism, lack of ability to sustain attention and solve complex problems, rigidity of thinking, bland affect, labile mood, personality change, and varying combinations of uninhibited motor activity, grasp and suck reflexes, decomposition of gait, and sphincteric incontinence.

SYNDROMES CAUSED BY LESIONS OF THE TEMPORAL LOBES

The sylvian fissure separates the superior and lateral surfaces of the temporal lobe from the frontal lobe and from the anterior part of the parietal lobe (Fig. 22-1). The temporal lobe merges posteriorly with the occipital lobe and superolaterally with the parietal lobe. The temporal lobe includes the superior, middle, and inferior temporal, fusiform, and hippocampal convolutions and, on its superior surface, the transverse gyri of Heschl, which constitutes the auditory receptive area. Hearing is represented bilaterally, so the Heschl gyri of both temporal lobes need to be affected to cause cortical deafness. The hippocampal convolution is of critical importance in learning and memory. A lesion in the superior convolution of the dominant temporal lobe (areas 41 and 42) results in a failure to understand the spoken word (auditory verbal agnosia) and is an important component of Wernicke aphasia (Chap. 23). Finally, the temporal lobes include a large part of the limbic system, which subserves the emotional and motivational aspects of behavior and vegetative functions ("visceral brain," Chap. 25). Less certain is its role, when diseased, in delirium, confusional states, and psychosis.

The lower fibers of the geniculocalcarine pathway (from the inferior retina) swing in a wide arc over the temporal horn of the ventricle en route to the occipital lobes, and lesions that interrupt them produce a contralateral upper homonymous quadrantanopia.

The effects of lesions in one or both temporal lobes are tabulated below:

I. Effects of unilateral disease of the dominant (left) temporal lobe
   A. Impaired comprehension of verbal material presented through the auditory sense (Wernicke aphasia)
   B. Dysnomia or amnesic aphasia
   C. Impaired reading and writing to dictation
   D. Impaired reading and writing of music
   E. Right superior quadrantanopia
II. Effects of unilateral disease of nondominant (right) temporal lobe
   A. Impairment in tests of visually presented nonverbal material
   B. Inability to judge spatial relationships in some cases
   C. Left superior quadrantanopia
   D. Aprosodia (lack of inflection and intonation of speech)
III. Effects of disease of either temporal lobe
   A. Auditory illusions and hallucinations
   B. Psychotic behavior and delirium
   C. Contralateral superior quadrantanopia
   D. Delirium with acute lesions
IV. Effects of bilateral disease
   A. Korsakoff amnesic defect (hippocampal formations)
   B. Apathy and placidity
   C. Increased sexual and oral exploratory activity (B and C constitute the Klüver-Bucy syndrome)
   D. Failure to recognize familiar tunes
   E. Failure to recognize faces (prosopagnosia) in some cases

SYNDROMES CAUSED BY LESIONS OF THE PARIETAL LOBES

This lobe is bordered anteriorly by the rolandic sulcus and inferiorly by the sylvian fissure; posteriorly, it has no definite boundary, but it abuts the occipital lobe. The postcentral convolution (areas 1, 3, and 5) is the terminus of somatosensory pathways from the opposite half of the body. However, destructive lesions here cause mainly a defect in sensory discrimination (position sense, stereognosis, localization of stimuli); impairment of primary sensation ("cortical sensory syndrome") occurs mainly with large lobar lesions. Also, with bilateral simultaneous stimulation, the patient may perceive only the stimuli from the unaffected side ("extinction").

With a large lesion of the *nondominant parietal lobe*, the patient is unaware of his hemiplegia and hemianesthesia and may even fail to recognize the left limbs as his own (*anosognosia*). Neglect of the left side of the body (as in grooming and dressing) and of extrapersonal space are related phenomena. There is great difficulty in copying figures or patterns and in constructing objects (constructional apraxia). These disorders are observed only infrequently with left-sided lesions.

With lesions of the *dominant angular gyrus*, the patient may lose the ability to read (alexia). Additionally, with large lesions, there is loss of ability to write (agraphia), to calculate (acalculia), to identify fingers (finger agnosia), and to distinguish the right from the left side. This constellation of abnormalities is known as the Gerstmann syndrome. Ideomotor and ideational apraxias (loss of ability to perform learned motor skills) result from left inferior parietal lesions.

The *effects of parietal lobe lesions* may be summarized as follows:

I. Effects of unilateral disease of the parietal lobe, right or left
   A. Cortical sensory syndrome and sensory extinction (or total hemianesthesia with large acute lesions of white matter)
   B. Mild hemiparesis, unilateral atrophy of limbs in children
   C. Homonymous hemianopia (incongruent) or inferior quadrantanopia
   D. Visual inattention and sometimes anosognosia, neglect of the opposite half of the body and of extrapersonal space (this constellation of symptoms has been referred to as amorphosynthesis and is far more evident with right than with left parietal lesions)
   E. Abolition of optokinetic nystagmus when a striped drum is rotated toward the side of the lesion
   F. Ataxia of contralateral limbs in rare cases

II. Effects of unilateral disease of the dominant parietal lobe (left hemisphere in right-handed patients); *additional* phenomena include
   A. Disorders of language (especially alexia)
   B. Gerstmann syndrome (see above)
   C. Tactile agnosia (bimanual astereognosis; see Chap. 9)
   D. Bilateral ideomotor and ideational apraxia

III. Effects of unilateral disease of the nondominant (right) parietal lobe
   A. Constructional apraxia
   B. Topographic memory loss
   C. Anosognosia and apractagnosia. These disorders may occur with lesions of either hemisphere but are observed more frequently with nondominant lesions.
   D. With posterior parietal lesions, there may be formed visual hallucinations, distortions of vision, hypersensitivity to contactual stimuli, or spontaneous pain.

SYNDROMES CAUSED BY LESIONS OF THE OCCIPITAL LOBES

The medial surface of the occipital lobe is demarcated from the parietal lobe by the parietal-occipital fissure; on the lateral surface, there is no sharp demarcation from the posterior temporal or parietal lobe. On the medial surface, the calcarine fissure, which courses in an anteroposterior direction, is the major landmark; the calcarine cortex on each side is the terminus of the geniculocalcarine pathways. The occipital lobe functions mainly as the receptive area for visual stimuli (area 17) and their recognition (areas 18 and 19). Perception of lines, figures, movement, and color—each has a specific localization in the occipital cortex. And for purposes of apperception (understanding the meaning of what is seen), each region connects with a widely distributed neuronal network. Like the other lobes of the cerebrum, the occipital lobe is connected through the corpus callosum with the corresponding lobe of the other hemisphere.

As indicated in Chap. 13, a destructive lesion in one occipital lobe results in a contralateral homonymous hemianopia—a loss of vision in part or all of the corresponding, or homonymous, fields (nasal field of one eye and temporal field of the other). Occasionally there may be a distortion of visually perceived objects (*metamorphopsia*) or illusory displacement of images from one side of the visual field to the other (*visual allesthesia*) or abnormal persistence of the visual image after the object has been removed (*palinopsia*). Visual illusions and elementary (unformed) hallucinations may also occur, but all of those experiences are as often the result of posterior temporal lobe disease. Bilateral occipital lesions cause "cortical blindness," a state of blindness without change in the optic fundi or pupillary reflexes and with preserved optokinetic response.

Lesions in Brodmann areas 18 and 19 of the dominant hemisphere surrounding the primary visual area, 17 (Fig. 22-2), cause an inability to recognize objects presented visually, even though, by tests of visual acuity, the individual appears to see sufficiently well to do so (visual object agnosia); such individuals are able to recognize objects by tactile or other nonvisual senses. *Alexia*, or inability to read, represents a visual verbal agnosia, or "word blindness"; patients can see letters and words but do not know their meaning, although they can still recognize them through tactile or auditory senses. Other types of agnosia—e.g., loss of color discrimination (*achromatopsia*), inability to recognize faces (*prosopagnosia*), visuospatial impairment, or failure to perceive simultaneously all the elements of a scene, with retained ability to recognize individual parts (*simultanagnosia*)—and the Balint syndrome (inability to look at and grasp an object, visual ataxia, and visual inattention) are observed with bilateral ventromesial occipitoparietal lesions.

These *occipital syndromes* are summarized below:

I. Effects of a unilateral lesion, either right or left
   A. Contralateral (congruent) homonymous hemianopia, which may be central (splitting the macula) or peripheral; also hemiachromatopsia (inability to identify colors in one field)
   B. Elementary (unformed) visual hallucinations—particularly with seizures and migraine

II. Effects of a left occipital lesion
   A. Right homonymous hemianopia
   B. If deep white matter or splenium of corpus callosum is involved, alexia and color-naming defect
   C. Visual object agnosia

III. Effects of right occipital disease
   A. Left homonymous hemianopia
   B. With more extensive lesions, visual illusions (metamorphopsias) and hallucinations (more frequent with right-sided than with left-sided lesions)
   C. Loss of visual orientation

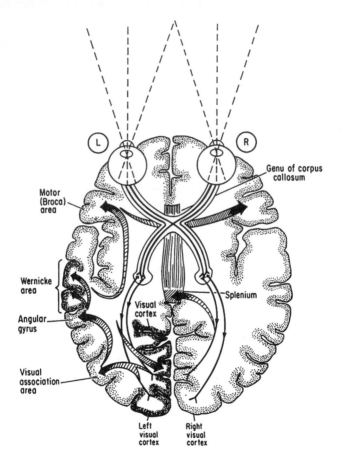

FIG. 22-4   The main proposed "disconnection" syndromes. Lesions in the left occipital lobe and adjacent posterior corpus callosum result in alexia without agraphia. The right hemianopia prevents information from the right visual field from reaching the angular gyrus and Wernicke area, and visual information from the left field cannot cross the corpus callosum to reach the speech areas.

Also depicted are disconnections between language areas that theoretically give rise to transcortical and conduction aphasias (Chap. 23), and anterior disconnection between the motor areas that may underlie a sympathetic left hand apraxia associated with a left frontal lesion (Chap. 3).

IV. Bilateral occipital lesions
   A. Cortical blindness (pupils reactive) with or without denial of blindness (Anton syndrome)
   B. Loss of perception of color
   C. Prosopagnosia, simultanagnosia, and other agnosias
   D. Balint syndrome (parietal-occipital borderzones, see text)

DISCONNECTION SYNDROMES

Focal lesions of cerebral white matter, which separate different parts of one hemisphere (*intrahemispheric*) or one hemisphere from another (*interhemispheric or commissural*), have certain definable but not always consistent effects. These are called disconnection syndromes, some of which are illustrated in Fig. 22-4.

For example, when the corpus callosum is sectioned surgically or destroyed (anterior four-fifths) by an anterior cerebral artery occlusion, the language and perceptual areas of the left hemisphere are isolated from those of the right. If blindfolded, such a patient is unable to match an object held in one hand with that in the other, nor can he match an object seen in the right half of the visual field with one in the left half. If given verbal commands, he performs correctly with the right hand but not with the left. Without vision, objects placed in the right hand are named correctly but not those in the left.

In lesions confined to the posterior fifth of the corpus callosum (splenium), visual disconnection syndromes occur. Occlusions of the left posterior cerebral artery provide the best examples. Infarction of the left occipital lobe causes a right homonymous hemianopia; as a consequence, all visual information needed for activating the language areas must come from the right occipital lobe. If, in addition, there is a lesion in the splenium or at some other point along the crossing fibers from the right occipital lobe, the patient cannot read or name colors because the visual information cannot reach the left angular gyrus (Fig. 22-4). There is no difficulty in copying words, although the patient cannot read what he has written (*alexia without agraphia*), or name colors. The patient can match colors without error but cannot name them.

Sympathetic limb apraxia with Broca aphasia represents yet another possible disconnection syndrome. Here, a lesion of the subcortical white matter, underlying the Broca area, separates the left and right premotor cortices, preventing the execution of commanded (spoken or written) movements of the left hand.

It is also thought that certain discrete aphasic disturbances, such as conduction aphasia and pure word deafness, are most readily explained by intrahemispheric disconnections. These are described in the next chapter, on aphasia.

For a more detailed discussion of this topic, see Victor and Ropper: *Adams and Victor's Principles of Neurology*, 7th ed, pp 464–498.

ADDITIONAL READING

Benson DF: *The Neurology of Thinking*. New York, Oxford University Press, 1994.

Critchley M: *The Parietal Lobes*. London, Arnold, 1953.

Damasio AR, Damasio H, van Hoesen GW: Prosopagnosia: Anatomic basis and behavioral mechanisms. *Neurology* 32:331, 1982.

Denny-Brown D, Banker B: Amorphosynthesis from left parietal lesion. *Arch Neurol Psychiatry* 71:302, 1954.

Feinberg TE, Farah MJ (eds): *Behavioral Neurology and Neuropsychology*. New York, McGraw-Hill, 1997.

Fuster JM: *The Prefrontal Cortex*, 2nd ed. New York, Raven Press, 1989.

Geschwind N: The clinical syndromes of cortical disconnections, in Williams D (ed): *Modern Trends in Neurology*, vol 5. London, Butterworth, 1970, p 29.

Lilly R, Cummings SL, Benson F, Frankel M: The human Klüver-Bucy syndrome. *Neurology* 33:1141, 1983.

Mesulam M-M (ed): *Principles of Behavioral and Cognitive Neurology*. Oxford, Oxford University Press, 2000.

23 | Disorders of Speech and Language

The human ability to substitute word symbols for objects and ideas is the basis of our extraordinary communicative skill, which, together with manual facility, sets us apart from all other members of the animal kingdom. Much of our thinking and other aspects of inner psychic life also take place in terms of word symbols, and literate men and women use them to record their ideas and experiences for others to read. In a much narrower sense, language is the means by which the patient makes known his complaints and the physician gathers information on the status of the nervous system and the manifestations of its diseases.

Speech and language depend on elaborate mechanisms that evolve over the first two decades of life and come to be localized in particular (perisylvian) parts of the left cerebral hemisphere (Fig. 23-1). Right-hand dominance usually develops in parallel. We know this from nature's experiments in humans, wherein speech and language functions are lost when these parts of the brain are destroyed. These statements require qualification only insofar as the right cerebral hemisphere is dominant for language in a small proportion of left-handed individuals (and a few right-handed ones), and lesions there cause aphasia. Some aspects of communicative speech—those utilizing *prosody* (melody, rhythm, pitch, and intonation of speech), vocalization, and gestures—are represented bilaterally. In either hemisphere, language functions have their sensory and motor aspects, and certain restricted lesions may interfere more with one than with the other, in which case the aphasia is referred to somewhat imprecisely as one of comprehension ("receptive") or of production ("expressive").

TERMINOLOGY

Aphasia or dysphasia is defined as a loss or impairment of comprehension or production of spoken or written language, or both, due to an acquired disease of the brain. A failure to name objects is called *anomia*. *Alexia*, or *visual verbal agnosia*, refers to an inability to read by a person who was literate. *Agraphia* is a loss of ability to write. *Auditory verbal agnosia*, or *word deafness*, specifies a loss of understanding of spoken words. *Dysarthria*, slurred speech (or the more severe *anarthria*), is purely a motor disorder of the muscles of articulation; language function remains intact. *Aphonia* or *dysphonia* signifies a loss or impairment of vocalization.

CLINICAL VARIETIES OF APHASIA

Despite the complexity of language mechanisms and the bewildering nomenclature that surrounds this subject, most instances of aphasia constitute a relatively small number of recurring, identifiable types, tabulated below. Moreover, more than 80 percent of all aphasias fall into the first

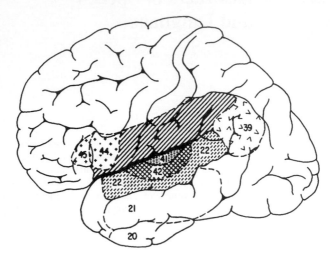

FIG. 23-1 Lateral surface of the left cerebral hemisphere, showing the classic language areas, numbered according to Brodmann. The Broca area, having to do with speech production, is centered in Brodmann areas 44 and 45. The auditory association areas of Wernicke (areas 41 and 42) actually lie on the superior surface of the temporal lobe, deep within the sylvian fissure. The elaboration of speech and language probably involves a much larger area of cerebrum, including all of the shaded zone of cortex and several subcortical areas. (The latter are not shown.)

(major) group. An overlapping of syndromes is frequent, and their localization, which has preoccupied neurologists for more than a century, is not altogether precise.

A. Major aphasic syndromes
   1. Global aphasia
   2. Broca aphasia
   3. Wernicke aphasia
   4. Anomic aphasia
B. Minor, or restricted (disconnection), syndromes
   1. Conduction aphasia
   2. Transcortical aphasias, motor and sensory
   3. Restricted and transient "mini-Broca"
   4. Modality-specific aphasias
      a. Pure word blindness (acquired dyslexia)
      b. Pure word deafness
      c. Pure word mutism (aphemia)
      d. Agraphia

Global, or Total, Aphasia

Here, all language functions, both receptive and expressive, are lost. Although awake, able to regard and follow the examiner with his eyes, move his tongue and lips, and swallow, the patient emits no words or at most a stereotyped, repetitive utterance or an expletive. Nor is there any understanding of words spoken or written by the examiner. Moreover, the patient is unable to express himself by writing with the left hand if the right is paralyzed (as it often is). The lesion is almost always left-sided, usually large, and there is typically a right hemiplegia and hemisensory defect and a tendency to turn and look to the left. Drowsiness, inattentiveness, and apathy (abulia) may also be present if the lesion is large.

The usual cause is an embolic occlusion of the stem of the left middle cerebral artery or occlusion of the internal carotid artery, affecting large portions of the frontal and temporal cortex. Large hemorrhages may have a similar effect but are more likely to cause stupor and coma, in which case the language disorder is less evident. Widespread tumor invasion, involving both the Broca and Wernicke areas (defined below), may also progress to the point of abolishing all language functions. Global aphasia of vascular cause tends to recover to some degree and may come to resemble Broca aphasia or some other type.

Broca, or Motor, Aphasia

Here the primary deficit is in language output or production; hence the synonym *motor*, or *expressive*, *aphasia*. The latter term is not entirely apt, since all aphasic patients have some difficulty expressing themselves.

Broca aphasia varies greatly in severity. In the milder forms, the capacity to speak (and to write) is moderately impaired, while the understanding of written and spoken words seems little affected. However, if the patient's comprehension is stringently tested (e.g., with complex spoken commands), it is found to be variably impaired, almost without exception. In some cases the patient may be transiently mute, despite preserved understanding of the written and spoken word, a condition that Broca originally referred to as "aphemia." This term is now used as a synonym for *pure word mutism* (see below). As a rule, the mutism gives way to a sparse, effortful, and frequently dysarthric speech and then to recovery, sometimes complete. Mohr and colleagues point out that the lesion in this recoverable type of aphasia ("mini-Broca") is relatively small and restricted to a zone in and immediately around the posterior part of the inferior frontal convolution—i.e., in Brodmann area 44 or 45 or what is conventionally referred to as the Broca area (see Figs. 23-1 and 22-2). Awareness of these difficulties frustrates the patient. Often there is an inability to execute commanded movements of the tongue and lips even though the patient can move these parts automatically (orobuccal "apraxia"). There is often weakness of the right lower face and sometimes the right arm and hand, reflecting damage to the adjacent motor cortex, but unlike the case in Wernicke aphasia, there is no visual field defect.

In the more severe form of Broca aphasia, the abolition of motor speech is more protracted and accompanied by greater difficulty in understanding spoken and written language. Recovery may be limited to a few stereotyped utterances that are repeated in response to all questions. Or there may be a gradual return to a slow, effortful, agrammatic, *nonfluent* speech, devoid of small words (articles, prepositions, conjunctions) and lacking all semblance of normal inflection and melody. In the severe form of Broca aphasia, the lesion extends well beyond the Broca area to involve the anterior insula, the frontal-parietal operculum and underlying white matter, and even the basal ganglia.

The common cause is an embolic occlusion of the upper (superior, or rolandic) division of the middle cerebral artery. Hemorrhage, a traumatic lesion, or an inflammatory, neoplastic or degenerative lesion in this anatomic territory may have the same effect, but such lesions are less frequent.

Wernicke, or Sensory, Aphasia

This syndrome comprises two main elements: (1) an inability to understand spoken or written words, even though hearing and vision are normal, and (2) a fluently articulated but paraphasic speech. By *paraphasia* is meant the distortion of words by substitution of unwanted phonemes or syllables—e.g., *frem* for *friend* (literal paraphasia)—or the substitution of one word for another in the same category, such as *father* for *brother* (verbal paraphasia). Neologisms (nonsense words that are not part of the language) may also appear. Despite the fluency and normal inflection of the patient's speech, it is devoid of meaning and may be entirely incomprehensible (jargon aphasia). The patient, however, is usually unaware or not fully aware of his deficit. In addition, there are invariable defects in reading, writing, naming, and repetition of the examiner's words or phrases—parallel in severity to the defect in comprehension. The lesion involves the posterior perisylvian region (superior temporal and supramarginal convolutions—Fig. 23-1). Varying degrees of right homonymous hemianopia may accompany the language disorder. The most frequent cause is an embolic occlusion of the posterior temporal branch or inferior division of the left middle cerebral artery, but hemorrhage, tumor, contusion, and encephalitis may involve the same region.

Anomic (Amnesic, Nominal) Aphasia

Some degree of word-finding and naming difficulty is observed in all forms of aphasia. Only when the patient's main deficit is in naming does the term *anomic aphasia* apply. Patients with such a disorder have little receptive or expressive difficulty and can immediately repeat a spoken word, but have lost the ability to name objects. The lost word, when supplied by the examiner, is usually recognized. There are also pauses in speech, groping for words, circumlocution, and the substitution of another word, phrase, or gesture to convey the meaning.

Anomic aphasia has been associated with lesions in disparate parts of the language area—deep in the basal portion of the posterior temporal lobe, in the frontal lobe, and in the angular gyrus. It may be a manifestation of early Alzheimer disease or of confusional states due to metabolic or infectious disease, in which case it has no localizing value. Finally, anomic aphasia may be the only residual abnormality after recovery from Wernicke, conduction, or transcortical aphasia (see below).

Disconnection, or Dissociative, Language Syndromes

This term denotes certain language disorders resulting not from lesions of the cortical language areas themselves but presumably from lesions that interrupt association pathways, thus separating primary receptive areas or the more strictly receptive parts of the language mechanisms from the motor ones (*conduction aphasia*) or separating the perisylvian language areas from other parts of the cerebral cortex (*transcortical aphasias*). The explanation of these disorders in terms of interruption of tracts that disconnect discrete language areas from one another is a useful heuristic device, as indicated in Fig. 22-4, but in the author's view it is a rather naïve postulation of cerebral organization of language function.

Conduction aphasia In this form (formerly called *central aphasia*), the patient comprehends spoken and written language with only minor flaws but is *unable to repeat* what is heard or read; spontaneous speech is fluent but paraphasic. The Wernicke language area in the temporal lobe is said to be separated from the Broca area, presumably by a lesion of the arcuate fasciculus, although such a lesion, strictly confined to this fasciculus, has not been demonstrated pathologically. Most examples of this aphasia have resulted from infarction in the angular gyrus.

Transcortical aphasias As a result of ischemic damage in the region between major vascular territories (watershed), the motor-sensory language areas may be isolated from the surrounding cortex. In the *sensory type* of transcortical aphasia, information from the damaged (parietal-occipital) cortex cannot be transferred to the Wernicke area for conversion into verbal form. The disorder of language is much like that of Wernicke aphasia, except for the remarkable *preservation of repetition*. In extreme degree, this takes the form of parrot-like echoing of words, phrases, and songs that are heard (*echolalia*). In *transcortical motor aphasia* (observed usually with subcortical lesions in the frontal lobe, partially recovered Broca aphasia, and abulic states due to frontal lobe damage), the patient, who spontaneously produces only a few grunts and syllables, can faultlessly repeat phrases that are heard or read, and even sentences of some length.

Several modality-specific aphasias have also been classified as dissociative or disconnection syndromes. In *pure word mutism*, a syndrome that also goes by many other names (including aphemia), the patient loses all capacity to speak while retaining perfectly the ability to write, to understand spoken words, and to read silently with comprehension.

In *pure word deafness*, the patient can hear but cannot comprehend spoken language. Expressive speech remains normal. This disorder has been attributed to a lesion of the dominant temporal lobe, undercutting the Wernicke area and separating it from the auditory receptive area (Heschl gyri) as well as from the contralateral auditory region (by interrupting fibers that cross in the corpus callosum). *Pure word blindness* (*visual verbal agnosia, alexia without agraphia*) has been alluded to in Chap. 22, with other commissural syndromes. *Pure agraphia* is a great rarity and its pathologic basis in the left frontal lobe is uncertain.

Subcortical Aphasias

On occasion, a lesion, usually vascular, that is seemingly confined to the dominant thalamus or striatocapsular region may cause an aphasia. These two aphasias—thalamic and striatocapsular—resemble but are not identical to the Broca and Wernicke types, respectively. With *thalamic aphasia,* the posterior nuclei are usually involved; complete recovery in a matter of weeks is the rule. In *striatocapsular aphasia,* the head of the caudate, anterior limb of the internal capsule, and anterior putamen are the critically involved structures; if the lesion extends laterally into the subcortical white matter, the prognosis is less favorable.

DISORDERS OF ARTICULATION AND PHONATION

Phonation, or the production of vocal sounds, is a function of the larynx, more particularly of the vocal cords. Articulation, i.e., the act of speaking, is effected through the modulation of vocal sounds by an intricate and highly coordinated sequence of contractions of the respiratory musculature, larynx, pharynx, palate, tongue, and lips. These structures are innervated by the phrenic, vagal, hypoglossal, and facial nerves; their nuclei, on each side of the brainstem, are under the control of both motor cortices through the corticobulbar tracts. As with all motor activity, there are also extrapyramidal influences from the basal ganglia and cerebellum.

Dysarthria and Anarthria

With pure disorders of articulation (dysarthria or anarthria), language functions are intact. The only exception occurs with a restricted left frontal lesion and "mini-Broca" aphasia (see above); with recovery from mutism, elements of both aphasia and dysarthria can be recognized. This aphasic dysarthria is distinguished from nonaphasic (upper motor neuron) dysarthria by its variability and normalization in the pronunciation of single sounds and automatic words and phrases. Defects in articulation are of several types, depending on the location of the causative lesion.

Lower motor neuron dysarthria (atrophic bulbar paralysis): This is due to a primary affection of the motor nuclei of the lower brainstem or their peripheral extensions. The tongue is weak and withered; there is difficulty speaking, vocalizing, and swallowing; lingual (la-la-la) and labial (mi-mi-mi) consonants are poorly enunciated. The usual cause is a progressive bulbar palsy (motor neuron disease). Disorders of one or more lower cranial nerves from diverse causes produce elements of this same syndrome. The same disorder of articulation can also be seen in a variety of myopathic disorders and in myasthenia gravis.

Spastic dysarthria: This is due to bilateral corticobulbar lesions and is characterized by slow slurred speech, spasticity of the masseter muscles, and other signs of pseudobulbar palsy—dysphonia, dysphagia, and hyperactive jaw jerk and facial reflexes—but no atrophy of the tongue. Outbursts of uncontrollable laughter or crying, as described in Chap. 25, may be associated. Usual causes are multiple strokes, amyotrophic lateral sclerosis, and progressive supranuclear palsy.

In *Parkinson disease* and *choreoathetotic disorders,* speech is also affected in characteristic ways. In the former, speech is rapid, cluttered, uninflected, and hypophonic. Choreoathetotic speech is slow, halting, uneven in volume, and accompanied by grimacing due to the superimposition of involuntary movements of the face, tongue, pharynx, and larynx.

Ataxic dysarthria: With cerebellar lesions, speech may be slow and slurred, but it is not strained, as with spastic dysarthria. Characteristic of some cases of cerebellar disease is a scanning speech pattern, in which there is an unnatural separation of syllables, much as a line of poetry is scanned for meter; in addition, words are of variable volume, some syllables being uttered with lesser or greater (explosive) force than intended.

Defects in phonation With paralysis of both vocal cords, the patient can speak only in whispers. There may be inspiratory stridor, due to failure of the vocal cords to separate during inspiration. Whispering speech is also a feature of advanced Parkinson disease, certain frontal lobe lesions, and stuporous states. With paralysis of only one vocal cord, the voice is low-pitched and rasping and its range is reduced. Myxedema produces a characteristic hoarseness.

A restricted dystonia of bulbar muscles underlies the strained, high-pitched, effortful speech of so-called *spastic* (or better termed *spasmodic) dysphonia.*

EXAMINATION OF SPEECH AND LANGUAGE

This begins with the first encounter with the patient—by listening to his spontaneous utterances and conversation. One takes note of his choice of words, the volubility and fluency of conversation or the lack of it, the inflection and melody of speech, and the speed of utterance. The inability to construct ideas in well-connected sequences is readily evident, as is any tendency to grope for words, to make grammatical errors out of keeping with the level of education, and to interject paraphasias and neologisms. A failure to understand questions and to give correct answers immediately raises questions as to defective hearing or the presence of a receptive aphasia.

One must then explore the language mechanism more pointedly by asking the patient to do the following:

1. Carry out one-, two-, and three-part spoken commands
2. Name common and uncommon objects, parts of objects, and parts of the body
3. Repeat words, phrases (e.g., "no ifs, ands, or buts"), and full sentences after the examiner
4. Read passages from a book or newspaper, and perform written commands
5. Write from dictation and copy printed passages

From these data, one should be able to determine the nature of the speech disorder (dysphonia, dysarthria, or aphasia) and, if an aphasia exists, whether any of the special language functions—speaking, writing, reading, understanding spoken words, repeating, and naming—is disproportionately affected.

Developmental language disorders are described in Chap. 27, on growth and development.

For a more detailed discussion of this topic, see Victor and Ropper: *Adams and Victor's Principles of Neurology*, 7th ed, pp 499–521.

ADDITIONAL READING

Benson DF: *Aphasia, Alexia, and Agraphia.* New York, Churchill Livingstone, 1979.
Damasio AR, Damasio H: The anatomic basis of pure alexia. *Neurology* 33:1573, 1983.
Damasio AR: Aphasia. *N Engl J Med* 326:531, 1992.

Geschwind N: Disconnection syndromes in animals and man. *Brain* 88:237, 585, 1965.

Gloning K: Handedness and aphasia. *Neuropsychologia* 15:355, 1977.

Kertesz A: *Aphasia and Associated Disorders*. Needham Heights, MA, Allyn and Bacon, 1989.

Kertesz A: Clinical forms of aphasia. *Acta Neurochir* 56(Suppl):52, 1993.

Mohr JP, Pessin MS, Finkelstein S, et al: Broca aphasia: Pathologic and clinical. *Neurology* 28:311, 1978.

Naeser MA, Alexander MP, Helm-Estabrooks N, et al: Aphasia with predominantly subcortical lesion sites. *Arch Neurol* 39:2, 1982.

Wise RJ, Greene J, Büchel C, Scott SK: Brain regions involved in articulation. *Lancet* 353:1057, 1999.

24 | Fatigue, Nervousness, Irritability, Anxiety, and Depression

These phenomena are more abstruse than the cognitive abnormalities described in the preceding chapters and, in their least complicated forms, represent only an exaggeration of normal reactions to all manner of life stresses and medical diseases. Yet they may be expressions of disturbed neurologic function and the forerunners of important medical or psychiatric diseases. Their proper place in the semiology of neuropsychiatry is difficult to judge. We have placed them in this section of the book, in juxtaposition to limbic, autonomic, and hypothalamic diseases, of which they are not infrequently a part. In any case, they are so ubiquitous in medical practice that all physicians must be familiar with their interpretation.

USE OF TERMS

These phenomena, by their very vagueness, require that special care be taken in their definition. Patients, in their attempts to describe these phenomena, use many different terms with various degrees of imprecision; the physician must determine what the patient means by these terms if he is to assess their seriousness intelligently.

Lassitude, *fatigue*, *lack of energy*, and *listlessness* are more or less synonymous terms, referring to weariness or a loss of the sense of well-being that is well known to persons who are otherwise healthy in mind and body. A lack of physical and mental *endurance* are components of most fatigue states. *Weakness*, which many patients call fatigue, is clearly a separate phenomenon, denoting a diminished power and endurance of muscle contraction, and is more appropriately considered in relation to neuromuscular diseases (Chaps. 46 and 48). *Nervousness* is the vaguest of all the terms in this group. It may be used by the patient to describe feelings of restlessness, tension, apprehension, and irritability or more serious psychiatric symptoms (obsessions, phobias, delusions, etc.) or even tics and tremors. *Anxiety* is defined as an intermittent or sustained emotional disturbance characterized by feelings of fear and apprehension, usually with a topical content and associated with signs of autonomic overactivity. *Depression* as a symptom simply refers to a state of sadness, dejection, hopelessness, and despair; frequently it is combined with anxiety or fatigue. The wider implications of anxiety and depression are considered in Chaps. 56 and 57.

In a great majority of patients, these complaints come and go without explanation. But at times they persist and are aggrandized to the point where they demand medical attention. It is a mark of high medical competence to recognize whether they are more or less normal reactions to transient circumstances or require further investigation and treatment.

FATIGUE AND LASSITUDE

Of all the symptoms in this group, these are the most frequent. More than half of all hospitalized patients register a direct complaint of fatigability or admit to it when questioned. Of course, patients have their own way of stating their complaints—"tired all the time," "exhausted," "no endurance," "pooped out," "no pep," etc. Often they speak of "weakness" when they mean fatigability. Indeed, the distinction between the two is not always easy. Loss of endurance and muscle aching may occur in a number of ill-defined neurologic and muscle diseases, described in Chap. 55, even though tests of maximum strength, or "peak power," show the muscles to be normal. Surprisingly, in a number of neuromuscular diseases that actually weaken muscles, fatigability is rarely a complaint.

In approaching this clinical problem, the physician begins with a survey of the patient's daily schedule. Long hours of sustained work—sometimes from necessity, at other times because of certain notions of duty—are one cause, but most people recognize this state and do not seek medical advice for it. Chronic infection, anemia, diabetes, hypothyroidism, sedative drugs, obesity, alcoholism, and neoplasia are other causes that must be sought medically. Physical fatigue may for a long time be the only manifestation of chronic infections such as tuberculosis, HIV or Epstein-Barr virus infection, viral hepatitis, and Lyme disease; a lack of fever may lower one's suspicion of an infective process. Less common diseases that should be sought in the patient with chronic fatigue are hypothyroidism, hypercalcemia, adrenal insufficiency, and brucellosis. Patients with certain chronic neurologic illnesses (notably multiple sclerosis and Parkinson disease) complain inordinately of fatigue.

However, the majority of patients who complain of chronic fatigue will, in our experience, be found to suffer some type of psychiatric illness. Formerly the condition was called *neurasthenia*. A modern euphemism is "chronic fatigue syndrome," with the implication that it represents the lingering effects of a viral infection. Here mental fatigue—inability to maintain concentration and to sustain long conversations or periods of reading and study—is combined with physical fatigue and poor endurance and is regularly associated with other symptoms such as headaches, muscle aches (fibromyalgia), irritability, insomnia, palpitation, trembling, feelings of hopelessness, etc., so that the condition comes to be recognized for what it usually is—anxiety neurosis or, most frequently, depression. Actually, this constellation of symptoms is no more frequent after viral infections than in the general population. The symptom complex has been observed in war veterans after each major war and is frequent following concussive head injury, especially if compensation is an issue.

NERVOUSNESS, ANXIETY, AND DEPRESSION

Complaints of nervousness, anxiety, and depression, like lassitude and fatigue, are remarkably common in office and hospital practice. Virtually everyone has experienced some degree of these symptoms when faced with a threatening event, a challenging task for which one feels inadequate, or some overwhelming personal problem. They should then be viewed as natural and transient reactions to the vicissitudes of life. Only when they occur without explanation or are unduly severe and prolonged are they brought to medical attention.

These symptoms are more likely to occur at certain times of life than at others. Adolescence rarely passes without a period of turmoil, as the young attempt to emancipate themselves from parental dominance and adjust to scholastic demands, a work situation, or the opposite sex. The menses are regularly accompanied by increased tension and moodiness, a state that is given its own name ("premenstrual syndrome"). In the postpartum period, it is exceptional for a new mother not to experience transient anxiety and depression ("postpartum blues"), possibly due to hyperprolactinemia. Menopause is another time when emotional stability may be threatened. The irritability and peevishness of the aged is an accepted fact of life.

Even in their simplest form, anxiety and depression reveal themselves in a number of behavioral changes. Headaches may increase in frequency, and sleep is disturbed. Often there is a mild somberness of mood, frequent sighing, and increased tendency to tears and anger or to irascibility, a fatigue that bears no proper relationship to activity and rest, and episodes of sweating, trembling, light-headedness, and palpitations. When the autonomic features are combined in acute episodes with a feeling of suffocation, dread, or impending demise, they constitute a *panic attack*. Some of the more prominent autonomic effects can be evoked by hyperthyroidism and hyper-adrenocorticism and, of course, by the ingestion of excessive amounts of caffeine.

All of these symptoms may seem trivial but deserve study, especially if they are persistent and distressing to the patient. Many of them are but a reaction to a major medical problem and require explanation and appropriate medical attention. More often they are identifiable as components of a chronic anxiety neurosis; sometimes they mask a depressive illness that ends in suicide. These latter conditions, which surely have a neurologic basis, are more fully described in Chaps. 56 and 57.

For a more detailed discussion of this topic, see Victor and Ropper: *Adams and Victor's Principles of Neurology*, 7th ed, pp 525–535.

ADDITIONAL READING

Cassidy WL, Flanagan NB, Spellman M, Cohen ME: Clinical observations in manic depressive disease. *JAMA* 164:1535, 1953.

Dawson DM, Sabin TD (eds): *Chronic Fatigue Syndrome*. Boston, Little, Brown, 1993.

Holmes GP, Kaplan JE, Glantz NM, et al: Chronic fatigue syndrome: A working case definition. *Ann Intern Med* 108:387, 1988.

Lader M: The nature of clinical anxiety in modern society, in Spielberger CD, Sarason IG (eds): *Stress and Anxiety*, vol 1. New York, Halsted, 1975, pp 3–26.

Snaith RP, Taylor CM: Irritability: Definition, assessment, and associated factors. *Br J Psychiatry* 147:127, 1985.

Straus S (ed): *Chronic Fatigue Syndrome*. New York, Dekker, 1994.

Swartz MN: The chronic fatigue syndrome—One entity or many? *N Engl J Med* 319:1726, 1988.

Weinberger DR: Anxiety at the frontier of molecular medicine. *N Engl J Med* 344:1247, 2001.

Wheeler EO, White PD, Reed EW, Cohen ME: Neurocirculatory asthenia (anxiety neurosis, effort syndrome, neurasthenia). *JAMA* 142:878, 1950.

25 | The Limbic Lobes and the Neurology of Emotion

In medical parlance, much license is taken with the terms *emotional problem* and *stress*, which are applied indiscriminately to states of anxiety and depression, strong reactions to distressing life events, so-called psychosomatic diseases, and many other conditions for which a ready explanation is not available. To some physicians, the terms are synonymous with *functional disorders*, the implication being that function of the brain can change without a physical basis. Our objections to this idea are set forth in the introduction to the section on psychiatric diseases.

By *emotion*, we mean a condition of the organism involving certain bodily changes (mainly visceral ones, under the control of the autonomic nervous system) in association with any of several mental states such as excitement or agitation, usually leading to an impulse to action or to a certain type of behavior. Happiness, love, hate, fear, and anger are examples of primary emotions; gloom, anxiety, and amiability are thought to represent lesser degrees of emotion. If emotion is intense, there may ensue a disturbance of intellectual functions—i.e., a measure of disorganization of ideas and actions—and a tendency toward a more automatic behavior of ungraded and stereotyped type. *Affect* refers to the outward manifestations of the emotional state, such as the associated facial expression.

The cerebral mechanisms that control the experience and expression of emotion are located in the limbic system. The latter comprises the medial parts of the temporal, frontal, and parietal lobes and their central connections with the amygdaloid nuclei, septal region, preoptic area, hypothalamus, anterior thalamus, habenula, and central midbrain tegmentum (Fig. 25-1). The peripheral effector apparatus is the autonomic nervous system and the visceral and other structures under its control.

NEUROLOGY OF EMOTIONAL DISTURBANCES

The most studied and best-known derangements of emotion are listed below. Emotional states that are associated with hallucinations and delusions are considered in Chaps. 57 and 58.

I. Disturbances of emotionality
   A. Due to perceptual abnormalities (illusions and hallucinations)
   B. Due to cognitive derangements (delusions)
II. Disinhibition of emotional expression
   A. Emotional lability
   B. Pathologic laughing and crying
III. Heightened irritability, rage reactions, and aggressivity
IV. Apathy and placidity
   A. Klüver-Bucy syndrome
   B. Other syndromes: abulia, akinetic mutism, psychomotor asthenia
V. Altered sexuality
VI. Endogenous fear, anxiety, depression, and euphoria

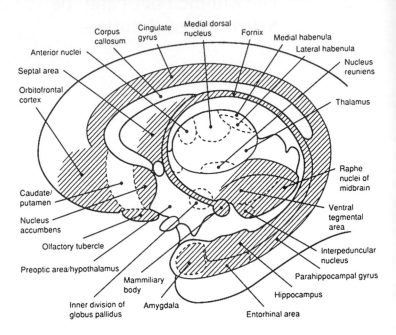

FIG. 25-1 Sagittal schematic of the limbic system. The major limbic structures and their relationship to the thalamus, hypothalamus, and midbrain tegmentum are shown. (*From Angevine and Cotman, with permission.*)

EMOTIONAL LABILITY

The emotions of the infant and child are easily provoked and little inhibited. Their control is achieved gradually, through maturation of the brain and through learning and conditioning. To be "grown up" implies an ability to inhibit one's emotions; not that there is less feeling with maturation, but rather the outward expression of it is suppressed. The acceptable display of emotion in adults varies between the sexes and in different cultures.

Any patient whose cerebrum has been damaged is prone to emotional lability. Tears come too easily; loud and prolonged laughter is evoked by mildly amusing events or remarks. A sentimental movie, meeting an old friend, or hearing the national anthem results in an embarrassing display of weeping. The response, while excessive, is more or less appropriate to the stimulus, and the affect is congruent with the visceral and motor components of emotional expression. The precise anatomic substrate is not known, except in the special case discussed below. To a lesser degree, aging alone loosens emotional control, but the condition is most prominent with diffuse degenerative and multifocal vascular lesions of the brain, which have so far not lent themselves to exact clinicoanatomic correlation.

PATHOLOGIC (FORCED, PSEUDOBULBAR) LAUGHING AND CRYING

In this state, as a consequence of cerebral disease, the patient is readily provoked to outbursts of uncontrollable laughter and, far more frequently, crying, sometimes continuing to the point of exhaustion. In general, the reaction is consonant with the stimulus situation and the feeling or affect is appropriate, although the provocative stimulus can be remarkably slight—for example, the mere mention of the patient's family or the sight of his doctor. In some patients, no relationship between stimulus, affect, and response can be discerned. Characteristic of both pathologic laughter and crying is the stereotypy of the response and its excessive nature (the expression of mild degrees of pleasure or sadness is not possible). All the facial, bulbar, and respiratory muscles, which participate in the demonstration of emotional expression and are innervated by the motor nuclei of the lower brainstem, appear to be liberated from cerebral control. The condition is often a part of *pseudobulbar* palsy due to multiple vascular, demyelinative (multiple sclerosis), or motor system disease (amyotrophic lateral sclerosis) in which corticobulbar tracts are interrupted bilaterally. However, forced laughing and crying may occasionally be observed without discernible weakness of faciobulbar muscles, and vice versa. These clinical observations suggest that the pontomedullary mechanisms involved in pseudobulbar palsy and in forced laughing and crying are under the control of two distinct supranuclear mechanisms, which may be affected separately or together.

The administration of antidepressants may lessen both spasmodic laughing and crying and the other emotionally labile states.

ANGER, AGGRESSIVITY, RAGE, AND VIOLENCE

The control of these reactions is also achieved during the processes of maturation and "civilization." Raw emotion is sublimated into socially acceptable behavior patterns. Tantrums, aggressivity, and rage are turned into competitiveness in sports, scholastic activities, and boldness in business ventures. The rate at which this developmental sequence proceeds varies from one person to another (Chap. 28). In some, especially males, the process is not complete until 25 to 30 years of age or even later; until that time, the abnormal behavior is called sociopathic or a manifestation of borderline psychiatric disorder (Chap. 57).

Persons with behavioral reactions of this type can, with little provocation, change from a calm demeanor to a state of wild rage, with blindly furious impulses to violence and destruction. They appear out of contact with reality and are impervious to all argument and pleading. What is obviously abnormal is the provocation of such behavior by some trifling event and a degree of reaction that is out of all proportion to the stimulus.

Rage reactions of this magnitude may also be encountered in the following medical settings: (1) as part of a psychomotor seizure; (2) as a transient phenomenon in acute metabolic derangements such as hypoglycemia; (3) as a manifestation of certain brain tumors or the aftermath of stroke or head injury, particularly of the temporal lobes; or (4) as a manifestation of mania or psychosis. As many as 70 percent of patients suffering severe brain injury are left in an irritable, aggressive state. Alcoholism may be an aggravating factor. The location of the lesions in the few cases in which they have been identified is shown in Fig. 25-2.

In treatment, behavior modification techniques reduce violent outbursts in as many as 75 percent of cases. When violent behavior is secondary to psychotic ideation, antipsychotic drugs are the favored treatment. Some authors have had success with propranolol and drugs of similar action.

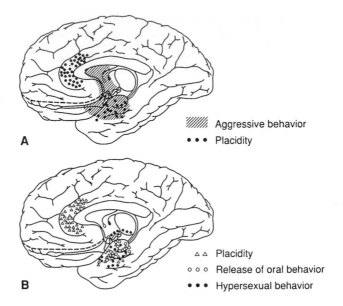

FIG. 25-2   *A.* Localization of lesions that, in humans, can lead to aggressive behavior and placidity. *B.* Localization of lesions that, in humans, can lead to placidity, release of oral behavior, and hypersexuality. (*From Poeck, with permission.*)

PLACIDITY AND APATHY

A quantitative reduction in all psychomotor activity is the most common behavioral alteration in patients with cerebral disease. There are fewer thoughts, fewer words, and fewer movements per unit of time ("psychomotor asthenia"). That this is not a pure motor deficit is disclosed in conversation with the patient, who shows a lack of ongoing psychic activity, a slowness in thinking, and a diminished perceptivity, inquisitiveness, and interest in his surroundings. Depending on one's theoretical view of this state, there is a heightened threshold to stimulation, reduced attentiveness, an inability to focus the mind and maintain an alert attitude, apathy, or a lack of drive or impulse (abulia).

By collating the data of several neurologists, Poeck charted the lesions associated with a state of placidity and apathy (Fig. 25-2).

ALTERED SEXUALITY

The normal pattern of sexual behavior may be altered with diseases of the limbic system. Lesions of the orbital parts of the frontal lobes may remove moral-ethical restraints, with indiscriminate hypersexuality. With superior prefrontal lesions, apathy and lack of impulse reduce sexual drive as well as other functions. We have observed an occasional case of marked hypersexuality in male and female patients with encephalitis and temporal lobe tumor, but the exact anatomy of the lesions could not be ascertained. Stimulation of the ventral septal area has evoked sensations of pleasure and lust, and sexual arousal has been reported with psychomotor seizures arising from medial temporal foci. Diminished libido and hyposexuality are common manifestations of depressive illness and, conversely, mania is an important cause of hypersexuality. Most persons with temporal lobe epilepsy prove to be hyposexual. Many medications, among them beta blockers and serotoninergic antidepressants, may reduce libido and sexual performance, and others, such as L-dopa, may cause hypersexuality.

ANXIETY, FEAR, AND DEPRESSION (see also Chaps. 56 and 57)

In relation to structural disease of the brain, these emotional states may occur episodically or persistently with lesions of the medial temporal lobe in the region of the amygdaloid body and its connections with the thalamus and hypothalamus. Williams observed such emotional disturbances as part of a seizure in 80 of 2000 epileptics. Fear and anxiety were three times more frequent than depression. Attacks of anger and rage have been induced by stimulation of the amygdala through depth electrodes, and destruction of the central part of this structure has allegedly abolished fear reactions. Some of the abnormal emotional effects of seizure activity can be abolished by the administration of valproate, carbamazepine, or other antiepileptic drugs (see Chap. 16).

For a more detailed discussion of this topic, see Victor and Ropper: *Adams and Victor's Principles of Neurology*, 7th ed, pp 536–549.

ADDITIONAL READING

Angevine JB Jr, Cotman CW: *Principles of Neuroanatomy*. New York, Oxford University Press, 1981, pp 253–283.

Geschwind N: The clinical setting of aggression in temporal lobe epilepsy, in Field WS, Sweet WH (eds): *The Neurobiology of Violence*. St. Louis, Warren H. Green, 1975.

Panksepp J: Mood changes, in Vinken PJ, Bruyn GW, Klawans HL (eds): *Handbook of Clinical Neurology*, vol 45. Amsterdam, North-Holland, 1985, pp 271–285.

Poeck K: Pathophysiology of emotional disorders associated with brain damage, in Vinken PJ, Bruyn GW (eds): *Handbook of Clinical Neurology*, vol 3: *Disorders of Higher Nervous Activity*. Amsterdam, North-Holland, 1969, pp 343–367.

Poeck K: Pathological laughter and crying, in Vinken PJ, Bruyn GW, Klawans HL (eds): *Handbook of Clinical Neurology*, vol 45. Amsterdam, North-Holland, 1985, pp 219–225.

Williams D: The structure of emotions reflected in epileptic experiences. *Brain* 79:29, 1956.

Disorders of the Autonomic Nervous System, Respiration, and Swallowing

The visceral and homeostatic functions of the human organism, which are essential to life and survival of the species, are involuntary and under the control of the autonomic nervous system acting in unison with the endocrine glands.

The autonomic nervous system consists of two parts: craniosacral (parasympathetic) and thoracolumbar (sympathetic). The cerebral control of these two systems resides in the hypothalamus. These features are illustrated in Figs. 26-1 and 26-2. The configuration of sympathetic fibers as they exit from the spinal cord and their distribution are illustrated in Fig. 26-3.

The diseases that affect the autonomic nervous system are summarized in this chapter, and the hypothalamic-pituitary syndromes, in Chap. 27.

TESTS FOR ABNORMALITIES OF AUTONOMIC FUNCTION

These tests are outlined in Table 26-1. The use of the simpler ones (listed in the table as noninvasive bedside tests and tests of pupillary innervation), coupled with clinical inquiry and examination, permits the diagnosis of the following disorders.

Idiopathic, or Primary, Orthostatic Hypotension

In this chronic condition there is a failure of reflex constriction of resistance and capacitance vessels in the lower extremities upon standing; as a result, there is excessive pooling of blood in large veins of the legs and pelvis, diminution of venous return and cardiac output, and the blood pressure falls precipitously, often with syncope (see Chap. 18). Corrective vasomotor reflexes are incompetent, and plasma catecholamine and renin fail to rise adequately.

Two types of primary orthostatic hypotension have been identified:

1. The first type (originally described by Bradbury and Eggleston) is believed to involve mainly the postganglionic sympathetic fibers, with sparing of the parasympathetic, somatosensory, and motor fibers. Orthostatic hypotension develops gradually, most often in middle-aged women. Cases are sporadic and the cause unknown.
2. The second type (Shy-Drager) involves mainly the preganglionic neurons that originate in the spinal cord and may develop in conjunction with or be followed by a parkinsonian syndrome due to striatonigral or olivopontocerebellar degeneration ("multiple system atrophy," as discussed in Chap. 39).

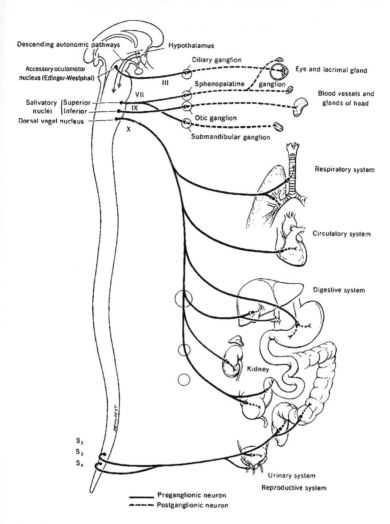

FIG. 26-1 The *parasympathetic (craniosacral)* division of the autonomic nervous system. Preganglionic fibers extend from nuclei of the brainstem and sacral segments of the spinal cord to peripheral ganglia. Short postganglionic fibers extend from ganglion cells to the effector organs. The lateral-posterior hypothalamus is part of the supranuclear mechanism for the regulation of parasympathetic activities. The frontal and limbic parts of the supranuclear regulatory apparatus are not indicated in the diagram (see text). *(From CL Noback, R Demarest, The Human Nervous System, 3rd ed, New York, McGraw-Hill, 1981, with permission.)*

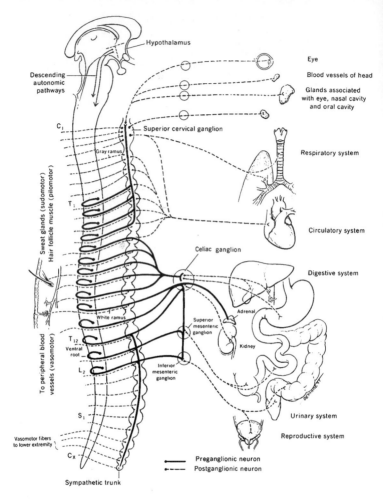

FIG. 26-2 The *sympathetic (thoracolumbar)* division of the autonomic nervous system. Preganglionic fibers extend from the intermediolateral nuclei of the spinal cord to the paraspinal autonomic ganglia (sympathetic chain), and postganglionic fibers extend from the ganglion cells to the effector organs, according to the scheme in Fig. 26-3. *(From CL Noback, R Demarest, The Human Nervous System, 3rd ed, New York, McGraw-Hill, 1981, with permission.)*

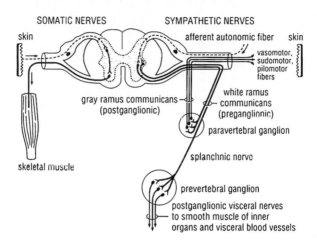

FIG. 26-3 Sympathetic outflow from the spinal cord and the course and distribution of sympathetic fibers. The preganglionic fibers are in heavy lines; postganglionic fibers are in thin lines. *(From Pick, with permission.)*

Anhidrosis, impotence, and atonicity of the bladder are common to both syndromes. Vagal paralysis with hoarseness and stridor is characteristic of the central (second) type. The two types can sometimes be distinguished pharmacologically. In the peripheral postganglionic type, resting plasma norepinephrine levels are subnormal and fail to rise on standing. In the central preganglionic type, plasma norepinephrine levels also fail to rise on standing, but resting levels are normal, as is the sensitivity to administered norepinephrine.

Treatment follows along the lines indicated in Chap. 18 (leg stockings, Florinef, Midodrine).

Secondary Orthostatic Hypotension

In clinical practice, the most common type of orthostatic hypotension is that induced by drugs (beta blockers, diuretics, central α-agonists, L-dopa, etc.). Prolonged bed rest and immobility are frequent causes of orthostasis in hospitalized and nursing home patients; there is a rise in pulse rate on assuming the upright posture. Blood loss and extreme dehydration are other common causes. In several types of polyneuropathy—diabetic, Guillain-Barré, amyloid, porphyric, toxic, alcoholic-nutritional—the autonomic fibers may be damaged, and some of the symptoms of disordered autonomic function (impotence, anhidrosis or hyperhidrosis, atonicity of the bladder, diarrhea or constipation, orthostatic hypotension) are then added to the more common neuropathic picture (see Chap. 46). In most of these polyneuropathies, affection of the vagus nerves prevents a tachycardia from compensating for the hypotension.

Table 26-1 Clinical Tests of Autonomic Function

Test	Normal response	Part of reflex arc tested
Noninvasive bedside tests		
BP response to standing or vertical tilt	Fall in BP ≤ 20/10 mmHg*	Afferent and sympathetic efferent limbs
Heart rate response to standing	Increase 11–29 beats per minute; 30:15 ratio ≥ 1.04*	Vagal afferent and efferent limbs
Isometric exercise	Increase in diastolic BP, 15 mmHg	Sympathetic efferent limb
Heart rate variation with respiration	Maximum–minimum heart rate ≥ 15 beats per minute; expiration-inspiration ratio ≥ 1.2*	Vagal afferent and efferent limbs
Sweat tests	Sweating over all body and limbs	Sympathetic efferent limb
Axon reflex	Local piloerection, sweating	Postganglionic sympathetic efferent fiber
Plasma norepinephrine level	Rises on tilting from horizontal to vertical	Sympathetic efferent limb
Plasma vasopressin level	Rise with induced hypotension	Afferent limb
Valsalva maneuver	Phase I: Rise in BP	Afferent and sympathetic efferent limbs
	Phase II: Gradual reduction of BP to plateau; tachycardia	
	Phase III: Fall in BP	
	Phase IV: Overshoot of BP, bradycardia*	
Baroreflex sensitivity	Slowing of heart rate with induced rise of BP*	Parasympathetic afferent and efferent limbs
Other tests of vasomotor control		
Radiant heating of trunk	Increased hand blood flow	Sympathetic efferent limb
Immersion of hand in hot water	Increased blood flow of opposite hand	Sympathetic efferent limb
Cold pressor test	Increased BP	Sympathetic efferent limb
Mental arithmetic	Increased BP	Sympathetic efferent limb
Tests of pupillary innervation		
4% cocaine	Pupil dilates	Sympathetic innervation
0.1% epinephrine	No response	Postganglionic sympathetic innervation
1% hydroxyamphetamine hydrobromide	Pupil dilates	Postganglionic sympathetic innervation
2.5% methacholine, 0.125% pilocarpine	No response	Parasympathetic innervation

Note: BP = blood pressure.
*Age-dependent response.
Source: Modified from McLeod and Tuck, with permission.

Pandysautonomia (Dysautonomic Polyneuropathy)

This is a relatively rare but instructive type of acute or subacute polyneuropathy characterized by the almost exclusive involvement of sympathetic and parasympathetic postganglionic fibers. The disease occurs sporadically in adults and children and is thought to represent an autoimmune or postinfectious disorder, similar to the Guillain-Barré syndrome. In a few cases it has been linked in some way to the Epstein-Barr virus or to HIV and rarely to an underlying neoplasm (paraneoplastic dysautonomia).

Over a period of a week or a few weeks, the patient develops orthostatic hypotension, an invariant pulse rate, paralysis of pupillary reflexes, anhidrosis, impaired bladder and bowel function, gastric anacidity and hypomotility (ileus and constipation), and loss of lacrimation, salivation, and pilomotor and vasomotor reflexes in the skin. Somatic sensory and motor functions and tendon reflexes are generally preserved, but some patients complain of acral paresthesias or pain. The entire syndrome may be a part of an otherwise typical case of Guillain-Barré polyneuropathy or may have some shared features, such as areflexia or distal sensory loss. The CSF protein is normal or elevated. Slow recovery is the rule.

Riley-Day Syndrome

This is a familial disease of the autonomic nervous system, inherited as an autosomal recessive trait and observed mainly in Jewish infants and children. Postural hypotension, impaired temperature regulation, hyperhidrosis, insensitivity to pain, cyclic vomiting, and denervation hypersensitivity of the pupils are the main clinical features. This disorder is described further in Chap. 46, with the inherited neuropathies.

PARTIAL OR RESTRICTED AUTONOMIC SYNDROMES

Horner and Stellate Ganglion Syndromes

The features of the Horner (Bernard-Horner) syndrome are listed in Table 14-2. The cardinal signs are unilateral ptosis, miosis, and impaired pupillary dilation in the dark. Depending on the site of the lesion, there may be unilateral facial anhidrosis. The lesion may occur at any of the following sites: descending sympathetic pathways in the lateral medullary tegmentum, the cervical spinal cord (see below), the T2 spinal root, the superior cervical ganglion, or the postganglionic fibers that course along the carotid artery. In most series approximately two-thirds of cases are due to brainstem strokes or other brainstem lesions. About 20 percent are preganglionic, due to trauma or tumors of the neck and upper thorax or to carotid dissection, and a lesser number are postganglionic, due to a variety of causes (see Table 14-2).

A lesion of the inferior cervical (stellate) ganglion produces a Horner syndrome in combination with a paralysis of sympathetic reflexes in the arm (hand and arm are dry and warm)—*the stellate ganglion syndrome.* The latter may involve the preganglionic fibers or the ganglion cells. If the ganglion cells and their postganglionic extensions are mainly affected, denervation hypersensitivity to norepinephrine can be demonstrated. The usual causes are trauma, metastatic tumor, radiation injury, and subclavian aneurysm.

Sympathetic and Parasympathetic Paralysis in Tetraplegia and Paraplegia

A complete spinal cord lesion at the level of C4 or C5 or uppermost thoracic segments of the spinal cord, in addition to abolishing all sensorimotor function below the lesion, interrupts all suprasegmental control mechanisms of the spinal sympathetic and sacral parasympathetic nervous system. (Lesions of the lower thoracic cord spare the descending sympathetic pathways to a large extent but interrupt the descending parasympathetic ones.) Hypotension that is accentuated by standing, loss of sweating and piloerection, gastric dilatation, paralytic ileus, and paralysis of bladder function are the initial effects. Plasma epinephrine and norepinephrine are reduced. This state has a time course similar to that of spinal shock: it subsides in a few weeks and is followed in some instances by hyperactivity of autonomic reflexes and automatic bladder function (see Chap. 44).

Disturbances of Bladder and Bowel Function

The storage and intermittent evacuation of urine are served by three components of the bladder: the large detrusor muscle, which forms the viscus; the functionally related internal sphincter, which is formed by the inner layer of the muscular coat around the internal opening of the urethra; and the external sphincter, which is composed of striated muscle (as is the external anal sphincter). Afferent and efferent innervation of these structures is provided through the pudendal nerves and sacral segments 2, 3, and 4. These segments give rise to preganglionic fibers, which synapse in the parasympathetic ganglia in the bladder wall. The hypogastric plexus, derived from T10, T11, and T12 segments, supplies sympathetic nerves to the dome of the bladder. The innervation of the bladder and its sphincters is illustrated in Fig. 26-4.

Suprasegmental control of the sacral segments comes from the pontomesencephalic tegmentum via reticulospinal tracts, which are both facilitatory and inhibitory, and from the medial frontal motor cortex via tracts that descend in apposition to the corticospinal tracts and are inhibitory.

Acute lesions of the spinal cord at levels above the sacral segments cause spinal shock, inhibiting detrusor function and resulting in urinary retention with overflow incontinence. As spasticity of the legs gradually supervenes, the detrusor also becomes "spastic" (overactive); the detrusor cannot be inhibited, and the patient is intermittently incontinent as the bladder empties automatically. *Deafferentation* of the bladder (as in diabetic autonomic neuropathy and tabes dorsalis) leaves it insensitive and hypotonic; the bladder distends and there is overflow incontinence. *Lower motor neuron lesions* (as in meningomyelocele) produce the same effects, except that bladder sensation may be intact. *Frontal lobe lesions*, particularly if bilateral, cause incontinence by decreasing voluntary inhibitory control; mental confusion is often an additional factor.

Disturbances of the colon and anal sphincters obey the same general principles as disturbances of bladder function.

Disturbances of Sexual Function

Sexual function in the male can be divided into several parts: (1) sexual impulse, drive, or desire (libido); (2) the ability to obtain and sustain penile

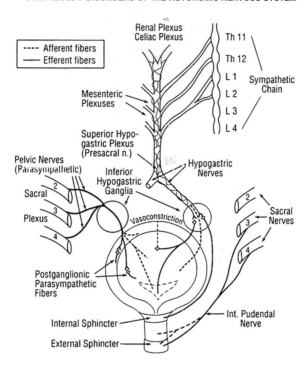

FIG. 26-4   Innervation of the urinary bladder and its sphincters.

erection, enabling the act of sexual intercourse (potency); and (3) ejaculation of semen (orgasm). Libido, receptive postures and secretory changes, and orgasm are corresponding functions in the female.

The reflex centers for these sexual functions reside in spinal sacral segments 3 and 4. There is also a sympathetic outflow from T12 and L1.

Sexual function may be affected in different ways. Loss of libido is the most complex and depends on both psychic and physical factors. It may become complete in old age and in a number of medical and endocrine diseases and is subject to alteration by certain medications. The inability to obtain or sustain an erection (impotence) while nocturnal erections during rapid-eye-movement (REM) sleep are preserved is commonly due to depression, drugs, or other psychologic factors. Diseases of the spinal cord may abolish psychic erections but leave reflex ones intact; in fact, the latter may be overactive and painful (priapism). Destructive lesions of the sacral segments and nerves (nervi erigentes and pudendal nerves) may abolish all genital sensation and response.

Loss of libido and inability to attain orgasm are more frequent in women than in men. Fecundity and fertility are usually unrelated to the other aspects of sexuality.

DISORDERS OF RESPIRATION

The respiratory rhythm in human beings is generated and maintained throughout life by three paired aggregates of neurons that are located in the tegmentum of the pons and medulla. The neuronal aggregates in the rostral ventrolateral medulla illustrated in Fig. 26-5 are of particular importance in the control of breathing. A dorsal respiratory group (DRG) containing mainly inspiratory neurons is located in the ventrolateral subnucleus of the nucleus of the tractus solitarius. A ventral respiratory group (VRG) is situated near the nucleus ambiguus and contains, in its caudal part, neurons that fire predominantly during expiration and, in its rostral part, neurons that fire synchronously with inspiration. The latter structure merges rostrally with the Botzinger complex, which is located just behind the facial nucleus and is active mostly during expiration. The pons contains a pair of nuclei (PRG), one of which fires in the transition between inspiration and expiration and the other between expiration and inspiration. The intrinsic rhythmicity of the entire system probably depends on interactions between all these regions, but the "pre-Botzinger" area in the rostral ventromedial medulla is believed to play a special role in generating the respiratory rhythm.

The voluntary act of breathing is governed by descending pathways from the motor and premotor cortex. During speech, breath-holding, or voluntary hyperventilation, the automaticity of the brainstem mechanisms of respiration is momentarily arrested to permit the conscious control of the diaphragm. When the descending tracts are interrupted, as in the "locked-in syndrome," the automatic respiratory system in the medulla is still capable of maintaining independent breathing at approximately 16 per minute, with uniform tidal volumes.

Respiratory drive is modulated by chemoreceptors in the carotid body and ascending aorta; the former are influenced by changes in pH, and the latter more by hypoxia. Chemoreceptor afferents from these structures course in the glossopharyngeal and vagus nerves and terminate in the nuclei of the tractus solitarius.

Aberrant Respiratory Patterns

These are observed mainly in comatose patients and have only an approximate value in localization (the main patterns are *central neurogenic hyperventilation*, *apneusis*, *ataxic breathing*; see Chaps. 17 and 19). *Cheyne-Stokes breathing*, the well-known waxing-and-waning type of cyclic ventilation, occurs most often with deep, bilateral hemispheral lesions. Centrally driven hyperventilation, which is seen on occasion with pontine lesions, has also been seen with brain lymphoma even without involvement of the brainstem.

A loss of automatic respiration during sleep with preserved voluntary breathing goes by the name of *Ondine's curse*. Patients with this disorder must have nighttime mechanical ventilation to survive. Selective interruption of the descending ventrolateral medullocervical pathways is the presumed pathologic basis, caused most often by brainstem infarction or hemorrhage. By contrast, lesions that cause *hyperventilation* are located widely in the brain, not only in the brainstem. *Persistent hiccup* (singultus) occurs as part of the lateral medullary syndrome or other medullary lesion or with metabolic encephalopathies, such as uremia, but it is most often an idiopathic and self-limited upper gastric reflex. Of the multitude of suggested remedies for hiccup, none has proved consistently effective.

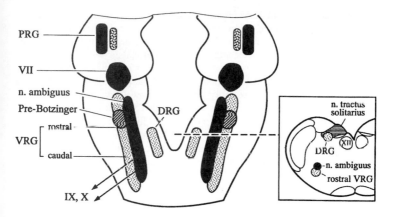

FIG. 26-5 The location of the main centers of respiratory control in the brainstem as currently envisioned from animal experiments and limited human pathology. See text for details. *(Adapted from Duffin et al.)*

Neuromuscular Diseases Affecting Ventilation

These diseases involve the respiratory nerves (phrenic and spinal), the neuromuscular junction at the diaphragm, or the muscles of respiration themselves. Respiratory failure is of overriding importance in diseases such as Guillain-Barré polyneuropathy, poliomyelitis, myasthenia gravis, motor neuron disease, and muscular dystrophy; often the main problem in the treatment of such patients is respiratory intensive care. The earliest indication of these neuromuscular diseases is at times the subacute onset of respiratory failure manifest by dyspnea and exercise intolerance. Motor neuron disease, myasthenia gravis, acid maltase deficiency, polymyositis, and Lambert-Eaton syndrome are the ones most likely to begin in this way, before there is manifest weakness in other regions. There are also instances of isolated unilateral or bilateral *phrenic nerve paresis* following surgery or an infectious illness. One type may be akin to brachial neuritis (Parsonage-Turner syndrome, Chap. 46).

DISORDERS OF SWALLOWING

The act of swallowing, like breathing, continues periodically through waking and sleeping, largely without conscious will or awareness. Swallowing occurs at a natural frequency of about five to six times per minute while an individual is idle and is suppressed during concentration and emotional excitement. Since the oropharynx is a shared conduit for breathing and swallowing, obligatory reflexes exist to assure that breathing is held in abeyance during swallowing. Because of this relationship and the frequency with which dysphagia and aspiration complicate neurologic disease, the neural mechanisms that underlie swallowing are of considerable importance.

A highly coordinated sequence of muscle contractions moves a bolus of food safely through the oropharynx. This programmed activity may be initiated voluntarily or reflexively. Swallowing begins as the tongue (cranial nerve XII) sweeps food to the posterior oral cavity and brings the bolus into contact with the posterior wall of the oropharynx. Tactile sensation carried through nerves IX and X triggers the contraction of numerous pharyngeal muscles, most innervated by nerve X, that propel the bolus and close the tracheal opening. At the same time, the upward movement of the larynx opens the cricopharyngeal sphincter and a wave of peristalsis begins in the pharynx, which pushes the bolus through the sphincter into the esophagus.

This tightly controlled sequence of muscle activity is organized in a region of the medulla that roughly comprises a swallowing center, located in the region of the nucleus tractus solitarius (NTS), and the adjacent reticular formation close to the respiratory centers. This juxtaposition ostensibly allows the refined coordination of swallowing with the cycle of breathing. Reflex swallowing requires only medullary functioning and occurs in the vegetative and locked-in states. As to the cortical regions involved in swallowing, it appears that the inferior precentral and the posterior inferior frontal gyri are active and lesions in these parts of the brain give rise to the most profound degree of dysphagia.

Dysphagia and Aspiration Weakness or incoordination of swallowing is manifest as dysphagia and aspiration. The patient is often able to discriminate one of several defects: (1) difficulty initiating swallowing, which leaves solids stuck in the oropharynx; (2) nasal regurgitation of liquids; (3) coughing and choking immediately after swallowing and a hoarse, "wet cough" following the ingestion of fluids; and (4) some combination of these. Difficulties with swallowing may begin subtly and express themselves as weight loss or as a noticeable increase in the time required to swallow. Nodding or sideways head movements to assist the propulsion of the bolus or the need to repeatedly wash food down with water are other clues to the presence of dysphagia. It should be noted that the tongue and the muscles that cause palatal elevation may appear to act normally on direct examination despite an obvious failure of coordinated swallowing. For this reason, the gag reflex has been inconsistently useful as a neurologic sign. Palatal elevation in response to touching the posterior pharynx only assures that cranial nerves IX and X and the related musculature are not paralyzed; however, the presence of the reflex does not assure smooth coordination of the act of swallowing.

The first type of swallowing defect is usually attributable to weakness of the tongue and may be a manifestation of myasthenia gravis, motor neuron disease, inflammatory muscle diseases, palsies of the 12th cranial nerve (metastases at the base of the skull or meningoradiculitis), and a number of other causes. There is usually an associated dysarthria with difficulty pronouncing lingual sounds. Nasal regurgitation of liquids indicates a failure of velopalatine closure and is characteristic of myasthenia gravis, 10th nerve palsy of any cause, or incoordination of swallowing due to bulbar or pseudobulbar palsy. A nasal pattern of speech with air escaping from the nose is a common accompaniment.

The symptoms of aspiration, such as choking, or of recurrent unexplained pneumonias ("silent aspiration"), have myriad causes that fall into three main categories: (1) weakness of the musculature due to lesions of the vagus on one or both sides, a myopathy (myotonic and oculopharyngeal dystrophies), or neuromuscular disease [amyotrophic lateral sclerosis (ALS) and myasthenia gravis are the common ones]; (2) a medullary lesion that affects the NTS or the cranial motor nuclei (lateral medullary infarction is the prototype, but also syringomyelia-syringobulbia and less often multiple sclerosis, polio, and brainstem tumors); and (3) a less well defined mechanism of dyscoordinated swallowing that arises either from corticospinal disease (pseudobulbar palsy, hemispheral stroke) or from diseases of the basal ganglia (mainly Parkinson disease); these alter the timing of breathing-swallowing and permit the airway to remain open as food passes through the posterior pharynx. In the parkinsonian syndromes, a decreased frequency of swallowing causes saliva to pool in the mouth (leading to drooling) and adds to the risk of aspiration. Aspiration and swallowing difficulty also occur in a surprisingly large number of patients after stroke. These effects last for 1 or 2 weeks and render the patient subject to pneumonia and fever even if only saliva is aspirated.

Videofluoroscopy is useful in demonstrating the presence of aspiration during swallowing and in differentiating the several clinical types of dysphagia. However, observation of the patient swallowing water and while eating can be equally informative. Swallowing water is a particularly effective test of laryngeal closure; the presence of coughing, wet hoarseness or breathlessness, or the need to swallow small volumes slowly is indicative of a high risk of aspiration. Based on bedside observations and videofluoroscopy, an experienced therapist can make recommendations regarding the safety of oral feeding, the appropriate consistency and texture of the diet, postural adjustments, and the need to insert a tracheostomy or feeding tube.

For a more detailed discussion of this topic, see Victor and Ropper: *Adams and Victor's Principles of Neurology*, 7th ed, pp 550–585.

ADDITIONAL READING

Bannister R, Mathias CJ (eds): *Autonomic Failure: A Textbook of Clinical Disorders of the Autonomic Nervous System*, 3rd ed. New York, Oxford University Press, 1992.

Blaivas JG: The neurophysiology of micturition: A clinical study of 550 patients. *J Urol* 127:958, 1982.

Bradbury S, Eggleston C: Postural hypotension: A report of three cases. *Am Heart J* 1:73, 1925.

Cohen J, Low P, Fealey R, et al: Somatic and autonomic function in progressive autonomic failure and multiple system atrophy. *Ann Neurol* 22:692, 1987.

Cohen MI: Neurogenesis of respiratory rhythm in the mammal. *Physiol Rev* 59:1105, 1979.

Duffin J, Kazuhisa E, Lipski J: Breathing rhythm generation: Focus on the rostral ventrolateral medulla. *News Physiol Sci* 10:113, 1995.

Hughes TA, Wiles CM: Neurogenic dysphagia: The role of the neurologist. *J Neurol Neurosurg Psychiatry* 64:569, 1998.

Keane JR: Oculosympathetic paresis: Analysis of 100 hospitalized patients. *Arch Neurol* 36:13, 1979.

Low PA (ed): *Clinical Autonomic Disorders: Evaluation and Management*, 2nd ed. Philadelphia, Lippincott-Raven, 1997.

McLeod JG, Tuck RR: Disorders of the autonomic nervous system. Part I: Pathophysiology and clinical features. Part II: Investigation and treatment. *Ann Neurol* 21:419, 519, 1987.

Newsom Davis J: An experimental study of hiccup. *Brain* 39:851, 1970.

Pick J: *The Autonomic Nervous System*. Philadelphia, Lippincott, 1970.

Young RR, Asbury AK, Corbett JL, Adams RD: Pure pandysautonomia with recovery: Description and discussion of diagnostic criteria. *Brain* 98:613, 1975.

27 | The Hypothalamus and Neuroendocrine Disorders

The hypothalamus serves as the "head ganglion" of both the autonomic nervous system and the endocrine system. The two are closely integrated and abundantly connected to the entire limbic brain.

The hypothalamic nuclei, by synthesizing and releasing specific neurotransmitter peptides, control the activities of the secretory cells of the anterior lobe of the pituitary body. Additionally, hormones secreted by cells of the supraoptic and paraventricular nuclei are transported, in the form of granules, to the posterior lobe of the pituitary; from there they are absorbed into the bloodstream. Also, there are nuclear aggregates in the hypothalamus that regulate appetite, body temperature, and sleep. Following the discovery of oxytocin and vasopressin, secreted in the anterior hypothalamus and transported to the posterior lobe of the pituitary, a number of specific hypophysiotropic peptide substances, called "releasing factors," were isolated for growth hormone (GRH), thyrotropin (TRH), corticotropin (CRF), prolactin (PRF), and luteinizing hormone, or gonadotropin (LHRH, or GnRH). Each is elaborated by a particular group of neurons and is carried by venules to the anterior pituitary, where it activates specific cellular groups. For growth hormone and prolactin there are also release-inhibiting factors elaborated by the hypothalamus; in the case of prolactin, the inhibitor is dopamine.

Under conditions of disease, the neurotransmitter peptides may be quantitatively increased, decreased, or in some way made defective; the neurons that synthesize these peptides or their glandular targets may fail to function or become overactive. Thus, with respect to these neuroendocrine symptoms or syndromes, one may have difficulty in deciding whether the lesion is in the pituitary gland or hypothalamus. However, there are often derangements of other functions, unique to the hypothalamus or the pituitary, that help resolve this clinical problem.

The nuclei of the hypothalamus are conventionally divided into three paired groups: the anterior group, including the preoptic, supraoptic, and paraventricular nuclei, which are mainly *neurohypophysial* in their relationships; the middle group, including the tuberal, arcuate, ventrolateral, and dorsomedial nuclei; and the posterior group, including the mammillary and posterior nuclei. The anatomic relationships of these small aggregates of cells, which lie between the thalamus and optic chiasm, are illustrated in Fig. 27-1. The cells that regulate the *anterior lobe of the pituitary* are clustered around the median eminence, or infundibulum, and are in contact with the hypophysial portal veins. The infundibulum extends into the pituitary stalk, which contains the axons of the anterior hypothalamic nuclei en route

HYPOTHALAMIC-NEUROHYPOPHYSIAL
SYSTEM

HYPOTHALAMIC-ADENOHYPOPHYSIAL
SYSTEM

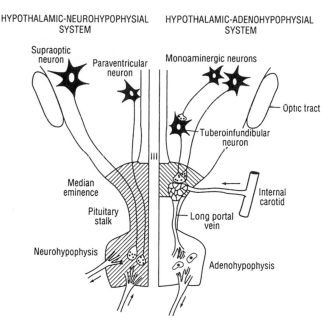

FIG. 27-1   Diagram of the hypothalamic-pituitary axis. Indicated on the left is the hypothalamic-neurohypophysial system, consisting of supraoptic and paraventricular neurons, axons of which terminate on blood vessels in the posterior pituitary (neurohypophysis). The hypothalamic-adenohypophysial system is illustrated on the right. Tuberoinfundibular neurons, believed to be the source of the hypothalamic regulatory hormones (releasing factors), terminate on the capillary plexus in the median eminence. *(Courtesy of Dr. JB Martin.)*

to the neurohypophysis. The highly vascular stalk joins the medial-basal hypothalamus and the *pituitary body*, or *hypophysis*.

As mentioned above, the hypophysis is divided into two lobes: (1) the anterior, or *adenohypophysis*, which is derived from the buccal endoderm (Rathke's pouch), and (2) the posterior, or *neurohypophysis*, which forms as a diverticulum from the base of the hypothalamus. There are no recognizable neurons in the posterior lobe of the pituitary, only a matrix of specialized glia. The glandular cells of the anterior pituitary were formerly classified as acidophil, basophil, and chromophobe on the basis of their staining qualities. Now they are classified by specific markers for the precursors of the hormones that they form. Asa and Kovacs have identified seven cell types, each of which may form an adenoma. For details of the histology of these structures, the reader is referred to the monograph of Martin and Reichlin.

The following is a brief description of (1) neurohypophysial diseases, (2) adenohypophysial diseases, and (3) other mixed hypothalamoendocrine and nonendocrine hypothalamic disorders.

NEUROHYPOPHYSIAL DISEASES

Diabetes Insipidus

Diabetes insipidus (DI), the best known of the hypothalamic syndromes, is characterized by polyuria (the excretion of large quantities of urine) and polydipsia (increased thirst and drinking of water). Greatly increased serum sodium and osmolality result from the urinary loss of water and lack of its replacement. DI is caused by lesions that prevent granules of *vasopressin* (antidiuretic hormone, or ADH), which are formed in the cells of the supraoptic and paraventricular nuclei, from being transported and released into the posterior lobe of the pituitary body, from which they are normally transferred into the bloodstream and carried to the renal tubules. The renal tubule cells control the amount of water that is excreted, and a congenital abnormality or destruction of the tubular cells (nephrogenic DI) has the same effect as a hypothalamic lesion. The cells of these hypothalamic nuclei also elaborate *oxytocin*, the principal hormonal stimulant to lactation and uterine contraction.

The diagnosis of DI is suggested by the presence of dilute polyuria (urine specific gravity <1.005 even under conditions of fluid restriction) and polydipsia (drinking >3000 mL of fluid daily). Proof that the patient has DI and is not a compulsive water drinker is obtained by observing the patient under controlled conditions of water deprivation and documenting a progressive polyuria and hypernatremia or by the injection of 2 µg of desmopressin (an ADH analogue) subcutaneously, which will diminish urine output and decrease the osmolality of blood.

As to the causes of DI, a small number of cases are congenital or familial, existing for a lifetime; both central and renal forms are known. Others are traceable to cerebral metastases, neurosurgery, head trauma, Hand-Schüller-Christian disease, and granulomatous lesions (e.g., sarcoid), all involving the hypothalamus. In 25 percent of cases of DI, or more, no cause is found; an autoimmune destruction of hypothalamic cells has been suggested. In neurologic practice, nephrogenic DI is seen with the use of lithium and with polycystic kidney disease (associated with cerebral aneurysms). DI can be corrected by the administration of a long-acting vasopressin compound such as desmopressin given subcutaneously or intramuscularly (2 to 4 µg every 12 h) or intranasally (10 to 20 µg daily). Polydipsia may occasionally be psychogenic (compulsion to drink water), and polyuria has many causes, including diabetes mellitus.

Hypodipsia or adipsia, much less common than polydipsia, may result from lesions of the lateral hypothalamus. It leads to marked hyperosmolality and hypernatremia.

Syndrome of Inappropriate ADH Secretion (SIADH)

The maintenance of blood volume and osmolality, which is the normal function of the antidiuretic hormone (ADH), may also be deranged by neurologic disease. The normal serum osmolality is 280 mosmol/L ± 1.8. A rise above 287 mosmol/L stimulates the osmoreceptors in the hypothalamus to secrete more ADH; lowering osmolality below 273 mosmol/L suppresses ADH secretion. The thirst mechanism is likewise stimulated or inhibited by changes in osmolality.

This delicate mechanism becomes unbalanced in a number of clinical circumstances. When there is "inappropriate secretion" or ectopic production of ADH, blood volume rises and serum osmolality falls, accompanied by a fall in serum sodium levels. If the level falls below approximately 120 meq/L, hyponatremia poses a danger and should be corrected—but cautiously (see Chap. 40). The rapidity of development of hyponatremia as well as the absolute serum sodium level determine the likelihood of the patient developing convulsions and encephalopathy. The diagnosis of SIADH is supported by a disproportionately concentrated urine in the face of hyponatremia for which no other cause is found. Merely reducing water intake to 400 to 600 mL/day is usually sufficient to counteract milder degrees of hyponatremia. The usual causes are lung tumors (ectopic ADH production), nontumorous pulmonary diseases, positive-pressure ventilation, certain drugs (carbamazepine, chlorothiazide, chlorpromazine, meperidine, vincristine), and a variety of acute intracranial diseases (e.g., subarachnoid hemorrhage, meningitis)—not necessarily ones that affect the hypothalamus directly; the Guillain-Barré syndrome is an occasional cause.

Cerebral Salt Wasting

A salt-wasting syndrome that may be mistaken for SIADH causes a reduction in serum sodium *and* in plasma volume. It may occur with a number of different intracranial diseases. An increased secretion of atrial natriuretic factors (peptides that were first identified in the cardiac atria but are also present in the brain) promotes diuresis and sodium excretion and may be responsible for this derangement. It occurs most often as a transient feature of subarachnoid hemorrhage or head injury. The distinction of a salt-wasting syndrome from SIADH is important, because treatment consists of the administration of intravenous fluid and sodium rather than fluid restriction.

ADENOHYPOPHYSIAL DISEASES

Panhypopituitarism (Simmonds Disease)

This is among the most frequent adenohypophysial syndromes; it comprises multiple glandular deficiencies. Most of the patients have a nonsecretory or a prolactin-secreting pituitary adenoma. Lying within the sella turcica, the adenoma compresses normal glandular tissue, destroying many of the cells and diminishing the function of others. The resultant endocrine failures, in order of their usual appearance, are those of growth hormone, ACTH, TSH, and FSH-LH. A combination of hypothyroidism, adrenal insufficiency, and gonadal failure is therefore the most frequent clinical presentation, but earlier there may be a failure of only one endocrine function. The tumor may greatly enlarge the sella and extend upward, pressing against the optic chiasm and optic nerves.

A prolactin-secreting adenoma in a woman is expressed by irregular menses or amenorrhea, infertility, and galactorrhea. The mechanism in most cases is a disinhibition of prolactin-secreting cells by compression of dopamine pathways in the pituitary stalk. In girls, puberty may be prevented or delayed. In men, there is loss of libido and impotence. Headache is variable. The diagnosis is confirmed by the finding of a serum prolactin level greater than 200 ng/mL (normal <5). Bromocriptine, a dopamine analogue, suppresses the tumor activity and reduces the prolactin level. A number of drugs may indirectly raise the prolactin level, but usually to <100. The main features of the various types of pituitary adenomas are summarized in Table 31-4 (p. 265) and further on in this chapter.

Another cause of hypopituitarism is infarction of the pituitary during parturition (Sheehan syndrome). Symptoms occur only if the destruction exceeds 70 percent. It may leave an "empty sella," but there are also other causes of the latter. Involution of an adenoma, other tumors (including metastases), aneurysms, granulomas, and Hand-Schüller-Christian disease are documented causes of pituitary insufficiency.

A distressing and dangerous complication of large tumors is *pituitary apoplexy*. The tumor appears to outgrow its blood supply and becomes hemorrhagic and necrotic, giving rise to acute hypothalamic, pituitary, and visual symptoms and changes in the cerebrospinal fluid.

Abnormalities of Growth

A deficiency of growth hormone releasing factor (GRH) and therefore of GH may cause *growth retardation*. Or it may be caused by an inherently inactive GH molecule, in which case plasma levels of GH are actually high, as in some forms of dwarfism. Growth retardation may occur as a separate entity or in association with other hypothalamic defects (e.g., Froelich syndrome). The opposite condition—*gigantism*—may occur if an excess of GH is produced before closure of the epiphyses.

Acromegaly Hypersecretion of GH after epiphyseal closure results in *acromegaly*. These disorders are usually related to pituitary adenomas or, very rarely, to a hypothalamic gangliocytoma. This leads to enlargement of hands, feet, jaws, cranium, and viscera. Headache is frequent and in some instances severe. Hypertension, menstrual irregularities, diabetes mellitus, muscle weakness, and hypotonia are other symptoms. GH levels are increased and may be combined with hyperprolactinemia.

Cushing Disease and Cushing Syndrome

The clinical features of *Cushing disease*, described in Cushing's classic monograph, are familiar to everyone in medicine: truncal obesity, with reddish-purple cutaneous striae, hypertension, rounded plethoric facies, acne, hirsutism, easy bruising, osteoporosis, menstrual irregularity, proximal leg and hip weakness, and psychiatric symptoms. Cushing's cases were due to basophilic pituitary adenomas, which seldom enlarged the sella. Adrenal tumors, ectopic ACTH production by carcinoma of the lung, and corticosteroid therapy, more appropriately referred to as *Cushing syndrome*, duplicate the clinical picture. Cortisol concentrations in the blood are elevated in Cushing disease and in the syndrome. Some patients, after the removal of an adrenal tumor, develop a persistent elevation of ACTH and become diffusely hyperpigmented (*Nelson syndrome*).

Transsphenoidal surgery is the usual approach for the treatment of intrasellar tumors. An alternative is one form or another of stereotactic radiosurgery, provided that vision is not threatened. Tumors that expand beyond the sella are more difficult. Intracranial surgery and radiation are then usually required. The endocrine deficiencies need to be replaced.

Pituitary tumors are considered further in Chap. 31.

OTHER HYPOTHALAMIC SYNDROMES

Precocious Puberty

This disorder in males or females always prompts a neurologic and endocrinologic investigation. In males, the most frequent cause is a teratoma of the pineal gland (Chap. 31). In females, one should suspect an ovarian estrogen-secreting tumor or hypothalamic hamartoma (a tumor-like collection of cells due to a developmental abnormality). The latter is often associated with neurofibromatosis or polyostotic fibrous dysplasia. Diagnosis is greatly facilitated by magnetic resonance imaging.

Adiposogenital Dystrophy (Froelich Syndrome)

This consists of obesity, growth retardation, and delayed sexual development. The nuclei in the medial part of the hypothalamus (tuberal nuclei) fail to stimulate the production of GH and FSH in the adenohypophysis. A profound apathy may be added. The usual causes are craniopharyngioma (suprasellar cyst), pituitary adenoma, cholesteatoma, and sometimes other rare tumors.

Disturbances in Regulation of Temperature, Appetite, and Sleep

Lesions of the posterior part of the hypothalamus result in hypothermia or poikilothermia and those of the anterior hypothalamus, in severe hyperthermia. The hypothalamus also plays an important role in the regulation of appetite. However, only seldom is hyperphagia and extreme obesity related to lesions of satiety centers in the medial part of the hypothalamus, or aphagia and inanition to lesions in the lateral hypothalamus.

Sleep disturbances, usually hypersomnia, can sometimes be traced to lesions at the junction of the posterior hypothalamus and the midbrain.

The Pineal Gland and Melatonin

The pineal gland, or pineal body, is a small glandular structure that projects from the dorsal diencephalon and lies just posterior to the third ventricle. The identification of the pineal hormone melatonin (by Lerner in the 1950s)—along with the recognition of its role in maintaining biologic rhythms and the modulating effects on its secretion by the circadian light/dark cycle—revived scientific interest in the gland. Ablation of the pineal in humans, with the loss of most of the circulating melatonin, leads to few clinical changes, even though the hormone has an indirect effect on several other neuroendocrine systems.

In humans, the pineal has no direct ability to transduce light, as it does in amphibians. Nonetheless, it receives input from the retina through a pathway that traverses the suprachiasmatic nucleus, the descending sympathetic tracts, and superior cervical ganglion cells and their noradrenergic terminals on the pinealocytes.

Although arginine vasopressin (ADH), and other peptides in smaller amounts are found in the pineal, the main product of pinealocytes is melatonin—an indoleamine derived from serotonin. The secretion of this hormone is cyclic, under hypothalamic control. Decreased serum melatonin concentration has been found in some cases of depression and the hormone may be active in the modulation of the hypothalamic-gonadal axis, but not in an obligatory manner. Pineal tumors do not secrete melatonin, but the loss of serum melatonin may be used as a marker for the completeness of surgical excision of the gland. Most interest in the past several years has centered around melatonin as a therapeutic soporific agent, its role in late-life depression, and its potential to reset sleep rhythms.

For a more detailed discussion of this topic, see Victor and Ropper: *Adams and Victor's Principles of Neurology*, 7th ed, pp 586–601.

ADDITIONAL READING

Asa SL, Kovacs K: Histological classification of pituitary disease. *Clin Endocrinol Metab* 12:567, 1983.

Breningstall GN: Gelastic seizures, precocious puberty and hypothalamic hamartoma. *Neurology* 35:1180, 1985.

Lamberts SWJ, deHerder WW, van der Lely AJ: Pituitary insufficiency. *Lancet* 352:127, 1998.

Martin JB, Reichlin S: *Clinical Neuroendocrinology*, 2nd ed. Philadelphia, Davis, 1987.

Orth DN: Cushing's syndrome. *N Engl J Med* 332:791, 1995.

Reichlin S: Neuroendocrinology, in Wilson JD, Foster DW, Kronenberg HM, Larsen PR (eds): *Williams Textbook of Endocrinology*, 9th ed. Philadelphia, Saunders, 1998, pp 165–248.

PART III | GROWTH AND DEVELOPMENT OF THE NERVOUS SYSTEM AND THE NEUROLOGY OF AGING

28 | Development of the Nervous System

Disease must always be judged by comparing the patient's condition with standards of normality. Only when a given function falls outside the range of natural individual variation does it become pathologic. This poses a problem for the neurologist because, at each period until adulthood, as development and maturation of the nervous system proceed, the standards change. These changes are most marked during embryonic and fetal life, but they continue at a rapid rate during infancy and early childhood and are not completed until late adolescence. Senescence—the process of growing old— proceeds for an even longer period provided that it is not interrupted by disease. Thus, for more than half the average life span, the standards of normal neurologic functioning are in inclination or declination. What is normal at one age is abnormal at another.

In order to evaluate the status of the nervous system intelligently, the neurologist must be familiar with the normal standards of nervous system functioning for each epoch of life. This is especially difficult in infancy and early childhood. Indeed, in these age periods, failures in attaining certain milestones of motility, language, and general behavior are far more useful indicators than the conventional signs of neurologic disease. Also, age is a factor in determining the incidence of a disease; the neurologist must know which diseases are more likely to appear at any given age.

NORMAL AND ABNORMAL DEVELOPMENT OF THE NERVOUS SYSTEM

In the normal neonatal, infantile, and childhood periods (as defined in Table 28-1), neurologic functions emerge in a reasonably predictable sequence. By examining large numbers of normal infants, pediatric neurologists and psychologists have been able to construct a developmental timetable with due allowances for individual variations. By comparing the patient's age at the time of attainment of certain behaviors with the standard performance at a given chronological age, one can derive a developmental quotient. Of course, due allowance must be made for the effects of intercurrent illness and social neglect. The main milestones are itemized in Tables 28-2 and 28-3.

Exogenous and endogenous agents may exert their adverse effects on the nervous system long before birth. One can judge the time of their occurrence and to some extent the nature of the intrauterine diseases only after birth by comparing the physical findings and functional capacities with normal standards of brainstem and spinal reflex function for the neonate. Some knowledge of embryology helps in this regard—recognition of the stage at which development was arrested indicates the point at which the disease struck. The timing and nature of major morphologic milestones in the development of the fetal nervous system form the basis of *teratology* (the science of congenital malformations).

229

TABLE 28-1 Time Scale of Stages in Human Growth and Development

Growth period	Approximate age
Prenatal	0–280 days
Ovum	0–14 days
Embryo	14 days–9 weeks
Fetus	9 weeks–birth
Premature infant	27–37 weeks
Birth	Average 280 days
Neonate	First 4 weeks after birth
Infancy	First year
Early childhood (preschool)	1–6 years
Late childhood (prepubertal)	6–10 years
Adolescence	Girls, 8 or 10 to 18 years; boys, 10 or 12 to 20 years
Puberty (average)	Girls, 13 years; boys, 15 years

From Lowrey, with permission.

The adaptations required of the fetus are most demanding during the parturitional period, when the newborn is suddenly thrust into the outside world and forced to exist independently. At this time, the brain is subjected to unusual forces as it passes through the birth canal. Once the umbilical cord is severed, the heart must circulate enough oxygenated blood to sustain the organs. This blood supply may prove to be inadequate, however, most often because of prematurity and respiratory difficulty and sometimes because of failure of closure of the foramen ovale or ductus arteriosus, so that the brain suffers irreversible hypoxic-ischemic damage. Later, such infants are observed to manifest so-called cerebral palsy and mental retardation.

Departures from normal development take the form of either (1) a slowness or an arrest of development or (2) a regression from a functional level that had been achieved earlier. The former is an expression of a developmental failure of genetic type or the result of a nonprogressive disease. The latter—regression after a period of normal development—stands as the most reliable indicator of an ongoing disease process. The only exceptions to this principle are cases in which injury or disease strikes when the nervous system is insufficiently developed to manifest neurologic signs. At such a time, examination may disclose no abnormalities; the latter appear only at a later stage of development, when the injured structures come to be required for normal functions. A congenital hemiplegia, for example, will usually not be evident until 5 to 6 months of age, when the corticospinal tract has become sufficiently myelinated and functional.

Delays in Motor Development

The most severe forms of delayed motor development, spasticity and athetosis, are usually manifestations of prenatal and perinatal diseases of the brain that are commonly subsumed under the term "*cerebral palsy*," as discussed in Chap. 38. Mental retardation is a usual accompaniment. In distinction to these gross deficits in motor development, there is a relatively small but distinct group of young children who exhibit only mild abnormalities of muscle tone, clumsiness or unusual postures of the hands, tremor, and ataxia (*fine motor deficit*). Such mild developmental deficits in the somewhat older

TABLE 28-2 Neurologic Functions and Their Disturbances in Infancy

Age	Normal functions	Pathologic signs
Newborn period	Blinking, tonic deviation of eyes on turning head, sucking, rooting, swallowing, yawning, grasping, brief extension of neck in prone position, incurvation response, Moro response, flexion postures of limbs; biceps reflexes present and others variable; infantile type of flexor plantar reflex; stable temperature, respirations, and blood pressure; periods of sleep and arousal; vigorous cry	Lack of arousal (stupor or coma); high-pitched or weak cry; abnormal (incomplete or absent) Moro response; opisthotonus; flaccidity or hypertonia; convulsions; tremulous limbs; failure of tonic deviation of eyes on passive movement of head or of head and body
2–3 months	Supports head; smiles; makes vowel sounds; adopts tonic symmetric neck postures (tonic neck reflexes); large range of movements of limbs, tendon reflexes usually present; fixates on and follows a dangling toy; suckles vigorously; periods of sleep sharply differentiated from awake periods; support and stepping unelicitable; vertical suspension (legs flex, head up)	Absence of any or all of the normal functions; convulsions; hypotonia or hypertonia of neck and limbs; vertical suspension (legs extend and adduct)
4 months	Good head support, minimal head lag; coos and chuckles; inspects hands; tone of limbs moderate or diminished; turns to sounds; rolls over from prone to supine; grasping, sucking, and tonic neck reflexes subservient to volition	No head support; motor deficits; hypertonia; no social reactions; tonic neck reflexes present; strong Moro response; absence of symmetric attitude

(continued)

TABLE 28-2 *(cont.)* Neurologic Functions and Their Disturbances in Infancy

Age	Normal functions	Pathologic signs
5–6 months	Babbles; reaches and grasps; vocalizes in social play; discriminates between family and strangers; Moro response and grasp disappear; tries to recover lost object; begins to sit, no head lag on pull to sit; positive support reaction; tonic neck reflexes gone; Landau response (holds head above horizontal and arches back when held horizontally); begins to grasp objects with one hand, holds bottle	Altered tone; obligatory posture; cannot sit or roll over; hypo- or hypertonia; persistent Moro response and grasp; persistent tonic neck reflexes; no Landau response
9 months	Creeps and pulls to stand, stands holding on; sits securely; babbles "Mama," "Dada," or equivalent; sociable, plays "pat-a-cake," seeks attention; drinks from cup; Landau and parachute responses present; grasps with thumb to forefinger	Failure to attain these motor, verbal, and social milestones; persistent automatisms and tonic neck reflexes or hypo- or hypertonia
12 months	Stands alone; may walk, or walks if led; tries to feed self; may say several single words, echoes sounds; plantar reflexes definitely flexor; throws objects	Retardation in attaining these milestones; functions at earlier level; persistence of automatisms
15 months	Walks independently (9–16 months), falls easily; moves arms steadily; says several words, scribbles with crayon; requests by pointing; interest in sounds, music, pictures, and animal toys	Retardation at earlier age level; persistent abnormalities of tone and posture; sensory discriminations defective

(continued)

TABLE 28-2 *(cont.)* Neurologic Functions and Their Disturbances in Infancy

Age	Normal functions	Pathologic signs
18 months	Says at least 6 words; feeds self; uses spoon well; may obey commands; runs stiffly, seats self in chair; hand dominance; throws ball; plays several nursery games; uses simple tools in imitation; removes shoes and socks; points to two or three parts of body, common objects, and pictures in book	Cannot walk; no words (may or may not be pathologic)
24 months	Says 2- or 3-word sentences; scribbles; runs well, climbs stairs one at a time; bends over and picks up objects; kicks ball; turns knob; organized play; builds tower of 6 blocks; sometimes toilet trained	Retarded in all motor, linguistic, and social adaptive skills

Modified from Gesell.

child have been referred to as *soft signs*. Like speech delay and dyslexia, they are more frequent in males.

The detection of gross delays or abnormalities of motor development in the neonatal or early infantile period of life is aided little by tests of tendon and plantar reflexes. Arm reflexes are always rather difficult to obtain in infants, and a normal neonate may have a few beats of ankle clonus. The plantar response tends to be wavering and uncertain in pattern. However, a consistent extension of the great toe and fanning of the toes on stroking the side of the foot is abnormal at any age.

In assessing developmental abnormalities of the motor system in the neonate and young infant, several maneuvers that elicit certain postures and reflexive movements are particularly useful (see also Table 28-2):

1. The *Moro response*—elevation and abduction of the arms followed by clasping movements to the midline—is the infant's reaction to startle and can be evoked by suddenly withdrawing support of the head and allowing the neck to extend. A loud noise or jerking one leg will have the same effect. It is present in all newborns and infants up to 4 or 5 months of age, and its absence indicates a profound disorder of the motor system. An inadequate Moro response on one side is found in infants with hemiplegia, brachial plexus palsy, or a fractured clavicle. Persistence of the Moro response beyond 4 or 5 months of age indicates a neurologic defect.

2. The *tonic neck reflex*—extension of the arm and leg on the side to which the head is passively turned and flexion of the opposite limbs ("fencing posture")—if obligatory and sustained, is a sign of pyramidal or extrapyramidal motor abnormality. Fragments, such as a brief extension of one

TABLE 28-3 Developmental Achievements of the Normal Preschool Child

Age	Observed items	Useful clinical tests
2 years	Runs well; goes up and down stairs, one step at a time; climbs on furniture; opens doors; helps to dress self; feeds well with spoon; puts 3 words together; listens to stories with pictures	Pencil-paper test: scribbles, imitates horizontal stroke; folds paper once; builds tower of 6 blocks
2 1/2 years	Jumps on both feet; walks on tiptoes if asked; knows full name, asks questions; refers to self as "I"; helps put away toys and clothes; names animals in book, knows 1 to 3 colors; can complete 3-piece form board	Pencil-paper test: horizontal and vertical line; builds tower of 8 blocks
3 years	Climbs stairs, alternating feet; talks constantly, cites nursery rhymes; rides tricycle; stands on one foot momentarily; plays simple games; helps in dressing; washes hands; identifies 5 colors	Builds 9-cube tower; builds bridge with 3 cubes; imitates circle and cross with pencil
4 years	Climbs well, hops and skips on one foot, throws ball overhand, kicks ball; cuts out pictures with scissors; counts 4 pennies; tells a story, plays with other children; goes to toilet alone	Copies cross and circle; builds gate with 5 cubes; builds a bridge from model; draws a human figure with 2 to 4 parts other than head; distinguishes short and long lines
5 years	Skips; names 4 colors, counts 10 pennies; dresses and undresses; asks questions about meaning of words	Copies square and triangle; distinguishes heavier of 2 weights; more detailed drawing of a human figure

arm, are found in 60 percent of normal infants at 1 to 2 months and may be adopted spontaneously by the infant up to 6 months of age.

3. The *placing reaction*—wherein the foot or hand, brought passively into contact with the edge of a table, is lifted automatically and placed on the flat surface—is present in normal newborns. Its absence or asymmetry under 6 months of age indicates a motor abnormality.

4. In the *Landau maneuver*, the infant, if suspended horizontally in the prone position, will extend the neck and trunk and will break the trunk extension when the neck is passively flexed. This reaction is present by 6 months; its delayed appearance in a hypotonic child is indicative of a faulty motor apparatus.

5. If an infant is held prone in the horizontal position and is then dropped toward the bed, an extension of the arms is evoked, as if to break the fall, known as the *"parachute response"*; it is elicitable in most 9-month-old infants. An asymmetry indicates a unilateral motor abnormality.

The early detection of "cerebral palsy" is hampered by the fact that the corticospinal tract is not fully myelinated until 18 months of age, allowing only quasivoluntary movements up to this time. For this reason, a *congenital hemiparesis* may not be evident until many months after birth. Even then it is manifest only by subtle signs, such as holding the hand in a fisted posture or clumsiness in reaching for objects and in transferring them from one hand to the other. Later, the leg is seen to be less active as the infant crawls, steps, and places the foot. Early hand dominance should always raise the suspicion of a motor defect on the opposite side.

Developmental motor delay and other abnormalities are present in a large proportion of infants with *hypotonia*. When the *"floppy infant"* is lifted and its limbs are passively manipulated, there is little muscle reactivity. In the supine position, the weakness and laxity result in a "frog-leg" posture, along with an increased mobility at the ankles and hips. Hypotonia, if generalized and accompanied by an absence of tendon reflexes, is most often due to Werdnig-Hoffmann disease, although the range of possible diagnoses is large and includes diseases of muscle, nerve, and the central nervous system.

Delays in Sensory Development

Failure to see and to hear are the most important sensory defects affecting the infant and child. When *both* senses are affected, a severe cerebral defect is usually responsible; only at a later age, when the child is more testable, does it become apparent that the trouble is not with the peripheral sensory apparatus but with the central integrating mechanisms of the brain.

Failure of development of visual function is usually revealed by a disorder of ocular movements. Any defect of the refractive apparatus or integrity of the central visual pathways results in wandering, jerky movements of the eyes. The optic discs may be atrophic, but it should be pointed out that the discs in infants tend naturally to be paler than those of an older child.

With respect to hearing, there is the difficulty in evaluating this function in an infant. Normally, after a few weeks of life, alert parents notice a brisk startle to loud noises and a response to other sounds. A tinkling bell brought from behind the infant usually results in hearkening or head turning and visual searching, but a lack of these responses warns only of the most severe hearing defects. The elicitation of slight degrees of deafness, enough to interfere with auditory learning, requires special testing. To make the problem even more difficult, both a peripheral and a central disorder may be present in some conditions, such as kernicterus. Brainstem auditory evoked responses (BAER) are particularly helpful in confirming peripheral abnormalities. After the first few months, impaired hearing becomes more obvious and interferes with the development of language.

RESTRICTIVE OR SELECTIVE DEVELOPMENTAL DISORDERS

In the course of early development, a large number of abnormalities become evident in the spheres of acquisition of speech and language, in learning ability and scholastic achievement, and in behavior and social adaptation. A single complex function may be retarded in its development; except for this one abnormality, the rest of the nervous system seems to be functioning normally. Since these shortcomings can also be influenced by the patient's social and cultural surroundings, there is an ongoing controversy about the relative importance of purely genetic and environmental factors ("nature versus nurture"). Both are important, but the genetic aspect dominates current thinking on this subject.

Disorders of Speech and Language

The acquisition of speech and language begins in the first months of postnatal life with babbling and lalling; it progresses successively through the stages of articulated words, phrases, and sentences to reading and writing, enlargement of vocabulary, knowledge of grammar, and rhetorical skill. The process is not finalized until adulthood. Each successive stage depends on the continued maturation of the brain. For example, not until the sixth year of age are most children ready to be taught reading and writing—i.e., to become literate. Educational opportunity is necessary for the full realization of these capacities.

In a considerable number of children, particularly those with family histories of speech defect, ambidexterity, and left handedness, there are specific types of delay in the timetable of language development. These restricted abnormalities appear more frequently in males than in females (in a proportion of 4:1). Table 28-4 lists the common types of developmental speech and language disorders in children who are otherwise normal (i.e., are neither deaf nor mentally retarded or impaired in any other way). In the most common of these, the child has difficulty in reading, spelling, or writing (developmental dyslexia, or congenital word blindness). Presumably—and there is some histologic evidence for this—an aberration of normal cerebral cortical development of the planum temporale or perisylvian region has deranged the timetable of language and speech acquisition. In all developmental disorders of speech and language, the child's intelligence, vision and hearing, and control of labial, lingual, palatal, and laryngeal movements should be tested in order to determine if a defect in one of these is responsible.

Mixed forms of speech impairment are frequent in children (stuttering, lisping, cluttering, etc.). They tend to lessen with maturation, and milder forms may disappear in late adolescence and adulthood. These disorders are not psychogenic, but some children may develop a sense of inferiority or other neurotic tendencies because of the speech disorder. Special drills and educational methods are helpful in correcting these maturational defects.

The Development of Intelligence

Intelligence is defined as the capacity to assimilate new information, to think, and to solve problems. Most psychologists view it as a unitary mental capacity dependent on the proper functioning of the diencephalon and entire cerebral cortex. Closer analysis of intelligent behavior discloses that

TABLE 28-4 Developmental Disorders of Speech and Language

Type	Clinical manifestations
Developmental speech delay	Failure to speak words and short phrases by age 2 years (delay may be up to 3–4 years); normal understanding of spoken word and normal communication by gestures; speech later becomes normal or nearly so
Congenital word deafness (developmental receptive dysphasia)	Despite adequate hearing (response to sounds), an inability to distinguish word patterns or reproduce them in speech; idioglossia develops
Congenital inarticulation	Impaired ability to coordinate vocal, articulatory, and respiratory movements for speaking; normal understanding of spoken words; lisping, lallation, cluttered speech (special types of articulatory defect)
Congenital word blindness (developmental dyslexia and dysgraphia)	Impaired ability to read, spell, and write words, despite ability to recognize letters; normal understanding of spoken word and meaning of objects and diagrams; difficulty in copying and color naming; many variants thereof
Dyscalculia	Impaired ability to learn basic arithmetic; may be combined with dyslexia
Stuttering-stammering	Intermittent, involuntary repetition of syllables or blocking; worse with excitement or stress; disappears or improves with maturity except in severe forms
High-level semantic and syntactic disorders	Ability to comprehend single words but not complex phrases. Difficulty in formulating language

it incorporates a number of separate factors, such as attention, motivation, facility with language, arithmetic skills, memory, etc., which are relatively localized, as pointed out in Chap. 22. General intelligence and these several components mature slowly from birth to late adolescence. Although the rate of development and levels of attainment are to a large extent genetically determined (probably polygenetic), the quality of the home environment and education certainly facilitate the development of intelligent behavior.

It is apparent that humans vary greatly in intelligence. When measured by standard verbal or nonverbal intelligence tests, the scores (intelligence quotients, or IQs) obtained by a large population of children are distributed in accordance with a normal Gaussian (bell-shaped) curve. It is also known that intelligent parents beget intelligent children. The existence of several X-linked forms of mental retardation (see Chap. 38) suggests that a heritable component of intelligence resides on the X chromosome. Genius is found among those with the very highest IQs, and the lowermost scores set apart a group with subnormal intelligence; they make up 1 to 3 percent of the population. To a large extent, their parents have similar low levels of intelligence. But since these parents are in the lowest economic group in society and often live in an impoverished environment, the influences of genes and environment are difficult to distinguish. These individuals are euphemistically referred to as sociocultural retardates. They must be distinguished from the severely retarded, as discussed in Chap. 38.

Learning Disorders

The preceding remarks about sociocultural retardation are relevant to learning problems in children and their capacity for academic achievement. In most public school systems, approximately 15 percent of the students do not measure up to the normal level. Psychosocial factors such as lack of scholastic opportunity and a bad home environment and neighborhood may play a role. In many instances, however, borderline intelligence or a particular inability to process information or marginal defects in reading and calculation are more important. The hyperkinetic state, common to boys (attention deficit hyperactivity disorder), may also interfere with learning. Affected children are overactive, impulsive, inattentive, distractible, impatient, and easily frustrated. This, too, is a specific abnormality—a restricted, genetically determined developmental delay.

Correction of learning disorders requires the concerted effort of family and special educators. Drugs such as methylphenidate, 5 to 10 mg tid, or dextroamphetamine, 2.5 to 5 mg tid, may be helpful in some cases of hyperactivity, but they must be used judiciously.

Sexual Development

Physicians are often confronted with problems relating to sexual behavior. Like that of the menarche, the timetable of sexual development is not uniform, and there is considerable individual variation. Some 10 percent of the population fail to gain the biologically favorable heterosexual orientation. The largest of this group is the homosexual, whose members are motivated in adult life by a preferential erotic attraction to members of their own sex. By recent estimates, the incidence of homosexuality, in both men and women, ranges from 1 to 5 percent.

The origins of homosexuality are unsettled. The most cogent hypothesis is that differences or variations in genetic patterning of the immature nervous system (hypothalamus) set the sexual predilection during early life. Of significance is the observation that the preoptic zone is larger in heterosexual males than it is in females and in homosexual males. Also, an aggregate of neurons in the interstitial nucleus of the hypothalamus has been said to be between two and three times larger in heterosexual than in homosexual men. These findings, which must be confirmed, would support the view that homosexuality has a biologic basis. Genetic studies point in the same direction. About 57 percent of identical twins (and 13 percent of brothers) of homosexual men are also homosexual. The inheritance of male homosexuality would appear to be from the maternal side, implicating a gene on the X chromosome.

The Development of Personality

Personality encompasses all the psychologic traits that distinguish one individual from every other. A great difference between individuals can be recognized in energy, capacity for effective work, intellectual power, sensitivity, temperament, emotional responsivity, aggressivity or passivity, strength of character, and tolerance to change, to risk, and to stress. The composite of these qualities constitutes the human personality.

In the formation of personality, especially the part concerned with feeling and emotional sensitivity, basic temperament surely plays a part. By nature, some children from the beginning seem to be happy, cheerful, and unconcerned about immediate frustrations; others are the opposite. By the third month of life, there is an emergence of individual differences in activity/passivity, intensity of action, approach/withdrawal, adaptivity/unadaptivity, threshold of response to stimulation, positive/negative mood, selectivity, and distractibility. Ratings at this early age have been found to correlate with the results of examinations made at 5 years and even later in life. The more common aspects of adult personality— i.e., worry about one's health and other matters, anxiety or serenity, timidity or boldness, the power of instinctual drives and needs for satisfaction, sympathy for others, sensitivity to criticism, and degree of disorganization resulting from adverse circumstances —are presumed to be genetically determined. Identical twins raised apart are remarkably alike in these and many other personality traits. These observations are supported by the finding that certain aspects of personality, such as thrill seeking and risk taking, have been linked in part to allelic differences at specific gene loci. Nonetheless, the effects of early experiences, child rearing, and peer exposure have modulatory influences on the development of personality.

Impaired Social Development

Here the retardation is in the sphere of social adaptation, a long process that includes the successive harmonious adaptation to mother, family, teachers, and social peers. Easy frustration, disobedience, persistent tantrums, and inability to accept authority and curb one's impulses are flagrant manifestations of maladaptation. This may lead to truancy, family discord, unlawful conduct, fire setting, etc. (sociopathy; see Chap. 56). With maturation there is usually some degree of improvement.

MENTAL RETARDATION

The symptom complex of incomplete or insufficient development of mental capacities and associated behavioral abnormalities combines many of the developmental abnormalities already discussed. Mental retardation stands as the single largest neuropsychiatric disorder in every civilized society, estimated to affect 3 percent of the population. Using any one of a number of indices of social and psychologic failure, two somewhat overlapping groups are recognized: (1) The mildly impaired (IQ 45 to 70), corresponding to what in the past had been called high-grade imbecile and "feeble-minded," and (2) the severely impaired, corresponding to the categories that were formerly called idiot (IQ <20) and low-grade imbecile (IQ 20 to 45). A third category that might be added encompasses *autism* and related disorders discussed in Chap. 38. It has been recognized that aspects of autism may be present in children with normal or virtually normal cognitive ability (Asperger syndrome); however, the severe form (Kanner syndrome) creates a disability equivalent to the severe forms of retardation. The first (mildly impaired) group is now referred to as having *subcultural*, *physiologic*, or *familial mental retardation*; it is much larger than the group with *pathologic mental retardation*. Because of the opprobrious implications of the terms *idiot*, *imbecile*, and *moron*, the American Association on Mental Deficiency proposed that the mentally retarded be grouped instead into four categories: (1) *profound deficiency*, incapable of self-care (IQ 1 to 25); (2) *severe deficiency*, incapable of living an independent existence and essentially untrainable (IQ 25 to 39); (3) *moderate deficiency*, trainable to some extent (IQ 40 to 54), and (4) *mild deficiency*, impaired but trainable and to some extent educable.

It is important to emphasize that only a small proportion of cases of mental retardation—representing those with profound and severe deficiency—can presently be traced to congenital abnormalities of development and diseases reviewed in Chap. 38. The most acceptable view of the mildly affected group of retarded persons is that it represents the proportion of the population that is the opposite of genius. Lewis was one of the first to call attention to this large group of simple mental retardates, and he referred to them by the ambiguous term *subcultural*. Two clinical types can be recognized. In the first, the essential characteristic is that, almost from birth, the infant is backward in all aspects of development. There is a tendency to sleep more, to be less demanding of nourishment, to move less than normal, and to suck poorly and regurgitate. Parents often comment on how good their baby is, how little he troubles them by crying. As the months pass, every expected achievement is late. The baby is usually more hypotonic and turns over, sits unsupported, and walks later than the normal infant. These babies do not smile at the usual time and take little notice of the mother or other persons or objects in their environment. They are inattentive to visual and often to auditory stimuli, to the point where questions are raised about blindness or deafness. Mouthing (putting everything in the mouth) and slobbering, which should end by 1 year of age, also persist. There are only fleeting signs of interest in toys, and the impersistence of attention becomes increasingly prominent. Vocalizations are scant, often guttural, piercing, or high-pitched and feeble. Babbling is not replaced by attempts at word formation.

In the second type, early motor milestones (supporting the head, rolling over, sitting, standing, and walking) may be attained at their normal times, yet the infant is later inattentive and slow in learning the usual nursery tricks. It seems as though motor development had somehow escaped the retardation process. There may, however, be aimless overactivity and persistence of rhythmic movements, grinding of the teeth (bruxism), and hypotonia.

Members of both groups exhibit a high incidence of minor congenital anomalies of the eyes, face, mouth, ears, and hands; they tend to be sickly, and the more severely retarded among them have poor physiques and are often undersized. Abandonment, neglect, and child abuse are frequent in this group. The majority of children with deviant behavior need to be placed in special classes or schools, and special measures must be taken to reduce their tendency to truancy, sociopathy, and criminality.

An endless debate is centered on matters of causation—whether the so-called subcultural or physiologic retardates are products of a faulty genetic influence, which prevents successful competition and adaptation, or of societal discrimination and lack of training and education, coupled with the effects of malnutrition, infections, or other exogenous factors. Surely both environmental and genetic factors are at work, although the relative importance of each has proved difficult to measure.

In the first year or two of life, suspicion of mental retardation is based largely on clinical impression, but it should always be validated by psychometric procedures. Most pediatric neurologists utilize some of the criteria laid down by Gesell and Amatruda or the Denver Developmental Screening Scale, from which a developmental quotient (DQ) is calculated.

For testing of preschool children, the Wechsler Preschool and Primary Scale of Intelligence is used, and for school-age children, the Wechsler Intelligence Scale for Children. IQ tests for preschoolers must be interpreted with caution, since they have had less predictive validity for school success than the tests that are used after 6 years of age. In general, normal scores for age eliminate mental retardation as a cause of poor school achievement and learning disabilities, but special cognitive defects may be revealed by low scores on particular subtests. Retarded children not only have low scores but exhibit more scatter of subtest scores. Also, they achieve greater success with performance than with verbal items. It is essential that the physician know the conditions of testing, for poor scores may be due to fright, inadequate motivation, lapses in attention, dyslexia, or a subtle auditory or visual defect rather than a developmental lag.

For a more detailed discussion of this topic, see Victor and Ropper: *Adams and Victor's Principles of Neurology*, 7th ed, pp 605–638.

ADDITIONAL READING

Barlow C: *Mental Retardation and Related Disorders*. Philadelphia, Davis, 1977.

Capute AJ, Accardo PJ: *Developmental Disabilities in Infancy and Childhood*. Baltimore, Brookes, 1991.

Fox P, Ingham R: Commentary on stuttering. *Science* 270:1438, 1995.

Galaburda AM, Sherman CF, Rosen GD, et al: Developmental dyslexia: Four consecutive patients with cortical anomalies. *Ann Neurol* 18:222, 1985.

Gesell A (ed): *The First Five Years of Life: A Guide to the Study of the Pre-school Child*. New York, Harper & Row, 1940.

Hynd GW, Semrud-Clikeman M, Lorys AR, et al: Brain morphology in developmental dyslexia and attention deficit disorder/hyperactivity. *Arch Neurol* 47:919, 1990.

Hill JC, Schoener EP: Age-dependent decline of attention deficit hyperactivity disorder. *Am J Psychiatry* 153:1143, 1996.

Kanner I: Early infantile autism. *J Pediatr* 25:211, 1944.

Kinsbourne M: Disorders of mental development, in Menkes JH (ed): *Textbook of Child Neurology*, 5th ed. Baltimore, Williams & Wilkins, 1995, pp 924–964.

LeVay S, Hamer DH: Evidence for a biological influence in male homosexuality. *Sci Am* 270:44, 1994.

Lowrey GH: *Growth and Development of Children*, 8th ed. Chicago, Year Book, 1986.

Rapin I: Autism. *N Engl J Med* 337:97, 1997.

Rosenberger PB: Learning disorders, in Berg B (ed): *Principles of Child Neurology*. New York, McGraw-Hill, 1996, pp 335–369.

Shaywitz SE: Dyslexia. *N Engl J Med* 338:307, 1998.

Zametkin AJ, Ernst M: Problems in the management of attention-deficit hyperactivity disorder. *N Engl J Med* 340:40, 1999.

29 | The Neurology of Aging

At the other end of the life cycle, there is a predictable decline in neurologic functioning. The aging process is based on neuronal loss in many systems, beginning in midlife and proceeding until death. In many systems of neurons, the most obvious morphologic changes are neuronal lipofuscinosis, gradual cell loss, and replacement gliosis. A volumetric change in the cerebrum with age is regularly displayed in computed tomography (CT) scans and magnetic resonance imaging (MRI), which show widened sulci and enlarged ventricles. At a later stage, senile plaques and Alzheimer neurofibrillary changes are added, but there still is not full agreement on whether this simply represents an aging effect or the development of an age-linked disease. We have taken the latter standpoint, and for this reason we discuss Alzheimer dementia with the degenerative diseases (Chap. 39).

Neurologic Signs of Aging

There are a number of neurologic abnormalities for which no cause can be discerned other than the effects of aging itself. The following are the most consistent ones:

1. Neuro-ophthalmic signs: progressive smallness of pupils and decreased reactions to light and accommodation, insufficiency of convergence, restricted upward conjugate gaze, diminished dark adaptation, and increased sensitivity to glare.
2. Progressive perceptive hearing loss (presbycusis), especially for high tones, and a commensurate decline in speech discrimination due mainly to a diminution in the number of hair cells in the cochlea.
3. Diminution in the sense of smell and, to a lesser extent, the sense of taste.
4. Motor signs: reduced rate and amount of motor activity, slowed reaction time, impairment of fine coordination and agility, reduced muscular power (legs more than arms and proximal muscles more than distal ones), and thinness of muscles, particularly the dorsal interossei, thenar, and anterior tibial muscles. A progressive decrease in the number of anterior horn cells is largely responsible for these changes, although muscles also atrophy with age.
5. Changes in tendon reflexes: depression of tendon reflexes at the ankles in comparison with those at the knees is observed frequently, and a loss of Achilles reflexes is often found in those above age 80. The snout or palmomental reflex, which can be detected in mild form in a small proportion of healthy adults, is a frequent finding in the elderly (in as many as half of normal subjects over 60 years of age). However, other so-called cortical release signs, such as suck and grasp reflexes, are indicative of frontal lobe disease and are not to be expected simply as a result of aging.

6. Impairment or loss of vibratory sense in the toes and ankles. Proprioception, however, is impaired very little or not at all. These changes correlate with a loss of sensory fibers in sensory nerves and probably loss of dorsal root ganglion cells.
7. The most notable aging changes—those of stance, posture, and gait—are described in Chap. 7 and further on in this chapter.

Also, old age is often thought to carry a liability to tremulousness; indeed, one sees this association with some frequency. The hands particularly but also the head and chin may tremble and the voice may quaver, yet there is not the usual slowness and poverty of movement, facial impassivity, or flexed posture that would stamp the condition as parkinsonian. Some instances are clearly familial, having appeared or worsened only late in life.

Spastic, or spasmodic, dysphonia, a disorder of late life characterized by spasm of all the throat muscles on attempted speech, is discussed with the dystonias on page 49. Blepharoclonus or blepharospasm, another involuntary movement of the eyelids, is described on page 124.

The common neurologic signs of aging and their frequency in each epoch are summarized in Table 29-1.

Effects of Aging on Memory and Other Cognitive Functions

There is a steady decline in cognitive function starting at age 30 and progressing into the senium. Apparently all forms of cognitive function partake of this decline, although certain elements of the verbal scale (vocabulary, fund of information, and comprehension) withstand the effects of aging better than those of the performance scale (block design, reversal of digits, picture arrangement, object assembly, and the digit-symbol task). The most definite effects of age are in learning and memory and in problem solving—cognitive impairments probably attributable to a progressive reduction in the speed of processing information.

The ability to memorize, acquire, and retain new information, recall names, and avoid distraction once set on a course of action diminishes with advancing age, particularly in those more than 70 years old. Moreover, memory function may be disturbed despite the relative intactness of other intellectual abilities. Characteristically, there is difficulty with recall of a name or the specific date of an experience despite a preservation of memory for the experience itself or for the many features of a person whose name is momentarily elusive ("tip-of-the-tongue syndrome"). Also characteristic is an inconsistent retrieval of the lost name or information at a later date. This type of memory disturbance is referred to as *benign senescent forgetfulness*, or *age-associated memory impairment*. The latter, in distinction to Alzheimer disease, worsens very little or not at all over a period of many years and does not interfere significantly with a person's work performance or daily activities.

The changes of benign senescent forgetfulness, present in varying degree in most elderly individuals, may sometimes pose a clinical problem—how to decide whether they are part of the aging process per se or the early manifestations of Alzheimer disease. The differentiation can usually be made by careful testing of the mental status over months or years, as described in Chap. 21. Repetition of spoken items such as a series of digits, orientation as to place and time, capacity to learn and to retain several items, tests of

TABLE 29-1 Frequency of Certain Neurologic Signs in Uncomplicated Aging (in Percent)

Sign	65–69 years	70–74 years	75–79 years	>80 years
Glabellar sign (inability to inhibit blink in response to tapping the brow)	10	15	27	37
Snout reflex	3	8	7	26
Limited upgaze	6	15	27	29
Limited downgaze	8	15	26	34
Abnormal visual tracking	8	18	22	32
Paratonic rigidity	6	10	12	21
Unable to recall 3 words	24	28	25	55
Unable to spell "world" backward	10	12	18	21

Adapted from Jenkyn and Reeves by permission.

arithmetic and calculation (concentration), and specific tests for memory (particularly tests of delayed recall or forgetfulness) reveal that normal aging persons invariably perform at a significantly higher level than patients with Alzheimer disease. High intelligence, well-organized work habits, and sound judgment compensate for many of the progressive deficiencies of old age.

Personality Changes in the Aged Many old people become more opinionated, repetitive, and rigid and conservative in their thinking; the opposite qualities—undue pliancy, vacillation, and the uncritical acceptance of ideas—are observed in others. Often these changes can be recognized as exaggerations of lifelong personality traits. Elderly persons tend to become increasingly cautious; many of them seem to lack self-confidence and require a strong probability of success before undertaking certain tasks. These changes may impair their performance on psychologic testing. Studies of senescent monozygotic twins suggest that genetic factors are more important than environmental ones in molding these traits. Aggressive individuals with much energy and a diversity of interests, leading to a wide range of social interactions, appear to resist the ravages of age better than those with the opposite traits. Those with depressive tendencies are more easily overwhelmed by prospects of the senium and adopt an attitude of hopelessness, fear, suspicion, and worry. This may explain the threefold increase in suicides in late middle life and old age. *Certainly an agitated depression is the most frequent psychiatric disease in these periods of life.*

Effects of Aging on Stance and Gait and Related Motor Impairments

These are among the most conspicuous manifestations of aging. Gradually, steps shorten, walking becomes slower, and there is a tendency to stoop. The older person becomes less confident and more cautious in walking and habitually reaches for the handrail in descending stairs, to prevent a misstep. All movements become less graceful, more inelastic. Putting on pants while standing alternately on one leg and the other becomes difficult. Handwriting tends to worsen, and all arm and hand movements become more clumsy. Choking on food is more frequent. Urinary incontinence is a surprisingly common occurrence in the elderly. Doubtless this complex of motor impairments is based on neuronal losses in the spinal cord, cerebellum, and cerebrum as well as a loss of muscle fibers.

The ubiquitous and subtle changes in gait of the "normal" aged population must be distinguished from a more rapidly evolving and inordinate deterioration of gait that afflicts a small proportion while they remain relatively competent in other ways. In all likelihood, the latter disorder represents an age-linked degenerative disease of the brain, since most instances of it are sooner or later accompanied by mental changes. The patient looks to the ground and finds it difficult to walk and converse at the same time. The body assumes a flexed posture. Gradually, as the steps shorten, the feet barely clear the ground (a state referred to as marche á petit pas); finally the feet are merely shuffled forward. Later still, the patient, upon standing up from a lying or sitting position, finds it difficult to initiate the first step, even though there is no difficulty in moving the legs while lying in bed. Taking the patient's arm or walking alongside and urging him to keep step with a marching cadence may improve the gait disorder at this stage. In the most advanced form of this condition, the capacity for upright stance and walking is completely lost and the patient lies in bed, unable to turn over and eventually curled up in a posture of cerebral paraplegia in flexion. The inexperienced physician may suspect a psychologic disorder. The basis of the aforementioned gait disorder is probably a combined frontal lobe–basal ganglionic degeneration, the anatomy of which has never been fully clarified. It does not respond to the administration of L-dopa or to any other therapeutic measures.

Also, the partially remediable condition *normal-pressure hydrocephalus (NPH)* is responsible for a sizable proportion of such cases (Chap. 30). One recognizes in NPH a mild ataxia as well as several elements of the Parkinson syndrome, and, of course, Parkinson disease is yet another treatable cause of walking difficulty (Chap. 39). In the analysis of gait disorders, one should search for evidence of *posterior column or vestibular disorder, cerebellar ataxia, and the spastic ataxia of cervical spondylosis,* all of which may unbalance the patient. These are discussed in detail in Chaps. 7 and 39.

Falls in the Elderly Among elderly persons without apparent neurologic disease, falls constitute a major health problem. For such persons living in the community, about 30 percent suffer one or more falls each year; this figure rises to 40 percent among those over the age of 80 and to more than 50 percent among elderly persons living in nursing homes.

Several factors, some mentioned above in regard to deterioration of gait, are responsible. Impairment of vision and particularly of vestibular function with normal aging are important contributors. The failure to make rapid postural adjustments, which is a product of aging alone, accounts for the occurrence of falls in the course of usual activities such as walking, changing position, or descending stairs. Postural hypotension, often due to antihypertensive agents and the use of sedative drugs, is another important cause of falling among the elderly. It should be emphasized that falling is an even more prominent feature of certain age-related neurologic diseases: stroke, Parkinson disease, NPH, and progressive supranuclear palsy, among others.

Age-Related Neurologic Disease

Among the *age-linked degenerative diseases of the nervous system,* the nonhereditary form of Alzheimer disease is the most common and important. Dementia as a cardinal manifestation of cerebral disease is considered in Chap. 21; Alzheimer disease and other age-linked degenerative diseases are described in Chap. 39.

Cerebral atherosclerosis is, of course, a frequent finding in the elderly, but it does not parallel aging with any consistency, being severe in some 30- to 40-year-old individuals and practically absent in some octogenarians. In addition to atherosclerotic disease, the basilar arteries become somewhat larger and more tortuous and opaque in the elderly.

Most *neoplasms of the nervous system* occur with increasing frequency in early and middle adult life. Only in advanced old age does the incidence tend to fall. One class of endocrine tumors appears to form during periods of intensified functional demands—e.g., hypophysial adenomas with atrophy of gonads and adrenals during late adult life.

The high incidence of *adverse drug reactions* in the elderly is related to several factors—the increased duration and severity of drug effects, the frequent failure to adjust drug dosage to diminished body weight, a reduction in hepatic detoxification and in renal clearance, and, most importantly, the unmasking by certain drugs, sedatives in particular, of an underlying mild dementia.

Often in the elderly, the exigencies of disease cannot be met efficiently because of a combination of organ inadequacies, no single one of which is of sufficient severity to be manifest clinically. The sum total of these organ deficits constitutes a kind of gestalt of senility. The long list of diseases found in the elderly at autopsy reflects the individual's increasing susceptibility to disease with aging. However, the contributing effects of the aging processes are relatively inapparent, which is why the medical student so often asks, after the autopsy of an elderly person, "But what was the cause of death?"

For a more detailed discussion of this topic, see Victor and Ropper: *Adams and Victor's Principles of Neurology*, 7th ed, pp 639–651.

ADDITIONAL READING

Albert ML, Knoefel JE (eds): *Clinical Neurology of Aging*, 2nd ed. New York, Oxford University Press, 1994.

Critchley M: Neurologic changes in the aged. *J Chronic Dis* 3:459, 1956.

Drachman DA: Aging and the brain: A new frontier. *Ann Neurol* 42:819, 1997.

Duckett S, DeLaTorre JC: *Pathology of the Aging Human Nervous System*, 2nd ed. New York, Oxford University Press, 2001.

Fisher CM: Hydrocephalus as a cause of disturbances of gait in the elderly. *Neurology* 32:1358, 1982.

Jenkyn LR, Reeves AG: Neurologic signs in uncomplicated aging (senescence). *Semin Neurol* 1:21, 1981.

Kemper TL: Neuroanatomical and neuropathological changes during aging and dementia, in Albert ML, Knoefel JE (eds): *Clinical Neurology of Aging*, 2nd ed. New York, Oxford University Press, 1994, pp 3–67.

Kral VA: Senescent forgetfulness: Benign and malignant. *J Can Med Assoc* 86:257, 1962.

Tinetti ME, Speechley M: Prevention of falls among the elderly. *N Engl J Med* 320:1055, 1989.

Weiner WJ, Nora LM, Glantz RH: Elderly inpatients: Postural reflex impairment. *Neurology* 34:945, 1984.

PART IV | THE MAJOR CATEGORIES OF NEUROLOGIC DISEASE

Disturbances of CSF Circulation and Intracranial Pressure

The cerebrospinal fluid (CSF) serves as a kind of water jacket in which the brain is suspended and thereby protected from blows to the head. It also acts as a "sink" from which waste products of cerebral metabolism—such as CO_2, lactate, NH_3, and H^+ ions—are absorbed into the bloodstream and as a conduit for the distribution of various substances throughout the nervous system. Approximately 500 mL/day of CSF are formed, predominantly by the choroid plexuses of the lateral ventricles. The fluid flows to the third and fourth ventricles, exiting through the foramina of Luschka and Magendie at the base of the medulla and then circulating upward via the brainstem cisterns to the subarachnoid space overlying the convexities of the cerebral hemispheres. It is absorbed into the blood through the arachnoid villi that line mainly the sagittal sinus. In the adult, the volume of intracranial contents is roughly 1700 mL, comprising the brain itself (1450 mL), the CSF (estimated to be about 140 mL), and intravascular blood (150 mL). The relative volumes of CSF in the ventricles, the various cisternal spaces, and the subarachnoid spaces of the cerebrum and spinal column vary with age. CSF pressure, normally 90 to 150 mmH_2O (6 to 11 mmHg), is maintained largely by vascular (venous) pressure, for which reason there is a pulsatile intracranial pressure (ICP) waveform that follows the cardiac cycle.

Due to the rigidity of the cranium and the relative inelasticity of the dura, an increase in the volume of brain, blood, or CSF must be at the expense of the other components (Monro-Kellie doctrine; Fig. 30-1). This accommodative pressure-volume relationship is termed *compliance*; increments of intracranial volume are tolerated initially, but further expansion causes an exponential rise in ICP and, eventually, interference with cerebral blood flow.

INCREASED INTRACRANIAL PRESSURE

There are five mechanisms whereby ICP is raised:

1. An *increase in intracranial volume* (mass effect), the most important and frequent causes of which include cerebral tumor, abscess, hemorrhage, massive contusion or infarction; epidural or subdural hematoma; or acute diffuse brain swelling as occurs in anoxic states, hypertensive encephalopathy, some types of encephalitis, water intoxication, cerebral trauma, and Reye syndrome.
2. *Increased venous pressure* from sagittal sinus thrombosis, heart failure, or superior vena cava obstruction, which increases the volume of blood in pial veins and dural sinuses and probably also interferes with CSF absorption.

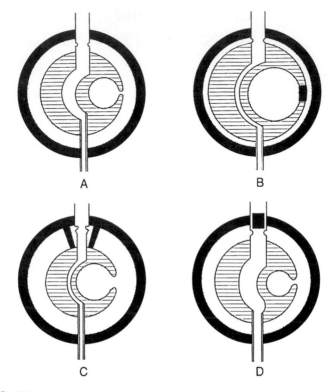

FIG. 30-1 *A.* Schematic representation of the three components of the intracranial contents: the incompressible brain tissue *(shaded)*; the vascular system, open to the atmosphere; and the CSF *(white)*. *B.* With ventricular obstruction. *C.* With obstruction at or near the points of outlet of the CSF. *D.* With obstruction of the venous outflow. *(Redrawn, with permission, from Foley.)*

3. *Obstruction to the flow and absorption of CSF, causing hydrocephalus*: Obstruction may be within the ventricular system, at absorption sites on the arachnoid villi, or around the base of the brain. The main causes are tumor, meningitis, and subarachnoid hemorrhage.
4. An *expanded CSF compartment*, also causing *hydrocephalus*, is rarely caused by excess CSF production due to a choroid plexus papilloma or to the acute addition to CSF volume by subarachnoid hemorrhage.
5. *A pseudotumor state of diffuse cerebral swelling* develops if there is no pressure differential between the ventricles and the CSF space over the cerebral convexity. Most cases are idiopathic.

These forms of increased ICP are discussed below.

With the head and trunk elevated to 45°, the pressure is normally only 2 to 5 mmHg. An increased ICP is present when the CSF pressure exceeds 200 mmH$_2$O (14 mmHg), but steady levels up to 30 mmHg are harmless. Above that level, clinical signs of increased ICP appear—headache, nausea and vomiting, and drowsiness, followed by lateral rectus palsies, papilledema, visual obscurations, and eventually blindness. Signs that are due to shifts of cerebral structures within the cranium, such as pupillary dilatation, abducens palsies, drowsiness/stupor, raised systolic blood pressure, and bradycardia (Cushing response from medullary compression), do not bear a direct relationship to the ICP. Patients maintain normal mental function and adequate cerebral circulation at intracranial pressures up to 30 to 40 mmHg provided the blood pressure is maintained. At 40 to 50 mmHg, cerebral blood flow is reduced; rhythmic rises in CSF pressure (Lundberg plateau waves) are superimposed, and coma supervenes.

Preventing a persistent rise in ICP above 15 to 20 mmHg appears to be associated with a better outcome in diseases that cause increased ICP. Effective measures to reduce ICP are elevation of the head and shoulders to 15 to 20° or more; restriction of free water by the use of intravenous normal saline; mechanical hyperventilation to reduce P_{CO_2}; and the use of hyperosmolar agents or diuretics (to maintain an osmolality above 290 mOsm/L). Reduction of P_{CO_2} by hyperventilation causes vasoconstriction, which reduces cerebral blood volume and in turn reduces ICP, albeit for only an hour or less. Mannitol, given as an IV bolus of 0.25 to 0.5 g/kg every 3 to 4 h, is the favored hyperosmolar agent. Some neurosurgeons prefer to use furosemide, glycerol, or hypertonic saline, particularly in the operating room. The use of large doses of barbiturate to lower ICP is controversial, since it carries the risk of causing hypotension, and most studies have failed to demonstrate clinical benefit. In many cases, the surgical removal of a focal mass lesion (subdural, epidural, parenchymal hematoma; tumor) or decompression of infarctive brain swelling by hemicraniectomy are the most effective means of reducing ICP.

HYDROCEPHALUS

This is due to an obstruction to the flow of CSF at some point between its main site of formation (within the lateral ventricles) and the basilar subarachnoid space. Because of the obstruction, CSF accumulates within the ventricles, dilating them, compressing the periventricular tissues, and slightly expanding the cerebral hemispheres. In general, the ventricle just proximal to the point of obstruction is the one that enlarges the most (Ayer's rule); obstruction to the flow of CSF at the base of the brain (caused usually by neoplastic or infectious meningitis) produces enlargement of the lateral, third and fourth ventricles. If the block is at the sites of CSF absorption, over the superior surfaces of the cerebral hemispheres, the pressure of the accumulated CSF outside the cerebrum ("external hydrocephalus") counteracts the internal hydrocephalus, and despite high ICP the ventricles may remain normal in size or enlarge only slightly. In all surviving hydrocephalic patients, the obstructions are only partial; complete obstruction is fatal within a few days unless relieved by shunting. In an infant or young child (up to 2 years) whose cranial sutures are not fully closed, the head enlarges as well (*manifest or overt hydrocephalus* or *macrocephaly*). Some degree of suture separation (diastasis) is also possible in slightly older children.

Unfortunately, the term *hydrocephalus* is sometimes used when the ventricles enlarge passively, as a result of brain atrophy (*hydrocephalus ex vacuo*). It is preferable to use the qualifying adjective *tension* for the obstructive type of hydrocephalus, in which the CSF is or has been under increased pressure. The term *tension hydrocephalus* also obviates the need for the ambiguous concept of a "communicating" versus a "noncommunicating" (obstructive) hydrocephalus. All forms of tension hydrocephalus are obstructive at some level, and an appropriate prefix indicates the site of the obstruction—e.g., *aqueductal, third-ventricular,* or *meningeal* tension hydrocephalus.

Four hydrocephalic syndromes are recognized:

1. *Congenital or infantile overt hydrocephalus* The common causes are matrix hemorrhages (in premature infants), fetal and neonatal meningitis, Chiari malformation, aqueductal stenosis or atresia, and the Dandy-Walker syndrome (atresia of the foramina of Luschka with a greatly dilated fourth ventricle). The head enlarges rapidly after birth, soon exceeding the 97th percentile for age. The fontanels are tense. The infant is fretful, feeds poorly, and becomes torpid and uninterested in his surroundings. Later there is lid retraction and paralysis of upward gaze ("setting sun" sign). The forehead is prominent (bossed). The older child is feeble, cannot manage the large head, and cannot stand or walk. There is no papilledema.

2. *Acquired tension hydrocephalus* The usual causes are a posterior fossa mass (tumor, hemorrhage, abscess, or parasitic cyst); the late effects of meningitis, ependymitis, or subarachnoid hemorrhage; Paget disease and other bony abnormalities around the foramen magnum; and decompensation of a congenital hydrocephalus from aqueductal stenosis. Bifrontal and biooccipital headaches, nausea, and vomiting are frequent manifestations. Papilledema is present. Slowness of response (abulia), inattentiveness, poverty of mental activity, perseveration, and sometimes grasp reflexes develop gradually. Gait becomes progressively impaired, which may eventually result in the inability to stand.

3. *Normal-pressure (occult) hydrocephalus* As a high-pressure, occult hydrocephalus corrects itself (compensates) or as a *relatively* normal-pressure (150 to 200 mmH$_2$O) hydrocephalus gradually develops, the enlarged ventricles continue to exert undue force against the tracts in the cerebral white matter. Headache, if present originally, recedes, and there is no papilledema. *A subacutely or slowly developing unsteadiness of gait with shortened steps is the most prominent manifestation,* followed by blunting of the intellect and urinary incontinence. The most commonly recognized causes are the late fibrosing effects of meningeal inflammation and subarachnoid hemorrhage from trauma or ruptured aneurysm. Intraventricular tumors and meningeal carcinomatosis are less common causes. Most often, however, a cause cannot be established. The CT and MRI scans show disproportionate enlargement of the lateral ventricles in comparison to the degree of cortical atrophy (Fig. 30-2), although this may be difficult to judge.

FIG. 30-2 CT scan of a patient with normal-pressure hydrocephalus. There is enlargement of all the ventricles, particularly of the frontal horns of the lateral ventricles *(top),* which is disproportionate to the extent of cortical atrophy *(bottom).* Ventriculoperitoneal shunting resulted in an improvement in gait.

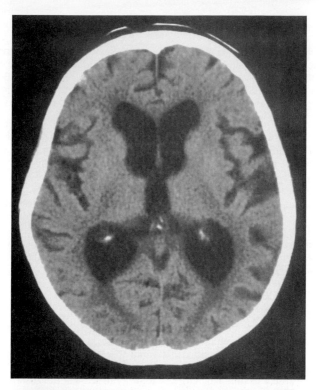

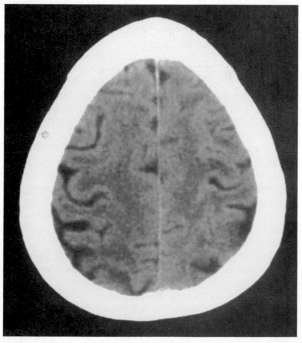

4. *Acute hydrocephalus* With subarachnoid hemorrhage or hemorrhage into the cerebellum, the ventricles may enlarge suddenly and cause coma with small pupils, increased muscle tone in the legs, and bilateral Babinski signs. Milder cases are characterized by drowsiness, laconic responses, and grasp reflexes.

The *treatment* of all forms of persistent symptomatic hydrocephalus is ventriculoatrial or ventriculoperitoneal shunting with a one-way valve, or with temporary external shunting. Lumbar puncture is also a temporizing maneuver if there is no obstruction within the ventricular system. Lumboperitoneal shunts may be used for the treatment of meningeal-obstructive (communicating) hydrocephalus.

The complications of shunting are mechanical shunt failure (obstruction of the valve or tubing or disconnection); infection (septicemia, endocarditis, glomerulonephritis); subdural hematoma formation; and, rarely, "slit-ventricle syndrome," with headaches on standing and low intraventricular pressure. Newer shunt valves with externally programmable pressure settings may reduce the latter complications.

BENIGN INTRACRANIAL HYPERTENSION (PSEUDOTUMOR CEREBRI)

This is a syndrome of obscure origin observed most frequently but not exclusively in obese young women. Over a period of weeks, the patient develops headaches and papilledema in the absence of ventricular enlargement or any other evidence of an intracranial mass lesion. Other neurologic signs are absent or minimal. There is some evidence that the absorption of CSF is impaired, possibly because of raised venous pressure, but no consistent pathophysiology has emerged to explain the illness. Excess vitamin A levels may contribute in some cases and toxic levels of the vitamin have long been known to produce pseudotumor cerebri.

The sustained high CSF pressure, unless controlled, threatens vision and may result in blindness. In some patients, the pressure can be reduced by lumbar punctures repeated every few days or weeks. Gradually the pressure may stabilize at a lower safe level (200 to 250 mmH$_2$O). Weight reduction may also be helpful but is difficult to accomplish. Prednisone (40 to 60 mg/day) or oral hyperosmotic agents such as glycerol (15 to 60 mg qid) or acetazolamide (500 mg bid) may be of short-term value in some cases but should not be depended upon to save failing vision. Patients who do not respond to any of these measures and are threatened with visual loss sometimes respond to lumbar thecoperitoneal shunting, but this procedure is not without risk (mainly infection) and has a high rate of failure due to closure or dislodgement of the shunt. Fenestration of the sheath of one optic nerve is a favored procedure in most centers; it decompresses the nerve locally and appears to have a salutary effect on intracranial pressure, possibly through leakage of CSF, but the long-term results are inconsistent.

In addition to idiopathic pseudotumor cerebri, there are several pseudotumor syndromes in which a cause can be identified: excessive doses of tetracycline and vitamin A in children, lead encephalopathy, hypo- and hyperadrenalism, and withdrawal of corticosteroid treatment. Yet another group of nontumorous cases of raised ICP have a venous basis. Sagittal and lateral sinus thromboses are known to increase intracranial pressure without enlarging the ventricles and are, in effect, instances of symptomatic pseudo-tumor. These cases can be visualized by angiography or magnetic resonance venography (MRV). Hypertensive encephalopathy, large arteriovenous malformations, hypercarbia from chronic lung disease, and occasionally heart failure are other uncommon causes.

INTRACRANIAL HYPOTENSION

The most frequent cause is lumbar puncture, which allows persistent leakage of CSF. Upon sitting or standing, which increases the negative intracranial pressure, a generalized headache develops within minutes, accompanied by pain and stiffness of the neck and sometimes by nausea and vomiting. Sixth nerve palsy (lateral rectus) and a self-audible venous bruit occur in a few patients. The most characteristic feature is relief of these symptoms by recumbency. The leak stops after a few days (occasionally longer). In recalcitrant cases, the injection of several milliliters of autologous blood into the spinal epidural space closes the leak and relieves symptoms (blood patch).

A syndrome of spontaneous intracranial hypotension may follow a strain or hurtful fall, or it may have no discernible explanation. The CSF may contain a few white blood cells, and the craniospinal meninges enhance with gadolinium on MRI. If the site of leakage is found to be in the spinal arachnoid, a blood patch may hasten recovery. A similar syndrome may occur in patients with ventricular shunts; usually the valve pressure setting is too low, and readjustment of the pressure setting relieves the symptoms.

For a more detailed discussion of this topic, see Victor and Ropper: *Adams and Victor's Principles of Neurology*, 7th ed, pp 655–675.

ADDITIONAL READING

Adams RD, Fisher CM, Hakim S, et al: Symptomatic occult hydrocephalus with "normal" cerebrospinal fluid pressure: A treatable syndrome. *N Engl J Med* 273:117, 1965.

Black PM: Idiopathic normal pressure hydrocephalus: Results of shunting in 62 patients. *J Neurosurg* 53:371, 1980.

Corbett JJ, Thompson HS: The rational management of idiopathic intracranial hypertension. *Arch Neurol* 46:1049, 1989.

Fisher CM: Hydrocephalus as a cause of disturbances of gait in the elderly. *Neurology* 32:1358, 1982.

Fishman RA: *Cerebrospinal Fluid in Diseases of the Nervous System*, 2nd ed. Philadelphia, Saunders, 1992.

Foley J: Benign forms of intracranial hypertension—"Toxic" and "otitic" hydrocephalus. *Brain* 78:1, 1955.

Ropper AH: Treatment of intracranial hypertension, in *Neurological and Neurosurgical Intensive Care*, 3rd ed. New York, Raven, 1993, pp 29–52.

Schievink WI, Meyer FB, Atkinson JL, Mokri B: Spontaneous spinal cerebrospinal fluid leaks and intracranial hypotension. *J Neurosurg* 84:598, 1996.

Cerebral neoplasms are of two main types: (1) *primary tumors*, made up of astrocytes, oligodendrocytes, ependymocytes (together called *gliomas*), and special arachnoidal fibroblasts (*meningiomas*); neuroblasts-medulloblasts; and pineocytes; and (2) *secondary tumors*, which are metastatic carcinomas from lung, breast, etc., and lymphomas. The second type is more common in general practice and brain lymphoma has become particularly frequent, in large part because of its association with AIDS. All of these tumors cause symptoms by infiltrating, displacing, and compressing brain tissue and by provoking seizures. Cerebral neoplasms need to be distinguished from *hamartomas*, which are tumor-like formations that have their basis in maldevelopment and undergo no significant growth. A diversity of intracranial tumors have been classed as hamartomas—lesions of tuberous sclerosis, the central lesions of neurofibromatosis, teratomas of the pineal gland, suprasellar craniopharyngiomas, certain vascular malformations, lipomas, and cholesteatomas. Well-differentiated neurons do not become neoplastic.

Etiology

Little is known about causation. Familial occurrence is low but not insignificant, notably in tumors that are associated with neurofibromatosis, tuberous sclerosis, von Hippel–Lindau disease, and carotid body tumors. It was formerly thought that most glial tumors were derived from primitive nerve and glial cells, but it is now generally accepted that neoplastic transformation can occur in relatively mature elements. The age of the patient is also a factor; medulloblastoma, pilocytic astrocytoma, pinealoma, optic glioma, and brainstem glioma are essentially tumors of childhood. Certain viruses (e.g., the Epstein-Barr virus) appear to have the capacity to transform the cellular genome from its normal reproductive cycle into an unrestrained replicative cycle (oncogenes). This mechanism has been implicated in lymphomas of the brain.

A number of genetic aberrations are found in primary cerebral tumors (particularly of the p53 gene) but it is likely that these are secondary changes. Certain mutations, however, appear to be directly responsible for tumor genesis (e.g., the RB retinoblastoma gene).

Classification Intracranial tumors are classified according to the types of cells that constitute the nervous system and its coverings. The frequency of the different types is indicated in Table 31-1. Of these tumors, the most common are derived from glial cells (astrocytes, oligodendrocytes, and microglia); others arise from ependymal cells. The most common of this group are *astrocytic tumors (gliomas)*, categorized as astrocytoma, anaplastic astrocytoma, and glioblastoma multiforme. In modern classifications

TABLE 31-1 Types of Intracranial Tumor in the Combined Series
of Zülch, Cushing, and Olivecrona, Expressed in Percentage
of Total (Approximately 15,000 Cases)

Tumor	Percentage of total
Gliomas*	
Glioblastoma multiforme	20
Astrocytoma	10
Ependymoma	6
Medulloblastoma	4
Oligodendroglioma	5
Meningioma	15
Pituitary adenoma	7
Neurinoma (schwannoma)	7
Metastatic carcinoma[†]	6
Craniopharyngioma, dermoid, epidermoid, teratoma	4
Angiomas	4
Sarcomas	4
Unclassified (mostly gliomas)	5
Miscellaneous (pinealoma, chordoma, lymphoma)[‡]	3
	100

*In children, the proportions differ: astrocytoma, 48%; medulloblastoma,
44%; ependymoma, 8%.
[†]In autopsy series from general hospitals, 20 to 50% of tumors are metastatic.
[‡]Incidence of lymphoma has increased markedly since these series were
collected, largely because of their association with AIDS.

favored by neuropathologists these are denoted as grades 1, 2, and 3. The
higher grade represents an increased growth potential (degree of nuclear
atypia, cellularity, mitoses, and vascular changes) and poorer prognosis. The
glioblastomas (Fig. 31-2) are set apart from high-grade (anaplastic) astrocy-
tomas (Fig. 31-3) by the added features of vascular proliferation resulting in
hemorrhage and necrosis and on the basis of earlier age of onset and greater
malignancy. The cells of a diffusely infiltrating type of glioma, called
gliomatosis cerebri, do not conform to any one of the conventional classes.

Ependymomas are subdivided by cell type into cellular, myxopapillary,
clear-cell, and mixed types; anaplastic myxopapillary tumor and the
subependymoma are given separate status.

Meningiomas (Fig. 31-4) are classified on the basis of their cytoarchitec-
ture and genetic origin into three categories: the common meningothelial or
syncytial type, the anaplastic or malignant type, and atypical forms. Tumors
of the pineal gland comprise pineocytomas, pineoblastomas, and embryonal
forms. The *medulloblastoma* is classified with other tumors of presumed
neuroectodermal origin, namely the neuroblastomas, retinoblastomas, and
ependymoblastomas. Tumors of cranial and peripheral nerves are believed
to differentiate into three types: schwannomas, neurofibromas, and neurofi-
brosarcomas. Given separate status are intracranial midline germ-cell
tumors, such as germinoma, teratoma, choriocarcinoma, and endodermal
sinus carcinoma. A miscellaneous group comprises lymphoma, hemangioblastoma, chordoma, hemangiopericytoma, and ganglioneuroma.

Pathophysiology

As a group, the *gliomas* arise in one or a few foci in the cerebral white matter, central gray matter, brainstem, or cerebellum. Their borders are ill defined, and only rarely can they be completely excised. The well-differentiated tumor cells of an astrocytoma and oligodendroglioma infiltrate and displace the normal cells and myelinated fibers. Undifferentiated glial cells (glioblastoma multiforme) proliferate more rapidly, often outstripping their blood supply and becoming necrotic and hemorrhagic in places. They are among the most malignant tumors with which humans are afflicted.

With tumor growth there is compression of venules in the adjacent cerebral white matter and a disruption of the blood-brain barrier. Plasma proteins seep into the cerebral white matter, causing *vasogenic* or *localized cerebral edema*. This is evidenced by increased protein levels in the cerebrospinal fluid (CSF), decreased attenuation on computed tomography (CT), and an increase in T2 and FLAIR signal intensity in MR images. Edematous brain may initially cause few or no symptoms except in relation to its mass effect and the distortion and displacement of other central brain structures.

As the mass in the cerebrum or cerebellum increases in size, intracranial pressure rises and adjacent normal brain is displaced. Because of the compartmentalization of the cranial cavity by sheaths of dura (falx, tentorium), pressure from a mass in one compartment causes a shift of brain tissue into another compartment, where the pressure is lower (Fig. 31-1). The deficits produced by these displacements, which appear late in the course of tumor growth, are added to those of the tumor itself. Summarized below are the main features of these secondary effects, commonly referred to as herniations, of which the temporal lobe–tentorial, cerebellar–foramen magnum, and subfalcial are the most common. (See Chap. 17.)

Lateral displacement of the temporal lobe and transtentorial herniation
These displace the thalamus and upper midbrain, causing drowsiness and stupor, and force the medial part of the temporal lobe (including the uncus) medially and downward through the tentorial opening. The cerebral peduncle opposite the mass may be pressed against the margin of the tentorium (Kernohan-Woltman phenomenon), causing hemiparesis and a Babinski sign ipsilateral to the mass. Most of the associated signs can be accounted for by lateral displacement of deep structures. The ipsilateral oculomotor nerve may be compressed, resulting in pupillary enlargement, and one or both posterior cerebral arteries may be occluded, with occipital lobe infarction, and, in the terminal stages, secondary (Duret) hemorrhages form in the midbrain and upper pons.

Centrally placed cerebral masses may compress the deep structures from above and depress the upper brainstem below the plane of the tentorium (*central herniation*). Drowsiness, stupor, and coma, with small symmetrical pupils and cyclic breathing, result.

Cerebellum–foramen magnum herniation The medulla and inferomesial parts of the cerebellum (mainly the tonsils) are thrust downward into the cervical canal by a posterior fossa or central cerebral mass. Stiff neck may be an early sign, progressing to decerebrate posturing, coma, respiratory irregularity, and finally respiratory arrest.

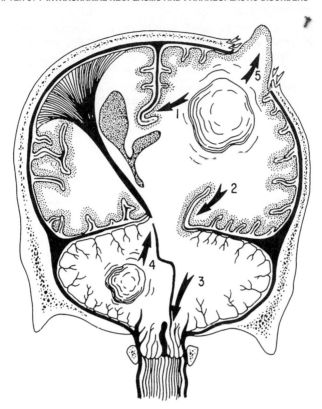

FIG. 31-1   Brain herniations. 1, The cingulate gyrus is displaced under the falx, toward the opposite side. 2, The inferomedial parts of the temporal lobe are forced into the posterior fossa through the tentorial opening, alongside the brainstem. 3, The cerebellar tonsils are pressed into the foramen magnum, displacing the medulla caudally. Less common: 4, Upward herniation of the cerebellum, through the tentorial opening, and 5, transcalvarial herniation.

Subfalcial herniation   The medial part of one cerebral hemisphere, mostly the cingulate gyrus, is pushed contralaterally under the falx, sometimes compressing the anterior cerebral artery and causing infarction of the medial frontal lobe. This effect is more readily recognized with MRI and arteriography than from its clinical manifestations.

CLINICAL MANIFESTATIONS

In general, patients with brain tumors are likely to present clinically in one of three ways:

1. A generalized cerebral disorder (mental impairment, headaches), seizures (focal or generalized), and slowly worsening focal neurologic signs (aphasia, hemiparesis, etc.), occurring singly or in various combinations

2. With evidence of increased ICP (headache, vomiting, drowsiness, papilledema) as a result of the mass or of meningeal spread (carcinomatous meningitis)
3. By one of several specific intracranial tumor syndromes

The intracranial tumors that are most likely to cause each of these syndromes, along with their main clinical features, are summarized in Tables 31-2 to 31-4 and shown in Figs. 31-2 to 31-5. Special diagnostic procedures and treatment are considered separately.

Diagnostic Tests

CT scanning and MRI demonstrate virtually all intracranial tumors and should be the initial investigative procedures when the patient exhibits progressive symptoms or signs of diffuse or focal cerebral disease or one of the specific tumor syndromes. Occasionally, it is difficult to distinguish a tumor from an abscess or other process. Plain films of the chest and other routine studies should always be obtained to help rule out metastatic disease, which may present as single or multiple brain nodules. Examination of the CSF may disclose tumor cells or related chemical markers in cases of meningeal carcinomatosis, but the test is not routinely performed in patients with a large brain mass. In general, a histologic diagnosis by biopsy is required. The main distinction to be made is from an infectious mass (abscess).

Treatment

Surface tumors such as meningiomas and acoustic neuromas are amenable to complete surgical removal. Meningiomas of the base of the brain (sphenoid wing, olfactory groove, tuberculum sellae, and posterior fossa) may infiltrate bone and can be excised only partially. Radiation therapy is then added.

For gliomas, the common practice is biopsy with partial excision, radiation therapy up to 5000 cGy over 3 to 4 weeks, and, in selected cases, antitumor drug therapy. In the case of glioblastoma multiforme, this regimen prolongs useful life by only several months. Dexamethasone is used to control cerebral edema.

Primary cerebral lymphoma may be treated with intravenous methotrexate and may respond for a variable time to radiation therapy. Corticosteroids effect a marked but brief improvement in the clinical state and the radiologic appearance of the tumor—this itself may be diagnostically helpful. In patients with AIDS, there is often difficulty in determining whether a cerebral lesion is a primary lymphoma or a toxoplasmal abscess; antibody tests and treatment of the latter with antimicrobial drugs usually settle the question.

Special therapeutic skill is demanded if the dire effects of radiation damage to arteries, brain, cranial nerves, and pituitary gland are to be avoided. Each of the antineoplastic drugs also has its neurotoxic complications (see *Adams and Victor's Principles of Neurology*, 7th ed., and Additional Reading).

Tumors that cause hydrocephalus or a specific regional syndrome require a special combination of surgical and radiation therapy.

TABLE 31-2 Tumors Presenting with Impairment of Mental Function, Headaches, Seizures, or Focal Neurologic Signs: Increased Intracranial Pressure a Late Development

Glioblastoma multiforme and anaplastic astrocytoma (Fig. 31-2)	20% of all intracranial tumors, 55% of all gliomas; mainly cerebral but may affect all parts of brain and cord, widely infiltrative; survival about 12 months in most cases
Astrocytomas (low grade; Fig. 31-3)	25–30% of cerebral gliomas; in adults, common sites are cerebral hemispheres; in children, brainstem and cerebellum; slowly growing, tendency to form cysts; survival for many years
Oligodendroglioma	5–7% of intracranial gliomas; frontal lobes are most common sites; slowly growing; survival for many years if low-grade; may calcify; often mixed with astrocytoma; chemotherapy responsive
Ependymoma	Common sites are fourth ventricle (particularly in children), conus medullaris, and filum terminale; survival depends on degree of anaplasia
Meningioma (Fig. 31-4)	15% of all primary intracranial tumors; highest incidence in seventh decade; more frequent in women; common sites are sylvian region, superior parasagittal surfaces, olfactory groove, lesser wing of sphenoid, tuberculum sellae, cerebellopontine angle, spinal canal; very slow growing; symptoms depend on tumor site; amenable to surgical removal
Primary cerebral lymphoma (Fig. 31-5)	May arise in any part of the brain (monofocal or multifocal), often near ventricles, usually in adult life; lymphocytes, mononuclear and tumor cells often found in CSF; immunosuppressed patients at risk, particularly those with AIDS; median survival less than 30 months; treated with corticosteroids, radiation, and methotrexate
Metastatic carcinoma	Three main patterns; (1) *brain*, one or several cerebral or other foci, from lung, breast, melanoma, colon, kidney; (2) *skull and dura*, from carcinoma of breast and prostate, and multiple myeloma; may compress spinal cord, cranial nerves, and pituitary; (3) *meningeal* carcinomatosis or leukemic infiltration of leptomeninges and cranial and spinal nerve roots; average survival 3 months with meningeal carcinomatosis; patients with bony metastases survive longer

TABLE 31-3 Tumors Causing Mainly Increased Intracranial Pressure and Hydrocephalus, Focal or Lateralizing Signs Less Conspicuous

Medulloblastoma and cystic astrocytoma of cerebellum	Mainly in children 4 to 8 years; begins with listlessness, vomiting, headaches; later, squint, ataxic gait, falling, and papilledema
Ependymoma and papilloma of choroid plexus	Clinical syndrome similar to medulloblastoma but more protracted; two-thirds of patients present with increased ICP, others with vomiting, dysphagia, paresthesias of extremities, vertigo, head tilt
Hemangioblastoma of cerebellum (von Hippel–Lindau disease)	Dominant inheritance; retinal angioma and polycythemia often conjoined; may also develop multiple spinal cord lesions and syringomyelia
Pinealoma (includes pineal germinoma and teratoma)	Onset in adolescence and adulthood; symptoms and signs of increased ICP; paralysis of upward gaze and pupils fixed to light (Parinaud syndrome)
Colloid (paraphysial) cyst of third ventricle	Signs of intermittent or persistent increased ICP (headache) and hydrocephalus
Craniopharyngioma	In children and adolescents, delayed sexual maturation and growth, diabetes insipidus combined with visual loss from chiasmatic–optic nerve lesions; in adults, visual loss, signs of hydrocephalus, mild corticospinal and hypothalamic signs
Gliomatosis cerebri	Diffuse infiltration of cerebral hemispheres, spreading across corpus callosum; apathy, dementia, late focal frontal signs

PARANEOPLASTIC DISORDERS

This is a group of neurologic disorders that occur without invasion or compression of the nervous system by tumor in patients with carcinoma or other types of neoplasia. Presumably, tumors that induce these effects elaborate enzymes, hormones, or antibodies or dispose the patient to a viral agent capable of invading or cross-reacting with the nervous system. Several antibodies have been identified that are diagnostic of these disorders and some of these are pathogenic. The antibodies most often associated with certain syndromes are noted below. It should be emphasized that these neurologic syndromes are often identified before the primary cancer becomes evident. The most familiar of these remote effects and the chapters in which they are discussed are listed below:

1. *Polyneuropathy* This most often takes the form of a subacute distal sensory loss and hyporeflexia (Chap. 46). Lung cancer underlies most cases and the anti-Hu antibody is frequently detected in the serum. One variant seen with lymphoma and occasionally other cancers is a *sensory ganglionopathy (neuronopathy)* that causes ataxia and a rapid loss of all forms of sensation in the trunk and limbs.

TABLE 31-4 Distinctive Tumor Syndromes: Local Signs Predominate and General Cerebral Deficits and Increased ICP Are Late or Absent

Acoustic neuroma (schwannoma)	Usually solitary; may be part of neurofibromatosis, either solitary (type I) or bilateral (type II, autosomal dominant); unilateral neurosensory deafness, loss of balance, later facial weakness and loss of sensation, ataxia of ipsilateral limbs and gait and raised intracranial pressure
Carotid body tumor	Painless mass at bifurcation of common carotid, below angle of jaw; grows slowly; compresses cranial nerves IX to XII and sympathetic nerves; rarely familial and bilateral

Pituitary adenomas (with enlarged sella, rule out empty-sella syndrome by CT-MRI). See also page 224.

Prolactinomas (usually achromatic chromophobe, sometimes acidophilic adenoma)	Increased incidence with age; headache, bitemporal hemianopia, or mixed chiasmatic–optic nerve changes; sella turcica expands; hypothyroidism, hypoadrenalism; in females, amenorrhea, galactorrhea, serum prolactin increased (>100 ng/mL); in males, impotence
Acromegaly-gigantism (eosinophilic adenoma)	Oversecretion of growth hormone (GH); before closure of the epiphyses, gigantism; after closure, acromegaly
Cushing disease (basophil or nonbasophil adenoma)	Oversecretion of ACTH; sella not enlarged; truncal obesity, striae, hirsutism; hypertension; glycosuria; amenorrhea; osteoporosis; proximal muscle weakness; mental changes
Meningioma of sphenoid ridge	Mainly in women, average age 50 years; unilateral exophthalmos, slight temporal bulge, anosmia, ocular palsies, monocular blindness
Meningioma of olfactory groove	Older adults; anosmia and frontal lobe signs; high CSF protein
Meningioma of tuberculum sellae	Older adults, mainly women; bitemporal hemianopia with normal-sized sella
Glioma of brainstem	Onset mainly in childhood; progressive cranial nerve and long tract signs; increased ICP late; prognosis varies with degree of anaplasia
Glioma of optic nerve and chiasm	Mainly in children and adolescents, sometimes with neurofibromatosis; progressive loss of vision with optic atrophy or chiasmal field defect
Chordoma	Common sites are clivus and sacrococcygeal region; cauda equina syndrome or successive multiple cranial nerve signs, with conduction deafness, facial pain, and ataxia
Nasopharyngeal or sinus tumors	Multiple upper cranial nerve abnormalities; nasopharyngeal mass; erosion base of skull
Tumors of foramen magnum	Pain in occiput and posterior neck; combination of lower cranial nerve, cervical cord, and cerebellar signs

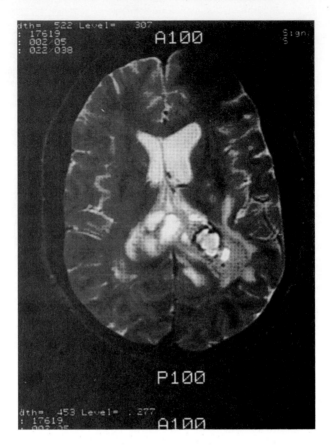

FIG. 31-2 Malignant astrocytoma (glioblastoma multiforme). T2-weighted MRI illustrates a large tumor deep within the left cerebral hemisphere and extending through the corpus callosum to the right hemisphere. The black rim around a portion of the tumor represents hemorrhage. The patient was a 59-year-old male who presented with seizures.

2. *Polymyositis* and *dermatomyositis* These inflammatory diseases of muscle are usually idiopathic, but cancer is associated in some cases, mostly those with dermatomyositis (Chap. 49). The syndrome is one of progressive proximal weakness and elevated serum CK concentration. There is no identifiable antibody.

3. *Myasthenic syndrome of Lambert and Eaton* Lung cancer underlies most cases. Weakness of muscle contraction affecting mainly the proximal limb muscles, diminished reflexes, and autonomic features characterize this syndrome (Chap. 53). On electromyography (EMG), the finding of an incremental response to repetitive stimulation of muscle (the opposite of what occurs in myasthenia gravis) is diagnostic. The presence of anti-

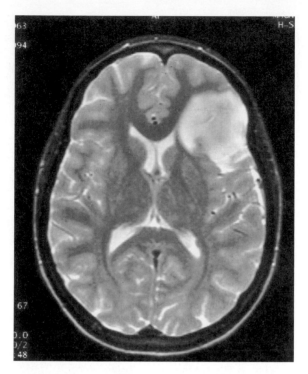

FIG. 31-3   Astrocytoma of the left frontal lobe; the T2-weighted MRI shows an infiltrating tumor with minimal mass effect and slight edema. The degree of enhancement of these tumors varies.

bodies against calcium channels of the presynaptic muscle membrane is the underlying pathophysiologic abnormality.

4. *Cerebellar degeneration*   This is a relatively common paraneoplastic disease. It is characterized by subacute ataxia that becomes quite severe and disabling. Mainly it occurs with ovarian and breast cancer, and over half of the cases are associated with anti-Purkinje cell antibodies, called anti-Yo, in the serum. The *opsoclonus-myoclonus syndrome* is highly characteristic of childhood neuroblastoma but may be found in adults with lung and other cancers, particularly breast cancer, in which case the anti-Ri antibody is often found.

5. *Brainstem* and *"limbic" (medial temporal) encephalitis*   These are focal inflammatory processes characterized by confusion and memory loss and associated with various types of systemic neoplasms. Limbic encephalitis appears most often with breast cancer and the anti-Hu antibody mentioned earlier. Lesions in the brainstem produce a variety of syndromes, often with early oculomotor signs. The anti-Hu antibody or, in the case of testicular and other cancers, the newly described anti-Ma antibody

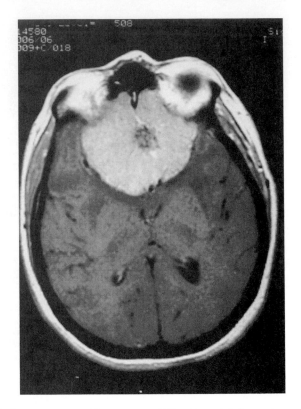

FIG. 31-4   Meningioma. T1 sequence MRI with gadolinium enhancement showing a large subfrontal mass with central calcification and prominent surrounding vasogenic edema.

may be detected; these syndromes can coexist and may be associated with paraneoplastic sensory neuropathy.

6. *Necrotizing myelopathy* and *motor neuronopathy* These are quite rare syndromes of obscure nature, associated with several types of cancers. The first of these needs to be differentiated from an intramedullary spinal cord metastasis, which is more common; the latter resembles amyotrophic lateral sclerosis.

For a more detailed discussion of this topic, see Victor and Ropper: *Adams and Victor's Principles of Neurology*, 7th ed, pp 676–733.

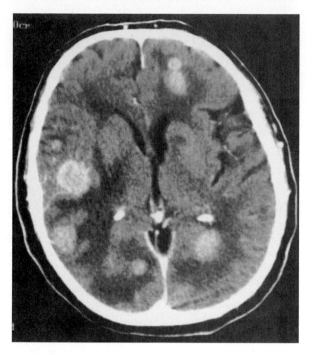

FIG. 31-5 Contrast-enhanced CT scan showing multiple metastases from bronchogenic carcinoma. Each lesion is surrounded by edema.

ADDITIONAL READING

Dawson DM: Antineoplastic drugs, in Asbury AK, McKhann GM, McDonald WI (eds): *Diseases of the Nervous System*, 2nd ed. Philadelphia, Saunders, 1992, pp 1121–1129.

DeAngelis LM: Current management of primary central nervous system lymphoma. *Oncology* 9:63, 1995.

DeAngelis LM: Brain tumors. *N Engl J Med* 344:114, 2001.

Glantz MJ, Rottenberg DA: Harmful effects of radiation on the nervous system, in Asbury AK, McKhann GM, McDonald WI (eds): *Diseases of the Nervous System*, 2nd ed. Philadelphia, Saunders, 1992, pp 1130–1143.

Henson RA, Urich H: *Cancer and the Nervous System*. Oxford, UK, Blackwell, 1982.

Levine AJ, Schmidek HH (eds): *Molecular Genetics of Nervous System Tumors*. New York, Wiley-Liss, 1993, pp 357–369.

Posner JP: *Neurologic Complications of Cancer*. Philadelphia, FA Davis, 1995.

Russell DS, Rubinstein LJ: *Pathology of Tumors of the Nervous System*, 5th ed. Baltimore, Williams & Wilkins, 1989.

Bacterial, Spirochetal, Fungal, and Parasitic Infections of the Nervous System, and Sarcoidosis

BACTERIAL INFECTIONS

The most important members of this group of diseases, in decreasing order of their frequency, are meningitis, brain abscess, subdural empyema, dural sinus septic thrombophlebitis, and focal bacterial encephalitis. In all of these and other conditions, bacteria reach the brain in one of several ways: by hematogenous spread (i.e., septicemia or infected emboli), extension from infected cranial structures (ears, sinuses, osteomyelitic foci), penetrating cranial injuries, or surgical invasion.

Bacterial Meningitis

This is a bacterial infection of the pia and arachnoid and the cerebrospinal fluid (CSF) that they enclose. Since the subarachnoid space is continuous around the brain, spinal cord, and optic nerves, an infective agent (or blood or tumor cells) gaining entry to any part of the space spreads to all of it. Thus *meningitis is always cerebrospinal*. Infection also reaches the ventricles and their ependymal lining by reflux from the subarachnoid space. All structures bathed by the CSF—ependyma, choroid plexuses, intra-arachnoidal portions of the cranial and spinal nerves, cerebral and cerebellar cortices, and surface veins and arteries—are exposed to the meningeal infection.

Epidemiology Streptococcus pneumoniae, Neisseria meningitidis, *Haemophilus influenzae*, and *Listeria monocytogenes*—the most common bacteria causing meningitis—have a worldwide distribution and a more or less even incidence throughout the year. Meningococcal meningitis tends to occur in epidemics, in roughly 10-year cycles. This form of meningitis is most frequent in children and adolescents but can occur throughout adult life. *H. influenzae* meningitis affects mainly children between the ages of 2 months and 5 years but is being reported increasingly in adults over 50 years of age; its incidence in children is diminishing in developed countries as a result of vaccination programs. Pneumococcal meningitis predominates in the very young and old and has a predilection for patients with sickle cell anemia and those who have had a skull fracture or splenectomy. *Escherichia coli*, *Staphylococcus aureus*, group A streptococci, *Klebsiella*, *Pseudomonas*, *Proteus*, and *Listeria monocytogenes* are associated with immunodeficiency states, trauma, and neurosurgical procedures, including ventricular shunts.

Pathogenesis and pathology The usual routes by which bacteria reach the meninges have been indicated above.

Once bacteria enter the CSF, they excite an acute inflammatory reaction, mainly in the vascular pia. Hyperemia, exudation of blood proteins, and migration of neutrophils occur within hours. This exudate continues to accumulate for the next few days. Thereafter, lymphocytes and then plasma cells begin to appear in the pia as part of an immune response. Veins in the pia may thrombose and cause brain infarction. As the meningeal exudate blocks the subarachnoid space around the brainstem and the foramina of Luschka and Magendie, tension hydrocephalus develops. There is also an ependymitis at an aqueductal level, which may contribute to the obstruction of CSF flow. Cranial nerve roots, as they pass through purulent exudate in the subarachnoid space, may be involved. Although the brain is not invaded by bacteria, their endotoxins diffuse through the pia and along the Virchow-Robin spaces and excite a subpial edema and even a superficial focal noninflammatory necrosis. The thin arachnoid, especially in infants, may be transgressed, with development of a subdural inflammatory reaction and a sterile hygroma (see further on). If the meningitis is not treated successfully, arteritis and thrombosis, cerebral infarction, and hydrocephalus may result.

Clinical features Fever, severe headache and neck stiffness, generalized convulsions, and various degrees of drowsiness and confusion sometimes progressing to coma are the usual manifestations in adults and older children. Seizures occur more often in infants and young children. Signs of meningeal irritation—stiffness of the neck on forward flexion, with flexion of the knees and hips (Brudzinski sign) and inability to completely extend the legs (Kernig sign)—become evident. In infants and newborns, in whom meningitis is often lethal, the infection expresses itself by fever and bulging of the fontanels, vomiting, drowsiness, and, in some instances, convulsions; stiff neck may not be evident.

Certain clinical clues may indicate the type of meningitis:

1. Petechial and purpuric rash and circulatory collapse—meningococcal meningitis with Waterhouse-Friderichsen syndrome (a similar rash may be seen with certain enteroviral infections)
2. Ventriculoatrial or peritoneal shunt, cranial trauma, or neurosurgical procedure—coagulase-negative *Staphylococcus* or other nosocomial organisms
3. Upper respiratory and ear infections in children—*H. influenzae*
4. Immunocompromised host—*Strep. pneumoniae*, *L. monocytogenes*, *E. coli*, mycobacteria
5. Infection of ears, sinuses, lung, heart valves in adults—*Strep. pneumoniae* or mixed infections, including anaerobic organisms

Ancillary examinations The one indispensable laboratory procedure is lumbar puncture (LP) and examination of the spinal fluid. The CSF is usually under increased pressure (200 to 400 mmH$_2$O); is cloudy, owing to the presence of cells, mainly polymorphonuclear (a few hundred, or even less, up to 10,000 per mm^3); and contains bacteria seen on Gram stain, increased protein (100 to 500 mg/dL), and decreased glucose (<40 mg/dL or <40 percent of the blood glucose, which should be measured simultaneously). The fluid needs to be cultured. The CSF latex agglutination tests and the polymerase chain reaction (PCR) for detection of bacterial antigens are especially useful in cases of partially treated meningitis. Also, throat and blood cultures and a chest film should be obtained. The peripheral white blood cells are increased with a shift to the left.

Similarly, computed tomography (CT) and magnetic resonance imaging (MRI) can be performed to exclude brain abscess and subdural empyema. Actually, brain abscess rarely complicates meningitis. In infants, ultrasound examination is preferred for the detection of subdural empyema (see below) or sterile effusion because anesthesia is not required.

Treatment *Acute bacterial meningitis is a medical emergency.* Every hour of delay in starting antibacterial therapy increases the risk of complications and permanent neurologic residua. Treatment with broad-spectrum antibiotics should be started immediately after the LP, while identification of the organism is awaited. In Tables 32-1, 32-2, and 32-3 are listed the recommended antibiotics at each age and the dosages for different types of meningitis. LP pressure above 400 mmH$_2$O warns of cerebellar herniation and requires treatment with mannitol. The administration of dexamethasone to children with meningitis reduces the incidence of deafness. Antibiotic treatment should continue for 10 to 14 days. Persistent and recurrent subdural hygromas usually respond to repeated aspiration or shunting.

Preventive measures should not be neglected. All household contacts of patients with meningitis, particularly children, should receive rifampin, 10 mg/kg every 12 h by mouth daily for 2 days. Immunization against *Neisseria meningitidis* is effective and should be given during epidemics. Children after 2 months of age should be vaccinated against *H. influenzae* with the new protein-conjugate vaccine.

Bacterial Encephalitis

In acute and subacute bacterial endocarditis (SBE), the brain is seeded with bacteria-laden emboli; in subacute endocarditis, the bacteria are characteristically of low virulence and do not produce brain abscesses. Instead, sterile meningeal reactions and small infarcts, some with blood in the CSF, are the usual complications; mycotic aneurysms may form but are rare. The emboli of acute bacterial endocarditis give rise to miliary abscesses, infarcts, small hemorrhages, and bacterial meningitis; large abscesses are rare. Treatment in both acute and subacute types is directed to the endocarditis and septicemia.

Legionnaires' disease as well as infections due to *Mycoplasma pneumoniae* and *L. monocytogenes* may cause a more generalized direct infection of the brain—strictly speaking, a bacterial encephalitis, the nature of which is poorly understood. The clinical picture may be one of a confusional state, seizures, brain swelling, cerebellar ataxia, or, in the case of *Listeria*, lower cranial nerve palsies coupled with meningitis (rhomboencephalitis). Lyme disease probably belongs in this category as well (see p. 280).

Subdural Empyema

This is a purulent infection of the subdural space, stemming usually from disease of the frontal or ethmoid sinuses or middle ears and mastoid cells. Pus accumulates over one cerebral hemisphere (occasionally interhemi-

TABLE 32-1 Empiric Therapy of Bacterial Meningitis

Age of patient	Antimicrobial therapy*
0–4 weeks	Cefotaxime plus ampicillin
4–12 weeks	Third-generation cephalosporin plus ampicillin (plus dexamethasone)
3 months–18 years	Third-generation cephalosporin plus vancomycin (±ampicillin)
18–50 years	Third-generation cephalosporin plus vancomycin (±ampicillin)
>50 years	Third-generation cephalosporin plus vancomycin plus ampicillin
Immunocompromised state	Vancomycin plus ampicillin and ceftazidime
Basilar skull fracture	Third-generation cephalosporin plus vancomycin
Head trauma; neurosurgery	Vancomycin plus ceftazidime
CSF shunt	Vancomycin plus ceftazidime

*For all ages from 3 months onward, an alternative treatment is meropenem plus vancomycin. For severe penicillin allergy consider: vancomycin and chloramphenicol (for meningococcus) and trimethoprim/sulfamethoxazole (for *Listeria*). A high failure rate has been reported with chloramphenicol in patients with drug-resistant pneumococcus.

spherically). The arachnoid prevents organisms from entering the subarachnoid space in sufficient numbers to induce a bacterial meningitis. There is, however, a polymorphonuclear pleocytosis (50 to 1000 cells per mm^3) and an elevated CSF protein; the glucose is normal. Meningeal veins that underlie the empyema become thrombosed and give rise to cortical infarction, which is the cause of the cerebral symptoms.

Diagnosis is based on the presence of a known sinus or ear infection, generalized headache and fever, rapid accession of focal seizures, hemiparesis, hemisensory loss and aphasia, and a sterile CSF under increased pressure. CT and MRI disclose the extracerebral accumulation of pus.

Treatment consists of surgical drainage and administration of large doses of broad-spectrum antibiotics (20 to 24 million units of penicillin per day plus a third-generation cephalosporin and metronidazole, modified according to bacteriologic findings).

Cranial Extradural Abscess

This is usually a complication of osteomyelitis of a cranial bone. Local pain and tenderness, purulent discharge from an ear or sinus, palsies of cranial nerves V and VI (Gradenigo syndrome), and a normal CSF (except for a few cells) are the usual manifestations. *Staph. aureus* is the most common agent. An intensive course of antibiotics and, later, surgical removal of the infected bone are the recommended therapeutic measures.

Spinal epidural abscess is considered in Chap. 44.

TABLE 32-2 Recommended Dosages of Antimicrobial Agents for
Bacterial Meningitis in Adults with Normal Renal and Hepatic Function*

Antimicrobial agent	Total daily dose	Dosing interval, hours
Amikacin[†]	15 mg/kg	8
Ampicillin	12 g	4
Cefotaxime	8–12 g	4–6
Ceftazidime	6 g	8
Ceftriaxone	4 g	12–24
Chloramphenicol[‡]	4–6 g	6
Gentamicin[†]	3–5 mg/kg	8
Nafcillin	9–12 g	4
Oxacillin	9–12 g	4
Penicillin G	24 million units	4
Rifampin[§]	600 mg	24
Tobramycin[†]	3–5 mg/kg	8
Trimethoprim-sulfamethoxazole[¶]	20 mg/kg	6–12
Vancomycin[†‖]	2–3 g	8–12

*Unless indicated, therapy is administered intravenously.
[†]Peak and trough serum concentrations must be monitored.
[‡]Higher dose recommended for pneumococcal meningitis.
[§]Oral administration.
[¶]Dosage based on trimethoprim component.
[‖]CSF concentrations may have to be monitored in severely ill patients.

Septic Intracranial Thrombophlebitis

The *lateral sinus* may become thrombosed in the course of an ear infection and block cerebral venous drainage sufficiently to cause a rise in CSF pressure without enlargement of ventricles. Facial and nasal infections may lead to thrombosis of the anterior part of the *cavernous sinus* on one or both sides, manifest by orbital edema and involvement of cranial nerves III, IV, and VI, ophthalmic division of V, and sometimes, inexplicably, blindness. Thrombosis of the *superior longitudinal (sagittal) sinus* and its draining veins gives rise to headache, seizures, and unilateral or bilateral paralysis, mainly of the legs. In sagittal and lateral sinus thromboses there may be papilledema. The occurrence of these conditions should always be suspected in the presence of some other form of intracranial suppuration—meningitis, sinus or ear infection, subdural empyema, and extradural or brain abscess. Thrombosis of major venous sinuses can often be detected by MRI, which may also demonstrate an area of hemorrhagic infarction adjacent to the occluded sinus. The diagnosis can be corroborated by failure of the superior sagittal or lateral sinuses to fill during the late phase of carotid arteriography.

Treatment In intracranial thrombophlebitis, treatment consists of large doses of antibiotics, after which surgery of the affected ear or sinus may be necessary. The role of anticoagulation, shown to be of some value in aseptic venous occlusion, is still uncertain.

Brain Abscess

The brain is resistant to abscess formation, but this will occur under conditions that cause necrosis of tissue with simultaneous bacterial infection. The

TABLE 32-3 Specific Antimicrobial Therapy for Acute Meningitis

Microorganism	Standard therapy	Alternative therapies
Bacteria		
Haemophilus influenzae		
B-lactamase-negative	Ampicillin	Third-generation cephalosporin*; chloramphenicol
B-lactamase-positive	Third-generation cephalosporin*	Chloramphenicol; cefepime
Neisseria meningitidis	Penicillin G or ampicillin	Third-generation cephalosporin*; chloramphenicol
Streptococcus pneumoniae		
Penicillin MIC <0.1 μg/mL (sensitive)	Penicillin G or ampicillin	Third-generation cephalosporin*; chloramphenicol; vancomycin plus rifampin
Penicillin MIC 0.1–1.0 μg/mL (intermediate sensitivity)	Third-generation cephalosporin*	Vancomycin; meropenem
Penicillin MIC ≥2.0 μg/mL (highly resistant)	Vancomycin plus third-generation cephalosporin	Meropenem
Enterobacteriaceae	Third-generation cephalosporin*	Meropenem; fluoroquinolone; trimethoprim/sulfamethoxazole
Pseudomonas aeruginosa	Ceftazidime[†]	Meropenem; fluoroquinolone[†]
Listeria monocytogenes	Ampicillin or penicillin G[†]	Meropenem; trimethoprim/sulfamethoxazole
Streptococcus agalactiae	Ampicillin or penicillin G[†]	Third-generation cephalosporin*; vancomycin
Staphylococcus aureus		
Methicillin-sensitive	Nafcillin or oxacillin	Vancomycin
Methicillin-resistant	Vancomycin	
Staphylococcus epidermidis	Vancomycin[‡]	

*Cefotaxime or ceftriaxone or cefepime.
[†]Addition of an aminoglycoside should be considered.
[‡]Addition of rifampin should be considered.
Key: MIC = Minimal inhibitory concentration.

275

disease states that are conducive to the formation of brain abscess are chronic pulmonary infections (pneumonitis, bronchiectasis, lung abscess); chronic and recurrent sinusitis, otitis, or mastoiditis; congenital heart disease or pulmonary vascular malformation; distant infection of skin, bone, and kidney; and acute bacterial endocarditis. In a considerable proportion of cases, the source of the abscesses cannot be determined.

The abscess, as it forms over a period of several weeks, passes through several stages—from localized suppurative encephalitis to complete encapsulation. There may be a solitary abscess or several abscesses, depending on the cause. Those secondary to ear and sinus infection are single, with one or more daughter abscesses, and are localized in the part of the brain nearest the source. Thus, with frontal-ethmoidal sinusitis, the abscess tends to form in the frontal lobe; with sphenoid sinusitis, in the frontal or anterior temporal lobe; with otitis media, in the middle or posterior temporal lobe; and with mastoiditis, in the cerebellum.

The most common organisms causing brain abscess are streptococci, many of which are anaerobic or microaerophilic, and staphylococci; these are often found in combination with other anaerobes or with enterobacteria. The special cases of abscess due to toxoplasmosis, fungi, and tuberculosis are considered further on.

Clinical manifestations Headache is the most frequent presenting symptom, followed by drowsiness, confusion, focal or generalized seizures, and focal motor, sensory, visual field, and language disorders. The focal signs vary with the location of the abscess. With frontal abscess, frontal headache, hemiparesis, and unilateral contraversive seizures are the most prominent manifestations; with temporal lobe abscess, frontotemporal headache, upper homonymous quadrantanopia, dysnomia, and other aphasic symptoms if left-sided; and with cerebellar abscess, postauricular headache, ipsilateral ataxia, and paresis of gaze to the side of the lesion with gaze-paretic nystagmus.

In all types of abscess, the CSF pressure is elevated and there is usually a pleocytosis with elevated protein but normal glucose. CT and MRI reveal the lesion(s) as round, contrast "ring" enhancing masses (Fig. 32-1). If the pressure effects are not controlled, temporal lobe–tentorial or cerebellar herniations may terminate life. Ventricular rupture also proves fatal as a rule.

Treatment Bacterial brain abscess in all its forms requires the administration of a combination of ceftriaxone 4 g IV and metronidazole 2 to 4 g daily in divided doses or 20 to 24 million units of penicillin G and 4 to 6 g of chloramphenicol daily IV in divided doses. The initial elevation of intracranial pressure (ICP) is managed by IV mannitol, followed by dexamethasone 6 to 12 mg every 6 h. Early abscess formation and an incipient form, "cerebritis," can be treated by these measures alone, but a subacute or chronic abscess will usually not respond and requires aspiration for precise bacteriologic diagnosis or open surgical drainage. If the abscess is deep, it should be managed by aspiration and local injection of antibiotics, which may have to be repeated, coupled with the IV administration of antibiotics. Multiple abscesses can be treated only by parenteral antibiotics.

Tuberculous Meningitis

Once frequent, the incidence of tuberculous meningitis (and pulmonary tuberculosis) had decreased steadily in recent decades in both the United

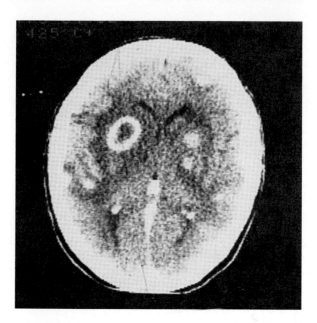

FIG. 32-1   Multiple brain abscesses associated with bacterial endocarditis *(Staphylococcus aureus)* in a 55-year-old man. The large abscess in the left hemisphere shows a characteristic ring enhancement.

States and western Europe. However, since 1985, there has been a dramatic surge in the incidence, which increased at a 16 percent annual rate, compared with an average annual decline of 6 percent in the preceding 30 years. In the past 3 to 4 years, the incidence of tuberculosis has resumed its pre-1985 rate of decline in the United States—attributable to the intensive public health measures undertaken by the Centers for Disease Control. In India, sub-Saharan Africa, parts of Central and South America, and other medically underdeveloped countries, tuberculosis is still very common.

The usual causal agent, *Mycobacterium tuberculosis*, generally reaches the brain via the bloodstream, the bacteremia occurring intermittently with pulmonary tuberculosis. The meningitis may be a manifestation of miliary tuberculosis or may occur in association with one or more tuberculomatous foci in the brain, from which infection spreads to the meninges. Otitic, bowel, renal, or vertebral sources do occur but are rare.

The *pathologic reaction* differs from that of other meningitides in that the meningeal exudate is concentrated at the base of the brain (its undersurface), and there are myriads of small tubercles (foci of caseation, epithelioid cells, and Langhans giant cells) on the meninges and external surface of the brain and ependyma. Hydrocephalus is usually present. Brain infarction is relatively frequent because of meningeal arteritis.

Clinical and laboratory features Fever, headache, confusion, and lethargy evolve less acutely than in other forms of bacterial meningitis, and cranial nerve palsies are more frequent. Occasionally, the disease presents with some focal cerebral sign or seizure or with signs of increased ICP.

The CSF formula is diagnostic: Increased pressure, pleocytosis (100 to 500 cells per mm^3, with lymphocytes predominating after a few days); protein content increased to 100 to 200 mg/dL or more, and low glucose (<40 mg/dL). When this spectrum of changes is found in a febrile patient and fungal infections and meningeal carcinomatosis can be excluded, antituberculous therapy should be instituted. Tubercle bacilli are often difficult to find in smears of CSF, and cultures do not become positive for 3 to 4 weeks or longer. These problems are being overcome by the use of the polymerase chain reaction, a method of DNA amplification to detect small amounts of tubercle bacilli. Also, new culture techniques may allow identification of the organism within a week.

Chest films may demonstrate the presence of healed or active pulmonary lesions, and CT and MRI may reveal hydrocephalus, tuberculomas, gadolinium enhancement of the basal meninges, or zones of infarction.

Treatment If unrecognized and untreated, tuberculous meningitis is invariably fatal. Treatment consists of administration of a combination of drugs: (1) isoniazid (5 mg/kg daily for adults and 10 mg/kg for children); (2) rifampin (600 mg daily for adults and 15 mg/kg for children); and (3) a third and sometimes a fourth drug, which may be ethambutol (15 to 25 mg/kg per day), ethionamide (750 to 1000 mg daily in divided doses after meals), or pyrazinamide (20 to 35 mg/kg per day). The drugs need to be given for 18 to 24 months as a rule.

Ventricular shunting may be needed for patients who remain stuporous with large ventricles.

SARCOIDOSIS

This disease involves the peripheral or central nervous system in about 5 percent of patients. It may present as a solitary granulomatous mass, especially in or around the pituitary stalk, or elsewhere. Myelitis and polyradiculitis are being recognized with increasing frequency. Single or multiple cranial or peripheral nerves, particularly the facial nerve, are affected. A relatively common combination of abnormalities consists of chronic uveitis, parotitis, and facial nerve involvement (uveoparotid syndrome).

Diagnosis is based on the general medical findings (mediastinal adenopathy, restrictive lung disease, lesions of the uveal tract, skin, and bones); blood findings, including hypercalcemia, hyperglobulinemia, and increased concentration of angiotensin-converting enzyme; and biopsy of a pulmonary or other non-CNS lesion (noncaseating granuloma). Contrast-enhanced CT and MRI may show meningeal involvement (including dura) and white matter lesions.

Recent onset of symptoms requires treatment with corticosteroids given over a period of many months and sometimes the addition of immunosuppressive medications such as cyclosporin.

SPIROCHETAL INFECTIONS

Neurosyphilis

Treponema pallidum is the recognized cause of a wide range of neurologic syndromes, which include acute syphilitic meningitis, meningovascular syphilis, syphilitic meningoencephalitis (general paresis or paretic neurosyphilis), syphilitic lumbosacral radiculitis (tabes dorsalis), meningomyelitis, and optic neuritis. The incidence of these late forms of syphilis has decreased dramatically during the past three to four decades. However, there has been an increase in reported cases of early syphilis in recent years, in part due to the AIDS epidemic; the clinical picture in AIDS has been altered somewhat from the usual pattern.

As indicated in Fig. 32-2, all of these syndromes derive from a common, low-grade, often asymptomatic syphilitic meningitis. In fact, this is the most chronic of all known forms of meningitis and may be active for 10 to 15 years. In its more subacute phase (within 2 years of infection), it may present with headache, drowsiness, and cranial nerve palsies (*meningeal syphilis*). After 2 to 10 years, arterial inflammation may result in a stroke (*meningovascular syphilis*). *General paresis* is a gradual dementing menin-goencephalitis appearing 12 to 15 years after the onset of infection. *Tabes dorsalis* (literally a wasting of the dorsal funiculi of the spinal cord sec-ondary to lumbosacral radiculitis) presents, after 15 to 20 years, with a chronic syndrome of lancinating pains in the legs, crises of gastric pain, deep sensory loss and ataxia, impotence, hypotonia of the bladder with uri-nary retention and overflow incontinence, Charcot joints, and small, nonre-active (Argyll Robertson) pupils (page 124). *Optic neuritis* may be added; it consists of unilateral and later bilateral loss of vision and optic atrophy.

Diagnosis is based on a history of primary or secondary syphilis, the clin-ical characteristics of the neurologic syndrome, and the laboratory testing for reagin and treponemal antibodies (VDRL and FTA-ABS). The CSF is abnormal in all cases of active neurosyphilis (increase in lymphocytes and mononuclear cells, increased protein, especially gamma globulin, normal glucose, presence of syphilitis antibodies).

The *treatment* of all forms of neurosyphilis consists of administration of penicillin G, 18 to 24 million units IV daily in six divided doses, for 14 days. Erythromycin and tetracycline, 0.5 g every 6 h, for 20 to 30 days are suit-able substitutes in penicillin-sensitive patients. If symptoms recede and CSF

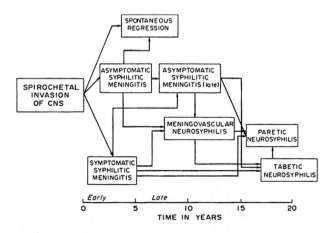

FIG. 32-2 Diagram of the evolution of neurosyphillis in the immune-competent host.

abnormalities are reversed (disappearance of cells and reduction in protein, gamma globulin, and serology titers), no further treatment is indicated. Relapse, which is revealed by the return of symptoms and reactivation of the CSF (pleocytosis), requires additional treatment, for which reason the CSF should be reexamined at 6 and 12 months after treatment.

Lyme Disease

This disease, known in Europe as *erythema chronicum migrans*, has been encountered with increasing frequency during the past few decades. The infective agent is the spirochete *Borrelia burgdorferi* and the vector in North America is the common ixodid tick. The initial manifestation, at the site of the tick bite, is an enlarging erythematous ring-shaped lesion, sometimes surrounded by satellites. The skin lesion may be overlooked or disregarded but is followed, weeks to months later, by arthritis (two-thirds of cases), cardiac manifestations (15 percent), and neurologic complications (8 percent). The disease is not fatal but can lead to prolonged disability if not recognized and treated. Neurologic involvement most often takes the form of a fluctuating meningoencephalitis (headache, stiff neck, nausea and vomiting, fatigue) with cranial or peripheral neuritis, particularly *facial palsy*. A meningoradiculitis involving the cauda equina particularly has long been known in Europe as the Bannwarth syndrome. Myelitic and cauda equina syndromes and a polymyositis are also documented. Meningeal symptoms are associated with a CSF lymphocytosis (up to 3000 cells per mm^3), an elevated protein content, but normal glucose.

A chronic lyme encephalopathy, characterized by profound fatigue and varying cognitive difficulties, has been documented, but this diagnosis should probably not be entertained unless the symptoms follow sequentially and clearly the typical early manifestations of the disease.

Diagnostic laboratory tests are the indirect immunofluorescence assay and the enzyme-linked immunosorbent assay (ELISA). The use of oral penicillin, tetracycline, or erythromycin in the initial stage of the disease will prevent the cardiac, arthritic, and neurologic manifestations. The onset of meningeal symptoms requires high doses of antibiotics—penicillin, 20 million units daily IV for 10 days, or probably better, ceftriaxone, 2 g/day for 30 days. Concomitant administration of prednisone is said to be helpful.

FUNGAL INFECTIONS OF THE CNS

These are much less common than bacterial infections. Cryptococcosis, candidiasis, aspergillosis, mucormycosis, coccidioidomycosis, blastomycosis, and actinomycosis have all been identified, but only the first three occur with any regularity. Mucormycosis is most often observed as a complication of diabetes. Candidiasis is associated with severe burns and other chronic illnesses. Coccidioidomycosis is a common, influenza-like disease of the southwestern United States, rarely causing meningitis. These infections may arise without obvious predisposing cause, but more often they complicate some other disease process, such as malignancy, AIDS, or other disease that suppresses the immune responses (*opportunistic infections*).

Cryptococcosis (formerly called torulosis) is the fungal infection seen most often in the United States. Its incidence has increased as a result of AIDS. It gives rise mainly to a subacutely evolving meningitis and meningoencephalitis, the symptoms of which are much the same as those of tuberculous meningitis. The CSF findings are also similar. Some cases are fatal within a few weeks; others are chronic over months or years, especially if treated. Specific diagnosis depends upon identifying *Cryptococcus neoformans* in India-ink preparations of the CSF, culturing the organism on Sabouraud glucose agar, or a positive latex agglutination test for the cryptococcal polysaccharide antigen in the CSF (90 percent reliable if negative in AIDS patients; 50 percent in others). Treatment consists of IV administration of amphotericin B. After a test dose of 5 mg, the drug is given in a dosage of 1.0 mg/kg daily or every second day to a total of 2 to 3 g. The addition of flucytosine (150 mg/kg per day) results in fewer failures and decreased nephrotoxicity, but the mortality is still about 40 percent and the patient must be monitored closely for bone marrow suppression. Small, deep brain infarctions may occur as a result of basal angiitis, similar to tuberculous meningitis. Cryptococcal brain abscesses (cryptococcoma) may simulate tumors.

INFECTIONS CAUSED BY PROTOZOA AND WORMS

Of the protozoal infections, only *toxoplasmosis* is observed with any frequency in the United States and Europe. Immunocompromised adults, notably those with AIDS, are particularly vulnerable. In healthy adults, the infection is usually asymptomatic, but an infected woman may transmit the disease to her unborn fetus. The disease takes the form of a multifocal encephalitis with inflammatory necrotic foci, large enough to be seen by CT and MRI. Diagnosis is established by elevation of specific serologic titers; it is rare to find the organism in the CSF. Treatment with sulfadiazine (4 to 6 g daily) and pyrimethamine (50 to 100 mg daily) with folinic acid should be continued for at least 4 weeks and should be lifelong in patients with AIDS. The main differential diagnostic consideration in AIDS patients is cerebral lymphoma (pages 263 and 290).

Cysticercosis and *schistosomiasis* are major infections in certain parts of the world, and involvement of the nervous system greatly worsens the outcome. Cysticercosis (the larval or intermediate stage of infection with the pork tapeworm *Taenia solium*) causes focal inflammatory lesions in the brain, which become encysted and calcified and often epileptogenic. Large intraventricular or cerebellar cysts may cause hydrocephalus. The chronic calcified lesions are readily seen on CT scans.

In rare instances, the ova of trematodes (schistosomiasis) cause necrotizing foci in the brain or spinal cord. Swimming in lakes or rivers known to harbor the intermediate hosts, infected snails, is the usual cause of infection. The illness is often preceded by a transient "swimmer's itch," which represents the transdermal entry of the parasite. Treatment of both cysticercosis and schistosomiasis has been greatly improved by the use of the antihelminthic agent praziquantel (50 mg/kg orally for 15 to 30 days) or albendazole (5 mg tid for 15 to 30 days).

Trichinosis presents essentially as a self-limiting polymyositis involving cranial muscles and the heart. Rarely, cerebral emboli complicate the myocarditis.

Cerebral malaria complicates about 2 percent of cases of malaria due to *plasmodium falciparum*. This is a rapidly fatal disease characterized by headache, seizures, and coma with diffuse cerebral edema and very rarely by hemiplegia, aphasia, hemianopia, ataxia, or other focal neurologic signs. Cerebral capillaries and venules are packed with parasitized erythrocytes and the brain is dotted with small foci of necrosis surrounded by microglia. Usually the neurologic symptoms appear in the second or third week of the infection, but they may be the initial manifestation. Children in hyperendemic regions are the ones most susceptible to cerebral malaria. Among adults, pregnant women and nonimmune individuals who discontinue prophylactic medication are most liable to involvement of the central nervous system. The CSF may be under increased pressure and sometimes contains a few white blood cells, but the glucose content is normal. With *Plasmodium vivax* infections, there may be drowsiness, confusion, and seizures without invasion of the brain by the parasite. Quinine, chloroquine, and related drugs are curative if the cerebral symptoms are not pronounced, but once coma and convulsions supervene, 20 to 30 percent of patients do not survive. It has been stated that large doses of dexamethasone, administered as soon as cerebral symptoms appear, may be lifesaving. Elevated CSF pressure should be relieved by appropriate measures.

For a more detailed discussion of this topic, see Victor and Ropper: *Adams and Victor's Principles of Neurology*, 7th ed, pp 734–782.

ADDITIONAL READING

Berenguer J, Moreno S, Laguna F, et al: Tuberculous meningitis in patients infected with the human immunodeficiency virus. *N Engl J Med* 326:668, 1992.

Coonrod JD, Dans PE: Subdural empyema. *Am J Med* 53:85, 1972.

Durand ML, Calderwood SB, Weber DJ, et al: Acute bacterial meningitis: A review of 493 episodes. *N Engl J Med* 328:21, 1993.

Feigin RD, McCracken GH Jr, Klein JO: Diagnosis and management of meningitis. *Pediatr Infect Dis J* 11:785, 1992.

Garcia-Monco JC, Benach JL: Lyme neuroborreliosis. *Ann Neurol* 37:691, 1995.

Nadelman RB, Wormser GP: Lyme borreliosis. *Lancet* 352:557, 1998.

Newton CR, Hien T, White N: Cerebral malaria. *J Neurol Neurosurg Psychiatry* 69:433, 2000.

Pomeroy SL, Holmes SJ, Dodge PR, Feigin RD: Seizures and other neurologic sequelae of bacterial meningitis in children. *N Engl J Med* 323:1651, 1990.

Quagliarello JJ, Scheld WM: Treatment of bacterial meningitis. *N Engl J Med* 336:708, 1997.

Reik L: Spirochetal infections of the nervous system, in Kennedy PGE, Johnson RT (eds): *Infections of the Nervous System*. Boston, Butterworth, 1987, pp 43–75.

Snider DE, Roper WL: The new tuberculosis. *N Engl J Med* 326:703, 1992.

Swartz MN: "Chronic meningitis"—Many causes to consider. *N Engl J Med* 317:957, 1987.

Tyler KL, Martin JB: *Infectious Diseases of the Nervous System*. Philadelphia, FA Davis, 1993.

33 | Viral Infections of the Nervous System

Viruses enter the body in many ways—via the respiratory passages (mumps, measles, varicella), by the oral-intestinal route (enteroviruses) or the genital-mucosal route (herpes), by inoculation (arboviruses, AIDS), transplacentally (rubella, cytomegalovirus), or along peripheral nerves (herpes, rabies). Once the nervous system is invaded, the virus multiplies in selective regions of the brain or spinal cord or in the choroid plexuses and meninges. Six neurologic syndromes are thus induced, occurring with such regularity that, if recognized, they not only stamp the infection as viral but also may indicate the identity of the virus. These syndromes are as follows:

1. Acute aseptic (nonpurulent) meningitis
2. Acute encephalitis and meningoencephalitis
3. Herpes zoster and simplex ganglionitis
4. Chronic infections due to "slow viruses" and unconventional agents (prions)
5. Acquired immunodeficiency syndrome (AIDS) encephalitis
6. Acute anterior poliomyelitis

A number of rarer special viral syndromes such as cauda equina neuritis [cytomegalovirus (CMV), Lyme disease] are discussed in *Adams and Victor's Principles of Neurology*, 7th ed.

THE SYNDROME OF ASEPTIC MENINGITIS

This term designates a common clinical syndrome consisting of fever, headache, and other signs of meningeal irritation, and a predominantly lymphocytic pleocytosis with normal cerebrospinal fluid (CSF) glucose and negative bacterial and fungal cultures. Photophobia and pain on movement of the eyes are other common complaints. Sometimes drowsiness and confusion are added, making it difficult to distinguish a pure meningitis from a meningoencephalitis. The CSF reaction is the same in both—pleocytosis, mainly lymphocytes (typically 100 to 300 per mm^3, sometimes more), increase in protein, but normal glucose. Rarely, the glucose level is reduced slightly.

Most cases of aseptic meningitis are due to viral infections, but there are important nonviral causes as well. Only a limited number of cases show signs of a preceding or concomitant respiratory or enteric infection.

Viral Causes of Meningitis

1. Enteroviral infections: echovirus, Coxsackie, and nonparalytic poliomyelitis. Peak incidence is in August and September. These viruses account for 80 percent of cases of established viral origin. Some cases in children are associated with an exanthem.

2. Mumps: Highest incidence is in late winter and spring. Male-to-female ratio is 3:1. Orchitis, parotitis, oophoritis, and pancreatitis may be associated.

3. Herpes simplex type 2, genital (rarely type 1), Epstein-Barr virus (EBV), and CMV.

4. Lymphocytic choriomeningitis: Lymphocyte count in CSF may be 1000 per mm^3 or higher. Infection is acquired by contact with infected hamsters and mice, mainly in late fall and winter.

5. Adenovirus infections.

6. HIV (AIDS) may cause an acute or chronic aseptic meningitis, sometimes soon after seroconversion, with fever and lymphadenopathy.

Most of these conditions are benign. Specific diagnosis requires viral isolation or detection of at least a fourfold rise in serum antibody titers during the acute and convalescent phases of the illness. A specific cause is not established in one-half or more of cases of presumed viral origin. The same holds true for many cases of suspected viral encephalitis (see below).

Nonviral Causes of Aseptic Meningitis

1. Spirochetal infections: The most important are *syphilitic* meningitis and *Lyme disease*, described in Chap. 32. *Leptospirosis*, with a peak incidence in August, is acquired by contact with contaminated urine of rats, dogs, swine, and cattle.

2. *Mycoplasma pneumoniae*: Cold agglutinins in the serum toward the end of the first week of illness or detection of the organism by the polymerase chain reaction (PCR) is diagnostic. *Legionella*, *Q fever*, and other rickettsial illnesses may also give rise to aseptic meningitis and meningoencephalitic syndromes, also with atypical pneumonia.

3. Bacterial infections lying adjacent to the meninges (Chaps. 31 and 32).

4. Neoplastic invasion of the meninges by lymphoma or carcinoma.

5. Chemical irritation of the meninges by blood, by contents of a craniopharyngioma, or by substances injected intrathecally.

6. Recurrent and chronic inflammatory meningitides of obscure origin—Vogt-Koyanagi-Harada syndrome (iridocyclitis, depigmentation of skin, deafness); sarcoidosis; meningitis with serum sickness and connective tissue disease such as systemic lupus erythematosus; Behçet disease (relapsing meningitis, iridocyclitis, ulcers of mouth and genitalia); and so-called Mollaret's recurrent meningitis (which is in some cases due to the herpes simplex virus).

In the diagnosis of aseptic meningitis, it is important to *exclude tuberculosis, cryptococcosis, Lyme disease, neurosyphilis, fungal infection, and inadequately treated bacterial meningitis*, all potential causes of lymphocytic meningitis that require urgent treatment.

SYNDROME OF ACUTE ENCEPHALITIS

In this class of viral diseases, a febrile illness is expressed by meningitis, often mild, to which are added the following neurologic abnormalities in various combinations: impairment of consciousness (confusion, stupor, and coma); seizures; mutism or aphasia; hemiparesis, with asymmetry of reflexes and Babinski signs; involuntary movements, cerebellar ataxia, and polymyoclonus; and cranial nerve palsies. The arboviral and some of the enteroviral encephalitides have a strong seasonal incidence. Viral encephalitis is in effect a *meningoencephalitis*, and mild forms of encephalitis, in which the meningeal symptoms and CSF abnormalities predominate, cannot be distinguished from viral (aseptic) meningitis, as mentioned in the preceding section.

The causes of acute viral meningoencephalitis in their approximate order of frequency are as follows:

1. Herpes simplex, zoster, CMV, and EBV
2. Mumps virus
3. Arboviruses: eastern, western, and Venezuelan equine; La Crosse, St. Louis, California, and Colorado tick fever, West Nile, Murray Valley, Russian spring-summer viruses; Japanese B (outside the United States)
4. Lymphocytic choriomeningitis virus
5. Enteroviruses (Coxsackie, echoviruses)
6. Adenoviruses
7. Rabies virus

Herpes Simplex Encephalitis

This, the most serious of the viral encephalitides, occurs sporadically throughout the year, in patients of all ages and in all parts of the world. It is caused by type 1 herpes simplex virus, very rarely by type 2 (genital herpes).

The symptoms—consisting of fever, headache, confusion, stupor, and coma—evolve over a period of several days. Additional acute symptoms in some patients include olfactory and gustatory hallucinations, temporal lobe or motor seizures, changes in personality and behavior, and aphasia. While a single convulsion or a flurry of seizures is common, status epilepticus almost never occurs. The symptoms reflect the highly characteristic localization of the disease process in the inferior and medial parts of the temporal lobes and orbital parts of the frontal lobes. The lesions are intensely inflammatory, often hemorrhagic, and show pannecrosis of nearly all tissue elements. The virus can be detected in brain tissue by antibody staining; intranuclear eosinophilic inclusions are found in neurons and glial cells.

The destructive temporal lobe lesions can be seen with computed tomography (CT) and magnetic resonance imaging (MRI), often asymmetrically in the two hemispheres (Fig. 33-1). The CSF findings are like those of other encephalitides (predominantly mononuclear pleocytosis, elevated protein, normal glucose) except that in some cases there may be as many as several thousand red cells and a few early cases show a predominance of polymorphonuclear cells. Certain electroencephelographic (EEG) findings (periodic high-voltage sharp waves and slow-wave complexes at 2- to 3-s intervals in the temporal leads) should suggest the diagnosis. *If the diagnosis is reasonably certain, it is best to proceed at once with treatment.* Diagnostic brain biopsy carries a greater risk than the inappropriate use of antiviral agents. Moreover, there is now a relatively sensitive PCR technique to detect the virus in the CSF during the early phase of the illness.

About half the patients with this disease (those who are stuporous or comatose when first seen) do not survive, and many of those who do are left with an amnesic state and seizures. However, the survival rate is 90 percent

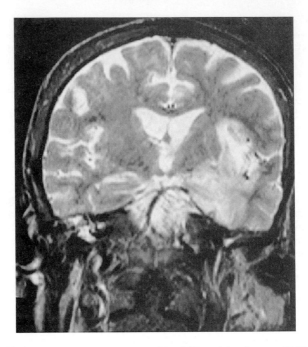

FIG. 33-1   Herpes simplex encephalitis. A T2-weighted coronal MR image in the axial plane taken during the acute stage of the illness. There is increased signal from practically all of the left inferior and deep temporal lobe and the insular cortex.

in patients who are awake or drowsy and are treated within the first 4 days of illness.

Treatment consists of the administration of *acyclovir* (30 mg/kg per day for 14 days). Initiation of treatment early in the illness (before the onset of stupor and coma) significantly reduces mortality and the severity of the residual neurologic deficits.

Nonviral Forms of Encephalitis

Numerous bacterial, fungal, parasitic, and noninfectious diseases may simulate the viral encephalitides and need to be distinguished from them. These nonviral diseases, many of which require urgent therapeutic intervention, are listed in Table 33-1. Postviral immune-mediated disseminated encephalomyelitis (ADEM) is particularly difficult at times to differentiate from acute viral encephalitis (see Chap. 35).

SYNDROME OF HERPES ZOSTER

This well-known disorder (also called zona or "shingles") is caused by the varicella-zoster (VZ) virus. It has an overall incidence of 3 to 5 cases per 1000 patients per year and is considerably more frequent in the elderly, in those with malignancies, particularly lymphoma and Hodgkin disease, and

TABLE 33-1 Diseases Simulating Viral Encephalitis

Bacterial encephalitides
  Mycoplasma pneumoniae
  Leptospirosis
  Lyme disease
  Syphilis (secondary or meningovascular)
  Listeriosis
  Cat-scratch disease (*Bartonella henselae*)
  Brucellosis (particularly *Brucella melitensis*)
  Tuberculosis
  Legionella
  Typhoid fever
  Nocardiosis
  Actinomycosis
  Parameningeal infections (epidural, petrositis)
  Partially treated bacterial meningitis
  Brain abscess
Fungal
  Cryptococcosis
  Coccidioidomycosis
  Histoplasmosis
  North American blastomycosis
  Candidiasis
Rickettsial
  Rocky Mountain spotted fever
  Typhus
  Q fever
Parasitic
  Toxoplasmosis
  Cysticercosis
  Echinococcosis
  Trypanosomiasis
  Plasmodium falciparum
  Amebiasis (*Naegleria* and *Acanthamoeba*)
Neoplastic
  Carcinomatous and lymphomatous meningitis
  Gliomatosis cerebri
  Paraneoplastic limbic encephalitis
  Intravascular lymphoma
Vascular
  Granulomatous angiitis
  Systemic lupus erythematosus
Others
  Sarcoid
  Behçet syndrome
  Oculocephalic syndromes (e.g., Stevens-Johnson, Vogt-Kayanagi-
    Harada)

in immunosuppressed patients. Herpes zoster probably represents a reactivation of varicella virus infection that has been latent in sensory ganglia following the primary childhood infection with chickenpox.

Clinical features The characteristic manifestations are radicular pain, a vesicular cutaneous eruption involving one or two dermatomes on one side of the body, and in some cases sensory and motor deficits in the segments bearing the skin lesions. The vesicular eruption is preceded for 3 to 4 days (sometimes as long as 7 days) by dysesthesias in the involved dermatomes, or there may be severe localized pain suggestive of lumbar disc herniation, pleurisy, or an acute abdominal condition.

Any part of the body may be affected, but thoracic lesions are the most frequent. Zoster of multiple dermatomes should always suggest an underlying immunocompromised state.

Involvement of cranial ganglia is associated with two special syndromes, both with prominent paralytic features: (1) *ophthalmic herpes*, with pain and eruption in the distribution of the first division of the trigeminal nerve, ophthalmoplegia, and risk of corneal ulceration, and (2) so-called *geniculate herpes* (Ramsay Hunt syndrome), with facial paralysis, vertigo, deafness, and otic-palatal vesiculation (sometimes restricted to a small region of the concha of the ear). A third type, *herpes occipitocollaris*—with involvement of palate, pharynx, neck, and retroauricular region—is caused by herpetic infection of the ganglia of cranial nerves IX and X and upper cervical roots. The CSF in all the zoster syndromes contains 10 to 100 cells, mainly lymphocytes, and a slightly increased protein. A delayed cerebral arteritis and ischemic stroke complicate some cases of cranial zoster and an encephalitis, usually mild, may occur in elderly patients after a dermatomal eruption.

Pain and dysesthesia last for 1 to 4 weeks in most cases, but in as many as one-third of patients, pain persists for months or even years and creates a difficult therapeutic problem.

Pathologically, there is an intense inflammation in two or three adjacent dorsal root or cranial nerve ganglia and in corresponding posterior and anterior roots, adjacent meninges, and gray matter of the spinal cord on one side. The latter lesion is a veritable poliomyelitis, but the neuronal destruction is more in the posterior than in the anterior horn. Myelitis and the above-mentioned encephalitis are rare complications.

A course of acyclovir (800 mg five times daily for 7 days), if begun within 48 h after the appearance of the rash, shortens the period of acute pain and hastens the healing of the vesicles; however, it does not prevent the occurrence of *postherpetic neuralgia*. In nonimmunosuppressed patients, prednisone (45 to 60 mg/day for 7 days, then tapered) does appear to decrease the incidence of postherpetic neuralgia. The latter disorder is best treated by a combination of carbamazepine or neurontin and amitriptyline, beginning with small doses that are gradually increased to 400 to 800 and 75 to 150 mg/day, respectively. Lidocaine, aspirin-chloroform, or capsaicin topical creams and nerve root blocks are effective in some cases. Intrathecal injection of methylprednisolone has also been suggested but is infrequently required, since in most instances postherpetic pain subsides over weeks or months.

HERPES SIMPLEX

The most important nervous system complication of herpes simplex infection is the encephalitis (described above) due usually to the type 1 virus. However, there are other examples of nervous system involvement by the herpes simplex virus, usually type 2—infection of the facial nerve, probably the main cause of Bell's palsy; localized infection of the trigeminal ganglion, giving rise to a unilateral facial sensory loss; genital herpes that may lead to a lumbosacral ganglionitis and painful radiculopathy with urinary retention; meningitis, sometimes recurrent (Mollaret meningitis); rare instances of transverse myelitis; and an encephalitis (in adults) due to the type 2 virus.

In the newborn, herpes simplex infection can be a devastating and rapidly fatal disease. It is usually contracted in the birth canal from a mother with type 2 (genital herpes). The results of antiviral treatment are unclear.

CHRONIC INFECTIONS DUE TO "SLOW VIRUSES"

Subacute sclerosing panencephalitis (SSPE) This is a slowly evolving inflammatory disease, now very rare, appearing in children and adolescents several years after an attack of measles. It is characterized by dementia, focal or generalized seizures, ataxia of gait, and polymyoclonus. It evolves over a period of months to several years and leaves the child virtually decerebrate. The EEG is typical—periodic bursts of high-voltage slow waves followed by a flat pattern. Gamma globulin and measles antibodies are greatly elevated in the CSF. Since measles vaccine has come to be widely used, this neurologic disease has virtually disappeared.

A somewhat similar subacute progressive panencephalitis, also very rare and occurring many years after congenital rubella, has also been identified.

Progressive multifocal leukoencephalopathy (PML) This disease is usually associated with AIDS, Hodgkin disease, lymphoma, or chronic leukemia and less often with tuberculosis, sarcoid, or other states of immunosuppression. It develops over a 3- to 6-month period, with focal cerebral, brainstem, and cerebellar signs. The lesions are demyelinative and well delineated by MRI. Inclusion bodies are seen in oligodendrocytes; astrocytes are gigantic and show tumor-like mitoses. A polyomavirus—designated JC virus—has been isolated from the lesions. Remission has occurred in AIDS patients treated with an aggressive retroviral regimen. There is no effective treatment for the others.

CHRONIC INFECTIONS DUE TO UNCONVENTIONAL AGENTS (PRIONS)

This group of diseases is considered here for the want of a more suitable chapter in which to include them. It must be understood, however, that they are due not to any of the known viruses but to infectious proteinaceous particles that lack the DNA, RNA, and morphologic attributes of conventional viruses. These particles appear to be infectious by virtue of their ability to induce a conformational change in normal brain proteins. Although an example of prion disease was originally appreciated among cannibals in New Guinea who ingested infected brains and a rare form has been transmitted from cattle to humans, the mode of transmission is not clear in the more common sporadic cases. Certain forms may also be inherited as a result of mutations in the genes coding for these same proteins.

Subacute spongiform encephalopathy (SSE) This disease, referred to commonly as *Creutzfeldt-Jakob disease*, is characterized by a rapidly progressive dementia in association with cerebellar ataxia, heightened startle reaction, diffuse myoclonic jerks, and cortical blindness in some cases. Among variant presentations are cases that begin with subacute ataxia, cortical disorders of vision, or both. A related illness, contracted by the ingestion of meat from infected cattle (bovine spongiform encephalopathy or "mad-cow disease"), while rare, has become a matter of great concern in Great Britain and western Europe. It is characterized by psychiatric and sensory symptoms. The CSF in all these types is normal. Usually, after one or two months of illness, the EEG is diagnostic—high-voltage slow and sharp waves, occurring almost periodically at 1- to 3-Hz intervals, on an increasingly disorganized and low-voltage background. The lenticular nuclei often display subtle signal changes on MRI.

As the disease advances, the patient becomes totally unresponsive and the outcome is invariably fatal, usually in months.

The disease affects principally the cerebral and cerebellar cortices, in which there is a diffuse loss of neurons, gliosis, and a striking vacuolation of the tissues. Inflammatory changes are absent, and no inclusion bodies have been observed. The disease is due to an unconventional agent mentioned above—a proteinaceous infectious particle, called a *prion*, which lacks the structure of a virus and can be transmitted to chimpanzees, with an incubation period of more than a year. In some cases, the diagnosis can be confirmed by the detection of the prion protein in the CSF or by the presence of a particular peptide fragment (14-3-3) of a normal brain protein. Also, the content of enolase and of neopterin in the CSF are increased. Pathologically and epidemiologically, SSE resembles a disease first recognized among natives of New Guinea and known as kuru. Gerstmann-Sträussler disease is an inherited form of SSE that results in spinocerebellar degeneration; fatal familial insomnia is another rare variant attributed to prion infection.

There is no known treatment. Precautions need to be taken in the medical care of these patients and the handling of their tissues.

THE ACQUIRED IMMUNODEFICIENCY SYNDROME (AIDS)

This viral disease is characterized by an acquired and unusually profound depression of cell-mediated immunity, reversal of T-helper/T-suppressor cell ratio (CD4/CD8), and depressed in vitro lymphoproliferative response to various antigens. The causative virus, originally called human T-cell lymphotropic virus (HTLV-3), is now generally referred to as human immunodeficiency virus (HIV or HIV-1). The diseases it induces, due to the effects of the virus itself and a wide array of complicating opportunistic infections and neoplasms, are designated as AIDS (acquired immunodeficiency syndrome).

Epidemiology AIDS is mainly a disease of homosexual or bisexual men (56 percent) and of male and female drug users (19 percent)—these figures are for North America. A smaller group at risk are hemophiliacs (and other patients who receive transfusions or injections of blood products) and infants born of women with AIDS. There is a small group of heterosexual men who appear to have been infected by prostitutes, and heterosexual transmission is rampant in portions of Africa and the Far East. Four-fifths of the reported cases in the United States have been from New York, California, New Jersey, and Florida.

Clinical manifestations These range from the asymptomatic seroconversion state to widespread lymphadenopathy, diarrhea, and weight loss (AIDS-related complex, or ARC) to full-blown AIDS, comprising some or all of the complications listed in Table 33-2. In approximately one-third of

TABLE 32-2 Neurologic Complications in HIV-1–Infected Patients

Brain
Predominantly nonfocal
AIDS dementia complex (subacute-chronic HIV encephalitis)
Acute HIV-related encephalitis
Cytomegalovirus encephalitis
Herpes simplex virus encephalitis
Predominantly focal
Cerebral toxoplasmosis
Progressive multifocal leukoencephalopathy
Varicella-zoster virus encephalitis
Tuberculous brain abscess/tuberculoma
Neurosyphilis (meningovascular)
Vascular disorders—notably nonbacterial endocarditis and cerebral
hemorrhages associated with thrombocytopenia; also cerebral
vasculitis
Primary CNS lymphoma
Spinal cord
Vacuolar myelopathy
Herpes simplex or zoster myelitis
Meninges
Aseptic meningitis (HIV)
Cryptococcal and other fungal meningitis
Tuberculous meningitis
Syphilitic meningitis
Lymphomatous meningitis
Peripheral nerve and root
Herpes zoster
Cytomegalovirus cauda equina polyradiculopathy
Acute and chronic inflammatory HIV polyneuritis
Mononeuritis multiplex
Sensorimotor demyelinating polyneuropathy (Guillain-Barré syndrome)
Distal painful sensory polyneuritis
Dysautonomic neuropathy
Muscle
Polymyositis and other myopathies
AZT and other treatment-induced myopathies

---

patients, the central nervous system (CNS) or peripheral nervous system
(PNS) is clinically involved by the time of death, and on postmortem examination nearly all patients prove to have CNS lesions.

The neurologic manifestations are too numerous and varied to describe in
detail. They are listed in Table 33-2 and are addressed in the appended references as well as in appropriate chapters throughout this book.

Laboratory tests Many screening tests are now available, all of them based
on an enzyme-linked immunosorbent assay (ELISA). While these are highly
sensitive, there is a small incidence of false positives. The Western blot test,
which identifies antibodies to viral proteins, is more specific and is used to
confirm a positive screening test.

A reversal of the usual CD4/CD8 ratio is found and can be used as an
imprecise surrogate for AIDS testing.

Treatment The treatment of AIDS is evolving rapidly. The addition of transcriptase inhibitor drugs (AZT and 3-TC) to the newer protease inhibitors (such as indinavir) has greatly decreased the amount of active virus and prolonged survival in many patients, but the influence on the neurological complications—with the exception of PML, which improves—is uncertain.

The frequently occurring opportunistic infections and the lymphomas are treated individually (Chap. 31).

Tropical Spastic Paraparesis (TSP)

This spinal cord disorder, which is endemic in many tropical and subtropical countries, also occurs sporadically elsewhere. Originally thought to be nutritional, it is now known to be due to the human T-cell lymphotropic virus type 1 (HTLV-1).

The clinical picture is one of a slowly progressive spastic paraparesis, with increased reflexes, Babinski signs, and a disorder of sphincteric control. Paresthesias, reduced vibratory and position sense, and sensory ataxia are variably present, usually only in the lower limbs. There may be a sensory level on the trunk. The CSF contains 10 to 50 lymphocytes per mm^3. Total protein and glucose content is normal, but IgG is increased, with antibodies to HTLV-1. Neuropathologic study has documented an inflammatory and vacuolated myelitis involving mainly the corticospinal pathways and posterior columns, not dissimilar to AIDS myelopathy.

TSP needs to be differentiated from the heredofamilial and degenerative forms of progressive spastic paraplegia, cervical spondylosis, and the spinal form of multiple sclerosis, with which it can easily be confused.

Other Subacute Encephalitides (Possibly Viral)

Rasmussen encephalitis This is an idiopathic meningoencephalitis in children characterized by intractable focal epilepsy usually in association with a hemiparesis. Both features are progressive over months to years and are resistant to treatment with anticonvulsant drugs, although corticosteroids, if started early in the course of the illness, may be beneficial. There is extensive focal destruction of the cortex and underlying white matter (visualized on MRI) with intensive gliosis and lingering inflammatory reactions. Recently an autoimmune causation has been suggested.

Limbic encephalitis This is a well-known subacute paraneoplastic syndrome, involving the brainstem and cerebellum as well as limbic structures. The neuropathologic changes resemble those of a viral encephalitis, but a virus (or any other organism) has not been isolated (see page 267).

SYNDROME OF ACUTE ANTERIOR POLIOMYELITIS

In the past, this syndrome was almost invariably due to one of the three types of poliovirus. Vaccines have practically eliminated the disease, but occasional cases still occur in unvaccinated children and in adults exposed to a recently vaccinated child. A similar though more benign syndrome can be caused by other enteroviruses, such as Coxsackie viruses A and B and echoviruses.

Clinical features Fever, malaise, headache, nausea and vomiting, and stiffness and aching of muscles are followed, in 3 to 4 days, by pain in the back and neck and signs of mild meningeal irritation and then by weakness or paralysis of muscles. In most cases, the disease arrests in the preparalytic phase and cannot be distinguished from other viral diseases that give rise to aseptic meningitis.

Paralysis, when it develops, usually attains its maximum severity in 48 h or less. Its distribution is quite variable. Weakness of one or both legs or an arm and both legs is the most common form. Trunk muscles may be severely affected, or the paralysis may be purely bulbar, with fatal respiratory failure. Tendon reflexes are lost in weakened limbs. Paresthesias and muscle pain are frequent complaints, but very seldom can sensory loss be demonstrated. Bladder and other smooth muscles are usually spared. The CSF shows a modest increase in cells, mainly mononuclear, and in protein, but the glucose concentration is normal.

The final outcome is an atrophic, areflexive paralysis in some of the initially affected parts, always less severe than the acute paralysis. A gradual increase in weakness may occur 20 to 30 or more years after the acute paralytic illness ("postpolio syndrome") and probably represents the additive effect of anterior horn cell loss that occurs with aging.

Destruction of anterior horn cells with phagocytosis of cell remnants by microgliacytes, gliosis, and perivascular meningeal infiltrates of lymphocytes and monocytes compose the principal neuropathologic changes. Nerve cells in the bulbar motor nuclei, dentate nuclei, and motor cortex are also involved.

Treatment is essentially preventive. The Sabin vaccine, which consists of attenuated live virus, is administered orally to infants in two doses 8 weeks apart, with boosters at 1 year and 4 years of age. Poliomyelitis may follow vaccination (0.02 to 0.04 cases per million doses).

Treatment of paralytic poliomyelitis is purely supportive, utilizing respiratory assistance and physical therapy.

For a more detailed discussion of this topic, see Victor and Ropper: *Adams and Victor's Principles of Neurology*, 7th ed, pp 734–782.

ADDITIONAL READING

Antel JP, Rasmussen T: Rasmussen's encephalitis and the new hat. *Neurology* 46:9, 1996.

Bell JE: The neuropathology of adult HIV infection. *Rev Neurol* 154:816, 1998.

Berger JR, Levy RM (eds): *AIDS and the Nervous System*, 2nd ed. Hagerstown, MD, Lippincott-Raven, 1997.

Gilden DH, Klein Schmidt-DeMasters BK, Laguardia JS, et al: Neurologic complications of the reactivation of varicella-zoster virus. *N Engl J Med* 342:635, 2000.

Holland NR, Power C, Mathews VP, et al: Cytomegalovirus encephalitis in acquired immunodeficiency syndrome (AIDS). *Neurology* 44:507, 1994.

Johnson RT: *Viral Infections of the Nervous System*, 2nd ed. New York, Raven Press, 1998.

Leehey M, Gilden D: Neurologic disorders associated with the HIV and HIV-1 viruses, in Appel SH (ed): *Current Neurology*, vol 10. St. Louis, Mosby–Year Book, 1990.

Manji H, Miller RF: Progressive multifocal leucoencephalopathy: Progress in the AIDS era. *J Neurol Neurosurg Psychiatry* 69:569, 2000.

Prusiner SB, Hsiao KK: Human prion disease. *Ann Neurol* 35:385, 1994.

Richardson EP Jr: Progressive multifocal leukoencephalopathy. *N Engl J Med* 265:815, 1961.

Rodgers-Johnson PE. Tropical spastic paraparesis/HTLV-1 associated myelopathy: Etiology and clinical spectrum. *Mol Neurobiol* 8:175, 1994.

Smith JE, Aksamit AJ: Outcome of chronic idiopathic meningitis. *Mayo Clin Proc* 69:548, 1994.

Tyler K, Martin JB: *Infectious Diseases of the Nervous System*. Philadelphia, FA Davis, 1993.

Whitley RJ: Viral encephalitis. *N Engl J Med* 323:242, 1990.

Zerr I, Bodemer M, Recker S, et al: Diagnosis of Creutzfeldt-Jakob disease by two-dimensional gel electrophoresis of cerebrospinal fluid. *Lancet* 348:846, 1996.

Zajicek JP, Scolding NJ, Foster O, et al: Central nervous system sarcoidosis—Diagnosis and management, *Q J Med* 92:103, 1999.

34 | Cerebrovascular Diseases

Next to heart disease and cancer, cerebrovascular disease is the most frequent cause of death in the western world. And at least one-half of all neurologic patients in general hospitals have some type of cerebrovascular disease. The medical student and house officer are well advised to concentrate on this group of diseases, since they have traditionally provided one of the most instructive approaches to neurology.

The term *cerebrovascular disease* denotes any abnormality of the brain resulting from a pathologic process of blood vessels—arteries, arterioles, capillaries, veins, or sinuses. The main pathologic change in the vessels takes the form of occlusion by thrombus or embolus, or of rupture of the vessel wall. The resulting abnormalities in the brain are of two types: ischemic, with and without infarction, and hemorrhagic. Other forms of cerebrovascular disease are those due to altered permeability or inflammation of the vascular wall, hypertension, and increased viscosity or other changes in the quality of blood. The latter changes underlie the strokes that complicate diseases such as sickle cell anemia and polycythemia vera. Altered vascular permeability accounts for the headache, brain edema, and convulsions of hypertensive encephalopathy. There are many more types of cerebrovascular disease; these are listed in Table 34-1, and the relative frequency of the main types is indicated in Table 34-2.

THE STROKE SYNDROME

The distinctive mode of presentation of cerebrovascular disease is the stroke, defined as any sudden or acute nonconvulsive focal neurologic deficit. In its most severe form, the patient becomes hemiplegic or falls senseless, an event so dramatic that it is given its own names—apoplexy, cerebrovascular accident, stroke, or, colloquially, "shock." If death does not follow within hours or days, there is nearly always some degree of recovery of function. This temporal profile of neurologic events, whether condensed into several minutes, as in a transient ischemic attack, or into hours or days, is diagnostic of stroke. Variations in the temporal profile reflect the type of vascular lesion. Embolic strokes characteristically begin with absolute suddenness, and their effects may recede rapidly or persist. Thrombotic strokes may have a similarly abrupt onset, but more often they evolve somewhat more slowly, over a period of minutes to hours or even days. Cerebral hemorrhage usually causes a severe deficit of rapid but not necessarily instantaneous onset; it is sometimes steadily progressive for hours or longer.

TABLE 34-1 Types of Cerebrovascular Disease

1. Atherosclerotic thrombosis
2. Transient ischemic attacks
3. Embolism (cardiogenic, carotid and aortic arch origin, paradoxical)
4. Primary (hypertensive) intracerebral hemorrhage and lobar nonhypertensive hemorrhage (anticoagulation, amyloid, AVM)
5. Ruptured or unruptured saccular aneurysm or AVM
6. Arteritis
   a. Meningovascular syphilis; arteritis secondary to pyogenic, fungal, and tuberculous meningitis; rare infective types (typhus, schistosomiasis, malaria, trichinosis, mucormycosis, etc.)
   b. Connective tissue diseases (polyarteritis nodosa, lupus erythematosus), Behçet disease, Wegener arteritis, temporal arteritis, Takayasu disease, granulomatous or giant-cell arteritis of the aorta, primary giant-cell granulomatous angiitis of cerebral arteries, intravascular lymphoma, and arteritis of AIDS
7. Cerebral thrombophlebitis: antiphospholipid antibody syndrome; secondary to infection of ear, paranasal sinus, face, etc.; with meningitis and subdural empyema; phlebothrombosis in postpartum and postoperative states; cardiac failure; cachexia; oral contraceptives (high-estrogen)
8. Hematologic disorders: polycythemia, sickle-cell disease, thrombotic thrombocytopenic purpura, thrombocytosis, cholesterol emboli, homocystinuria, etc.
9. Trauma and dissection of carotid, vertebral, and intracranial arteries
10. Dissecting aortic aneurysm
11. Systemic hypotension with arterial stenoses: intraoperative hypotension, sepsis, acute blood loss, myocardial infarction, Stokes-Adams syndrome, traumatic and surgical shock
12. Complications of arteriography
13. Neurologic migraine with persistent deficit
14. Vascular compression from tentorial, foramen magnum, and subfalcial herniations
15. Miscellaneous types: fibromuscular dysplasia, excessive irradiation, territory infarction in closed head injury (usually arterial dissection), pressure of unruptured saccular aneurysm, complication of oral contraceptives, vasospasm from subarachnoid hemorrhage
16. Undetermined cause in children and young adults: moyamoya; homocystinuria, CADASIL; Takayasu disease, MELAS

Key: AVM, arteriovenous malformation; CADASIL, cerebral autosomal dominant arteriopathy with leukoencephalopathy; MELAS, mitochondrial encephalomyopathy, lactic acidosis, and stroke.

The major neurovascular thrombotic and embolic syndromes, their symptoms and signs, and the corresponding cerebral structures that are involved are shown in Figs. 34-1 to 34-7.

ATHEROSCLEROTIC-THROMBOTIC INFARCTION

The large intracranial arteries, like the aorta and coronary arteries, are predisposed to atherosclerotic changes. Favored sites are the proximal and distal common and internal carotid (at its origin), the vertebral and basilar, and the proximal segments (stems) of the major cerebral arteries, mainly the middle cerebral. Factors enhancing this atheromatous process are hyperten-

TABLE 34-2 Major Types of Cerebrovascular Diseases and Their Frequency

	Harvard stroke series (756 successive cases)*	BCH autopsy series (179 cases)†
Atherosclerotic thrombosis	244 (32%)	21 (12%)
Lacunes	129 (18%)	34 (18.5%)
Embolism	244 (32%)	57 (32%)
Hypertensive hemorrhage	84 (11%)	28 (15.5%)
Ruptured aneurysms and vascular malformations	55 (7%)	8 (4.5%)
Indeterminate		17 (9.5%)
Other‡		14 (8%)

*Compiled by J Mohr, L Caplan, D Pessin, P Kistler, and G Duncan at Massachusetts General Hospital and Beth Israel Hospital, Boston.
†Compiled by CM Fisher and RD Adams in an examination of 780 brains during 1949 at Mallory Institute of Pathology, Boston City Hospital.
‡Hypertensive encephalopathy, cerebral vein thrombosis, meningovascular syphilis, and polyarteritis nodosa.

sion, diabetes mellitus, smoking, and hyperlipedemia. This type of stroke results from the superimposition of a thrombus on an artery severely narrowed by atherosclerosis.

Clinical Manifestations

More than one-half of patients who develop a thrombotic stroke have one or more brief warning episodes, called transient ischemic attacks (TIAs), the diagnosis and treatment of which may prevent an oncoming stroke (see further on). The thrombotic stroke, whether or not it is preceded by warning attacks, develops in one of the following ways: most often there is an abrupt onset of the neurologic deficit, evolving over a few minutes to a few hours; or there may be a stuttering onset and intermittent progression over several hours or a day or longer; or symptoms may regress for several hours and then advance again. More perplexing still is the rare stroke in which the deficit advances in a series of steps over a period of several days or more. Often the onset is during sleep; the patient awakens paralyzed.

The pattern of the neurologic deficit is determined by the site of arterial occlusion and the available anastomotic arrangements as shown in Figs. 34-1 through 34-7. It needs to be emphasized that partial and overlapping syndromes are more common than the strictly demarcated ones depicted.

Ancillary Examinations

Noninvasive blood flow procedures, such as carotid and transcranial Doppler studies, may reveal a stenotic or occluded artery. This can be verified by angiography, a procedure that carries a small risk of worsening the neurologic deficit. These methods have been in part replaced by magnetic resonance angiography (MRA) and spiral, or helical, computed tomography (CT), which are noninvasive. With these several techniques, one can see both stenotic segments or occlusion of arteries and sometimes mural thrombi that may become embolic (artery-to-artery embolism).

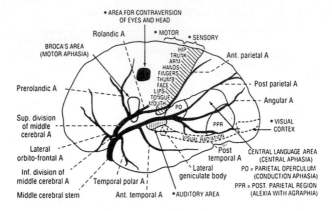

FIG. 34-1 Middle Cerebral Artery Diagram of the left cerebral hemisphere, lateral aspect, showing the branches and distribution of the middle cerebral artery and the principal regions of cerebral localization. Following is a list of the clinical manifestations of infarction in the territory of this artery and the corresponding regions of cerebral damage.

Signs and symptoms	Structures involved
Paralysis of the contralateral face and arm, greater than leg	Somatic motor area for face and arm and the descending fibers from the leg area in the corona radiata and internal capsule
Sensory impairment over the contralateral face, arm, and leg (pinprick, touch, vibration, position, two-point discrimination, stereognosis, tactile localization, cutaneographia)	Somatic sensory area for face and arm and thalamoparietal projections
Motor speech disorder	Broca's area and frontal operculum of the dominant hemisphere
Elements of Wernicke aphasia and Gerstmann syndrome	Central language area and dominant parietal cortex
Elements of asomatagnosia and amorphosynthesis	Nondominant parietal lobe
Inaccurate localization in the half field, impaired ability to judge distance, visual illusions; inattention and confusion usually associated	
Homonymous hemianopia (often superior homonymous quadrantanopia)	Optic radiation deep to second temporal convolution
Paralysis of conjugate gaze to the opposite side	Opposite frontal eye field or fibers projecting from it
Avoidance reaction of opposite limbs	Parietal lobe

(continued)

FIG. 34-1 *(continued)* Middle Cerebral Artery

Signs and symptoms	Structures involved
Miscellaneous:	
Ataxia of contralateral limb(s)	Parietal lobe
So-called Bruns ataxia or apraxia of gait	Frontal lobes (bilateral)
Agitated delirium	Right or left temporal
Loss or impairment of optokinetic nystagmus	Supramarginal or angular gyrus
Limb-kinetic apraxia	Premotor or parietal
Mirror movements	Precise location of responsible lesions not known
Cheyne-Stokes respiration, contralateral hyperhidrosis, mydriasis (occasionally)	Precise location of responsible lesions not known
Pure motor hemiplegia	Posterior limb of the internal capsule and the adjacent corona radiata

Treatment

Opinion is divided on whether the administration of IV heparin and oral warfarin, begun as early as possible, is capable of arresting a propagating thrombotic process. Surgical or thrombolytic revascularization of an accessible neck vessel may be effective if done within a few hours, but this is feasible in only a small proportion of stroke victims. Thrombolytic agents administered intravenously, such as tissue plasminogen activators (t-PA), have had some success in patients treated within 3 h of onset of the stroke with neither very minor nor very large infarcts and with blood pressure controlled. (See p. 308 for the dose of t-PA.) Intra-arterial thrombolytic treatment may be successful in recanalizing an occluded vessel up to 6 h or more after the stroke. With thrombolytic drugs, a cerebral hemorrhage complicates treatment in at least 3 to 6 percent of patients.

The long-term therapy of patients with completed thrombotic infarcts is equally uncertain. Anticoagulant or antiplatelet drugs (e.g., aspirin, ticlopidine, clopidogrel) in the prevention of further strokes or heart attacks have advocates and appear to be equivalent in most circumstances. Physiotherapy and speech therapy assist patients in coping with their disabilities but do not convincingly hasten the return of function.

Prognosis When the disease is seen at the onset, prediction of the outcome is difficult, since it depends on whether the stroke is still progressing or has been completed. The mortality is high in comatose patients. In every group of stroke patients there is, over a period of years, a rising mortality from coronary thrombosis, and this is as much of a hazard as recurrent cerebral thrombosis. There is an advantage to reducing risk factors for atherosclerosis.

Transient Ischemic Attacks (TIAs)

These are defined as transitory neurologic defects due to ischemia in a particular angioanatomic territory, lasting for minutes to hours and followed by complete restoration of function. Literally hundreds of attacks may occur or,

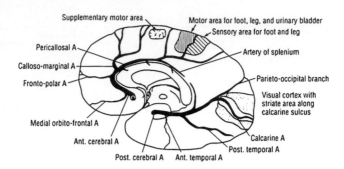

FIG. 34-2 Anterior Cerebral Artery Diagram of a cerebral hemisphere, medial aspect, showing the branches and distribution and the principal regions of cerebral localization. Following is a list of the clinical manifestations of infarction in the territory of this artery and the corresponding regions of cerebral damage.

Signs and symptoms	Structures involved
Paralysis of opposite foot and leg	Motor leg area
"Cortical" sensory loss over toes, foot, and leg	Sensory area for foot and leg
Urinary incontinence	Posteromedial part of superior frontal gyrus and anterior cingulate gyrus and their connections (bilateral)
Contralateral grasp reflex	Premotor and supplementary motor areas
Abulia (akinetic mutism), slowness, delay, lack of spontaneity, whispering, motor inaction, reflexive distraction by sights and sounds	Uncertain localization—probably deep medial-orbital (usually bilateral)
Impairment of gait and stance (gait "apraxia")	Inferomedial frontal-striate
Mental impairment (perseveration and amnesia)	Localization unknown
Miscellaneous: Dyspraxia of left limbs Cerebral paraplegia	Corpus callosum Motor leg area bilaterally (due to bilateral occlusion of anterior cerebral arteries)

Note: Hemianopia does not occur; transcortical aphasia occurs rarely (see Chap. 23).

more often, one or only a few. As remarked above, such attacks may anticipate an oncoming thrombotic stroke.

TIAs that are referable to the arteries arising from the carotid (middle and anterior cerebral) take the form of transient monocular blindness (TMB, amaurosis fugax), hemiparesis, hemisensory syndromes, aphasia, dyscalculia, confusion, and rarely a contralateral movement disorder. Vertebrobasilar

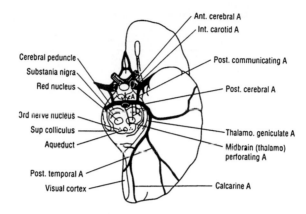

FIG. 34-3 Posterior Cerebral Artery Inferior aspect of the brain showing the branches and distribution and the principal anatomic structures supplied. Listed below are the clinical manifestations produced by infarction in its territory and the corresponding regions of damage.

Signs and symptoms	Structures involved
Peripheral territory	
Homonymous hemianopia (hemiachromatopsia may be present; macular or central vision is preserved if striate area is spared)	Calcarine cortex or optic radiation
Bilateral homonymous hemianopia, cortical blindness, unawareness or denial of blindness; achromatopsia; inability to perceive and touch objects not centrally located; apraxia of ocular movements (Balint syndrome)	Bilateral occipital lobe, possibly with involvement of parieto-occipital region
Dyslexia without agraphia, color anomia	Dominant calcarine cortex and posterior part of corpus callosum
Memory defect	Inferomedial temporal lobe (hippocampus) bilaterally
Topographic disorientation	Calcarine and lingual gyri
Prosopagnosia	Inferomedial temporo-occipital, usually bilateral
Simultanagnosia	Dominant visual cortex, sometimes bilateral
Unformed visual hallucinations, metamorphopsia, teleopsia, illusory visual spread, palinopsia, distortion of outlines, photophobia	Calcarine cortex

(continued)

FIG. 34-3 *(continued)* Posterior Cerebral Artery

Signs and symptoms	Structures involved
Central territory	
Thalamic syndrome: sensory loss (all modalities), spontaneous pain and dysesthesias, choreoathetosis, intention tremor, mild hemiparesis	Ventral posterolateral nucleus of thalamus in territory of thalamogeniculate artery; involvement of the adjacent subthalamic nucleus or its pallidal connections results in hemiballismus and choreoathetosis
Thalamoperforate syndrome: (1) superior, crossed cerebellar ataxia; (2) inferior, crossed cerebellar ataxia with ipsilateral third nerve palsy (Claude syndrome)	Dentatothalamic tract and issuing third nerve
Weber syndrome—third nerve palsy and contralateral hemiplegia	Issuing third nerve and cerebral peduncle
Contralateral hemiplegia	Cerebral peduncle
Paralysis or paresis of vertical eye movements, skew deviation, sluggish pupillary responses to light, slight miosis and ptosis (retraction nystagmus and "tucked-in" eyelids may be associated)	Supranuclear structures in high midbrain tegmentum ventral to superior colliculi (interstitial nucleus of medial longitudinal fasciculus, posterior commissure)
Contralateral ataxic or postural tremor	Dentatothalamic tract (?) after decussation; precise site of lesion unknown
Decerebrate attacks	Damage to motor tracts between red and vestibular nuclei
Peduncular hallucinosis (formed, colored)	Pars reticulata of substantia nigra (bilateral)

attacks consist of blindness, hemianopia, diplopia, vertigo, dysarthria, dysphagia, facial weakness or numbness, hemiplegia or quadriplegia, and sensory syndromes, in various combinations. In our experience, seizures and so-called drop attacks rarely if ever resemble and do not represent TIAs.

Single TIAs that are long-lasting (several hours to a day) or of diverse pattern are nearly always embolic. Those reflecting stenosis of the internal carotid artery are almost always briefer than 1 h, most lasting less than 10 min, and almost all repetitive stereotyped TIAs fall in this category. Despite wide-ranging speculation, the precise pathophysiology of most TIAs is not known. Certainly a single TIA may be due either to an embolus that causes an evanescent deficit or to carotid or basilar stenosis.

Treatment Patients who present with TIAs should be investigated with Doppler ultrasound flow studies of the appropriate cervical trunk artery (internal carotid or vertebrals), and, in selected cases, with MRA or arteriography. If the lesion is localized to the proximal internal carotid artery in the neck [high-grade stenosis (lumen diameter < 1.5 mm, equivalent to greater than 90 percent reduction in diameter, or a large ulcerated plaque)], endarterectomy (or angioplasty with deployment of a stent in patients who

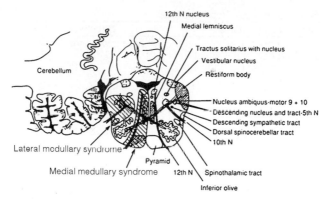

FIG. 34-4 Upper Medulla

Signs and symptoms	Structures involved
1. Medial medullary syndrome (occlusion of vertebral artery or branch of vertebral or lower basilar artery)	
a. On side of lesion: paralysis with atrophy of half the tongue	Twelfth nerve nucleus or issuing fibers
b. On side opposite lesion	
(1) Paralysis of arm and leg, sparing face	Pyramidal tract
(2) Impaired tactile and proprioceptive sense over half the body	Medial lemniscus
2. Lateral medullary syndrome (occlusion of any of five vessels—vertebral, posterior inferior cerebellar, or superior, middle, or inferior lateral medullary arteries)	
a. On side of lesion	
(1) Pain, numbness, impaired sensation over half the face	Descending tract and nucleus of fifth nerve
(2) Ataxia of limbs, falling to side of lesion	Possibly restiform body, cerebellar hemisphere, olivocerebellar fibers, spinocerebellar tract (?)
(3) Vertigo, nausea, vomiting	Vestibular nuclei and connections
(4) Nystagmus, diplopia, oscillopsia	Vestibular nuclei and connections
(5) Horner syndrome (miosis, ptosis, decreased sweating)	Descending sympathetic tract
(6) Dysphagia, hoarseness, paralysis of vocal cord, diminished gag reflex	Ninth and tenth nerve nuclei or their issuing fibers
(7) Loss of taste (rare)	Nucleus and tractus solitarius
(8) Numbness of ipsilateral arm, trunk, or leg	Cuneate and gracile nuclei
(9) Hiccup	Uncertain

(continued)

FIG. 34-4 *(continued)* Upper Medulla

Signs and symptoms	Structures involved
b. On side opposite lesion: impaired pain and thermal sense over half the body, sometimes face	Spinothalamic tract
3. **Total unilateral medullary syndrome** (occlusion of vertebral artery); combination of medial and lateral syndromes	
4. **Basilar artery syndrome** (the syndrome of the lone vertebral artery is equivalent); a combination of the various brainstem syndromes and those arising in the posterior cerebral artery distribution; the clinical picture comprises bilateral long-tract signs (sensory and motor) with cerebellar and cranial nerve abnormalities	
a. Paralysis or weakness of all extremities, plus all bulbar musculature	Corticobulbar and corticospinal tracts bilaterally
b. Diplopia, paralysis of conjugate lateral and/or vertical gaze, internuclear ophthalmoplegia, horizontal and/or vertical nystagmus	Ocular motor nerves, pathways for conjugate gaze, medial longitudinal fasciculus, vestibular apparatus
c. Blindness or impaired vision, various visual field defects	Visual cortex
d. Bilateral cerebellar ataxia	Cerebellar peduncles and cerebellar hemispheres
e. Coma	Tegmentum of midbrain, thalami
f. Sensation may be intact in the presence of almost total paralysis; sensory loss may be syringomyelic or involve all modalities	Medial lemniscus, spinothalamic tracts or thalamic nuclei

are poor surgical risks) reduces modestly the incidence of subsequent stroke. Here the medical condition of the patient, the state of the intracranial portion of the carotid artery, the configuration of the circle of Willis, the state of the other cerebral arteries, and the operative record of the surgeon are important in making the decision. If the disease is most apparent in the intracranial portion of the carotid artery or in the vertebrobasilar system, one resorts to long-term warfarin or aspirin therapy.

EMBOLIC INFARCTION

Cerebral embolism is considered to be the single most frequent cause of stroke. If one adds the strokes of indeterminate origin (most of which are probably embolic as well) to those of presumed embolism, 40 percent or more of all strokes will prove to be embolic, compared with 32 percent of thrombotic origin (see Table 34-2).

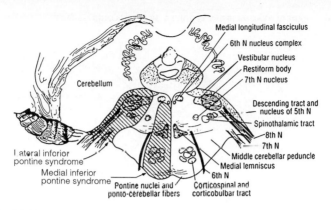

Medial longitudinal fasciculus
6th N nucleus complex
Vestibular nucleus
Restiform body
7th N nucleus

Cerebellum

Descending tract and
nucleus of 5th N
Spinothalamic tract
8th N
7th N
Middle cerebellar peduncle
Medial lemniscus
6th N
Corticospinal and
corticobulbar tract

Lateral inferior
pontine syndrome
Medial inferior
pontine syndrome
Pontine nuclei and
ponto-cerebellar fibers

FIG. 34-5 Lower Pons

Signs and symptoms	Structures involved
1. Medial inferior pontine syndrome (occlusion of paramedian branch of basilar artery)	
a. On side of lesion	
(1) Paralysis of conjugate gaze to side of lesion (preservation of convergence)	Pontine "center" for lateral gaze (PPRF)
(2) Nystagmus	Vestibular nuclei and connections
(3) Ataxia of limbs and gait	Middle cerebellar peduncle (?)
(4) Diplopia on lateral gaze	Abducens nucleus or exiting fibers
b. On side opposite lesion	
(1) Paralysis of face, arm, and leg	Corticobulbar and corticospinal tracts in lower pons
(2) Impaired tactile and proprioceptive sense over half of the body	Medial lemniscus
2. Lateral inferior pontine syndrome (occlusion of anterior inferior cerebellar artery)	
a. On side of lesion	
(1) Horizontal and vertical nystagmus, vertigo, nausea, vomiting, oscillopsia	Vestibular nuclei and their connections with oculomotor nucleus
(2) Facial paralysis	Seventh nerve nucleus or exiting fibers
(3) Paralysis of conjugate gaze to side of lesion	Pontine "center" for lateral gaze (PPRF)
(4) Deafness, tinnitus	Auditory nerve or cochlear nucleus
(5) Ataxia	Middle cerebellar peduncle and cerebellar hemisphere
(6) Impaired sensation over face	Descending tract and nucleus fifth nerve
b. On side opposite lesion: impaired pain and thermal sense over half the body (may include face)	Spinothalamic tract
3. Total unilateral inferior pontine syndrome (occlusion of anterior inferior cerebellar artery); lateral and medial syndromes combined	

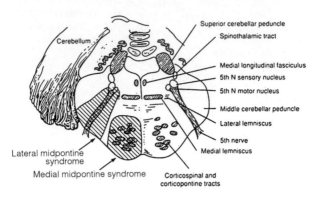

FIG. 34-6 Midpons

Signs and symptoms	Structures involved
1. Medial midpontine syndrome (paramedian branch of mid-basilar artery)	
a. On side of lesion: ataxia of limbs and gait (more prominent in bilateral involvement)	Middle cerebellar peduncle
b. On side opposite lesion	
(1) Paralysis of face, arm, and leg	Corticobulbar and corticospinal tracts
(2) Deviation of eyes	
(3) Variably impaired touch and proprioception when lesion extends posteriorly; usually the syndrome is purely motor	Medial lemniscus
2. Lateral midpontine syndrome (short circumferential artery): On side of lesion:	
a. Ataxia of limbs	Middle cerebellar peduncle
b. Paralysis of muscles of mastication	Motor fibers or nucleus of fifth nerve
c. Impaired sensation over side of face	Sensory fibers or nucleus of fifth nerve

Most cerebral emboli arise in the heart in relation to atrial fibrillation, myocardial infarction with mural thrombi, akinetic segment of heart wall, endocarditis, etc. Others come from the aorta or large cranial arteries or through a patent foramen ovale. Unlike a thrombus, which adheres to the vessel wall, the embolic particle is friable and migratory. Emboli tend to lodge in distal medium-size branches of brain arteries; hence there are many more partial syndromes than there are with thrombosis. The embolus may disintegrate before tissue necrosis can occur or, if the tissue is already infarcted, it may become hemorrhagic as circulation is restored.

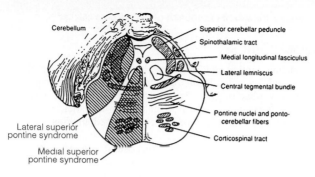

Labels on figure:
Cerebellum
Superior cerebellar peduncle
Spinothalamic tract
Medial longitudinal fasciculus
Lateral lemniscus
Central tegmental bundle
Pontine nuclei and ponto-cerebellar fibers
Corticospinal tract
Lateral superior pontine syndrome
Medial superior pontine syndrome

FIG. 34-7 Upper Pons

Signs and symptoms	Structures involved
1. Medial superior pontine syndrome (paramedian branches of upper basilar artery)	
a. On side of lesion	
(1) Cerebellar ataxia	Superior and/or middle cerebellar peduncle
(2) Internuclear opthalmoplegia	Medial longitudinal fasciculus
(3) Rhythmic myoclonus of palate, pharynx, vocal cords, diaphragm, ocular-motor and shoulder-girdle muscles, face	Central tegmental tract
b. On side opposite lesion	
(1) Paralysis of face, arm, and leg	Corticobulbar and corticospinal tracts
(2) Touch, vibration, and position senses are occasionally affected	Medial lemniscus
2. Lateral superior pontine syndrome (syndrome of superior cerebellar artery)	
a. On side of lesion	
(1) Ataxia of limbs and gait, falling to side of lesion	Middle and superior cerebellar peduncles, superior surface of cerebellum, dentate nucleus
(2) Dizziness, nausea, vomiting, horizontal nystagmus	Vestibular nuclei
(3) Paresis of conjugate gaze (ipsilateral)	Uncertain
(4) Loss of optokinetic nystagmus	Uncertain
(5) Skew deviation	Uncertain
(6) Miosis, ptosis, decreased sweating over face (Horner syndrome)	Descending sympathetic fibers
b. On side opposite lesion	
(1) Impaired pain and thermal sense on face, limbs, and trunk	Spinothalamic tract
(2) Impaired touch, vibration, and position sense, more in leg than arm	Medial lemniscus (lateral portion)

(Items 2 through 5 bracketed together: Territory of descending branch from superior cerebellar artery)

Clinical Manifestations

Of all ischemic strokes, the embolic type develops most rapidly, literally within several seconds. While the brain is the most frequent site of embolism of cardiac origin, other organs (spleen, kidney, gastrointestinal tract, legs) may also be involved. Again, the stroke pattern accords more or less with the neurovascular syndromes displayed in Figs. 34-1 to 34-7. Branches of the middle cerebral arteries are the most frequently affected (Fig. 34-8), followed in frequency by the posterior cerebral artery, branches of the vertebral and basilar arteries, and the anterior cerebral artery. About one-third of embolic infarcts become hemorrhagic, a phenomenon that can be exposed by serial CT scans or MRI.

The immediate prognosis for a patient with embolic infarction is much the same as for a patient with thrombotic infarction except that recession of the neurologic deficit tends to be more rapid in the former. Always there is a threat of recurrent embolism.

Treatment

Nothing except perhaps thrombolysis in certain cases (discussed below) can be done about an infarct that has already occurred, and treatment is directed to the prevention of recurrent embolism. The prevention of embolic strokes, more than any other, is amenable to long-term anticoagulation with warfarin and antiplatelet drugs. However, early heparinization of a potentially hemorrhagic infarct, particularly if the infarct is large and the patient is hypertensive, carries a slightly increased risk of bleeding. Approximately 30 percent of all embolic cerebral infarcts become hemorrhagic, but it may require 3 to 4 days for that aspect to become apparent. For this reason, some neurologists prefer to wait for this length of time before initiating heparinization, particularly if thrombolytic agents have been used. There is, of course, a danger, however slight, of recurrent embolism during this brief waiting period. If there is no evidence of hemorrhage, we generally proceed with IV heparin on the first day, a bolus of 5000 U to begin with and a continuous infusion at a rate of about 1000 U/h for several days. A safe target is to establish a partial thromboplastin time (PTT) of 2 to 2½ times the control value. It must be acknowledged, however, that there is little firm evidence to support the early use of heparin in cases of embolic stroke, and many centers forgo its use. If a source of embolus is established or strongly suspected, warfarin is introduced at the same time and given for 6 to 12 months or indefinitely. In cases of *atrial fibrillation*, a dosage (usually 2.5 to 7.5 mg daily) is used to maintain a prothrombin time of 1½ times the control value or an international normalized clotting ratio (INR) of 2 to 3.

As indicated earlier, there are special circumstances, applicable to relatively few patients, in which the development of an infarct can be mitigated by the administration of *thrombolytic agents* (t-PA, 0.9 mg/kg, 10 percent as an IV bolus and the remainder over 1 h). To be effective, therapy must be instituted within 3 h of the onset of symptoms and must be avoided in patients who are excessively hypertensive or taking anticoagulants. Under the best of circumstances, 6 percent of cases are accompanied by a cerebral hemorrhage. The risk of hemorrhage appears to be even higher, and the anticipated degree of improvement more limited in patients who present

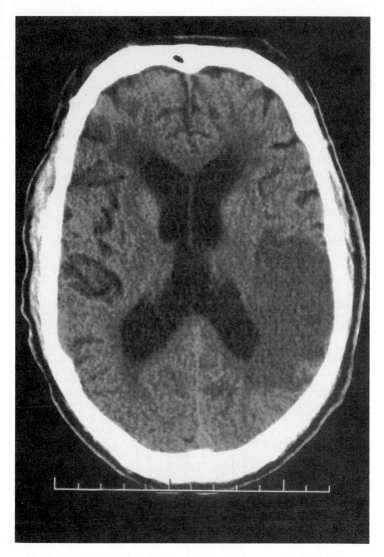

FIG. 34-8   CT scan showing a recent embolic infarction in the inferior division of the left middle cerebral artery. The well-demarcated region of low density may not appear on CT images for a day or more after the stroke.

with signs and radiologic evidence of massive infarction—those with minor neurologic deficits probably also benefit little; t-PA is not recommended under these circumstances. Intra-arterial administration of thrombolytics, while difficult to accomplish, may have benefit up to 6 h or longer in selected patients.

LACUNAR INFARCTION

Occlusion of small penetrating vessels in the putamen, caudate, internal capsule, thalamus, pons, and white matter of the corona radiata (in descending order of frequency) leads to small infarcts ranging from 3 to 4 mm to 1.5 to 2.0 cm in diameter. This happens most often in patients with atherosclerosis, on the basis of hypertension and diabetes. Fisher, who studied the affected vessels by serial section, observed the larger ones (400 to 900 μm) to be occluded by atheroma or emboli near their origins and the smaller ones (less than 200 μm) by a special type of atherosclerotic lesion, called *lipohyalinosis*, in their course through the brain. The resulting infarcts eventually cavitate, hence the term lacunes. CT scans may appear normal for a week or more, but most lacunar infarcts can be visualized by MRI within several hours of the stroke (Fig. 34-9).

Lacunar infarcts may be silent clinically or cause one of several characteristic restricted deficits such as *pure motor hemiplegia* (internal capsule or base of pons), *pure hemisensory deficit* (ventrolateral thalamus), *dysarthria and a clumsy hand* (pons or internal capsule), or *weakness and ataxia* on one side (capsule or pons). Lacunar strokes are occasionally preceded by TIAs. Multiple lacunar infarcts may eventually induce a pseudobulbar palsy.

Aspirin or another platelet antiaggregant is often used. A low-fat, low-cholesterol diet and antihypertensive medication are recommended as therapy, but there are no data on their efficacy. Anticoagulation seems to be of little benefit and may be risky in the hypertensive patient; the reported improvements with thrombolytic therapy are difficult to interpret.

INTRACRANIAL HEMORRHAGE

The many causes of intracranial hemorrhage are listed in Table 34-3. The most important of these are primary intracerebral hemorrhage, ruptured saccular aneurysm, arteriovenous malformation (AVM), anticoagulation or bleeding diathesis, and trauma, including epidural and subdural hematomas.

Primary Intracerebral Hemorrhage

This is also called hypertensive because most cases occur in patients with an elevated blood pressure, although in these cases hemorrhage does not necessarily correlate in occurrence with the presence or degree of chronic hypertension. Excitement or strain, or adrenergic drugs, may be provocative. In an unknown proportion of cases, amyloidosis of cerebral arteries appears to be the underlying cause.

Of all the cerebrovascular diseases, this is the most dramatic and most deserving of the name *apoplexy*. The patient is felled in his tracks or is seized with a headache and rapidly sinks into coma. With massive hemorrhage, death follows in hours or days. At autopsy, hemispheral clot swells the brain and bloodies the ventricular and subarachnoid fluid.

A lesser magnitude of hemorrhage is also possible. In 20 to 30 percent of cases, the headache is mild, and a focal neurologic deficit may occur without loss of consciousness and be indistinguishable clinically from an infarct. Only with CT scanning is a discrete hemorrhage recognized. All gradations between large and small hemorrhages may be observed.

The common sites of primary brain hemorrhage in order of their frequency are (1) putaminal-capsular (50 percent), (2) lobar (within the white

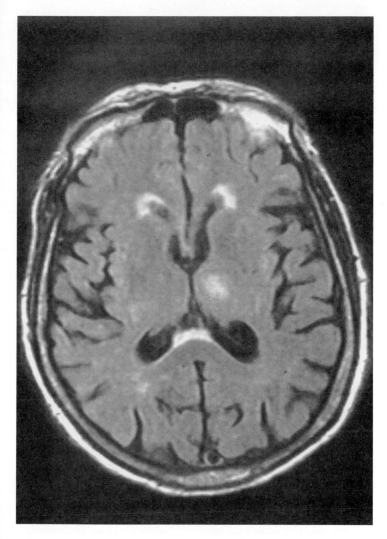

FIG. 34-9   MRI of an acute lacunar infarction in the left thalamus that caused a pure sensory syndrome. This FLAIR image highlights the bright edema in the region of the stroke. A small cavitary lesion follows.

matter of one of the lobes of the brain), (3) thalamic, (4) cerebellar, and (5) pontine. All but the second type, which has an association with antico-agulation, have a consistent relationship to chronic hypertension.

With large *putaminal hemorrhages*, patients quickly lapse into stupor and coma with hemiplegia. The onset may be with headache and vomiting, and hemiplegia may evolve over a period of 5 to 30 min, with deviation of the eyes to the side of the lesion, followed by progressive confusion, stupor, coma, increasing hypertension, and signs of upper brainstem compression,

TABLE 34-3 Causes of Intracranial Hemorrhage (including Intracerebral, Subarachnoid, Ventricular, and Subdural)

1. Primary (hypertensive) intracerebral hemorrhage
2. Ruptured saccular aneurysm
3. Ruptured AVM
4. Amyloid angiopathy
5. Hemorrhagic infarction
6. Trauma, including posttraumatic delayed apoplexy
7. Hemorrhagic disorders: warfarin anticoagulation, leukemia, aplastic anemia, thrombocytopenic purpura, liver disease, complication of thrombolytic therapy, hyperfibrinolysis, hypofibrinogenemia, hemophilia, Christmas disease, etc.
8. Hemorrhage into primary and secondary brain tumors
9. Septic embolism, mycotic aneurysm
10. With inflammatory disease of the arteries and veins
11. Miscellaneous rare types: after vasopressor drugs, on exertion, during arteriography, during painful urologic examination, as a late complication of early-life carotid occlusion, complication of carotid-cavernous AV fistula, with anoxemia, migraine, teratomatous malformations; herpes simplex encephalitis and acute necrotizing hemorrhagic encephalopathy may be associated with up to 2000 red blood cells or more and many white blood cells per cubic millimeter in the CSF; tularemia, anthrax, and *Pseudomonas* meningitis and snake venom poisoning may cause bloody CSF
12. Undetermined (normal blood pressure; no coagulopathy, AVM, or aneurysm)

Key: AVM, arteriovenous malformation; CSF, cerebrospinal fluid.

mainly enlargement of the pupils (Fig. 34-10). A smaller putaminal-capsular hemorrhage may behave clinically like an embolic or thrombotic ischemic stroke, its true nature being disclosed by CT scan.

The clinical picture of *lobar hemorrhage* will depend on its location: occipital (pain around ipsilateral eye and homonymous hemianopia), temporal (pain in or anterior to ear, incomplete homonymous hemianopia, fluent aphasia), frontal (contralateral hemiplegia and frontal headache), or parietal (anterior temporal headache and contralateral hemisensory defect). The occurrence of one of these syndromes in conjunction with headache, vomiting, and stupor is diagnostic, and CT scanning is corroborative. Warfarin or heparin anticoagulation and the presence of an underlying saccular aneurysm, arteriovenous malformation (AVM), bleeding disease, amyloid angiopathy, or metastatic tumor are other causes that need always to be considered, but many cases have no clear origin; a history of hypertension is present in only half of patients and its role in causation is usually unclear.

In *thalamic hemorrhage*, a complete hemisensory defect may be the most prominent feature. Hemiparesis is usually conjoined because of rupture into the internal capsule. Aphasia may be present with dominant lesions and amorphosynthesis (page 186) with nondominant ones. Ocular abnormalities are frequent, particularly downward deviation of the eyes and small, poorly reactive or nonreactive pupils. The prognosis relates closely to the size of the hemorrhage.

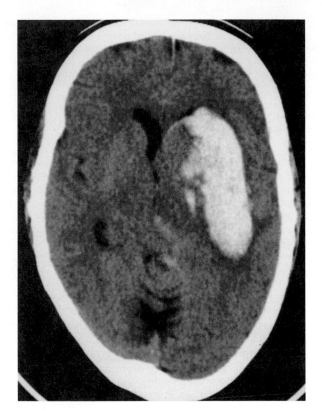

Figure 34-10   An unenhanced CT scan showing a typical primary (hypertensive) hemorrhage in the basal ganglia. The third ventricle and opposite lateral ventricle are compressed and displaced by the expanding mass (12 h after onset of stroke).

Pontine hemorrhage is characterized by the rapid evolution of coma and total paralysis, decerebrate rigidity, and small but reactive pupils. Survival is possible with small hemorrhages that do not cause coma.

With *cerebellar hemorrhage*, vomiting, occipital headache, vertigo, inability to stand, and forced deviation of the eyes to the side opposite the lesion are the usual manifestations. Ataxia of the limbs and nystagmus may not be evident, so examination of stance and gait is of special importance. Loss of consciousness at the onset is unusual unless the clot is massive or it blocks the fourth ventricle, causing acute hydrocephalus.

Treatment and prognosis Approximately half of patients with primary intracerebral hemorrhage and nearly all comatose ones succumb. Clots larger than 60 mL are almost invariably fatal. Survival is likely with clots smaller than 30 mL, sometimes with striking regression of focal signs. Patients with amyloidosis of cerebral vessels may suffer recurrent hemorrhages.

Surgical removal of the clot is seldom successful in saving life, although a few patients with a lobar hemorrhage and a large proportion of those who are not comatose with a cerebellar hemorrhage may be salvaged. In the acute stage, control of intracranial pressure and hypertension, by measures outlined in Chaps. 17 and 30, should be undertaken. Any abnormality of coagulation must be corrected immediately.

Spontaneous Subarachnoid Hemorrhage Due to Ruptured Saccular Aneurysm

This is the fourth most frequent cerebrovascular disease. The aneurysm consists of a small (2 mm to 2 cm, average 8 to 10 mm), berry-shaped dilatation of a surface artery of the brain. Most of these aneurysms lie in the crotch of a bifurcating artery on or near the circle of Willis. Some 80 to 90 percent are found on the intracranial branches of the internal carotid arteries; the rest, on vertebral and basilar arteries or their branches (Fig. 34-11). In most instances, they are small and clinically silent until the patient reaches 35 to 65 years of age, when they rupture and give rise to a subarachnoid hemorrhage. Chronic hypertension is not an essential preceding factor.

There may be one or several aneurysms (multiple in 20 percent of patients), but with subarachnoid hemorrhage only one will be found to have bled. Why the aneurysm forms in the first place is not certain. A congenital defect of the internal elastic lamina and media of the vessel wall is the most widely accepted theory. The occurrence of such aneurysms in 5 percent of patients with AVMs (see below) supports a theory of congenital origin.

Clinical manifestations Most aneurysms are recognized only when they rupture and cause a subarachnoid hemorrhage. This produces severe headache of acute onset, nausea, vomiting, and signs of meningeal irritation. *The occurrence of these symptoms in an adult who is not febrile and has no focal or lateralizing neurologic signs is virtually diagnostic of a ruptured saccular aneurysm.* In most cases, the bleeding remains confined to the subarachnoid space and causes no signs of cerebral damage, but a jet of blood may enter the brain and add a focal deficit to the syndrome. Occasionally the aneurysms may, by a process of expansion and by oozing and accretion of surface clots, reach a large size (3 to 4 cm) and compress cranial nerves or other structures.

Rupture of an aneurysm sometimes follows intense physical effort or Valsalva maneuver (heavy lifting, sexual intercourse). In some cases of hemorrhage, focal signs are an accurate indicator of the site of the aneurysm. An aneurysm at the junction of the internal carotid and posterior communicating arteries, as it enlarges, compresses the adjacent oculomotor nerve, with pupillary enlargement; one at the anterior-middle cerebral junction may compress the nearby optic nerve or bleed into inferomedial parts of the frontal lobe; and one at the bifurcation of the middle cerebral artery may bleed into the frontal lobes and cause hemiplegia.

A large subarachnoid hemorrhage may be immediately fatal—the only form of cerebrovascular disease that results in sudden death—but most patients reach the hospital in a conscious state. The diagnosis is established by CT scanning (Fig. 34-12) or by a lumbar puncture that is performed if the CT is normal. Angiography visualizes the aneurysm in 95 percent of cases. MRA and spiral CT scanning are increasingly being used to complement or supplant conventional angiography.

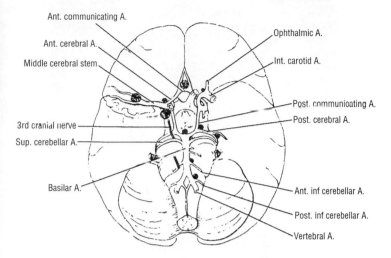

Figure 34-11 Diagram of the circle of Willis to show the principal sites of saccular aneurysms. Approximately 90 percent of aneurysms are on the anterior half of the circle.

Some 30 to 40 percent of untreated bleeding aneurysms *rerupture* within 2 months (most of them within the first week), and many of these prove fatal. The second major complication of ruptured aneurysm is vascular spasm (*vasospasm*) and cerebral infarction, occurring usually in the territory of the artery harboring the aneurysm, most often during the first and second weeks. Vasospasm often occurs in vessels that are surrounded by clotted blood, which can be visualized on the CT scan. *Hydrocephalus*, due to blockage of the cerebrospinal fluid (CSF) pathways by blood, may develop acutely or weeks after rupture. Cerebral salt wasting and the syndrome of inappropriate diuretic hormone (SIADH) may also be observed (see Chap. 27).

Treatment and prognosis Early diagnosis, definition of the vascular anatomy by angiography, direct surgical exposure of the aneurysm, and obliteration of it by a clip placed on its neck constitute the only sure treatment. As experience is being gained with newer endovascular techniques, they may gradually replace conventional surgical clipping, particularly for aneurysms that are difficult to reach, such as those on the basilar artery.

Early surgery, within 48 h of rupture, is practical in most patients and obviates rerupture. However, if the patient is in deep stupor or coma, the surgical mortality becomes so high as to be unacceptable. The preference then is to control the blood pressure and prevent convulsions until consciousness is regained. There is no certain method of preventing vascular spasm and subsequent infarction; intravascular volume expansion may do so, but this measure can only be used safely in the postoperative period. Evidence in recent years indicates that the use of calcium channel blockers (nimodipine, 60 mg every 4 h for 21 days) may be helpful in preventing infarction from vasospasm.

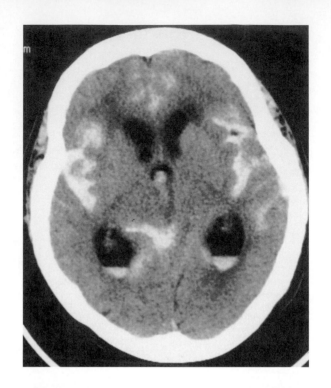

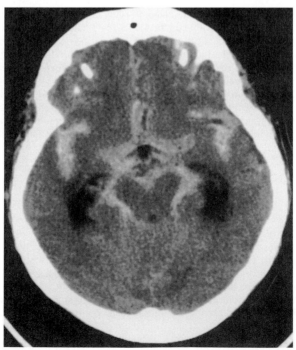

316

In some cases, the aneurysm cannot be seen angiographically, even when the procedure is repeated after the vascular spasm has subsided. In such patients, the risk of rebleeding is less than in patients with an untreated demonstrable aneurysm. A special group of patients with limited perimesencephalic hemorrhage tend not to have demonstrable aneurysms. Their prognosis also is favorable. Very small unruptured aneurysms, < 3 to 4 mm, found incidentally by an imaging procedure can usually be followed by serial imaging rather than requiring surgery.

Arteriovenous Malformation (AVM)

These hamartomatous malformations are about one-third as frequent as saccular aneurysms. They may be only 1 cm or even less in size or so large as to occupy the major portion of a lobe of a cerebral hemisphere or a large part of the brainstem or cerebellum. They consist of a mass of small vessels fed by large arteries and drained by large veins. In most instances, they are asymptomatic until they bleed into the subarachnoid space, brain, or ventricle. In a significant number of cases, there are focal seizures or a migraine syndrome, which should prompt one to initiate a search for the AVM by an enhanced CT scan or MRI. A small proportion of AVMs are manifested by a progressive neurologic deficit due to their gradual enlargement or to shunting of blood through enlarged vascular channels ("intracerebral steal"). Hemorrhage, the feared complication, may be recurrent and fatal, but the risk of death is less than with bleeding from ruptured aneurysm.

Cavernous angiomas constitute a separate group of vascular malformations, made up of a cluster of thin-walled veins. Often these are angiographically invisible, but they may have a characteristic appearance in MRI in which hemosiderin (black on T1 images) is deposited within or surrounding a small irregular nodule. They bleed frequently but the hemorrhages tend to be small in size, causing only minor deficits unless they are located in the brainstem. In some cases, they are multiple and familial.

If an AVM is small and accessible in a "quiet zone" of the brain, it can be extirpated surgically with an acceptably low mortality and morbidity. With large and complicated AVMs, preoperative embolization of large feeding vessels is a valuable adjuvant procedure and sometimes is alone adequate for treatment of smaller lesions. If AVMs are inoperable, focused gamma or proton radiation will obliterate small ones in 80 to 90 percent of cases and probably help the management of large ones as well.

Figure 34-12 Subarachnoid hemorrhage due to rupture of a basilar artery aneurysm. (*Top*) Axial CT scan image at the level of the lateral ventricles showing widespread blood in the subarachnoid spaces and layering within the ventricles with resultant hydrocephalus. (*Bottom*) At the level of the basal cisterns blood can be seen surrounding the brainstem, in the anterior sylvian fissures and the anterior interhemispheric fissure. The temporal horns of the lateral ventricles are again enlarged, reflecting acute hydrocephalus.

LESS COMMON TYPES OF CEREBROVASCULAR DISEASE

1. *Dissection of the carotid and vertebral arteries*: Carotid dissection may occur without explanation in a relatively young person (more often a woman) or following cervical, cranial, or thoracic trauma or even following forceful coughing or sneezing. Blood ruptures into the vessel wall, dissecting between its coats. The lumen is visibly narrowed in an arteriogram (string sign), sometimes to the point of occlusion. The clinical manifestations are craniofacial or neck pain and Horner syndrome on the side of the dissection, to which cerebral symptoms of ischemia in the carotid territory and lower cranial nerve palsies may be added. The vertebral or basilar artery may also be the site of dissection. There is risk of embolism from the upper end of the narrowed artery; hence, anticoagulant medication should be given while one is awaiting spontaneous recanalization.

2. *Fibromuscular dysplasia*: This is a segmental nonatheromatous, noninflammatory disease involving mainly the cervical arteries of middle-aged women. Radiologically, the affected artery is traversed by a series of ridges, imparting a "string of beads" appearance. It may be an unexpected finding during an arteriogram, or there may be neurologic symptoms consequent to a dissection, artery-to-artery embolism, or sometimes an associated saccular aneurysm. A similar condition occurs in the renal arteries, leading to hypertension.

3. *Moyamoya disease*: *Moyamoya* is the Japanese word for "cloud" or "haze" and refers to a network of fine anastomotic vessels at the base of the brain. The disorder is seen mainly in children who have suffered one or several inexplicable arterial occlusions. The cause of this finding is most often a fibrotic occlusion of the basal cerebral vessels, mainly the distal internal carotid artery. The condition may occur silently but is later revealed by seizures, focal cerebral symptoms, or a hemorrhage. There is no agreement on therapy. Many of the patients are of Asian extraction.

4. *Other causes of stroke in children and young adults*: Most have been traced to a hypercoagulable state (antiphospholipid antibody, sickle cell anemia, thrombocytosis, protein C and S deficiency, homocystinuria, etc.) or to moyamoya, paradoxical embolism through a patent foramen ovale, intra- or extracranial arterial dissection, MELAS (mitochondrial disorder—see further on), or inflammatory diseases of arteries or veins.

5. *Strokes occurring during pregnancy and postpartum*: Strokes occurring during pregnancy and in women taking oral contraceptives are mainly arterial. Strokes in the postpartum period (and postoperatively) are mainly venous and thought to be due to disorders of blood clotting.

6. *Binswanger subcortical infarction*: This is a predominantly white-matter disease of the elderly, manifest by symptoms of vascular dementia. The exact nature of the vascular lesions is unknown, and treatment is uncertain. Hypertension is almost invariable. A heritable condition termed CADASIL (defined in Table 34-1) causes similar subcortical confluent gliosis in the absence of hypertension.

7. *Hypertensive encephalopathy*: This term refers to an acutely or subacutely evolving syndrome of severe hypertension (diastolic pressure > 120 to 125 mmHg) associated with headache, nausea and vomiting, visual disturbances due to retinal hemorrhages, exudates, and

papilledema, convulsive seizures, and mental confusion. In addition, there may be signs of the more common cerebral complications (hemorrhage, infarction) of severe chronic hypertension. In *eclampsia* and *acute renal disease*, especially in children, similar encephalopathic symptoms and seizures develop at blood pressure levels lower than those indicated above. Histologically, there are widespread minute infarcts in the brain, the result of fibrinoid necrosis of arterioles and capillaries and occlusion by fibrin thrombi. These lesions are responsible for large exudative zones of cerebral edema most prominent in the occipital lobes, which imparts a characteristic CT and MR picture.

8. *Cranial arteritis*: Included under this title is a large and diverse group of inflammatory diseases of cranial arteries which can only be enumerated here. One group comprises the *giant-cell arteritides*: temporal arteritis, granulomatous arteritis of the brain, and aortic branch disease (Takayasu disease). A second group includes polyarteritis nodosa, arteritis of the Churg-Strauss type, Wegener granulomatosis, lupus erythematosus, Behçet disease, postzoster arteritis, and AIDS arteritis.

9. *Migraine with stroke:* A small number of patients with neurologic migraine (Chap. 10) will be left with residual defects. Furthermore, rare patients with a history of migraine develop TIA-like episodes in late life. These most often take the form of spreading paresthesias or aphasia followed by mild unilateral headache.

10. *Mitochondrial diseases:* Stroke and TIAs are core features of a syndrome that additionally includes myopathy, lactic acidosis, recurrent vomiting, focal and generalized seizures, and encephalopathy (MELAS). Most cases appear in childhood and result in growth retardation, but milder cases are seen in adults, with only migraine and stroke-like episodes.

CEREBRAL VEIN AND SINUS THROMBOSIS

Septic thrombophlebitis, usually in conjunction with meningitis or infections of the ear and paranasal sinuses, has been described in Chap. 32. Bland occlusion of cerebral veins and of the venous sinuses is far more common, giving rise to a number of important neurologic syndromes. Diagnosis is difficult except in certain clinical settings known to favor the occurrence of venous thrombosis, such as the taking of birth control pills or postpartum and postoperative states; hypercoagulable states in cancer and cyanotic congenital heart disease; cachexia in infants; sickle cell disease; antiphospholipid antibody syndrome, factor V Leiden mutation, protein S or C deficiency, antithrombin III deficiency, and resistance to activated protein C; primary or secondary polycythemia and thrombocythemia; and paroxysmal nocturnal hemoglobinuria. A few cases follow head injury or remain unexplained.

In general, a slow evolution of a focal frontoparietal deficit, the presence of multiple cerebral lesions not in typical arterial territories, early seizures, and a hemorrhagic tendency favor venous over arterial thrombosis. Certain syndromes occur with sufficient regularity to suggest thrombosis of a particular vein or sinus. In the case of *sagittal sinus thrombosis*, intracranial hypertension with headache, vomiting, and papilledema (without hydrocephalus) may constitute the entire syndrome or may be conjoined with hemorrhagic infarction; indeed, this is the main consideration in the differential diagnosis of pseudotumor cerebri (Chap. 30). A similar syndrome occurs with thrombosis of the jugular vein or lateral sinus. The main features of *thrombosis of cortical surface veins* are the presence of large cortical and subjacent white matter hemorrhagic infarctions and a marked tendency to seizures. To the extent that most of these cortical vein thromboses originate from clots in the sagittal sinus, the hemorrhagic infarctions tend to be parasagittal, characteristically biparietal, and less often bifrontal, with headache or paraparesis or hemiparesis predominantly of the leg. The variable location of the infarctions reflects the inconstant location of the main surface cerebral veins. Marked chemosis and proptosis—with findings referable to cranial nerves III, IV, VI, and the ophthalmic division of V— are indicative of *anterior cavernous sinus thrombosis*.

The radiologic picture of superior sagittal sinus occlusion is of superficial paramedian parietal hemorrhagic infarction, often bilateral. The enhanced CT scan, arteriography (venous phase), and MR venography greatly facilitate diagnosis by demonstrating directly the venous occlusion. In the case of CT scan with contrast infusion, a lack of dye in the posterior sagittal sinus can be observed with careful adjustment of the viewing window ("empty delta sign"). The spinal fluid pressure is increased and the fluid may be slightly sanguinous.

Anticoagulant therapy beginning with heparin for several days, followed by warfarin—combined with antibiotics if the venous occlusion is infectious (it rarely is in recent times)—has been lifesaving in some cases, but the overall mortality rate remains high due to large hemorrhagic venous infarctions. Thrombolytic therapy by local venous or systemic infusion has also been successful in several instances but is usually reserved for extreme cases with stupor or coma and greatly raised cerebrospinal fluid pressure.

APPROACH TO THE STROKE PATIENT

The physician is confronted by a diverse number of stroke problems, each of which needs to be managed in a particular way, depending on the clinical status of the patient and the underlying disease.

For the comatose stroke patient (massive hypertensive or subarachnoid hemorrhage, or massive cerebral or brainstem infarction), diagnosis and provision of symptomatic care are generally all that can be accomplished. Thrombolysis of a basilar artery occlusion or removal of a cerebellar or hemispheral hemorrhage or edematous cerebellar or hemispheral infarction will salvage some patients provided that deep coma has not supervened. Drainage of hydrocephalus after subarachnoid hemorrhage or cerebellar stroke may have dramatic results.

A recently completed or an evolving stroke in a noncomatose patient is a frequent clinical problem. The type of stroke needs to be determined by clinical and laboratory methods and the patient treated according to the methods outlined earlier.

Since most such patients survive, long-term plans need to be made for rehabilitation and the prevention of further strokes. Here the differentiation of thrombosis and embolism assumes importance. For embolism, one searches the heart, aorta, and great vessels for its source by using ultrasound, MRI, and Holter monitoring. For thrombosis of inapparent cause, one searches for abnormal clotting factors, arterial dissection, and arteritis.

The possibility of a stroke masquerading as another illness should be kept in mind—a small subarachnoid hemorrhage from a leaking aneurysm causing headache; a posterior cerebral artery occlusion with only a homonymous visual field defect (found by testing visual fields); a cerebellar hemorrhage not evident unless the patient is made to stand and walk; a mild paraphasic difficulty that may be misinterpreted as a confusional state or a psychosis; or a lateral medullary infarction mistaken for a gastrointestinal illness, myocardial infarction, vestibular neuronitis, or labyrinthitis.

Finally, there is the patient who gives a history of a stroke but has fully recovered. Here a premium attaches to accurate diagnosis of the type of stroke (by assessment of cardiovascular status and heart rhythm, coagulative factors, ultrasound studies of carotid arteries, serum lipids, and MRA and MRI) and the application of measures that reduce the risk of recurrent stroke.

For a more detailed discussion of this topic, see Victor and Ropper: *Adams and Victor's Principles of Neurology*, 7th ed, pp 821–924.

ADDITIONAL READING

Amarenco P, Cohen A, Tzourio C, et al: Atherosclerotic disease of the aortic arch and the risk of ischemic stroke. *N Engl J Med* 331:1474, 1994.

Barnett HJM, Mohr JP, Stein BM, Yatsu FM (eds): *Stroke: Pathophysiology, Diagnosis and Management*, 3rd ed. New York, Churchill Livingstone, 1998.

Boston Area Anticoagulation Trial for Atrial Fibrillation Investigators: The effect of low-dose warfarin in the risk of stroke in patients with nonrheumatic atrial fibrillation. *N Engl J Med* 323:1505, 1990.

Caplan LR: *Posterior Circulation Disease: Clinical Findings, Diagnosis, and Management*. Cambridge, MA, Blackwell, 1996.

Chester EM, Agamanolis DP, Bankcr BQ, Victor M: Hypertensive encephalopathy: A clinicopathologic study of 20 cases. *Neurology* 28:198, 1978.

Crawford PM, West CR, Chadwick DW, et al: Arteriovenous malformations of the brain: Natural history in unoperated patients. *J Neurol Neurosurg Psychiatry* 49:1, 1986.

Executive Committee for the Asymptomatic Carotid Atherosclerosis Study: Endarterectomy for asymptomatic carotid artery stenosis. *JAMA* 273:1421, 1995.

Fisher CM: Lacunar strokes and infarcts: A review. *Neurology* 32:871, 1982.

Fisher CM: Late-life migraine accompaniments as a cause of unexplained transient ischemic attacks. *Can J Neurol Sci* 7:9, 1980.

Jacobs K, Moulin T, Bogousslavsky J, et al: The stroke syndrome of cortical vein thrombosis. *Neurology* 47:376, 1996.

Kase CS, Caplan LR: *Intracerebral Hemorrhage*. Boston, Butterworth-Heinemann, 1994.

Kubik CS, Adams RD: Occlusion of the basilar artery: A clinical and pathological study. *Brain* 69:73, 1946.

National Institute of Neurological Disorders and Stroke rt-PA Stroke Study Group: Tissue plasminogen activator for acute ischemic stroke. *N Engl J Med* 333:1581, 1995.

Neurology in practice: Cerebrovascular diseases. *J Neurol Neurosurg Psychiatry* 70(suppl 1):I1–22, 2001.

North American Symptomatic Carotid Endarterectomy Trial Collaborators: Beneficial effect of carotid endarterectomy in symptomatic patients with high-grade carotid stenosis. *N Engl J Med* 325:445, 1991.

Pessin MS, Duncan GW, Mohr JP, Poskanzer DC: Clinical and angiographic features of carotid transient ischemic attacks. *N Engl J Med* 296:358, 1977.

Qureshi A, Turhim S, Broderick JP, et al: Spontaneous intracerebral hemorrhage. *N Engl J Med* 344:1450, 2001.

Ropper AH, Davis KR: Lobar cerebral hemorrhages: Acute clinical syndromes in 26 cases. *Ann Neurol* 8:141, 1980.

Schievink WI: Intracranial aneurysms. *N Engl J Med* 336:28, 1997.

Shields RW Jr, Laureno R, Lachman T, Victor M: Anticoagulant-related hemorrhage in acute cerebral embolism. *Stroke* 15:426, 1984.

Swanson RA: Intravenous heparin for acute stroke: What can we learn from the megatrials? *Neurology* 52:1746, 1999.

Toole JF, Yuson CP, Janeway R: Transient ischemic attacks: A study of 225 patients. *Neurology* 28:746, 1978.

Wiebers DO, Whisnant JP, Sundt TM, O'Fallon WM: The significance of unruptured intracranial saccular aneurysms. *J Neurosurg* 66:23, 1987.

35 | Craniocerebral Trauma

Head injury is such a commonplace event that at any one time almost 1 percent of the population is suffering in some manner from its effects. Severe head injuries may require the care of a neurosurgeon, but often no more can be done than to clean the scalp wound or in the case of an intracranial hemorrhage, its removal. For the great majority of head-injured patients, the management is medical, and the neurologist should be prepared to share the responsibility for diagnosis and treatment. The neurologist and the generalist will be called upon to initiate the care of such patients, both at the scene of injury and in the hospital, for which reason they must be well versed in the diagnosis of the types of head injury and their treatment.

Definitions

Most head injuries in civilian life are nonpenetrating ("closed" or "blunt"). The term *concussion* implies a violent agitation of the brain from a blow to the head, resulting in a transient paralysis of neurologic function. The word *contusion* refers to bruising of the brain; if beneath the point struck, it is called a "coup" injury, and if on the opposite side,"contrecoup." However, contusional injury comprises a wide spectrum of pathologic changes, such as local edema, petechial or frank hemorrhage, and tearing of nerve fibers (shearing injury). Nearly always, this complex of changes requires that the injury be severe enough to cause transient or persistent unresponsiveness (i.e., concussion).

Mechanism of Concussion, Contusion, and Related Traumatic Changes

Two points deserve emphasis: *First*, the brain is capable of motion separate from the skull, owing to the fact that it virtually floats in cerebrospinal fluid (CSF). With a brisk blow that sets the head in motion (acceleration injury), movement of the brain lags. Or if the moving head strikes an immovable object (deceleration injury), motion of the head is arrested but not that of the brain. Moreover, the brainstem is anchored in the posterior fossa, beneath the tentorium, and moves very little. As a result, there occurs a torque or rotational movement of the cerebral hemispheres, with maximum deformation at the level of the high brainstem reticular formation and resulting in concussion. This is the most plausible explanation of the fact that a transient loss of consciousness (concussion) occurs only if the head is mobile when struck. *Second*, as the cerebral hemispheres undergo torsion, the surface convolutions are flung against bony prominences of the inner skull surface and folds of dura, causing both coup and contrecoup bruises, hemorrhages, and tearing of adjacent nerve fibers. Thus, contusion is a kind of epiphenomenon of the same mechanism that produces concussion. In some cases the rotational forces are believed to shear or rupture axons of nerve fibers in the white matter, particularly in parasagittal regions of the hemispheres, the corpus callosum, and the brainstem, quite apart from surface bruising. In any of these processes, the skull may or may not be fractured.

Skull Fractures

The severity of cerebral injury correlates only roughly with skull fracture. A seemingly slight injury may fracture a temporal bone (and at the same time lacerate a meningeal artery, producing an epidural hemorrhage); conversely, there may be severe concussion and contusion without skull fracture. Indeed, much of the energy of a blow to the head is dissipated by a fracture and therefore not transmitted to the intracranial contents. The fractures themselves, especially basilar ones, acquire significance because they may injure the optic or other cranial nerves and allow ingress of air (pneumocele) or bacteria, or egress of CSF from paranasal sinuses or ears (rhinorrhea, otorrhea). A fracture through the sphenoid bone or sella may tear a carotid artery, producing a carotid-cavernous fistula; or the pituitary stalk may be torn, with development of a hypothalamic-pituitary syndrome (particularly diabetes insipidus).

Concussion and Contusion

A blunt injury in which the head accelerates or decelerates at a critical velocity change of 27 to 30 ft/s (for a macaque but probably less for humans) results in an instantaneous loss of consciousness, which may last seconds, minutes, or hours. The longer the duration of unconsciousness, the greater the likelihood that some combination of shearing injury and contusion, laceration, hemorrhage, and localized edema has been added. These changes are responsible for hemiparesis, aphasia, and other focal signs, as well as for the signs of shift of central structures and temporal lobe–tentorial herniation (page 260).

In the first hours of severe injury, brain death may occur from failure of medullary-respiratory function. More frequently, patients when first seen are already conscious or rapidly regaining consciousness after a brief period of unresponsiveness (*minor head injury*). With purely concussive injury, the patient passes quickly through a state of drowsiness and confusion to full recovery (with the qualifications noted below). If the effects of contusion are added, the period of initial unconsciousness is more prolonged, and recovery varies in completeness. The sequelae of the various forms of blunt head injury are considered further on.

Acute Epidural Hematoma

This is caused by bleeding from a meningeal artery, occasionally a vein, torn by a temporal or parietal fracture. The patient may or may not have suffered a concussion and may have regained consciousness; but then, as the clot expands over a period of hours, the patient becomes hemiplegic and comatose. The computed tomography (CT) scan is diagnostic, showing a lens-shaped clot with an inner smooth surface over the cerebral convexity (Fig. 35-1). Early recognition is essential. Unless the clot is removed and the torn vessel ligated, death is almost invariable.

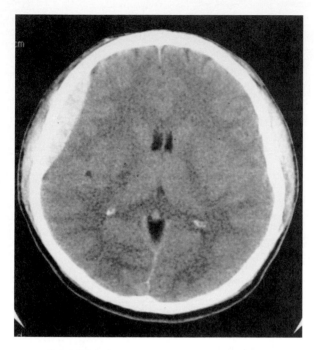

FIG. 35-1   Acute epidural hematoma; unenhanced CT scan showing a typical frontal lenticular epidural clot over the right hemisphere.

Acute and Chronic Subdural Hematomas

With the contusional type of injury, there is nearly always some degree of subarachnoid hemorrhage and, not infrequently, subdural hemorrhage as well. The latter, usually caused by rupture of the bridging veins between dura and brain, is readily detected with CT scanning (Fig. 35-2) and with less definition by magnetic resonance imaging (MRI). Acute subdural hematomas may cause only headache if small, or confusion, seizures, or coma if they are sizable. Often the venous bleeding is arrested by the intracranial pressure, allowing the condition to become chronic. Large subdural clots need to be removed surgically and the bleeding controlled.

Chronic subdural hematoma poses an entirely different problem. The head injury, particularly in the elderly and in those taking anticoagulant drugs, may have been trivial and even forgotten. A bridging vein, as it passes from the pia-arachnoid to a dural sinus, is torn, and this permits blood to accumulate under low pressure in the subdural space. The usual site is over one cerebral hemisphere (sometimes bilateral); occasionally the clot is interhemispheric, peritentorial, or subcerebellar. The clot elicits membrane formation from the dura; the membranes enclose the clot and attach it to the dura. Over 2 to 3 months, the fluid mass may enlarge, compressing and displacing the underlying brain. Headache, drowsiness, confusion, hemiparesis, seizure, and other focal abnormalities such as aphasia follow. The

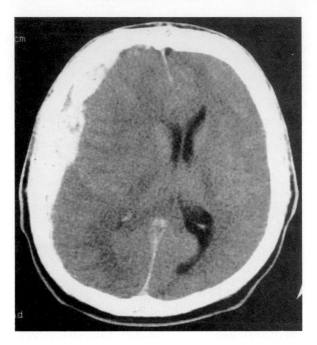

FIG. 35-2   Acute subdural hematoma over the right convexity with substantial mass effect (displacement) of brain tissue but little edema.

hematoma and its compressive effects are visible with MRI and CT (Fig. 35-3). If the symptoms are severe and progressive, surgical drainage is usually effective and recovery can be complete, but the fluid collection recurs in a proportion of patients, particularly the elderly. Small hematomas regress naturally and may respond as well to corticosteroids.

Penetrating Injuries

These are mainly due to gunshot wounds of the head, and if vital centers are struck or shock waves from the missile are of sufficient severity, death is instantaneous. Many patients reach the emergency department, where the physician's primary objective is to assure respiratory and cardiovascular stability. The wound needs to be cleaned and debrided. CT scanning will indicate whether a bullet or shell fragment or an expanding intracranial hemorrhage is an immediate threat to survival. The problem is mainly surgical, and the clinical status of the patient determines the timing of planned operative intervention. Immediate removal of the bullet or excision of shattered brain tissue is usually of no advantage.

TREATMENT OF THE HEAD-INJURED PATIENT

Patients with only transient unconsciousness Patients with an uncomplicated concussive injury who have already regained consciousness pose few

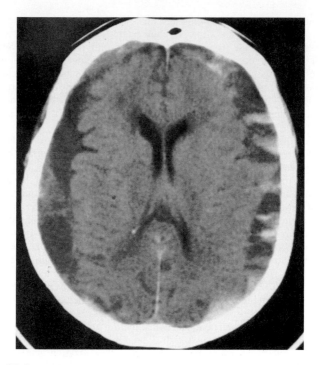

FIG. 35-3   Chronic subdural hematomas over both cerebral hemispheres without shift of the ventricular system. Chronicity results in hypodense appearance of the clots. Some old blood can still be seen within the collections. The bilaterally balanced masses result in an absence of horizontal displacement, but they may compress the upper brainstem.

difficulties in management. They should be observed until the capacity to form consecutive memories has been regained and arrangements have been made for observation by the family of signs of delayed complications (subdural and epidural hemorrhage, intracerebral bleeding, and edema).

Patients who recover but are left with persistent complaints of headache, dizziness, and nervousness are the most difficult to manage, as discussed further on. In some, the accident has provoked anxiety or an anxious depression. Another group with a premorbid neurotic or depressive personality type simply decompensate and are unable to function. The third and smallest number of patients, obviously the more severely injured, are found upon close examination to be suffering personality changes and subtle impairments of cognitive function. Treatment must be in accordance with the basic problem. There is endless medical controversy as to whether an athlete who has had a brief concussion should be permitted to resume competitive activity.

Severe head injury   If the physician arrives at the scene of the accident and finds an unconscious patient, a quick examination should be made before the patient is moved. Primarily, it must be determined that breathing, a clear airway, and pulse and blood pressure are established, and whether there is dangerous hemorrhage from a scalp laceration or injured viscera. Severe head injuries that arrest respiration are often soon followed by cessation of cardiac function; injuries of this magnitude are usually fatal. The likelihood of a cervical fracture-dislocation, which is occasionally associated with head injury, requires fixation of the cervical spine and precautions in moving the patient. It is best to assume that all such patients have had a neck injury.

In the hospital the first step is to clear the airway and ensure adequate ventilation by endotracheal intubation. A search for other injuries must be made, particularly of the abdomen, chest, spine, and long bones. Persistent hypotension should raise the suspicion of a ruptured viscus or of thoracic or abdominal internal bleeding, extensive fractures, or trauma to the cervical cord. It should be emphasized that sustained early hypotension (systolic blood pressure <90 mmHg) is associated with a doubling of mortality. If shock is present on admission to the emergency department, the mortality is around 65 percent. Initially, infused fluid should be normal saline, avoiding the administration of excessive free water because of its adverse effect on brain edema. Cervical spine films and cranial computed tomography (CT) scan should be obtained once vital functions are stable. If one is reassured that there is no subluxation of the cervical spine, including flexion and extension views, there is no longer a need to immobilize the neck.

A rapid survey can then be made, with attention to the depth of coma, size of the pupils and their reaction to light, ocular movements, corneal reflexes, facial movements during grimace, swallowing, vocalization, gag reflexes, muscle tone and movements of the limbs, predominant postures, reactions to pinch, and reflexes. Bogginess of the temporal or postauricular area (Battle sign), bleeding from the nose or ear, and extensive conjunctival edema and hemorrhage are useful signs of an underlying basal skull fracture. However, rupture of an eardrum or a blow to the nose may also cause bleeding from these parts. Fracture of the orbital bones may displace the eye, with resulting strabismus; fracture of the jaw results in malocclusion and discomfort on attempting to open the mouth.

CT scanning is of central importance at this juncture. A sizable epidural, subdural, or intracerebral blood clot is an indication for immediate surgery. The presence of contusions, brain edema, and displacement of central structures calls for measures to monitor progression of these lesions and to control intracranial pressure. These measures are best carried out in a critical care unit.

The *Glasgow Coma Scale* (Table 17-3) provides a practical means by which the state of impaired consciousness can be evaluated at frequent intervals, but it is not a substitute for a more complete neurologic examination. It registers three aspects of neurologic function: (1) eye opening (spontaneously, in response to command, and in response to pain); (2) verbal responsiveness (in terms of orientation, confusion, inappropriateness, and incomprehensibility); and (3) motor responsiveness (to command, to a localized stimulus, flexion and extension responses to pressure on the limb). It is useful in following the course and predicting the outcome of severe head injuries (a score of less than 8 is associated with a poor prognosis). A deteriorating score dictates a change in management.

Management of raised intracranial pressure It is the practice in many hospitals to insert one of several available devices that permits continuous recording of intracranial pressure (ICP) after moderate and severe head injury. Neither the neurologic examination nor the signs that constitute the Glasgow Coma Scale accurately reflect the pressure in the cranium. Monitoring warns of evolving hemorrhage and edema. However, there are few critical data to support the routine use of ICP monitoring, and the patient who is only drowsy or shows minimal mass effect on CT scanning is not likely to benefit.

The first step in lowering presumed or demonstrated high ICP is to control the secondary factors that raise pressure, particularly hypoxia, hypercarbia, hyperthermia, awkward head positions, and high airway pressures. If the intracranial pressure exceeds 15 to 20 mmHg, several measures can be instituted, such as inducing hypocarbia by controlled ventilation (maintaining P_{CO_2} at 28 to 34 mmHg) and the use of hyperosmolar dehydration (0.25 to 1.0 g of 20% mannitol every 3 to 6 h or 0.75 to 1 mg/kg of furosemide) to maintain serum sodium above 138 meq/L and osmolality between 290 and 300 mosmol/L. Intravenous fluids with free water should be avoided so as not to intensify cerebral edema; 5% dextrose in water, 0.5% saline, and 5% dextrose in 0.5% saline are avoided; lactated Ringer's solution is permissible and normal saline with or without dextrose is safe.

If the ICP continues to rise and brain swelling progresses despite these measures, the outlook for survival is bleak. Hypothermia and barbiturate anesthesia to reduce ICP have been used, but relatively few patients respond to such measures. Decompression craniectomy in cases of intractable brain swelling is possible and may salvage some younger patients.

In lowering high levels of blood pressure, diuretics, beta-adrenergic blocking agents, or angiotensin converting enzyme inhibitors should be used. The prophylactic use of anticonvulsant drugs is not generally favored. Only if there has been a seizure are anticonvulsants given.

SEQUELAE OF HEAD INJURY

Concussion invariably leaves the patient with a permanent gap in memory, extending from a point before the injury occurred until the time he was able to form consecutive memories. The duration of the retrograde and anterograde amnesia, particularly the latter, is a reliable index of the severity of the concussive injury.

Concussion and even more trivial injuries (in which there is no concussion) may also leave the patient with persistent headache, fatigue, irritability, dizziness (light-headedness), difficulty in concentration, disturbed sleep, anxiety, and depression. This syndrome is common and has been given many names—postconcussion syndrome, traumatic neurasthenia, and *posttraumatic nervous instability*, which is the one we prefer. These symptoms may persist for weeks, months, or a year or more. The syndrome is more frequent and prolonged when compensation or litigation is an issue. Settlement of the legal problem and reassurance are essential in the rehabilitation program. If there is mainly an anxious depression, antidepressants are often useful. Simple analgesics should be prescribed for the headache. Long periods of observation and repetition of a multitude of tests only reinforce the patient's fears and reduce the motivation to return to work. Concussive head

330 PART IV / THE MAJOR CATEGORIES OF NEUROLOGIC DISEASE

injury is thought, on the basis of clinical impressions, to increase the patient's vulnerability to subsequent concussions.

In respect to patients with contusional injury, all gradations in the severity of neurologic sequelae can be observed. There may be widespread hemorrhagic shearing and ischemic injuries that can be seen by MRI and to a lesser extent by CT scan. Death in the first few hours or days after the injury, or the vegetative state, is a frequent sequela. Some patients, following a protracted period of coma, maintain normal vital signs, open their eyes, and appear to be awake but betray no signs of cognition or responsiveness (*persistent vegetative state*, see Chap. 17). Other patients, in whom the symptoms fall short of those of the persistent vegetative state, function better but remain severely and permanently "brain-damaged."

In the majority of patients with contusion, the consequences of the brain damage recede, usually in the first 6 months and often to a surprising degree. Nevertheless, many patients are left with troublesome symptoms. Delayed onset of seizures is to be expected in 10 to 40 percent of patients with contusion (but not in those with pure concussion). Focal deficits—hemiparesis, dysphasia, frontal lobe disorder—may persist in mild form in patients with hemispheral injuries and cerebellar ataxia and various upper brainstem abnormalities in those who have had temporal lobe–tentorial herniations. Mental and personality changes may develop and cause serious problems in resuming employment and social adjustment; these demand expert neuropsychiatric care.

Other Problems due to Head Injury

Limitations of space preclude a full account of many problems based on head injury and the critical care of severely affected patients. We have omitted discussion of posttraumatic syncope; immediate traumatic epilepsy and the use of anticonvulsants; particular cranial nerve injuries with skull fractures; meningeal fibrosis, subarachnoid hemorrhage, and delayed tension hydrocephalus; acute swelling of the brain in children; traumatic dissection of the carotid and vertebral arteries; cavernous arteriovenous fistula; traumatic migraine; delayed cerebral hemorrhage; CSF rhinorrhea; dementia-pugilistica (the "punch-drunk" syndrome); and predictors of outcome of head injury (e.g., the Glasgow Coma Scale alluded to earlier).

Spinal cord trauma is described in Chap. 44.

> For a more detailed discussion of this topic, see Victor and Ropper: *Adams and Victor's Principles of Neurology*, 7th ed, pp 925–953.

ADDITIONAL READING

Adams JH, Graham DI, Murray LS, Scott G: Diffuse axonal injury due to nonmissile head injury in humans: An analysis of 45 cases. *Ann Neurol* 12:557, 1982.

Annegers JF, Hauser A, Coan SP, Rocca WA: A population-based study of seizures after traumatic brain injuries. *N Engl J Med* 338:20, 1998.

A Group of Neurosurgeons: Guidelines for initial management after head injury in adults. *Br Med J* 288:983, 1984.

Guerra WK, Gaab MR, Dietz H, et al: Surgical decompression for traumatic brain swelling: Indications and results. *J Neurosurg* 90:187, 1999.

Jennett B, Teasdale G: *Management of Head Injuries: Contemporary Neurology*, no. 20. Philadelphia, Davis, 1981.

Narayan RK, Wilberger JE, Povlishock JT: *Neurotrauma*. New York, McGraw-Hill, 1996.

Ommaya AK, Grubb RL, Naumann RA: Coup and contrecoup injury: Observations on the mechanisms of visible brain injuries in the rhesus monkey. *J Neurosurg* 35:503, 1971.

Ropper AH (ed): *Neurological and Neurosurgical Intensive Care*, 3rd ed. New York, Raven Press, 1993.

Strich SJ: The pathology of severe head injury. *Lancet* 2:443, 1961.

Symonds CP: Concussion and contusion of the brain and their sequelae, in Feiring EH (ed): *Brock's Injuries of the Brain and Spinal Cord and Their Coverings*, 5th ed. New York, Springer, 1974, pp 100–161.

The Traumatic Coma Data Bank. *J Neurosurg* 75(Suppl):S1–S66, 1991.

36 | Multiple Sclerosis and Related Demyelinative Diseases

In speaking of disease, the term *demyelinative*, as a defining adjective, is used in two ways. One, which is incorrect in our opinion, is to specify any disease that involves the white matter (myelin, oligodendrocytes), whether tumor, infarct, or whatever. The other and more correct usage is to denote a disease that affects mainly the myelin sheaths of nerve fibers, leaving axons and their cells of origin *relatively* intact. Other pathologic attributes of a true demyelinative process are a lack of secondary wallerian degeneration (because of relative sparing of axis cylinders), an infiltration of inflammatory cells in a perivascular distribution, and often a perivenous pattern of distribution of demyelination.

The diseases listed in Table 36-1 conform to this definition, and all share another attribute, that of being of presumed autoimmune causation. The most important one, by far, is multiple sclerosis. Omitted from this tabulation are a number of disorders such as subacute combined degeneration due to vitamin B_{12} deficiency, progressive multifocal leukoencephalopathy, and the cortical demyelination of hypoxic encephalopathy—each with prominent demyelination but with a readily defined and unique causative factor.

MULTIPLE SCLEROSIS

Multiple sclerosis (MS) is a disease of the central nervous system (CNS), beginning most often in late adolescence and early adult life and usually expressing itself by discrete and recurrent attacks of spinal cord, brainstem, cerebellar, optic nerve, and cerebral dysfunction. The underlying lesion is demyelinative, but axons and other structures may be damaged. The attacks are subacute in onset but may be acute and are often followed by remission of symptoms and even recovery. In many cases this relapsing-remitting course blends imperceptibly into a chronically progressive pattern.

Epidemiology

The geography of the disease is noteworthy. In the northern United States, Canada, Great Britain, and northern Europe, the prevalence is high—30 to 80 per 100,000 population. In the southern parts of Europe and the United States, the prevalence falls to 6 to 14 per 100,000, and in equatorial regions, to less than 1 per 100,000. Persons who migrate from a high- to a low-risk area (or vice versa) after the age of about 15 years are said to retain the risk of their place of origin. Before that age, they acquire the risk of the place to which they migrate. Familial incidence is low but several times higher than chance expectancy. Certain histocompatibility (HLA) antigens are more fre-

TABLE 36-1 Classification of the Demyelinative Diseases

I. Multiple sclerosis
  A. Chronic relapsing encephalomyelopathic form
  B. Acute multiple sclerosis
  C. Neuromyelitis optica (Devic disease)
II. Diffuse cerebral sclerosis (encephalitis periaxialis diffusa) of Schilder
   and concentric sclerosis of Baló
III. Acute disseminated (postinfections) encephalomyelitis and myelitis
  A. Following EBV, CMV, herpesvirus, *Mycoplasma*, or undefined
    infection
  B. Following measles, chickenpox, smallpox, and rarely mumps, rubella,
    influenza, or other obscure infection
  C. Following rabies or smallpox vaccination
IV. Acute and subacute necrotizing hemorrhagic encephalitis
  A. Acute encephalopathic form (hemorrhagic leukoencephalitis of Hurst)
  B. Subacute necrotic myelopathy

Key: EBV, Epstein-Barr virus; CMV, cytomegalovirus.

quent in the MS population (HLA-DR2, -DR3, -B7, and -A3). The occurrence of MS is rare in children. Women are more susceptible than men (1.7:1.0) and whites more than blacks. Trauma appears not to be causative, nor is pregnancy.

Clinical Manifestations

Rarely the disease occurs in asymptomatic form, the typical white matter lesions being found accidentally by MRI. Otherwise, the first attack comes without warning and may be mono- or polysymptomatic. In one-fifth of the cases, the onset is acute; i.e., the deficit attains its maximum severity in minutes or hours. Weakness or numbness of a limb, monocular visual loss, diplopia, vertigo, facial weakness or numbness, ataxia, and nystagmus are the most common presenting symptoms, and they occur in various combinations. Remission after the first attack is to be expected. Recurrences represent a recrudescence of earlier lesions or the effects of new ones, predominantly the former. Over a variable period, usually measured in years, the patient becomes increasingly handicapped, with an asymmetric paraparesis and obvious signs of corticospinal tract disease, sensory and cerebellar ataxia, urinary incontinence, optic atrophy, nystagmus, internuclear ophthalmoparesis, or dysarthria in some combination. Seizures occur in only 3 to 4 percent of patients. Mental changes are variable, depending on whether spinal or cerebral lesions predominate and whether the latter are numerous. The late established stage may not be reached until 20 or 25 years have elapsed. Once the advanced stage is attained, deterioration may be so slow as to suggest the presence of a degenerative disease. Other patients fail rapidly, within 3 to 4 years; in rare instances, the patient succumbs within months of onset (acute MS). Slow progression of the disease without episodes of relapse occurs, especially at more advanced ages. There are no systemic signs other than fatigue.

Retrobulbar optic neuritis A special form of demyelinative disease involves the optic nerve, which is an extension of the CNS, and proves to be the initial manifestation of MS in about 25 percent of patients. Monocular blurring of vision or blindness, eye pain with movement of the globe, and desaturation of red coloration evolve over several hours or days. The optic disc may appear normal (retrobulbar neuritis) or edematous (papillitis), depending on the location of the lesion within the nerve (see Chap. 13), and the afferent pupillary response is muted. One-half or more of patients who present with optic neuritis alone will develop other manifestations of MS, usually within several years but sometimes many years later.

Treatment of optic neuritis is with high doses of intravenous corticosteroids, which speed the recovery of visual loss but probably do not alter the eventual outcome, which is generally favorable for vision; orally administered steroids were found in one large study to actually increase the frequency of relapse.

Transverse myelitis This term is used somewhat loosely to describe a demyelinative lesion that involves all elements of the cord at one or several adjacent segments. It is one of the presenting syndromes of MS but has other causes, including a postinfectious process (page 404).

Pathology

Multiple discrete lesions of myelin destruction, called *plaques*, range in size from a few millimeters to several centimeters. The regions around the lateral ventricles are common sites, and the perivenous relationship of the lesions is most evident in this location, but the lesions can be anywhere in the CNS. The lesions also vary in appearance; fresh ones filled with macrophages are ivory- or cream-colored, and old gliotic ones are gray. Perivascular cuffs of lymphocytes (T cells of CD4 type) and mononuclear cells are more frequent in recent lesions. The neurons and many of the axis cylinders are spared. Cavitation of one or more old lesions with total destruction of myelin, axons, and even blood vessels may occur.

Pathogenesis

There is some evidence that favors an early-life viral or other infection as the initial event in the pathogenesis of MS. However, all attempts to isolate a virus have failed. Whatever the initial event, a cell-mediated inflammatory process focused on CNS myelin or some component thereof appears to be the basis of the recurrent attacks and plaque formation. The factor that provokes recrudescences is a mystery, although theories abound—masked infections with viruses or bacteria and a primary autoimmune disease being currently the most popular.

Diagnosis

Once there is evidence of multiple CNS lesions that have produced remitting and relapsing symptoms over a period of time—without evidence of syphilis or other infections, metastatic tumor, or cerebral arteritis (Behçet disease, lupus erythematosus)—the diagnosis becomes certain with a high degree of accuracy. A single lesion causing recurrent symptoms must be regarded with suspicion. Although it may be due to MS, certain other types of solitary lesions (vascular malformation of the brainstem, Chiari malformation, sarcoid, vasculitis, lymphoma or other tumor) may produce a clinical picture that closely mimics MS, particularly in its early stages. A syndrome linked with the antiphospholipid antibody and with systemic lupus may produce multifocal neurologic symptoms that remit, and magnetic resonance imaging (MRI) may show lesions that are difficult to distinguish from MS.

Laboratory Findings

In about 80 percent of established cases, the cerebrospinal fluid (CSF) is abnormal. There may be a mild mononuclear pleocytosis and a modest increase in total protein, but the gamma globulin fraction is often greatly increased (greater than 12 percent of the total protein). An even more sensitive index is the electrophoretic demonstration in the CSF of several discrete oligoclonal IgG bands. Lesions that are not clinically manifest may be revealed by visual, auditory, and somatosensory evoked potential studies and by MRI, providing proof that the lesions are truly multiple. The white matter lesions are most apparent on T2 and FLAIR images, and active, recently acquired ones may enhance with gadolinium. A periventricular distribution of demyelination, with foci oriented radially along the white matter tracts and veins, is a characteristic MRI finding (Fig. 36-1). Old gliotic lesions are hypodense on computed tomography (CT) and do not enhance after gadolinium infusion.

Treatment

The administration of corticosteroids, given over a period of days, appears to hasten the resolution of nascent lesions. IV methylprednisolone (500 mg daily for 3 to 5 days) is used in patients with acute symptomatic deterioration. It is not clear that this treatment is superior to oral corticosteroids. These drugs have not prevented or reduced the incidence of recurrences, nor do they halt the disease in the late deteriorative stage.

Administration subcutaneously, weekly or biweekly, of β-interferon or a polymer of myelin (copolymer I) lessens the frequency of attacks in relapsing-remitting cases and reduces the cumulative volume of cerebral white matter lesions on MRI if started early in the illness. Their effect on the chronic progressive phase of MS is less certain. Immunosuppression therapy with a drug such as azathioprine or cyclophosphamide, given over a period of years, has its advocates. Other methods of immunosuppression are under study.

OTHER FORMS OF DEMYELINATING DISEASE

Devic Disease (Neuromyelitis Optica, Necrotic Myelopathy)

This refers to the simultaneous or successive involvement of optic nerves and spinal cord by demyelinative lesions. Typically there is acute to subacute blindness in one or both eyes preceded or followed within days or weeks by signs of a transverse or ascending myelitis. The spinal cord lesions are often necrotizing rather than purely demyelinative in type, leading eventually to cavitation, and, as expected, the clinical effects are more likely to be permanent than those of demyelination.

Most patients have proved by subsequent clinical developments, and in a few instances by autopsy, to have chronic relapsing MS. Many cases of neuromyelitis optica, however, stand apart from MS by virtue of a number of

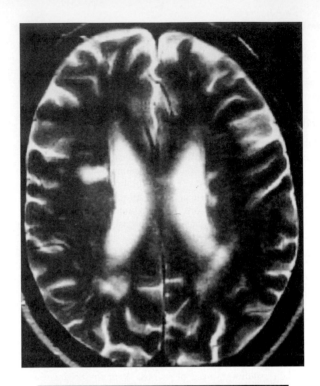

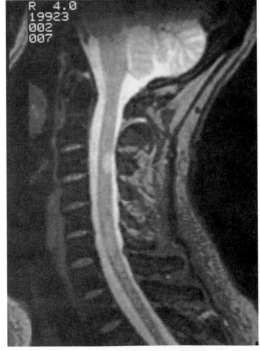

distinctive clinical and pathologic features, namely, failure to develop brainstem, cerebellar, or cerebral demyelinative lesions and normality of MRI of the cerebral white matter, even after years of illness; the almost uniform absence of oligoclonal bands in the spinal fluid; the necrotizing and cavitary nature of the spinal cord lesion, affecting both white and gray matter, with prominent thickening of vessels but with little or no inflammatory infiltrate. On the basis of these differences, several authorities favor the separation of Devic disease from MS. Insofar as the cause of neither disease is known, the relationship of these diseases cannot be resolved with finality. There also exists a progressive *subacute necrotic myelopathy* without optic neuritis that shares all the myelopathic features of Devic disease and probably represents the same process. The differential diagnosis is broader and includes arteriovenous malformation and infarction of the cord.

The treatment of neuromyelitis optica and of subacute necrotic myelopathy has been largely unsuccessful, most cases progressing despite aggressive therapy, including high-dose corticosteroids, plasma exchange, and cyclophosphamide.

Diffuse Cerebral Sclerosis (Schilder Disease)

The sporadic case of massive cerebral demyelination in one or several foci usually proves to be an example of cerebral MS. In addition to the large size of the lesions, this form of the disease, referred to as Schilder disease, differs from the usual form in being more frequent in childhood and adolescence and in the rapidity with which it may progress to a state of severe disability (weeks or months).

The clinical manifestations indicate that the lesions involve tracts of myelinated fibers (optic nerves, geniculocalcarine tracts, corticospinal tracts, posterior or lateral columns of spinal cord, lemnisci of brainstem, and cerebellar peduncles). The characteristic lesion is a large, sharply outlined demyelinative focus involving an entire lobe or hemisphere and extending to the opposite hemisphere across the corpus callosum, but careful examination usually discloses additional lesions of MS in the brainstem, optic nerves, or spinal cord. Some degree of remission and relapse under these circumstances and the laboratory findings mentioned above support the diagnosis of MS.

To be distinguished from Schilder disease are a number of other white matter diseases, not strictly demyelinative, called *leukodystrophies*. The known forms of leukodystrophy, distinguished by their histologic staining characteristics, are metachromatic leukodystrophy, globoid-body leukodystrophy (Krabbe disease), sudanophilic leukodystrophy, and adrenoleukodystrophy. These diseases are familial. Usually they begin in infancy and childhood, but each has been observed to have its onset in adult life, particularly *adrenoleukodystrophy*. The latter is essentially a male (sex-linked) disease diagnosed by finding evidence of adrenal insufficiency and very long chain fatty acids in cultured fibroblasts.

FIG. 36-1   Multiple sclerosis. T2-weighted MR images demonstrating multiple plaques in the periventricular white matter, some with a radial orientation (*top*), and in the spinal cord (*bottom*).

Progressive multifocal leukoencephalopathy is another disease that figures in the differential diagnosis of cerebral MS. The disease takes the form of a focal cerebral lesion, developing over a period of weeks, usually on a background of known lymphocytic leukemia, Hodgkin disease, lymphoma, AIDS, or immunosuppression of another type. Regional multifocality is demonstrated by CT scan and MRI. The CSF is usually normal (see Chap. 33).

Acute Disseminated Encephalomyelitis (ADEM, Postinfectious, Postexanthem, Postvaccinal Myelitis, and Encephalomyelitis)

All of these terms refer to a distinctive form of demyelinative disease, which evolves over a period of several hours or days in the setting of a viral disease, after certain vaccinations, or after some infection that often defies identification. The common viral precedents are Epstein-Barr virus (EBV), cytomegalovirus (CMV), and the exanthems (measles, rubella, chickenpox). Occasionally, ADEM follows *Mycoplasma* infections. Cerebral, cerebellar, or spinal cases (transverse myelitis) appear acutely, along with a CSF pleocytosis. In more aggressive cerebral cases, death may occur within days. With survival, however, there is often a gratifying recovery of function. The lesions are microscopic and consist of perivenous zones of demyelination with perivascular cuffing of lymphocytes and mononuclear cells. The changes are quite different from those of a viral infection, and a virus is not obtained from the cerebral tissue, but lesions may be difficult to separate from MS on purely pathologic grounds. An autoimmune reaction is postulated. Steroid therapy, plasma exchange, and intravenous immunoglobulin are of uncertain benefit. The widespread use of measles vaccine, the discontinuation of smallpox vaccination, and the introduction of new tissue culture vaccines for rabies have reduced the incidence of one form of this disease, but acute myelitis in relation to a postinfectious process continues to be common.

A more slowly evolving form of ADEM (over a period of weeks) is observed from time to time and has been referred to as "acute MS." The lesions are larger than those of classic ADEM and do indeed resemble the plaques of MS, but if the disease does not prove fatal in the initial attack, it usually does not recur.

Acute Necrotizing Hemorrhagic Encephalomyelitis (Leukoencephalitis of Hurst)

This is the most fulminant of the acute postinfectious demyelinative processes, affecting mainly adults who have had a recent respiratory infection, sometimes due to *Mycoplasma pneumoniae*. Within hours, there may be seizures, a massive hemiplegia or quadriplegia, and a polymorphonuclear pleocytosis up to 3000 per mm^3, with increased CSF protein but normal glucose. No virus or bacteria are seen or isolated by culture. In one of our cases, brain swelling and herniation ended the patient's life within 6 h. A slower form of the disease, developing over 1 to 2 weeks and with slight pleocytosis, has also been observed.

The lesions combine intense perivascular inflammation and demyelination with many small hemorrhages and meningeal inflammation. Only the white matter is affected. Corticosteroid therapy [IV dexamethasone, 6 to

10 mg every 6 h, or methylprednisolone (Solu-Medrol), 1 g/day] and plasma exchanges have apparently been beneficial in some cases of ADEM and Hurst disease.

A similar lesion may affect only the spinal cord (acute necrotizing myelitis) or the spinal cord and optic nerves (one type of *Devic neuromyelitis optica*).

For a more detailed discussion of this topic, see Victor and Ropper: *Adams and Victor's Principles of Neurology*, 7th ed, pp 954–982.

ADDITIONAL READING

Adams RD, Kubik CS: The morbid anatomy of the demyelinative diseases. *Am J Med* 12:510, 1952.

Barnes D, Hughes RAC, Morris RW, et al: Randomised trial of oral and intravenous methylprednisolone in acute relapses of multiple sclerosis. *Lancet* 349:902, 1997.

Beck RW, Cleary PA, Anderson MM Jr, et al: A randomized controlled trial of corticosteroids in the treatment of acute optic neuritis. *N Engl J Med* 326:581, 1992.

Berry I, Ranjeva J-P, Manelfe C, Clanet M: Visualisation I.R.M. des lésions de S.E.P. *Rev Neurol* 154:607, 1998.

Ebers GC: Optic neuritis and multiple sclerosis. *Arch Neurol* 42:702, 1985.

European Study Group on Interferon β-1b in Secondary Progressive MS. *Lancet* 352:1491, 1998.

Hughes RAC, Sharrack B: More immunotherapy for multiple sclerosis. *J Neurol Neurosurg Psychiatry* 61:239, 1996.

IFNβ Multiple Sclerosis Study Group: Interferon beta-1b is effective in relapsing-remitting multiple sclerosis. I. Clinical results of a multicenter, randomized, double-blind, placebo-controlled trial. *Neurology* 43:655, 1993.

Johnson RT, Griffin DE, Hirsch RL, et al: Measles encephalomyelitis: Clinical and immunologic studies. *N Engl J Med* 310:137, 1984.

Katz J, Ropper AH. Progressive necrotic myelopathy: Clinical course in 9 patients. *Arch Neurol* 57:355, 2000.

Lessel S: Corticosteroid treatment of acute optic neuritis. *N Engl J Med* 326:634, 1992.

McDonald WI: The mystery of the origin of multiple sclerosis. *J Neurol Neurosurg Psychiatry* 49:113, 1986.

Mathews WB, Acheson ED, Batchelor JR, Weller RO (eds): *McAlpine's Multiple Sclerosis*, 2nd ed. New York, Churchill Livingstone, 1991.

Noseworthy JH, Lucchinetti C, Rodriquez M. Weinsheinker BG: Multiple sclerosis. *N Engl J Med* 343:938, 2000.

Optic Neuritis Study Group: The five-year risk of MS after optic neuritis. *Neurology* 49:1404, 1997.

PRISMS Study Group: Randomized double-blind placebo-controlled study of interferon β-1a in relapsing/remitting multiple sclerosis. *Lancet* 352:1498, 1998.

Rudick RA, Cohen JA, Weinstock-Guttman B, et al: Management of multiple sclerosis. *N Engl J Med* 337:1604, 1997.

37 | Inherited Metabolic Diseases of the Nervous System

Advances in biochemistry and molecular genetics have made possible the discovery of more than two hundred inherited metabolic diseases of the nervous system; conversely, the study of many of these diseases has opened new fields of neurochemistry. The diseases that fall into this category are too numerous to describe individually. Because they vary in the time of life when they become clinically manifest, a logical way of grouping them is by the age period in which they are most likely to appear—i.e., in the neonatal period, in infancy, and in early and late childhood. Only when they tend to develop later in life do they present themselves with syndromes more familiar to adult neurologists—ataxia, myoclonus, rigidity, dementia, etc. Because of restrictions of space, it is possible to present only a few illustrative examples from each of these age periods. Information about the rest of them can be found in *Adams and Victor's Principles of Neurology*, 7th ed., and in the monographs of Scriver et al and of Lyon et al listed in the references.

The diseases being considered here are hereditary, and those appearing early are almost always transmitted as autosomal recessive traits. In other words, both the mother and father bear the abnormal gene but are themselves unaffected clinically; during intrauterine life, the mother's normal metabolism protects the fetus, which is then normal for a variable period postnatally. This fact is important because it offers the prospect of prevention. Indeed, biochemical screening of large populations at birth has identified those at risk for several inherited metabolic diseases, and in some instances it has been possible to prevent their effects on the nervous system.

METABOLIC DISEASES IN THE NEONATAL PERIOD

As indicated above, the infant appears normal at birth; only after several days or weeks do these diseases begin to express themselves. The clinical syndrome that ensues is relatively nonspecific because the immature nervous system has only a limited number of ways of expressing disorders of function. The usual clinical manifestations are reduced alertness and responsivity (stupor, coma), lack of normal support reactions of the body and neck, loss of the Moro and startle responses, quivering of the face and limbs and sometimes more overt seizure activity, hypo- or hypertonia, disturbances of ocular control (oscillations, nystagmus, loss of vestibulo-ocular reflexes), poor feeding, unstable temperature, and hyperventilation.

The most frequent inherited metabolic diseases of the neonatal period are cretinism, phenylketonuria (PKU), Hartnup disease, histidinemia, methylmalonic acidemia, galactosemia, arginosuccinic acidemia, biotin deficiency, homocystinuria, maple-syrup urine disease, ketotic and nonketotic hyperglycinemia, lactic acidemia, and the peroxisomal disorders.

340

Galactosemia is a typical example. The onset of symptoms is in the first days of life, after the ingestion of milk. Vomiting and diarrhea are followed by drowsiness, inattentiveness, hypotonia, diminished vigor of the normal neonatal automatisms, and a general failure to thrive. There is enlargement of the liver and spleen, jaundice, and anemia. Impaired psychomotor development, cataracts, visual impairment, and cirrhosis become manifest later. The biochemical abnormality is a defect in galactose-1-phosphate uridyl transferase (G-1-PUT). The diagnostic laboratory findings are increased galactose and diminished glucose concentrations in the blood, elevated blood galactose level, low glucose, galactosuria, and a deficiency of G-1-PUT in red and white blood cells. The treatment is dietary, using milk substitutes.

Diagnosis of neonatal inherited metabolic disorders   Serum NH_3 and glucose levels, measurement of T_3 and T_4, analysis of blood and urine for amino acids, and the finding of lactic acidemia (with clinical evidence of acidosis) will disclose the diagnosis in the majority of neonatal metabolic disorders. Magnetic resonance imaging (MRI) has proved to be a useful method for revealing development faults.

Nonhereditary metabolic disorders, notably *hypoglycemia* and *hypocalcemia*, need to be distinguished from hereditary ones. The former are readily recognized by simple biochemical tests and respond well to correction with glucose or calcium.

Parturitional *anoxic-ischemic encephalopathy* and *developmental anomalies*, the other major categories of neurologic disease at this time of life, can usually be distinguished by their earlier postnatal onset and other distinctive morphologic or neurologic findings.

HEREDITARY METABOLIC DISEASES OF EARLY INFANCY

Beyond the neonatal period diagnosis becomes easier, because by then there is evident psychosensorimotor regression after a period of normal development—the hallmark of hereditary metabolic disease. The common clinical manifestations are loss of vision, head control, and interest in the surroundings; impaired hand-eye coordination; regression of motor development, resulting in a failure to sit, stand, or walk; and the occurrence of seizures.

The most important members of this group are the lysosomal storage diseases, in which there is a genetic deficiency of enzymes necessary for the degradation of specific glycosides or peptides. As a result, the intracytoplasmic lysosomes become engorged with undegraded material, with eventual damage to nerve cells. Often the cells of other organs are similarly affected.

The lysosomal storage diseases are listed in Table 37-1. In addition to the sphingolipidoses, which are the ones most likely to occur in infancy, the table includes the storage diseases of childhood and adolescence, to be considered later.

GM_2 gangliosidosis (Tay-Sachs disease) is the best-known lysosomal storage disease of infancy. Mainly it affects Jewish infants of eastern European (Ashkenazi) background. The onset is usually by the fourth month of life, with an abnormal startle to acoustic stimuli, listlessness and irritability, and delay in psychomotor development (or regression if onset is at 4 to 6 months). These symptoms are followed by hypotonia and then spasticity

TABLE 37-1 Infantile and Childhood Hereditary Metabolic Diseases

Disorder	Primary deficiency	Accumulated metabolite
		Sphingolipidoses
GM$_1$ gangliosidosis	β-Galactosidase	G$_{M1}$ ganglioside, galactosyl oligosaccharides, keratan sulfate
GM$_2$ gangliosidoses		
Tay-Sachs disease	3-N-acetylhexosaminidase α subunit	G$_{M2}$ ganglioside
Sandhoff disease	β-N-acetylhexosaminidase β subunit	G$_{M2}$ ganglioside, oligosaccharides, glycosaminoglycans
Activator deficiency	G$_{M2}$ activator	G$_{M2}$ ganglioside (α and β subunits)
Metachromatic leukodystrophy	Arylsulfatase A (sulfatidase), sulfatide activator (saposin B)	Galactosyl sulfatide, lactosulfatide
Krabbe disease	Galactocerebrosidase	Galactosylceramide
Fabry disease	α-Galactosidase A	Ceramide trihexoside
Gaucher disease	Glucocerebrosidase	Glucosylceramide, glycopeptides
Niemann-Pick disease		
Types A and B	Sphingomyelinase	Sphingomyelin, cholesterol
Type C	Cholesterol esterification	Free cholesterol, bis-monoacylglycerophosphate
Farber disease	Ceramide	Ceramide
Schindler disease	α-Galactosidase B	α-N-acetylgalactosaminyl oligosaccharides and glycopeptides
		Neuronal ceroid lipofuscinoses
Infantile form (Haltia-Santavuori)	Palmitoyl-protein thioesterase	Granular osmiophilic deposits
Late infantile form (Jansky-Bielschowsky)	Tripeptidyl peptidase I	Curvilinear bodies, subunit C of mitochondrial ATP synthase
Juvenile form (Vogt-Spielmeyer-Sjögren)	438-amino acid membrane protein	Curvilinear and laminated (fingerprint) bodies, subunit C of mitochondrial ATP synthase
Adult form (Kufs disease)	Unknown	Mixed type osmiophilic deposits and lamellar inclusions
		Glycoproteinoses
Aspartylglucosaminuria	Aspartylglucosaminidase	Aspartylglucosamine
Fucosidosis	α-L-Fucosidase	Fucosyloligosaccharides
Galactosialidosis	Protective protein (β-galactosidase and α-neuraminidase)	Sialyloligosaccharides, galactosyloligosaccharides
α-Mannosidosis	α-Mannosidase	α-Mannosyl-oligosaccharides
β-Mannosidosis	β-Mannosidase	β-Mannosyl-oligosaccharides

Mucolipidoses

Sialidosis (mucolipidosis I)	α-Neuraminidase	Sialyloligosaccharides, sialylglycopeptides
Mucolipidosis II (I-cell disease)	UDP-N-acetylglucosamine: lysosomal enzyme, N-acetylglucosamine-1-phosphotransferase	Sialyloligosaccharides, glycoproteins, glycolipids
Mucolipidosis III (pseudo-Hurler polydystrophy)	Same phosphotransferase as above	Sialyloligosaccharides, glycoproteins, glycolipids
Mucolipidosis IV	Unknown	Gangliosides, phospholipids, mucopolysaccharides

Other lysosomal diseases

Acid lipase deficiency		
Woman disease	Acid lipase	Cholesterol esters, triglycerides
Cholesterol ester storage disease	Acid lipase	Cholesterol esters, triglycerides
Glycogenosis type II (Pompe disease)	α-Glucosidase (acid maltase)	Glycogen
Sialic acid storage disease		
Infantile form	Sialic acid transport	Free sialic acid
Salla disease	Sialic acid transport	Free sialic acid

Mucopolysaccharidoses

Hurler-Scheie syndrome	α-Iduronidase	Dermatan sulfate, heparan sulfate
Hunter disease	Iduronate sulfatase	Dermatan sulfate, heparan sulfate
Sanfilippo disease		
Type A	Heparan N-sulfatase	Heparan sulfate
Type B	α-N-Acetylglucosaminidase	Heparan sulfate
Type C	Heparan-N-acetyltransferase	Heparan sulfate
Type D	α-N-Glucosamine-6-sulfatase	Heparan sulfate
Morquio disease		
Type A	N-Acetylgalactosamine-6-sulfate sulfatase	Keratan sulfate
Type B	β-Galactosidase	Keratin sulfate
Maroteaux-Lamy disease	Arylsulfatase B	Dermatan sulfate
β-Glucuronidase deficiency (Sly disease)	β-Glucuronidase	Dermatan and heparan sulfate

343

of the axial musculature, visual failure, cherry-red spots in the retina, seizures, enlarging head (due to an enlarging brain), and death within a few years.

The abnormality here is a deficiency of hexosaminidase A, with accumulation of ganglioside in neurons and retinal ganglion cells. The enzyme defect can be found in serum, white blood cells, and cultured fibroblasts from amniotic fluid, permitting the detection of an affected fetus or a heterozygote carrier of the disease. The disease has been practically eradicated by screening of the ethnic group in which it occurs for the recessive enzyme defect.

INHERITED METABOLIC DISEASES OF LATE INFANCY AND EARLY CHILDHOOD

The following are the hereditary metabolic diseases that appear most often in this age period (1 to 4 years):

1. Many of the milder disorders of amino acid metabolism
2. Metachromatic, globoid-body (Krabbe), and sudanophilic leukodystrophies
3. Late infantile GM_1 gangliosidosis
4. Late infantile Gaucher disease and Niemann-Pick disease
5. Neuroaxonal dystrophy
6. The mucopolysaccharidoses
7. The mucolipidoses
8. Fucosidosis
9. The mannosidoses
10. Aspartylglycosaminuria
11. Ceroid lipofuscinosis
12. Cockayne syndrome

In this group, most attention has been given to the aminoacidurias, for which large-scale screening programs have been instituted in most parts of the western world. Phenylketonuria is the most familiar example.

The usual type of *phenylketonuria* (there are several milder variants) is transmitted as an autosomal recessive trait. Again, the baby is normal at birth and during the first year but then begins to lag in psychomotor development. By 5 to 6 years, the IQ has fallen to less than 50 and often to less than 20. Hyperactivity, aggressivity, clumsy gait, fine tremors of the hands and body, poor coordination, odd posturing, digital mannerisms, and rhythmias (e.g., hand waving) are the usual clinical manifestations. Many patients have a light complexion, and seizures occur in 25 percent. High serum levels of phenylalanine ($>$ 15 mg/dL) are diagnostic. The disease is due to a deficiency of the hepatic enzyme phenylalanine hydroxylase. A low-phenylalanine diet instituted at birth and continued for the first 5 to 10 years of life prevents the psychomotor decline. Severe mental retardation as a result of this disease has become a rarity. However, a homozygous mother with high phenylalanine level, if untreated during pregnancy, will invariably give birth to an abnormal infant that was affected in utero.

Diagnosis of metabolic disorders of infancy In distinguishing among the diseases of this group, it is useful to determine whether a particular syndrome is primarily one of white matter (oligodendrocytes and myelin) or gray matter (neurons). Indicative of the former (*leukodystrophies*) are early onset of spastic paralysis with or without ataxia, loss of tendon reflexes, and visual impairment with optic atrophy but normal retinas. Seizures and mental deterioration are late events. Gray matter diseases (*poliodystrophies*) are characterized by the early occurrence of seizures, myoclonus, blindness with retinal changes, and mental regression; spastic paralysis and sensorimotor tract signs occur later. The neuronal storage diseases, neuroaxonal dystrophy, and the lipofuscinoses conform to the pattern of gray matter disease. Metachromatic, globoid-body, and sudanophilic leukodystrophies exemplify white matter diseases.

The *mucopolysaccharidoses* are unique with respect to involvement of osseous and other connective tissues. In this group of diseases, there is abnormal storage of lipid in neurons and of polysaccharides in connective tissue. Each of the abnormalities accounts for the characteristic facies, visceral enlargement, skeletal changes, and the neurologic syndrome. Hunter and Hurler diseases are the classic types; in the first there is mental backwardness, corneal opacities, dwarfism, gargoyle facies, large head with synostoses, kyphosis, broad hands with stubby fingers, and hepatosplenomegaly. Hunter disease is similar but milder and lacking corneal clouding. In some types, mental function is relatively spared and survival to middle age is possible. The enzymatic defect that prevents the degradation of acid mucopolysaccharides (now called glucosaminoglycosans) or the storage products can be detected in tissue or urine by biochemical means.

INHERITED METABOLIC DISEASES OF LATE CHILDHOOD AND ADOLESCENCE

By this time of life, the hereditary metabolic diseases tend to be more selective in their effects on the nervous system and more chronic. Also, the maturational processes of the brain are nearing completion, so it has nearly the same capacity as the adult brain for the expression of clinical signs. Therefore the predominant syndrome often provides a clue to diagnosis.

Extrapyramidal Syndromes

The best-known disease that presents with this syndrome is *Wilson hepatolenticular degeneration*. This is an autosomal recessive disease of liver and brain that presents between 10 and 30 years of age with a syndrome of tremor, extrapyramidal rigidity, dystonia, dysarthria, and dysphagia and, in some cases, with cerebellar ataxia and dementia. Kayser-Fleischer (KF) rings of copper pigment gradually form in the deep layers of the corneas and are pathognomonic of the disease. The fundamental defect is probably a hepatic failure to incorporate copper into ceruloplasmin. Altered liver function is an invariable feature but is prominent in only some of the childhood cases. Hemolytic anemia and renal tubular acidosis are other important features.

Diagnostic findings in Wilson disease are KF rings, sometimes requiring slit-lamp examination for detection, low serum ceruloplasmin and copper, high copper content in urine and liver biopsy, and abnormal CT scan of the basal ganglia. Early diagnosis and control of copper levels (low dietary copper, D-penicillamine, 1 to 2 g/day orally, or zinc acetate or trientine) will prevent the development of neurologic symptoms or cause them to regress.

Other diseases inducing an extrapyramidal syndrome are Hallervorden-Spatz disease, childhood Huntington chorea, Leigh subacute encephalomyelopathy, and the juvenile type of Niemann-Pick disease.

Dystonia, Chorea, and Athetosis

This syndrome has been described in Chap. 4. Diseases that are most likely to express themselves by this syndrome are Lesch-Nyhan disease, familial calcification of the basal ganglia and cerebellum, ceroid lipofuscinosis, torsion dystonia (chemistry and pathologic basis unknown), late-onset Niemann-Pick disease, sulfite oxidase deficiency, and glutaric and D-glyceric acidemias.

Familial Polymyoclonias

Polymyoclonus as a symptom was described in Chap. 5. In late childhood and adolescence, it often occurs in conjunction with seizures, cerebellar ataxia, and intellectual deterioration and is characteristic of the following conditions: (1) Lafora-body polymyoclonus, (2) juvenile cerebroretinal (ceroid) degeneration, (3) the cherry-red spot–myoclonus syndrome (sialidosis or neuraminidosis), (4) the rare, juvenile-onset form of GM_2 gangliosidosis, (5) late-onset Gaucher disease, and (6) mitochondrial encephalopathy. A benign degenerative form is also known (dyssynergia cerebellaris myoclonica of Ramsay Hunt). There is also a familial syndrome of intermittent cerebellar ataxia and dystonia that responds to the administration of acetazolamide.

Bilateral Hemiplegia, Cerebral Blindness and Deafness, and Other Manifestations of Decerebration

Most of the hereditary leukodystrophies with onset during late childhood and adolescence present with this syndrome. The most familiar are leukodystrophy with bronzing of the skin and adrenal atrophy (adrenoleukodystrophy), globoid body (Krabbe), and metachromatic leukodystrophies of late onset.

Three of the hereditary metabolic diseases—homocystinuria, Fabry disease, and the mitochondrial disorder MELAS—may cause strokes in the juvenile period of life.

Personality, Behavioral, and Cognitive Disorders

Disorders of these types, beginning in late childhood and adolescence, may sometimes be an early expression of hereditary metabolic disease. Although these ailments are rare, diagnosis is possible if one keeps in mind that behavioral and personality disorders in these circumstances are usually accompanied by some decline in intellectual function. In this respect, the psychiatric disturbances of the hereditary metabolic diseases differ from those of schizophrenia and manic-depressive psychosis. Also, sooner or later, other neurologic abnormalities (spasticity of legs, foot deformity, ataxia, rigidity, choreoathetosis, polyneuropathy, seizures) make their appearance. Diagnosis is made more difficult if psychotropic drugs have been given, producing extrapyramidal symptoms.

Of the many hereditary metabolic diseases in this age period, the following are the most likely to demonstrate early regression of cognitive function in association with alterations of personality and behavior.

1. Wilson disease
2. Hallervorden-Spatz pigmentary degeneration
3. Lafora-body myoclonic epilepsy
4. Adolescent form of neuronal ceroid lipofuscinosis (Vogt-Spielmeyer)
5. Juvenile Gaucher disease (type III)
6. Some of the mucopolysaccharidoses
7. Schilder disease of multiple sclerosis, with or without adrenal atrophy (adrenoleukodystrophy)
8. Metachromatic leukodystrophy
9. Adult GM_2 gangliosidosis
10. Mucolipidosis I (type I sialidosis)
11. Nonwilsonian copper disorder with dementia, spasticity, and paralysis of vertical eye movements

ADULT FORMS OF INHERITED METABOLIC DISEASE

Exceptionally, one of the diseases mentioned above assumes a relatively mild and chronic form, or the disease may first appear in adult life. The hereditary metabolic diseases that we have observed in adults are listed below.

1. Metachromatic leukoencephalopathy
2. Adrenoleukodystrophy
3. Krabbe globoid body leukodystrophy
4. Kufs form of ceroid lipofuscinosis
5. GM_2 gangliosidosis
6. Wilson disease
7. Leigh disease
8. Gaucher disease
9. Niemann-Pick disease
10. Krebs cycle enzyme deficiencies (hyperammonemia)
11. Mucolipidosis, type I
12. Polyneuropathies (Andrade disease, porphyria, Refsum disease)

In summary, the reader must appreciate that the classification used in this chapter is somewhat arbitrary. Nearly every disease assigned to one age period may extend into another as a milder or more severe variant. Every disease that presents with one dominant manifestation may at times present with some other neurologic abnormality. The plan adopted here—of categorizing these diseases by age period and syndromic relationship—is intended merely to facilitate diagnosis.

MITOCHONDRIAL DISORDERS

The diseases included under this heading are so diverse and involve so many parts of the nervous system that they cannot easily be addressed in any one part of the book. In their heterogeneity and complex overlapping relationships they are unlike the more common, discrete clinical entities that are caused by nuclear genetic mutations of Mendelian inheritance. The neural damage in the mitochondrial diseases derives from defects in the energy-producing systems of many cells and organs. This diversity is evident not only in their clinical presentations but also in the differing ages at which symptoms first become apparent and the presence or absence of the signature features of dysmorphic physical development, lactic acidosis, and myopathy. The latter is characterized by a varying number of "ragged-red fibers," so-called because of the subsarcolemmal and intermyofibrillar collections of membrane (mitochondrial) material in the type 1 (red) fibers that are stained by the Gomori trichrome method. In some instances a mitochondrial disease presents abruptly in a child or adult who up to that point had developed normally.

Most of the variability in clinical presentation is understandable from the principles of mitochondrial genetics. Nonetheless, there are several recognizable core syndromes and a few variants that are discussed fully in *Adams and Victor's Principles of Neurology*, 7th ed. A number of acronyms, as indicated in the listing below of the better characterized mitochondrial diseases, are used to codify these syndromes.

1. Ragged-red fiber polymyopathy
2. Progressive external ophthalmoplegia (PEO) and Kearns-Sayre syndrome
3. Leigh disease (subacute necrotizing encephalomyelopathy)
4. Myoclonic epilepsy and ragged-red fiber myopathy (MERRF)
5. Mitochondrial encephalomyopathy, lactic acidosis, and stroke (MELAS)
6. Leber optic neuropathy
7. Myoneural-gastrointestinal encephalopathy
8. Neuropathy, ataxia, retinitis pigmentosa (NARP)

For a more detailed discussion of this topic, see Victor and Ropper: *Adams and Victor's Principles of Neurology*, 7th ed, pp 983–1049.

ADDITIONAL READING

Gray RGF, Preece MA, Green SH, et al: Inborn errors of metabolism as a cause of neurological disease in adults: An approach to investigation. *J Neurol Neurosurg Psychiatry* 69:5, 2000.

Johns DR: Mitochondrial DNA and disease. *N Engl J Med* 333:638, 1995.

Lyon G, Adams RD, Kolodny EH: *Neurology of Hereditary Metabolic Diseases of Children*, 2nd ed. New York, McGraw-Hill, 1996.

Menkes JH (ed): *Textbook of Child Neurology*, 5th ed. Baltimore, Williams & Wilkins, 1995.

Scriver CR, Beaudet AL, Sly WS, Valle D (eds): *The Metabolic and Molecular Bases of Inherited Disease*, 7th ed. New York, McGraw-Hill, 1995.

38 | Developmental Diseases of the Nervous System

Developmental diseases of the nervous system lie in the domain of pediatric neurology and are of particular interest to those concerned with mental retardation and cerebral palsy. These diseases are of two main types: one group has its basis in an intrauterine aberration of brain development. Some derailment of the process of neuronal formation, migration, or organization has occurred. The primary cause may be genetic, or some exogenous agent may have blighted the embryo or fetus. In the other category, something appears to have gone awry during the fetal period or during parturition, when the head and brain are exposed to forces never again duplicated. Whatever the cause, the final product is a deficient or malformed and malfunctioning brain with which the child must live for a lifetime and for which only inadequate substitutive or corrective measures are available. Identification and prevention of the pathogenic mechanisms are the primary medical goals.

The developmental anomalies of the brain assume many forms. Insofar as the size and shape of the cranium correspond closely to brain development in early life, it is not surprising that one group presents with craniospinal deformities. In another group, the phakomatoses—which includes neurofibromatosis, tuberous sclerosis, and cutaneous angiomatosis—an inherited disease affects both dermal structures and the brain in multiple foci; the lesions in the skin predict the pathologic changes in the brain. Chromosomal abnormalities, identifiable by karyotyping any cell in mitosis, are responsible for another group of developmental anomalies. Nevertheless, after careful analysis of any large group of mentally retarded and cerebral palsied children, the pathogenesis in approximately half of them is currently obscure.

NEUROLOGIC DISORDERS ASSOCIATED WITH CRANIOSPINAL DEFORMITIES

In many types of developmental disorder, the brain anomaly is associated with a malformation of the cranium. The most extreme example is anencephaly, in which major portions of both the brain and the cranial vault are absent. In another group, a particular brain anomaly can be traced to a mutant gene or chromosomal abnormality, but many are of unknown origin. In some cases, the head is strikingly small (<45 cm in circumference) and the brain weight is only a few hundred grams in adult life (*microcephaly vera*). Both autosomal recessive and sex-linked inheritance patterns have been verified in this undifferentiated type of microcephaly. Lesser degrees of smallness of the head and early closure of the fontanels also reflect the presence of cerebral disease of diverse type. *Enlargement and rapid growth of the head* are usually due to *hydrocephalus* (Chiari malformation, aqueductal stenosis) and less frequently to enlargement of the brain itself (Tay-Sachs disease, Alexander disease, spongy degeneration of infancy) or to subdural hematomas. Widespread destruction of the cerebrum, leaving only pial membranes in place of the hemispheres, also enlarges the head because of lack of resistance of the residual cerebral tissue to intraventricular pressure (*hydranencephaly*).

One of the most arresting types of cranial malformation, observed more frequently in males, is *craniostenosis*, in which the membranous junctions between the bones of the skull fuse prematurely, before the brain attains maximum growth. Early closure of the coronal suture causes the skull to be wide and short (*brachiocephalic*); closure of the sagittal suture results in a long, narrow skull (*scaphocephaly*); closure of the lambdoid and coronal sutures enlarges the skull in the vertical direction (tower skull, *oxycephaly* or *turricephaly*). In the latter, the orbits are shallow, the eyes bulge, and skull films show islands of bone thinning (lückenschädel). Syndactyly (fusion of fingers), seizures, and mental retardation may accompany the latter defect (Apert syndrome). If the malformation is recognized early, the neurosurgeon can create artificial sutures, a procedure that permits the skull to assume a more normal shape.

Many diseases that disrupt the development of the brain also deform the cranial and facial bones and the eyes, ears, nose, and fingers. The somatic stigmas serve as indicators of the cerebral abnormality. A catalog of these can be found in the monograph of Holmes and colleagues (see references).

Rachischisis (dysraphism) is another important developmental fault of the craniospinal bones. If, for any reason, the lower part of the neural tube fails to close, the baby is born with a lumbar meningomyelocele or meningocele; if the cephalic end remains deficient, a cranial encephalocele is formed. Familial coincidence of these conditions is known but is small; exogenous factors are also under suspicion. Folate deficiency appears to be a factor and the addition of folic acid early in pregnancy is preventative.

In the *Chiari malformation*, parts of the cerebellum and medulla are displaced into the cervical spinal canal. There are two main types: type II with a meningomyelocele; type I without. The resulting syndrome is a combination of hydrocephalus, palsy of lower cranial nerves, and high cervical cord compression. Syringomyelia is a frequent accompaniment (Fig. 44-4).

CHROMOSOMAL ABNORMALITIES

With the discovery of methods for displaying chromosomes in cells that are undergoing mitosis, several abnormalities of the autosomal chromosomes (triplication, deletions, or translocations) and a lack or excess of sex chromosomes were identified: *Down syndrome* (trisomy 21); one type of arrhinencephaly (*Patau syndrome*, trisomy 13); *Edwards syndrome* (trisomy 18); cri du chat syndrome (deletion of short arm of chromosome 5); *Klinefelter syndrome* (XXY); *Turner syndrome* (XO); and several others.

The *Down syndrome* is the most common, occurring once in every 700 births (mainly but not exclusively in older mothers). The round head, open mouth, broad stubby hands, upward slanting of the palpebral fissures with medial epicanthal folds, poorly developed nasal bridge, low-set oval ears, enlarged tongue, gray-white specks of depigmentation of the irides (Brushfield spots), short incurved little fingers (clinodactyly), single transverse palmar (simian) creases, and mental retardation (median IQ 40 to 50, range 20 to 70) constitute the characteristic syndrome. The chromosomal abnormality can be demonstrated in cells of the amniotic fluid. The brain of such an individual is rounded and approximately 10 percent lighter than normal. The frontal lobes are relatively small, with a simplified convolutional pattern, and the superior temporal gyri are thin. Lenticular opacities and cardiac septal defects are frequent. Alzheimer neurofibrillary changes and senile plaques are found in practically all Down patients who are more than 40 years of age. Translocation and mosaic patterns of chromosome 21 account for variants of the Down syndrome.

See *Adams and Victor's Principles of Neurology*, 7th ed., for details of the other chromosomal abnormalities.

THE PHAKOMATOSES (CONGENITAL ECTODERMOSES)

Encompassed by this term is a group of hereditary diseases affecting the skin and other organs as well as the brain. *Neurofibromatosis* and *tuberous sclerosis* are characterized by benign tumor-like formations in the central nervous system (CNS) (hamartomas), which have the potential of undergoing neoplastic change. *Cutaneous angiomatosis* with abnormalities of the CNS is the other member of this group.

Tuberous Sclerosis

This is an inherited disease (autosomal dominant) with a high spontaneous mutation rate (1 in 20,000 to 1 in 50,000) and a prevalence of 5 to 7 per 100,000. It accounts for 0.1 to 0.7 percent of mentally retarded patients in institutions. The abnormal gene has been localized on chromosome 9.

Characteristic skin lesions, seizures, and retarded mental development represent a diagnostic triad. The brain lesions have been seen at birth by computed tomography (CT). The seizures begin in infancy and change their pattern as the brain matures. The earliest skin lesions are white depigmented spots (amelanotic nevi), often shaped like an ash leaf. Later the facial adenomas (of Pringle) appear and also thickened zones of subepidermal fibrosis (shagreen patches). The cerebral lesions produce relatively few focal signs.

Postmortem examination discloses a variety of visceral lesions—rhabdomyoma of the heart and angiomyolipomas in many organs. In the brain, some of the convolutions are chalk white in color and are enlarged and firm to the touch. Whitish masses protrude into the ventricles. Under the microscope, these tuber-like structures, which give the disease its name, are composed of plump astrocytes. Those in the cortex contain nerve cells, some of giant proportions, mixed with calcium deposits. Neoplastic transformation of these abnormal cells into gliomas may occur later in life in a small proportion of the patients.

Of clinical importance is the fact that not all components of the clinical triad need to be present in any given patient. Some patients with seizures and skin lesions remain mentally normal. In others, a few trivial skin lesions or a rare retinal phakoma and a seizure or two may be the only manifestations to suggest the diagnosis, and some patients escape seizures altogether. Only the epilepsy can be treated, using anticonvulsant drugs selected in accordance with the seizure type.

Neurofibromatosis of Von Recklinghausen

In this hereditary disease, the skin, nervous system, bones, endocrine glands, and sometimes other organs are the sites of tumor-like masses of limited growth potential (i.e., hamartomas). Those of the skin and nerves are usually schwannomas. In the iris, the small hamartomas are called Lisch nodules. Prevalence of the disease is 40 per 100,000 population, or about one case in every 2500 to 3000 births. The disease is inherited as an autosomal dominant trait. The classic peripheral form (NF type I), with widespread skin lesions, is due to an abnormal gene located on chromosome 17. A milder central form with few skin lesions and often bilateral acoustic neuromas (NF type II) has been linked to chromosome 22.

Spots of skin hyperpigmentation (café au lait) and multiple cutaneous and subcutaneous tumors that increase in number during late childhood and adolescence are characteristic. Schwannomas and neurofibromas may form on spinal roots and cranial nerves, some in position to compress multiple nerve roots and the spinal cord. Often such lesions are asymptomatic for a long time. Meningiomas are occasionally added to the syndrome. A hamartoma or glioma of one optic nerve or both is another serious complication, mainly in NF type I. Some of the skin tumors, instead of extruding above the surface as papillomas, thicken the skin diffusely (plexiform neuroma) and disfigure the face or other parts of the body. In about 2 to 5 percent of cases, one or more of the neurofibromas undergo malignant degeneration. The treatment of the peripheral tumors, meningiomas, and gliomas is surgical excision, if possible, or radiation.

Cutaneous Angiomatosis with Abnormalities of the CNS

There are at least seven distinct conditions in which a cutaneous vascular anomaly is associated with an abnormality of the nervous system. Here only the most common one—meningofacial (encephalofacial) angiomatosis with cerebral calcification (Sturge-Weber syndrome)—is described. In this condition, a one-sided cutaneous hemangioma is seen at birth, extending from the forehead to the upper eyelid. The hemangioma may or may not be elevated. Other parts of the face or body are involved in some patients. Later in childhood, there may occur a progressive hemisensorimotor or visual field deficit and recalcitrant seizures, which are contralateral to the lesion. The vascular lesion in the brain lies in the meninges and is mainly venous. The underlying cortex undergoes a progressive laminar necrosis and calcification, the latter giving rise to characteristic double-contoured ("tramline") radiographic images. Surgical excision of the cortical vascular lesion arrests the progressive ischemic neurologic deficit in some cases.

CONGENITAL PARAPLEGIA AND OTHER MOTOR DEFICITS

Cerebral Palsy, Little Disease

Although hereditary forms of spastic paraplegia are well documented, most of the patients with this syndrome prove to have suffered parturitional or postparturitional damage to the brain. The latter conditions are much more frequent in premature infants. Hemiplegias at birth are usually of this type as well but may be due to intrauterine stroke. Quadriplegia may also be an expression of hydranencephaly or of spinal cord trauma during delivery (especially breech delivery). Birth injury with paraparesis or paraplegia (diplegia) or double athetosis is usually referred to as Little disease. The baby may have been born at term, but the greatest risk factors in every large series are birth weight below 2000 g, other fetal malformations in siblings, and maternal mental retardation, probably attesting to a multiplicity of causes, all subsumed under the term *cerebral palsy*.

Clinically, two main groups of cases have been recognized. In one, *spastic diplegia*, which gradually becomes apparent after 4 to 6 months of postnatal life, is associated with a slight diminution in head size and intelligence. Its frequency increases with the degree of prematurity. Matrix hemorrhages and periventricular leukomalacia are the most frequent types of neuropathologic change. In a second group, birth is difficult and severe intrapartum asphyxia and attendant fetal distress are evident. The difficulty may arise in either full-term or premature infants. Such infants will usually require resuscitation and have low Apgar scores at 5 and 15 min postpartum, which in this instance are of predictive value. The clinical picture, later to emerge, is tetraparesis and pseudobulbar palsy, with signs of bilateral corticospinal involvement, "double" athetosis, or both. A second group is characterized by extrapyramidal motor disorders (choreoathetosis, dystonia).

The pathologic lesions are those of hypoxia-ischemia in the distal arterial fields in gray and white matter (lobar sclerosis, or ulegyria) in the group with spastic paralysis or état marbré (a marbled appearance) due to gliosis of the lenticular nuclei and thalamus in those with choreoathetosis and dystonia.

Hemiplegia and, less often, double hemiplegia may also develop later in infancy or childhood, usually from embolic or thrombotic arterial occlusion or venous thrombosis. The resulting lesions are often epileptic.

Kernicterus

Erythroblastosis fetalis is secondary to Rh and ABO incompatibilities between mother and fetus. This results in a high postpartum concentration of bilirubin, which damages the brain, particularly the basal ganglia, thalamus, and brainstem nuclei (oculomotor and cochlear). At autopsy, dead neurons are stained a canary yellow color, hence the name of the lesion—*Kern* (nucleus) *icterus*. The clinical picture is one of double athetosis, gaze palsies, and deafness, often with relatively normal cognitive development. The condition can be prevented by immunizing the mother against the Rh antigen and by control of hyperbilirubinemia by phototherapy in the infant.

INTRAUTERINE AND NEONATAL INFECTIONS

The most frequent are toxoplasmosis, rubella, cytomegalic inclusion disease, and herpes simplex encephalitis (the so-called TORCH infections), *Listeria monocytogenes*, and neurosyphilis, although HIV infection may soon surpass them. Their clinical characteristics are summarized in Table 38-1. Bacterial meningitis (due mainly to *Escherichia coli, L. monocytogenes* and group B streptococcus) is common in the neonate and carries a high mortality. Many of the survivors remain mentally impaired.

TABLE 38-1 Intrauterine and Neonatal Infections of the CNS

Disease	Time of infection	Clinical manifestations	Diagnostic tests	Prevention and treatment
Rubella	First 10 weeks of intrauterine life	*Mother:* ± symptomatic *Infant:* mental retardation, cataracts, neurocochlear deafness, congenital heart disease, pigmentary degeneration of retina: cloudy cornea; hepatosplenomegaly	IgM antibodies or viral isolation in neonate	Vaccination of all women against rubella
Cytomegalic inclusion disease (CMV)	First trimester	*Mother:* asymptomatic *Infant:* jaundice, mental retardation, convulsions, sensorineural deafness, chorioretinitis, optic atrophy, microcephaly	↑ Cells and protein in CSF; cytomegalic changes in cells in urine	No treatment
Toxoplasmosis	Intrauterine: probably third trimester	*Mother:* usually asymptomatic *Infant:* foci of retinal destruction, spastic paralysis, severe retardation, hydrocephalus. Affects only one pregnancy	↑ Cells and protein in CSF; ↑ antibody titers in mother	Spiramycin or clindamycin to mother; pyrimethamine plus a sulfonamide to neonate
Neurosyphilis	Last half of pregnancy	*Mother:* recent primary or secondary syphilis *Infant:* stillbirth or syphilitic infection	Positive serology in mother; ↑ cells and protein and positive serology in CSF of neonate	Penicillin G to mother and infant
Herpes simplex	At or near birth	*Mother:* genital herpes infection *Infant:* skin lesions, salivary gland infection; encephalitis; diminished responsiveness and neonatal automatisms	↑ Antibodies in mother and fetus	Acyclovir
Neonatal bacterial meningitis*	First days after birth	*Mother:* usually infected *Infant:* fever, bulging fontanels, reduced responsivity; ↓ brainstem automatisms	↑ Cells and protein, ↓ glucose, and bacteria in CSF	Antibiotics
Viral infection: Coxsackie B. poliomyelitis, arboviruses	Late in pregnancy or at term	Signs of encephalitis or encephalomyelitis	↑ Cells and protein in CSF	
HIV	Intrauterine or during delivery	*Mother:* HIV seropositive *Infant:* clinical stigmas appear only after several months	↑ Maternally derived antibody to HIV	

Listeria monocytogenes, Escherichia coli, group B streptococci, etc.

FETAL ALCOHOL SYNDROME

See p. 388.

MENTAL RETARDATION

This is a condition of impaired psychomotor development of diverse etiology in which the most glaring defects are in learning and scholastic achievement and in adaptive behavior. Two groups are recognized. In the first, comprising the large majority of mentally retarded, the retardation is relatively mild, allowing some degree of benefit from training and education. As a rule, individuals in this group have no recognizable cerebral pathology. Also, early motor, sensory, visual, and auditory development may be more or less normal, and the mental retardation may not be fully appreciated until school age, when scholastic deficiency becomes apparent. For these reasons, an unfavorable environment (e.g., poverty and poor nutrition, lack of parental affection and social stimulation) has been blamed for the scholastic failure—a condition referred to as "subcultural retardation." Undoubtedly genetic factors are operative in this group. A noteworthy fact is that in this group, much more often than in the severely retarded, one parent or both are many times mentally impaired. At least one segment of this "subcultural" group lies at the lowest end of the Gaussian ("bell") curve of intelligence, the opposite of genius.

In the second smaller group (10 percent or less of all retarded individuals), the retardation is severe and with few exceptions is nonfamilial. The diagnosis in these patients is usually not difficult because of the frequently associated somatic and neurologic abnormalities, which are recognized soon after birth. (The congenital anomalies of development described in the preceding pages fall into this category.) In almost all cases of this type, pathologic changes can be found in the brain—hence the group is spoken of as the "pathologically retarded."

The main categories of disease that cause mental retardation are indicated in Table 38-2.

The pathologically retarded are of three broad types (see Table 38-3). In one, there are associated developmental abnormalities of nonnervous structures. A second type is characterized by prominent neurologic changes;

TABLE 38-2 Categories of Disease Causing Mental Retardation (in 1372 Patients at the W. E. Fernald State School)

Disease category	Number of patients		Percentage of all patients
	IQ < 50	IQ > 50	
Acquired destructive lesions	278	79	26.0
Chromosomal abnormalities	247	10	18.7
Multiple congenital anomalies	64	16	5.8
Developmental abnormality of brain	49	16	4.7
Metabolic and endocrine diseases	38	5	3.1
Progressive degenerative disease	5	7	0.9
Neurocutaneous diseases	4	0	0.3
Psychosis	7	6	1.0
Mentally retarded (cause unknown)	385	156	39.5

TABLE 38-3 Diseases Associated with Severe Mental Retardation*

I. Mental defect with associated developmental abnormalities in nonnervous structures
  A. Those affecting cranioskeletal structures
    1. Microcephaly
    2. Macrocephaly
    3. Hydrocephalus (including myelomeningocele with Chiari malformation and associated cerebral anomalies)
    4. Down syndrome (mongolism)
    5. Cretinism (congenital hypothyroidism)
    6. Mucopolysaccharidoses (Hurler, Hunter, and Sanfilippo types)
    7. Acrocephalosyndactyly (craniostenosis, Apert syndrome)
    8. Arthrogryposis multiplex congenita (in certain cases)
    9. Rare specific syndromes: e.g., de Lange
    10. Dwarfism, short stature: Russell-Silver dwarf, Seckel bird-headed dwarf, Rubinstein-Taybi dwarf, Cockayne-Neel dwarf, etc.
    11. Hypertelorism, median cleft face syndromes, agenesis of corpus callosum
  B. Those affecting nonskeletal structures
    1. Neurocutaneous syndromes: tuberous sclerosis, Sturge-Weber, neurofibromatosis
    2. Congenital rubella syndrome (deafness, blindness, congenital heart disease, small stature)
    3. Chromosomal disorders: Down syndrome, some cases of Klinefelter syndrome (XXY), XYY, Turner (XO) syndrome (occasionally), and others
    4. Laurence-Moon-Biedl syndrome (retinitis pigmentosa, obesity, polydactyly)
    5. Those associated with eye disorders: toxoplasmosis (chorioretinitis), galactosemia (cataract), congenital rubella
    6. Prader-Willi syndrome (obesity, hypogenitalism)
II. Mental defect without developmental anomalies in nonnervous structures, but with focal cerebral and other neurologic abnormalities
  A. Cerebral spastic diplegia, hemiplegia, tetraplegia
  B. Choreoathetosis
    1. Kernicterus
    2. Status marmoratus
    3. Hypoxia
  C. Congenital ataxia
  D. Syndrome resulting from hypoglycemia, trauma, meningitis, and encephalitis
  E. Associated with neuromuscular abnormalities (muscular dystrophy, Friedreich ataxia, etc.)
  F. Degenerative and metabolic diseases
  G. Neonatal infections
  H. Inborn errors of metabolism (Lesch-Nyhan syndrome, phenylketonuria, etc.)
III. Mental defect without signs of other developmental abnormality or neurologic disorder (epilepsy may or may not be present)
  A. X-linked simple mental retardation (Renpenning, fragile-X syndromes)
  B. Autism—Kanner and Asperger syndromes and autistic spectrum) with isolated retained cognitive abilities
  C. Rett syndrome (females)
  D. Williams syndrome (elfin facies, supravalvular aortic stenosis, retained language or musical abilities)

*Most forms of "mild mental subnormality" are not included in this classification.

cerebral diplegia, athetosis, and cerebellar ataxia are present in some combination. In a third group, there are neither somatic nor neurologic abnormalities, only an isolated nondysmorphic mental retardation with no visible abnormality of the brain. In some of these cases, a clinical diagnosis is possible but the pathologic basis is not fully known.

Among those with the latter types of pathologic retardation, *autism (Kanner-Asperger syndrome)* is unique. The retarded development does not pervade all aspects of mentation in autism. *Asociality*—a striking disregard for other persons—is the most evident behavioral abnormality, associated with a lack of communicative skills and a need (almost a compulsion) to engage in repetitive ritualistic activity. At the same time, there may be retention of certain intellectual capacities such as calculating, drawing, or musical ability ("idiot savant"). These defects occur in a spectrum of severity, but for many, the outlook is bleak.

Several other special heritable retardations with normal brain structure deserve mention. The *Renpenning* and *fragile-X* syndromes are X-linked mental retardations with few dysmorphic features. The fragile-X syndrome, in which there is an unstable chromosomal site that is prone to breakage, may account for 10 percent of mentally retarded males. The *Rett syndrome* is related to a dominant mutation on the X chromosome that is fatal in males; therefore only girls are affected. There is a regression of psychomotor development after a period of apparent normality up to ages 1 or 2 years. Withdrawn behavior and hand wringing or similar automatisms occur and may simulate autism. These are all of interest because of the implication that some aspect of intelligence is encoded on the X chromosome. The *Williams syndrome* produces mild mental retardation, often with preserved or precocious musical aptitude and writing facility. There is an associated supravalvular aortic stenosis. A microdeletion on chromosome 7 in a region that codes for elastin has been found.

Many of the developmental abnormalities and the acquired diseases of infants and young children are attended by seizures. These assume many forms not seen in adult life. They are described in Chap. 16.

For a more detailed discussion of this topic, see Victor and Ropper: *Adams and Victor's Principles of Neurology*, 7th ed, pp 1050–1105.

ADDITIONAL READING

Banker BQ, Larroche J-C: Periventricular leukomalacia of infancy. *Arch Neurol* 7:386, 1962.

Barlow CF: *Mental Retardation and Related Disorders*. Philadelphia, Davis, 1978.

Berg BO (ed): *Principles of Child Neurology*. New York, McGraw-Hill, 1996.

Fenichel GM: *Neonatal Neurology*, 3rd ed. New York, Churchill Livingstone, 1992.

Gomez MR: *Neurocutaneous Disease (A Practical Approach)*. Boston, Butterworth, 1987.

Hagberg V, Aicardi J, Dias K, et al: A progressive syndrome of autism, dementia, ataxia and loss of purposeful hand movements in girls: Rett's syndrome. *Ann Neurol* 14:471, 1983.

Holmes LB, Moser HW, Halldorsson S, et al: *Mental Retardation: An Atlas of Disease with Associated Physical Abnormalities.* New York, Macmillan, 1972.

Hutto C, Parks WP, Lai S, et al: A hospital based prospective study of perinatal infection with human immunodeficiency virus type 1. *J Pediatr* 118:347, 1991.

Jones KL: *Smith's Recognizable Patterns of Human Malformation*, 4th ed. Philadelphia, Saunders, 1988.

Kalter H, Warkany J: Congenital malformations: Etiologic factors and their role in prevention. *N Engl J Med* 308:424, 1983.

Martuza RL, Eldridge R: Neurofibromatosis 2 (bilateral acoustic neurofibromatosis). *N Engl J Med* 318:684, 1988.

Pulsifer MB: The neuropsychology of mental retardation. *J Int Neuropsychol Soc* 2:159, 1996.

Rapin I: Autism. *N Engl J Med* 337:97, 1997.

Short MP, Adams RD: Neurocutaneous diseases, in Fitzpatrick TB et al (eds): *Dermatology in General Medicine*, 4th ed. New York, McGraw-Hill, 1993, pp 2249–2289.

Volpe JJ: *Neurology of the Newborn*, 3rd ed. Philadelphia, Saunders, 1995.

39 | Degenerative Diseases of the Nervous System

The diseases subsumed under this heading answer to the following criteria: (1) they begin insidiously after a long period of normal nervous system function and pursue a gradually progressive course for many years, often a decade or longer; (2) some depend on genetic factors or at least appear in more than one member of the same family—i.e., they are *heredodegenerative*—but a large number occur sporadically; (3) the pathologic basis of the degenerative diseases is a gradual loss of neurons and replacement gliosis, and most often the neuronal loss is selective—i.e., it involves related functional systems such as the anterior horn cells and corticospinal tracts in ALS or the pigmented brainstem neurons in Parkinson disease; and (4) this system atrophy is more or less symmetrical once the disease has become fully established.

Why nerve cells that have functioned normally throughout most of a person's lifetime should waste away (atrophy) remains a biological mystery. Referring to the process as an *abiotrophy* (Gowers), or premature senescence, simply rephrases the same problem without shedding light on the pathogenesis. In recent years, newer methods of cytologic and molecular study have disclosed changes that are not at all compatible with simple aging. The term *apoptosis*, referring to programmed cell death in embryologic development, has been adopted to describe some of these changes, but it too may not be entirely apt.

In the ensuing discussion, the degenerative diseases are organized according to their main clinical feature (Table 39-1).

DEGENERATIVE DISEASES CHARACTERIZED MAINLY BY PROGRESSIVE DEMENTIA

Alzheimer Disease

This, the most frequent of all degenerative diseases, occurs in late life. Its prevalence between the ages of 60 and 69 years of age is less than 1 percent, but it increases strikingly to 11 percent or more in the eighties. The disease is familial in some 15 percent of cases and runs a progressive course that spans 5 to 10 years or more. The neuronal loss is mainly in the association areas of the frontal, temporal, and parietal cortices of both hemispheres; the primary motor, somatosensory, visual, and auditory cortices are spared. Apart from neuronal loss, the two most distinctive histopathologic features are the deposition of amyloid in senile (neuritic) plaques and a thickening and condensation of the neurofibrillary component of surviving and degenerating nerve cells (Alzheimer neurofibrillary change, or tangles) made up predominantly of tau protein. These two types of pathologic change are found in lesser amounts with increasing age, but they are immeasurably

TABLE 39-1 Classification of Degenerative Diseases of the Nervous System

I. **Syndrome of progressive dementia, other neurologic signs being absent or inconspicuous**
   A. Diffuse cerebral atrophy
      1. Alzheimer disease
      2. Diffuse cerebral cortical atrophy of non-Alzheimer type
      3. Some cases of Lewy body dementia
   B. Circumscribed cerebral atrophy
      1. Pick disease (lobar sclerosis)
      2. Frontotemporal dementia
II. **Syndrome of progressive dementia in combination with other neurologic abnormalities**
   A. Huntington chorea
   B. Lewy body disease
   C. Cortical-striatal-spinal degeneration (Jakob) and the dementia–Parkinson–amyotrophic lateral sclerosis complex (Guamanian and others)
   D. Dentatorubropallidoluysian degeneration (DRPLA)
   E. Cerebrocerebellar degeneration
   F. Familial dementia with spastic paraparesis, amyotrophy, or myoclonus
   G. Some cases of Parkinson disease
   H. Corticobasal ganglionic degeneration
III. **Syndrome of disordered posture and movement**
   A. Parkinson disease (paralysis agitans)
   B. Striatonigral degeneration with or without autonomic failure (Shy-Drager syndrome) and olivopontocerebellar atrophy (multiple system atrophy)
   C. Progressive supranuclear palsy (Steele-Richardson-Olszewski)
   D. Dystonia musculorum deformans (torsion spasm)
   E. Lewy body disease
   F. Corticobasal ganglionic degeneration
   G. Restricted dystonias, including spasmodic torticollis and Meige syndrome
   H. Familial tremors
   I. Multiple tic disease (Gilles de la Tourette syndrome)
   J. Acanthocytic chorea
IV. **Syndrome of progressive ataxia**
   A. Spinocerebellar ataxias (early onset)
      1. Friedreich ataxia
      2. Non-Friedreich, early-onset ataxia (with retained reflexes, hypogonadism, myoclonus, and other disorders)
   B. Cerebellar cortical ataxias
      1. Holmes type of familial pure cerebellar-olivary atrophy
      2. Late-onset cerebellar atrophy of Marie, Foix, and Alajouanine
   C. Complicated cerebellar ataxia (later-onset ataxia with brainstem and other neurologic disorders)
      1. Olivopontocerebellar degenerations (OPCA)
         a. Clinically pure (Déjerine-Thomas type)
         b. With extrapyramidal and autonomic degeneration (multiple system atrophy)
         c. Conjoined with spinocerebellar degeneration (Menzel type)
      2. Dentatorubral degeneration (Ramsay Hunt type)
      3. Dentatorubropallidoluysian atrophy (DRPLA)
      4. Machado-Joseph-Azorean disease (extrapyramidal)
      5. Other complicated late-onset, autosomal dominant ataxias with spastic paraparesis (Ferguson-Critchley), pigmentary retinopathy, ophthalmoplegia, slow eye movements, neuropathy, optic atrophy, deafness, extrapyramidal features, and dementia

(continued)

TABLE 39-1 *(continued)* Classification of Degenerative Diseases of the Nervous System

V. **Syndrome of slowly developing muscular weakness and atrophy (nuclear amyotrophy)**
   A. *Motor disorders with amyotrophy: motor system disease*
      1. Amyotrophic lateral sclerosis
      2. Progressive spinal muscular atrophy
      3. Progressive bulbar palsy
      4. Hereditary forms of progressive muscular atrophy and spastic paraplegia
   B. *Spastic paraplegia without amyotrophy*
      1. Primary lateral sclerosis
      2. Hereditary spastic paraplegia
VI. **Sensory and sensorimotor disorders (neuropathies)**
   A. Hereditary sensorimotor neuropathies—peroneal muscular atrophy (Charcot-Marie-Tooth); hypertrophic interstitial polyneuropathy (Déjerine-Sottas); Refsum disease; etc.
VII. **Syndrome of progressive blindness or ophthalmoplegia with or without other neurologic disorders**
   A. Hereditary optic neuropathy (Leber)
   B. Pigmentary degeneration of retina (retinitis pigmentosa)
   C. Stargardt disease
   D. Progressive external ophthalmoplegia with or without deafness or other system atrophies (Kearns-Sayre syndrome)
VIII. **Syndromes characterized by neurosensory deafness**
   A. Pure neurosensory deafness
   B. Hereditary hearing loss with retinal diseases
   C. Hereditary hearing loss with system atrophies of the nervous system

more pronounced in Alzheimer disease. Nevertheless, their ubiquity has led to the notion (incorrect in our view) that Alzheimer disease is merely an unusually advanced or premature senile change. There are also cases in which the features and course of dementia are indistinguishable from Alzheimer disease but in which the profusion of plaques and tangles is not evident. The blood flow to the atrophied cortex is reduced, but this is probably an adaptation to neuronal loss. The disease is not due to arteriosclerosis. Alzheimer changes are more frequent and occur earlier in patients with the Down syndrome, a finding that is explained by excess production of the amyloid precursor protein that is encoded on the triplicated chromosome 21. Familial disease, accounting for only a minority of cases, has been linked to chromosome 14 and rarely to chromosomes 1, 14, 19, and 21. The presence of the E4 variant of lipoprotein (and its allelic gene ϵ-4) also increases the risk of developing Alzheimer disease.

Clinical features The syndrome of dementia, described in Chap. 21, is most faithfully portrayed by Alzheimer disease. It begins insidiously, usually with an impairment of memory; as it worsens, other failures of cerebral function appear. Speech becomes halting, with groping for words; comprehension is less quick; errors in calculation become frequent; and visuospatial orientation becomes defective. With progression of the disease, testing of mental status confirms the presence of disorientation, amnesia, aphasia, apraxia, and agnosia (the four A's). In variants of the disease, any one of these deficits may precede or be more prominent than amnesia. By contrast, gait is usually preserved until late in the course of the illness; reflexes are normal, as are sensation, hearing, visual fields, ocular movements, and other brainstem functions. As the disease progresses, involuntary grasp and suck reflexes become prominent, the step is shortened, and mild rigidity (sometimes myoclonus or choreoathetosis) and slowness of movement are evident. Finally, the patient sits all day, idle and mute, or lies immobile in bed until an infection or other illness terminates his life.

The clinical picture, as it evolves over months and years, enables one to make the diagnosis with an accuracy of 80 to 85 percent. Computed tomography (CT) and magnetic resonance imaging (MRI) reveal a greater degree of cerebral atrophy than expected for age; this may be most pronounced in the medial temporal lobes and disproportionate enlargement of the temporal horns (Fig. 39-1). The electroencephalogram (EEG) late in the illness shows a diffuse slowing but is normal through most of the course. The cerebrospinal fluid (CSF) is normal.

One or more cerebrovascular lesions, which are to be expected in 25 percent of individuals in the Alzheimer age group, may complicate the clinical picture and appear to exaggerate the degree of dementia. Medical counseling and the use of drugs to counteract certain troublesome symptoms (e.g., insomnia, agitation, paranoia) are helpful to the patient and his family. Drugs that enhance central cholinergic activity may be of some limited value in slowing the progress of memory loss; vitamin E, estrogen, and monoamine oxidase-B (MAO-B) inhibitors may have slight benefits. The patient, being more or less unaware of his inadequacies, seldom complains.

Differentiation of Alzheimer disease from treatable forms of dementia is the prime diagnostic consideration, as indicated in Chap. 21.

Lobar Atrophy (Pick Disease and Frontotemporal Dementia)

These less common diseases consist of an extreme degree of atrophy (far greater than in Alzheimer disease) of the frontal or temporal lobes or both. Neurons are lost, and many of the surviving ones show a peculiar swelling and argentophilic intracytoplasmic inclusions (Pick bodies). Forms of lobar atrophy (frontal or frontotemporal dementia) without Pick bodies also occur. In one form, the neurons are filled with neurofibrillary tangles consisting of aggregated tau protein. Some are associated with disease of the basal ganglia (corticobasal ganglionic degeneration). The extreme loss of neurons and gliosis of the involved cortex are also associated with loss of myelinated nerve fibers in the central white matter.

A family history (autosomal dominant) and an early frontal lobe syndrome (marked apathy and psychomotor slowing; grasp and suck reflexes) or a syndrome of the convexity of the temporal lobes (severe, early impairment of language function) suggest the diagnosis of Pick disease. Some cases are sporadic. Otherwise, the clinical picture resembles that of Alzheimer disease. CT scanning and MRI reveal the extreme sulcal widening.

Lewy Body Disease

A dementia that may initially be indistinguishable from Alzheimer disease is one in which the cortical neurons contain Lewy bodies rather than neu-

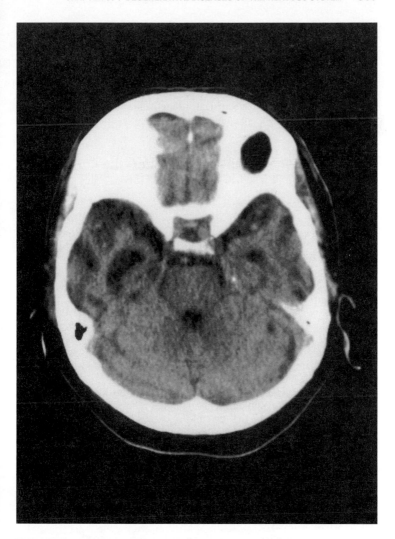

FIG. 39-1   CT scan in a case of advanced Alzheimer disease. There is generalized cerebral atrophy that is most pronounced in the temporal lobes. The temporal horns of the ventricles are greatly enlarged as a result of the loss of brain tissue.

rofibrillary tangles or amyloid plaques. Next to Alzheimer disease and diffuse (non-Alzheimer) cerebral atrophy. Lewy body disease is thought to be the most common form of diffuse cortical atrophy with dementia. The typical syndrome is of progressive dementia in an elderly patient with a later onset of parkinsonian signs. The movement disorder may be mild or prominent, and it may occur as an early manifestation. Almost half have tremor and some patients have orthostatic hypotension. The parkinsonian features may initially respond favorably to L-dopa. However, the most characteristic feature of the illness is an impressive fluctuation in behavior and cognitive function—episodic increases in confusion, hallucinations, and paranoid delusions. As the illness advances, amnesia, dyscalculia, visuospatial disorientation, aphasia, and apraxia do not differ from those of Alzheimer disease.

There are other forms of relatively pure dementing illnesses (the dementia of AIDS and so-called subcortical, frontal, and mesolimbic dementias), but their uncertain clinicopathologic specificity precludes further description here.

DISEASES IN WHICH DEMENTIA IS ASSOCIATED WITH OTHER NEUROLOGIC ABNORMALITIES

Huntington Chorea

This dominantly inherited neurologic disease usually begins in mid–adult life and progresses to death in 12 to 15 years. Either the characteristic choreoathetosis or intellectual decline may be the initial manifestation; later on, both are present. Often, emotional disturbances and disorders of behavior and personality precede the movement disorder and intellectual decline by several years. The abnormal movements embody elements of chorea, athetosis, and dystonia, described in Chap. 4. They are of wide range and arrhythmic, seemingly quasi-voluntary (like those of restlessness), involving limb, trunk, and cranial musculature. These abnormal movements are superimposed upon and interfere with gait and all voluntary activities. There may also be abnormalities of conjugate gaze. Variants consist of rigidity instead of chorea (Westphal form); in children, there may be seizures, ataxia, dystonia, and bradykinesia.

A loss of certain classes of neurons in the caudate nuclei and replacement gliosis are the main pathologic abnormalities. These changes are grossly evident in CT scans and MRI, which disclose a flattening of the normally rounded contour of the medial surfaces of the caudate nuclei. Less conspicuous neuronal loss is observed in the cerebral cortex. The underlying gene abnormality is an expanded (excessively long) "CAG trinucleotide repeat," localized to the short arm of chromosome 4. Genetic testing reveals the repeated CAG string to be longer than 39 in persons destined to become symptomatic or who already manifest the symptoms. Recently the abnormal protein product of the repeat sequence, huntingtin, has been found to accumulate within neurons.

Treatment is unsatisfactory. L-Dopa makes the choreoathetosis worse. Haloperidol in doses of 2 to 10 mg daily is moderately effective in suppressing the movement disorder, but it does not alter the course of the disease.

Special diagnostic problems are raised by nonfamilial cases of senile chorea and by paroxysmal choreoathetosis, acanthocytosis with chorea, acquired hepatocerebral degeneration, lupus-associated chorea, rheumatic choreas (Sydenham and gravidarum), dentatorubropallidoluysian atrophy, Wilson disease, and tardive dyskinesia (see Chap. 4).

Other diseases in which mental changes accompany a movement disorder are corticostriatospinal degeneration (Parkinson–dementia–ALS syndrome), corticobasal ganglionic degeneration of non-Huntington type, and familial dementia with spastic paraparesis. These are all well-recognized entities but are too rare to be described here. A proportion of patients with idiopathic

Parkinson disease (see below) also acquire a nondescript dementia in the late stages of illness.

DISEASES CHARACTERIZED MAINLY BY ABNORMALITIES OF POSTURE AND MOVEMENT

Parkinson Disease (Paralysis Agitans)

Hypokinesia, tremor at rest, rigidity, slowness of movement–bradykinesia (best seen in alternating movements of hands), "masked" facies and unblinking stare, stooped posture, and festinating gait (a hastening of steps) constitute the typical features. A central feature in many cases is the inability to regain normal posture and balance after being pushed or in response to assuming an eccentric body position, sometimes to the point of falling. Responsivity of the symptoms to L-dopa is another criterion for diagnosis. The disease usually appears late in life but sometimes as early as the fourth decade. About two-thirds of patients are disabled within 7 years, but the disease may drag on for 20 years or longer. Familial coincidence occurs in 10 to 15 percent of cases. There is no apraxia, aphasia, ataxia, or paralysis and no sign of corticospinal tract involvement. The proportions of akinesia, tremor, rigidity, and postural instability vary from case to case; the symptoms are at first asymmetrical; usually rigidity is not prominent until the late stages of the disease. The Parkinson patient is often fatigued or depressed. Also, dementia develops in a proportion of cases (10 to 15 percent) and is due mainly to an associated Alzheimer or Lewy body disease.

The distinguishing *pathologic features* are a loss of pigmented cells in the substantia nigra (pars compacta) and other pigmented nuclei in the brainstem and the presence of cytoplasmic inclusions—Lewy bodies—in the cells that remain. The Lewy bodies contain an aggregated form of alpha-synuclein, a synaptic protein. The population of nigral cells falls from about 425,000 to less than 200,000. As a result, there is a deficiency of dopamine, both in the nigral cells, in which dopamine is synthesized, and at the synaptic endings of nigral fibers, in the striatum.

Treatment   The many drugs that were used in past years to treat Parkinson disease have been superseded almost entirely by L-dopa, which replaces the depleted striatal dopamine, and by directly acting dopamine agonists. Ancillary treatment with selegiline, an MAO inhibitor, may slow the progress of disease by blocking the effect of an unidentified endogenous toxin. L-Dopa is usually given in combination with a decarboxylase inhibitor, to prevent its rapid destruction in the bloodstream before entering the nervous system. The usual dosage is 10 to 25 mg inhibitor with 100 to 250 mg L-dopa (Sinemet), three to four times daily. Nausea, hypotension, and depression are common side effects that can usually be managed medically. The most troublesome effect is the induction of involuntary movements, which force a reduction in dosage. Also useful are the dopamine agonists bromocriptine, pergolide, ropinirole, and others and the antiviral agent amantadine (50 to 100 mg tid). The directly acting agonists are most effective in the early stages of illness, during which they may be used instead of L-dopa for a time. They must be introduced very slowly in order to avoid hypotension. Marked fluctuations in rigidity ("on-off" phenomenon), which characterize the late stages of the illness, demand careful titration of drug dosages, literally hour by hour and by the use of combinations of the antiparkinson agents. L-dopa-induced hallucinosis can be ameliorated by newer antipsychosis drugs that lack parkinsonian side effects, such as olanzapine. If tremor is prominent, ethopropazine (50 mg qid) or long-acting propranolol (160 mg daily) may be helpful. Most of the patients who can sustain a low-protein diet (eliminating protein from breakfast and lunch) report some abatement in their symptoms. The tendency for some Parkinson patients to faint because of orthostatic hypotension can be ameliorated by fludrocortisone.

In recent years, the use of ablative surgical therapy has been revived and even more recently replaced by implanted electrode stimulation of various parts of the basal ganglia. Improved stereotactic techniques permit the precise placement of lesions or electrodes in the posterior and ventral part of the globus pallidus or the subthalmic nucleus, with improvement of contralateral tremor and rigidity and enhanced responsiveness to L-dopa for several years. Transplantation of fetal adrenal medullary or nigral cells, to instill dopamine into the brain, are under investigation but so far have given erratic results.

Striatonigral Degeneration and Multiple System Atrophy

In this disease, extensive loss of both putaminal and nigral neurons evokes the picture of Parkinson disease, although the typical parkinsonian tremor is usually lacking. These symptoms are sometimes combined with ataxia due to one type of olivopontocerebellar degeneration or more regularly with dysautonomia, due to degeneration of the lateral horn cells of the spinal cord (Shy-Drager syndrome). The central autonomic failure of Shy-Drager syndrome presents clinically with symptoms such as orthostatic fainting, stridor, urinary difficulties, and iridoplegia.

The complex syndrome that comprises these disorders in varying combinations has been termed *multiple system atrophy*. Nonspecific cytoplasmic and intranuclear glial cell inclusions are present in most cases, but there are no Lewy bodies in the neurons of the substantia nigra. Because of the degeneration of striatal neurons (loss of dopaminergic receptors), there is little or no response to L-dopa and related drugs. All the cases have been sporadic.

Progressive Supranuclear Palsy (Steele-Richardson-Olszewski Disease)

Here, supranuclear gaze palsy (especially of vertical saccades and later of vertical gaze) is combined with dystonia of the neck and trunk musculature, instability of balance with easy falling, pseudobulbar palsy, a fixed stare, and a number of other parkinsonian features that vary from case to case. Frequent, unexplainable falling may precede the changes in eye movements. Mental changes, usually mild, appear late in the course of the disease. The affected neurons of subthalamus, thalamus, and basal ganglia contain masses of tau-protein neurofilaments. There is only a slight and unsustained response to L-dopa.

Dystonia Musculorum Deformans (DMD; Torsion Spasm)

There are two main forms of this disease: An autosomal recessive form, which affects young children, usually of Jewish extraction, progresses slowly over a decade or longer. Limb, trunk, or cranial musculature is at first involved intermittently in tonic spasms, which later become widespread and persistent and cause grotesque deformities. Intellect is normal, and there are no other neurologic abnormalities. Stereotaxic ventrolateral thalamic surgery has been beneficial in some cases. In children, huge doses of Artane are said to alleviate the dystonia. A dominant form of DMD begins in later childhood or in adult life; it is generally milder and more slowly progressive than the recessive type, and it is not confined to a particular ethnic group.

In addition to DMD, a number of common, sporadic, restricted dystonic syndromes have been delineated. These are described in Chap. 6. One form of childhood dystonia with parkinsonism is remarkable in that it responds to low doses of L-dopa (Segawa disease).

SYNDROME OF PROGRESSIVE ATAXIA

A large number of heredodegenerative diseases fall into this category. No single classification of these diseases is entirely satisfactory, but the one presented in Table 39-1 (item IV), modified from Greenfield and from Harding, has proved clinically useful. Most cases begin in adolescence or early adult life, are slowly progressive, and are variably associated with ocular palsies, retinal degeneration, deafness, and peripheral neuropathy. One group affects mainly the Portuguese (Machado-Joseph disease). For a more complete account of the hereditary ataxias, the reader is referred to *Adams and Victor's Principles of Neurology*, 7th ed., and to the monographs of Greenfield and of Harding, listed in the references.

SYNDROME OF MUSCULAR WEAKNESS AND ATROPHY WITHOUT SENSORY CHANGES (MOTOR SYSTEM DISEASE)

The term *motor system disease* designates a progressive degenerative disorder of motor neurons of the spinal cord, brainstem, and motor cortex, manifest clinically by muscular weakness and atrophy (amyotrophy) and corticospinal tract signs in varying combinations. Mainly it is a disease of middle life and progresses to death in 2 to 5 years, sometimes longer. Several readily recognizable subtypes in both childhood and adult life have also been identified.

Amyotrophic Lateral Sclerosis (ALS)

This is the most common form of motor system disease, with an annual incidence rate of 0.4 to 1.76 per 100,000 population worldwide. In about 5 percent of cases, the disease is inherited as an autosomal dominant trait; in some of the hereditary cases, a deficiency of the enzyme superoxide dismutase has been found. The cause of the common sporadic form of ALS is not known.

The disease usually begins with weakness and wasting of hand muscles, associated with cramping and fasciculations in the arm muscles and then shoulder girdles. Less often, the symptoms begin in one leg as a foot drop, soon followed by weakness of plantar flexor and other leg muscles. Before long, the triad of atrophic weakness of the hands and forearms, slight spasticity of the legs, and generalized hyperreflexia with Babinski and Hoffman signs—all in the absence of sensory changes—leaves little doubt as to the diagnosis. Early or late in the illness, dysarthria, dysphagia, and dysphonia set in, and the tongue may wither and fasciculate; or a spastic bulbar paralysis (pseudobulbar palsy) may become prominent. ALS is the only common disorder in which progressive atrophic and spastic bulbar paralysis coexist. The disease is inexorably progressive, death resulting from aspiration pneumonia or inanition. There is no effective treatment, but the antiglutamate agent riluzole may delay the need for a respirator.

At any stage of the disease, the electromyogram (EMG) reveals the signs of widespread denervation, reinnervation changes, and reduced amplitude of compound muscle action potentials, while sensory and motor nerve conduction velocities are slowed only slightly or not at all. A cervical CT scan or MRI is often required to exclude spondylosis, which is a common cause of combined upper and lower motor neuron signs. The CSF is normal as a rule; serum CK is slightly elevated in rapidly progressive cases.

Neuropathologic examination discloses denervation atrophy of muscle and neurons in varying stages of degeneration in the anterior horns of the spinal cord motor nuclei of the lower brainstem and motor cortex, with secondary degeneration of corticospinal tracts.

Less Frequent Types of Motor System Disease

Weakness and atrophy may occur alone, without evidence of corticospinal tract dysfunction. These cases are referred to as *progressive muscular atrophy*. When weakness and wasting are more or less limited to the muscles innervated by the motor nuclei of the lower brainstem, the term *progressive bulbar paralysis* is used. In rare cases, the degenerative process remains confined to the corticospinal pathways, in which case it is designated *primary lateral sclerosis*.

There are in addition several inherited diseases of the anterior horn cells, most with their onset during infancy (Werdnig-Hoffman disease), childhood (Kugelberg-Welander spinal muscular atrophy), or adolescence. These are discussed in Chap. 52 with the congenital neuromuscular disorders. In adults, a unique X-linked amyotrophic disease involves the proximal shoulder and hip musculature and is accompanied by bulbar atrophy in most patients (Kennedy syndrome); facial fasciculations are characteristic. There is gynecomastia and oligospermia as a result of a disorder of androgen receptors; the genetic defect is a CAG repeat expansion that codes for this receptor.

Familial spastic paraplegia (Strumpell-Lorrain disease) without amyotrophy represents a special class of disease, to be distinguished from the forms of motor system disease described above. In the most common type of familial spastic paraplegia, only Betz cells and other cortical motor neurons and corticospinal tracts degenerate. The course spans decades. In some even rarer types of this syndrome, there may be optic atrophy or pigmentary retinal degeneration, polyneuropathy, or signs of extrapyramidal, cerebral (dementia), or cerebellar disorder.

SYNDROME OF PROGRESSIVE BLINDNESS

Three important degenerative diseases present in this way. These are the male sex–linked hereditary optic atrophy of Leber, now known to be a mitochondrial disorder; retinitis pigmentosa; and the tapetoretinal (macular) degeneration of Stargardt. Optic atrophy and retinitis pigmentosa overlap widely with other diseases, such as epilepsy, Refsum disease, Bassen-Kornzweig disease, Sjögren-Larsson syndrome, Kearns-Sayre syndrome, familial spastic paraplegia, and cerebellar degeneration, among others. The reader is referred to *Adams and Victor's Principles of Neurology*, 7th ed., for details.

HEREDITARY HEARING LOSS WITH DISEASES OF THE NERVOUS SYSTEM

There is also a very large number of degenerative neurologic disorders that are linked to hereditary progressive cochleovestibular atrophies. They have been described in detail by Konigsmark, whose review is listed in the references.

For a more detailed discussion of this topic, see Victor and Ropper: *Adams and Victor's Principles of Neurology*, 7th ed, pp 1106–1174.

ADDITIONAL READING

Greenfield JG: *The Spinocerebellar Degenerations*. Springfield, IL, Charles C Thomas, 1954.

Harding AE: *The Hereditary Ataxias and Related Disorders*. New York, Churchill Livingstone, 1984.

Kennedy WR, Alter M, Sung JH: Progressive proximal spinal and bulbar muscular atrophy of late onset. *Neurology* 18:671, 1968.

Konigsmark BW: Hereditary diseases of the nervous system with hearing loss, in Vinken PJ, Bruyn GW (eds): *Handbook of Clinical Neurology*, vol. 22. Amsterdam, North-Holland, 1975, pp 499–526.

Leenders KL, Frackowiak SJ, Lees AJ: Steele-Richardson-Olszewski syndrome. *Brain* 111:615, 1988.

Marsden CD: Parkinson's disease. *J Neurol Neurosurg Psychiatry* 57:672, 1994.

Martin JB: Molecular basis of the neurodegenerative disorders. *N Engl J Med* 340:1970, 1999.

Morris JC, Cole M, Banker BQ, Wright D: Hereditary dysphasic dementia and the Pick-Alzheimer spectrum. *Ann Neurol* 16:458, 1984.

Mulder DW, Kurland LT, Offord KP, Beard CM: Familial adult motor neuron disease: Amyotrophic lateral sclerosis. *Neurology* 36:511, 1986.

Neary D: Non-Alzheimer's disease forms of cerebral atrophy. *J Neurol Neurosurg Psychiatry* 53:929, 1990.

Pringle CE, Hudson AJ, Munoz DG, et al: Primary lateral sclerosis. *Brain* 115:495, 1992.

Rowland LP, Shneider NA: Amyotrophic lateral sclerosis. *N Engl J Med* 344:1688, 2001.

Shy GM, Magee KR: A new congenital non-progressive myopathy. *Brain* 79:610, 1956.

Silbermann M, Finkelbrand S, Weiss A, et al: Morphometric analysis of aging skeletal muscle following endurance training. *Muscle Nerve* 6:136, 1983.

Wenning GK, Ben-Shlomo Y, Magalhaes M, et al: Clinical features and natural history of multiple system atrophy: An analysis of 100 cases. *Brain* 117:835, 1994.

Wohlfart G, Fex J, Eliasson S: Hereditary proximal spinal muscular atrophy: A clinical entity simulating progressive muscular dystrophy. *Acta Psychiatr Scand* 30:395, 1955.

40 | Acquired Metabolic Diseases of the Nervous System

The nervous system is affected regularly, albeit indirectly, by diseases that cause failure of the heart, lungs, liver, kidneys, pancreas, and endocrine organs. This aspect of neurology obviously touches every branch of internal medicine, and the resulting syndromes must be familiar to internists and neurologists alike. In fact, recognition of the neurologic syndrome may lead to the diagnosis of the underlying medical disease.

Table 40-1 classifies the acquired metabolic disorders of the nervous system according to the syndrome by which they are most likely to present themselves clinically. As a rule, metabolic derangements that occur acutely are more prone to produce encephalopathy than those of long standing.

SYNDROME OF CONFUSION, STUPOR, AND COMA (METABOLIC ENCEPHALOPATHY)

Anoxic-Hypotensive Encephalopathy

Here the basic abnormality is a lack of oxygenation of the brain, caused by failure of the heart and circulation or of the lungs and respiration. The most frequent circumstances are cardiac arrest (myocardial infarction or ventricular arrhythmia); suffocation (drowning, smoke inhalation, strangulation, and tracheal obstruction); carbon monoxide poisoning; respiratory failure from cranial trauma and paralytic diseases (Guillain-Barré, poliomyelitis); and various other forms of circulatory collapse (external or internal hemorrhage, septic and traumatic shock). In all of these conditions, the mechanism can be reduced to insufficient perfusion or oxygenation of the brain; and since cerebral neurons have no capacity to store oxygen, they are destroyed when their oxygen supply is cut off (for more than 5 min if the anoxia is complete).

In the most severe form of ischemia-anoxia, the patient lapses rapidly into a state of deep, irreversible coma known as *brain death*, which is manifest by a complete lack of awareness of and responsivity to all manner of stimuli and abolition of all brainstem reflex activity, including respiration (see Chap. 17). The electroencephalogram (EEG) is isoelectric. Cardiac action and blood pressure are maintained, but nearly always, in these circumstances, circulatory failure follows within a few days. With lesser degrees of ischemia-anoxia, the patient survives, as happens when brainstem structures are preserved, but he may live on in a persistent vegetative or severely demented state.

Milder degrees of hypoxia may permit the restoration of consciousness, but with impairment of memory from selective destruction of hippocampal neurons. Even milder degrees of oxygen lack (*hypoxia*) induce only transient inattentiveness, impairment of judgment, and motor incoordination; if

TABLE 40-1 Classification of the Acquired Metabolic Disorders
of the Nervous System (Metabolic Encephalopathies)

I. Metabolic diseases presenting as a syndrome of episodic confusion,
stupor, or coma, sometimes with seizures
  A. Anoxia or hypoxia
  B. Hypercarbia
  C. Hypoglycemia
  D. Hyperglycemia
  E. Hepatic failure and Eck fistula
  F. Reye syndrome
  G. Uremia
  H. Sepsis, multiorgan failure, and burns
  I. Hypo- and hypernatremia and hyperosmolality
  J. Other metabolic encephalopathies: acidosis due to diabetes mellitus
     or renal failure (also inherited forms of acidosis, Chap. 37); Addison
     disease; hypercalcemia
II. Metabolic diseases presenting as an extrapyramidal syndrome
  A. Acquired hepatocerebral degeneration
  B. Hypoparathyroidism with calcification of basal ganglia
III. Metabolic diseases presenting as cerebellar ataxia
  A. Hypothyroidism
  B. Hyperthermia
  C. Hyperthyroidism
IV. Endocrine diseases causing psychosis or dementia
  A. Cushing disease and steroid encephalopathy
  B. Thyroid psychoses
  C. Hyperparathyroidism

consciousness was never lost, there are essentially no lasting effects. In all
these syndromes, anoxic or ischemic myoclonus is a common sequel.

In rare cases, recovery from anoxic encephalopathy appears to be complete, only to be followed after 1 to 4 weeks by a relapse, which in turn may
be reversible or followed by serious mental and motor disturbances. Widespread degeneration of cerebral white matter (delayed postanoxic leukoencephalopathy) has been reported in these cases.

Limited ischemia may also cause incomplete *infarction of vascular watershed* regions; several characteristic syndromes result, including shoulder-hip
weakness, agnosias, cortical blindness, and extrapyramidal disorders.

Often the period or degree of anoxia or ischemia is difficult to measure.
Although the patient may be pulseless or with blood pressure too low to
measure, there may still be some circulation to the brain. Cerebral function
may then be restored after a much longer period of apparent anoxia than
5 min. The attending physician, lacking these essential data, must therefore
be prepared to institute resuscitative measures (clear airway, artificial respiration, cardiovascular support) as quickly as possible.

Hypercapnia in Pulmonary Disease (Hypercarbia)

Chronic parenchymal lung disease, inadequacy of the respiratory centers, or
severe weakness of the muscles of respiration can cause a respiratory acidosis with elevation of P_{CO_2}. Secondary polycythemia and right-sided heart

failure (cor pulmonale) may accompany these disorders of ventilation, and there may be an added factor of pulmonary infection.

The neurologic syndrome comprises headache, papilledema, drowsiness, mental dullness, confusion, tremor, abrupt lapses in sustained muscle contraction (asterixis), and coma. In the fully developed state, the cerebrospinal fluid (CSF) is under increased pressure, and, with acute respiratory decompensation, arterial P_{CO_2} may exceed 75 mmHg. The pH of blood and CSF are lowered to 7.15 to 7.25. In this setting, the liberal administration of O_2 may be harmful, because the low arterial O_2 may be the only stimulus to the respiratory center, the latter having become insensitive to CO_2.

The essential therapeutic procedures are mechanical ventilation—to reduce CO_2 retention—using a volume-cycled intermittent positive-pressure device and providing supplemental oxygen if hypoxia is severe. Opioids and sedatives should be avoided until the patient is artificially ventilated because of their depressant effects on the respiratory centers.

Hypoglycemic Encephalopathy

The brain is largely dependent on glucose for its metabolism and has only a limited glucose reserve (1 to 2 g or 30 mol/100 g of tissue). This reserve will sustain cerebral activity for only about 30 min once no blood glucose is available. In conditions such as insulin overdose, islet cell tumor, severe hepatic destruction, Reye syndrome (page 374), glycogen storage disease, or an idiopathic state in infants, the blood glucose may fall to a critical degree. When it reaches a level of 30 mg/dL, hunger, sweating, headache, nervousness, and trembling develop; with a further drop in blood glucose, suck and grasp reflexes, muscular spasms, and decerebrate rigidity appear; in some patients, myoclonic twitching and seizures occur as well. At levels of 10 mg/dL or below, the patient becomes comatose, with dilated pupils, pale skin, shallow respiration, slow pulse, and hypotonicity of the limb musculature. Exceptionally, a relatively mild but persistent hypoglycemia, as occurs with islet cell tumors, may cause symptoms such as ataxia, chorea, rigidity, combativeness, drowsiness, and lethargy.

Infants tolerate marked reduction of blood glucose for a longer time than adults because of their higher glucose reserves.

The intravenous administration of glucose restores brain function completely if given before or at the very onset of coma. In nutritionally depleted patients, large doses of B vitamins should be given with the parenteral glucose in order to prevent Wernicke disease (see Chap. 41). If coma is prolonged, some degree of permanent damage results, and the patient then remains mentally impaired or shows other neurologic residua, like those that follow severe hypoxia.

Hyperglycemic Encephalopathy

Diabetic coma with hyperglycemia and ketoacidosis is correctible by proper medical measures. Usually in this condition the blood glucose is more than 400 mg/dL, the blood pH is less than 7.2, and P_{CO_2} is 15 mmHg or less. In *nonketotic hyperglycemia*, the blood glucose may reach extremely high levels, in the range of 1000 mg/dL, and be associated with seizures and focal cerebral signs (hemiparesis, aphasia, visual field defect), as well as stupor and coma, because of the extreme hyperosmolality (see further on under

Hypernatremia). Administration of isotonic solutions and insulin may result in full recovery, but the mortality in the elderly diabetic is distressingly high. Diabetic acidosis and the hyperosmolar state usually have no lasting effect on the brain provided that shock does not occur.

Hepatic Encephalopathy

This is a generic term for the several cerebral disorders that follow liver failure. An *acute encephalopathy* may complicate fulminant hepatitis and is lethal unless treated with liver transplantation; an acute nonicteric form, with raised intracranial pressure and coma, is associated with fatty infiltration of the liver and other organs (the now rare *Reye syndrome*). More common is the *subacute encephalopathy* that complicates all varieties of chronic liver disease; this is the type usually referred to as *hepatic stupor* or *coma* or *portal-systemic encephalopathy*. A chronic and irreversible syndrome (*acquired hepatocerebral degeneration*) may develop on a background of repeated attacks of hepatic coma, or it may develop independently (see below). There are also several *hereditary hyperammonemic syndromes* of infancy that cause episodic coma and seizures.

Probably all forms of hepatic encephalopathy have their basis in a disorder of nitrogen metabolism. Ammonia (NH_3) is formed in the bowel by the action of urease-containing organisms on dietary protein and is carried to the liver in the portal circulation. However, the NH_3 fails to be converted to urea because of hepatocellular disease or portal-systemic shunting of blood, usually both. As a result, excessive amounts of NH_3 reach the systemic circulation and interfere with cerebral metabolism in a way that is not fully understood. The ability of diazepine antagonists to partially reverse hepatic encephalopathy suggests that a disturbance of neurotransmitters is involved in the pathogenesis.

The *clinical syndrome of hepatic coma* consists essentially of a disorder of consciousness, ranging from confusion to stupor and coma, accompanied by a characteristic movement disorder and EEG abnormality. The disorder of movement, loosely referred to as a "flapping tremor," is in reality an intermittency of sustained muscle contraction termed *asterixis*. Asterixis is seen in several other metabolic encephalopathies, notably hypercapnia and anticonvulsant and other drug overdose, but it is most consistent and pronounced in liver failure. The EEG changes occur early in the evolution of hepatic coma and take the form of synchronous bursts of high-voltage slow (delta) waves, which appear first in the frontal regions and then replace all normal activity as coma deepens. A fluctuating rigidity of the limbs, reflex sucking and grasping, and sometimes Babinski signs and focal or generalized seizures round out the clinical picture. The blood NH_3 concentration, measured in arterial blood samples, usually exceeds 200 μg/dL and corresponds roughly to the depth of stupor and coma.

Hepatic coma is often precipitated by high protein intake or gastrointestinal hemorrhage. Hypoxia, hypokalemia, electrolyte depletion, and excessive diuresis are contributory factors. Measures that lower the blood NH_3—low-protein diet, oral neomycin and neomycin enemas (to reduce urease-producing bacteria in the gastrointestinal tract), and the use of lactulose (which acidifies the bowel contents)—are of therapeutic benefit and lend support to the ammonia intoxication hypothesis.

In the *Reye syndrome of children*, an acute viral infection (varicella, influenza B, and others) precipitates the rapid development of fever, vomiting, an enlarging fatty liver, convulsions, stupor, and coma, with decorticate or decerebrate rigidity, loss of brainstem reflexes, and death, all within a few days. The CSF is under high pressure but is acellular. NH_3 levels may exceed 500 mg/dL. SGOT levels are also high (several thousand units). At autopsy the liver cells are filled with fine droplets of fat, which are also present in renal tubules, myocardium, and skeletal muscle fibers. The brain is swollen and cerebral and cerebellar herniations are evident. The control of intracranial pressure by methods outlined in Chap. 30 may improve outcome. The use of aspirin in children with influenza-like illnesses appears to precipitate Reye syndrome; warnings to this effect have virtually eliminated the disease in recent years.

Uremic Encephalopathy

Two types of encephalopathy may develop in the course of renal failure and dialysis:

Uremic twitch–convulsive syndrome A variety of motor phenomena—twitching, tremor, myoclonus, convulsive seizures—may be associated with renal failure, sometimes when the patient is still mentally clear. The BUN is extremely high, but urea is not the responsible neurotoxin. Acidosis, hypocalcemia, and hypomagnesemia are added factors. Dialysis is the only effective treatment. Convulsions, which occur in about one-third of cases, respond to relatively low plasma concentrations of phenytoin and valproic acid.

In addition, there is a group of symptoms—headache, muscle cramps, agitation, drowsiness, and convulsions—observed in uremic patients during the third and fourth hours of dialysis or sometimes after completion of dialysis (*dysequilibrium syndrome*). Water intoxication and inappropriate ADH secretion are believed to cause a shift of H_2O into the brain, with brain swelling.

Hypertensive encephalopath (see page 318) This is a rapidly evolving syndrome that may occur with acute renal failure in which severe hypertension (diastolic >125 mmHg) is associated with headache, nausea and vomiting, visual disturbances, convulsions, confusion, stupor, and coma. Cautious lowering of blood pressure, anticonvulsant medication, and, in the eclamptic woman, immediate delivery of the infant are the essential elements in treatment.

Hypercalcemic Encephalopathy

Extremely high levels of serum Ca (>15 mg/dL) are associated with inattentiveness, confusion, drowsiness, and coma. Lower levels with a high fraction of ionizable Ca may have the same effects. Osseous carcinomatosis, multiple myeloma, vitamin D intoxication, sarcoidosis, and hyperparathyroidism are the usual causes.

Hypocalcemia, in addition to causing tetany, may result in convulsions and seizures.

Encephalopathy with Severe Sepsis and Burns

Attention has been drawn to a confusional state and drowsiness, without asterixis, in patients with bacterial sepsis and multiorgan failure. In the past, this encephalopathy was attributed to the metabolic effects of the failure of particular organs, to medications, or to electrolyte imbalance, but none of these provide an adequate explanation. Some immune or biochemical response to sepsis appears to be the unifying cause in most cases. A similar condition follows widespread burns.

Hypo- and Hypernatremia

These are among the most common of metabolic abnormalities encountered in a general hospital. As with other metabolic encephalopathies, the degree of central nervous system (CNS) disturbance is related to the rate at which the serum Na changes. Extremely high levels cause impairment of consciousness, myoclonus, asterixis, seizures, and, rarely, choreiform movements. Low levels are accompanied by a decrease in alertness, which progresses through stages of confusion to coma, often with convulsions.

Severe hypernatremic dehydration (Na > 155 meq/L) is observed in diabetes insipidus, nonketotic diabetic coma, protracted diarrhea, and in the stuporous patient who is not receiving fluids.

Among the causes of hyponatremia, the *syndrome of inappropriate antidiuretic hormone (SIADH) secretion* is of special importance, since it may complicate neurologic diseases—head trauma, meningitis and encephalitis, cerebral infarction, subarachnoid hemorrhage, neoplasm, and Guillain-Barré syndrome. The diagnosis is suspected when urine is hypertonic relative to plasma. Most instances respond to the restriction of fluid intake. Correction can also be effected by the intravenous infusion of hypertonic saline while inducing a diuresis, but excessively rapid restoration of the sodium level risks the development of pontine myelinolysis (see below).

A condition of "cerebral salt wasting" after subarachnoid hemorrhage and head trauma also leads to hyponatremia, but—in contrast to SIADH—with decreased blood volume. The distinction is of practical importance, insofar as fluid restriction to correct hyponatremia may be dangerous in patients with salt wasting.

Encephalopathy without Obvious Cause

In many patients, particularly elderly ones, in whom a metabolic encephalopathy is suspected, one searches in vain for a discrete cause. Usually a combination of factors is involved (fever, dehydration, drugs, etc.), and the patient improves over a period of a week or more. (See Chaps. 20 and 21 for a discussion of confusional states and "beclouded dementia.")

It should also be remarked that certain structural diseases of the brain are capable of producing a global encephalopathy that resembles the metabolic derangements described above. Examples are TTP, fat embolism, bilateral subdural hematomas, brain tumors (especially gliomatosis cerebri), and hydrocephalus. Likewise, the clinical state in the postconcussive and postconvulsive periods may be mistaken for a metabolic encephalopathy.

CENTRAL PONTINE MYELINOLYSIS (CPM)

In this disease, the center of the basis pontis and at times other parts of the brain undergo a more or less symmetrical noninflammatory demyelination. If the pontine lesion is large, the patient exhibits pseudocoma, i.e., is conscious but quadriplegic and pseudobulbar ("locked-in" syndrome). About one-half of the cases occur in alcoholics, the remainder in association with a wide spectrum of serious systemic diseases, severe and extensive burns, and following kidney and liver transplantation. MRI has greatly enhanced the ability to make a premortem diagnosis, although the lesion in the central pons may not be visualized for several days or for a week or more after the onset of symptoms.

The factor common to most cases of CPM is severe hyponatremia (95 to 120 meq/L). Although, as just noted, severe hyponatremia may be associated with symptoms of CNS dysfunction, it does not in itself cause CPM; the latter arises (but not in all cases) only *after rapid correction or overcorrection of hyponatremia*. Evidence from severely burned patients suggests that the production of hyperosmolality, rather than hypernatremia per se, is the critical pathogenetic factor. The optimum method for the correction of severe hyponatremia remains to be determined, but the best evidence to date indicates that this must be done cautiously, *at a rate not exceeding 12 meq in the first 24 h and not exceeding 20 meq in the first 48 h.*

See *Adams and Victor's Principles of Neurology*, 7th ed., for descriptions of other acquired metabolic encephalopathies produced by electrolyte imbalance.

ACQUIRED METABOLIC DISEASES PRESENTING WITH PROMINENT EXTRAPYRAMIDAL AND CEREBELLAR SIGNS

Chronic acquired hepatocerebral degeneration and *hypoparathyroidism* with calcification of the basal ganglia and cerebellum are the best-known examples. *Kernicterus*, a complication of *infanile erythroblastosis fetalis*, is another, now quite rare (p. 353). Chorea has been reported in *hyperthyroidism*.

As noted earlier, a patient with any type of cirrhosis, with or without preceding attacks of hepatic coma, may present with a slowly progressive syndrome of dysarthria, choreoathetosis, cerebellar ataxia, and mental deterioration. This acquired hepatocerebral degeneration correlates best with chronic hyperammonemia and may resolve to some extent when the latter is corrected.

In *hypoparathyroidism*, both choreoathetosis and ataxia, unilateral or bilateral, and parkinsonian symptoms have followed long after the early hypocalcemic manifestations of tetany and convulsions. The late neurologic effects appear to be related to basal ganglionic and cerebellar deposits of calcium, which are readily visible on CT scan.

Myxedema is said to produce a cerebellar ataxia, but we have had no experience with it. More convincing is the claim of experienced neurologists that the incoordination of gait and limb movements disappears with thyroid medication. There is no doubt that hypothyroidism is the basis of a slowness of movement, delayed relaxation of tendon reflexes, and, rarely, a sensorimotor polyneuropathy.

Extreme *hyperthermia*, as occurs with heat stroke, may damage Purkinje cells and may leave the patient with cerebellar ataxia.

ENDOCRINE DISEASES PRESENTING AS PSYCHOSIS AND DEMENTIA

Of these, the CNS effects of exogenous or endogenous adrenal and thyroid hormone are the most frequent and distressing. Large doses of adrenal corticosteroids regularly induce insomnia or an excited restless state, progressing sometimes to confusion and rarely to frank psychosis. *Cushing disease* may produce similar symptoms or be accompanied by a degree of dementia and brain shrinkage. Improvement follows reduction in the steroid dose or treatment of Cushing disease. Adrenal insufficiency may be attended by weakness, hypotension, and mild confusion.

Severe hypothyroidism leads to inattentiveness and drowsiness or a mildly demented state. *Thyrotoxicosis* may produce a tremulous and restless confusional state or at times psychosis. There is, as well, a curious myoclonic and stuporous encephalopathy associated with *Hashimoto thyroiditis*. High titers of antithyroid antibodies are found and there is a response to the administration of corticosteroids.

For a more detailed discussion of this topic, see Victor and Ropper: *Adams and Victor's Principles of Neurology*, 7th ed, pp 1175–1204.

ADDITIONAL READING

Adams RD, Foley JM: The neurological disorder associated with liver disease. *Res Publ Assoc Res Nerv Ment Dis* 32:198, 1953.

Cooper AJL, Plum F: Biochemistry and physiology of brain ammonia. *Physiol Rev* 67:440, 1987.

Laureno R, Karp BJ: Pontine and extrapontine myelinolysis following rapid correction of hyponatremia. *Lancet* 1:1439, 1988.

Levy DE, Bates D, Caronna JJ: Prognosis in nontraumatic coma. *Ann Intern Med* 94:293, 1981.

Plum F, Posner JB: *Diagnosis of Stupor and Coma*, 3rd ed. Philadelphia, Davis, 1980.

Raskin NH, Fishman RA: Neurologic disorders in renal failure. *N Engl J Med* 294:143, 204, 1976.

Rosenblum JL, Keating JP, Prensky AI, Nelson JS: A progressive neurologic syndrome in children with chronic liver disease. *N Engl J Med* 304:503, 1981.

Victor M, Adams RD, Cole M: The acquired (non-wilsonian) type of chronic hepatocerebral degeneration. *Medicine* 44:345, 1965.

Victor M, Rothstein J: Neurologic complications of hepatic and gastrointestinal disease, in Asbury AK, McKhann G, McDonald WI (eds): *Diseases of the Nervous System*, 2nd ed. Philadelphia, Saunders, 1992, pp 1442–1455.

Wright DG, Laureno R, Victor M: Pontine and extrapontine myelinolysis. *Brain* 102:361, 1979.

Young GB, Ropper AH, Bolton CF: *Coma and Impaired Consciousness*. McGraw-Hill, New York, 1998.

41 | Diseases of the Nervous System due to Nutritional Deficiency

Included here are diseases in which the nervous system suffers injury from the lack of an essential nutrient in the diet or from some conditioning factor that increases the need for such nutrients. The vitamins, and particularly the water-soluble B vitamins—thiamine, nicotinic acid, pyridoxine, pantothenic acid, riboflavin, folic acid, and cobalamin (vitamin B_{12})—are the most important as far as the nervous system is concerned. With the exception of subacute degeneration of the spinal cord (due solely to vitamin B_{12} deficiency), and certain other malabsorptive states (vitamin E deficiency), most deficiency states are associated with a lack of multiple vitamins. In western society, alcoholism is the condition that most often leads to B vitamin deficiency. Starvation itself is usually not responsible except in some infants and children who suffer the harmful effects of calorie-protein deprivation.

Nutritional deficiencies give rise to the following disorders of the nervous system:

1. The Wernicke-Korsakoff syndrome
2. Polyneuropathy (neuropathic beriberi)
3. Optic neuropathy
4. Syndrome of amblyopia, painful neuropathy, and orogenital dermatitis (Strachan syndrome)
5. Subacute combined degeneration (vitamin B_{12} deficiency)
6. Pellagra
7. Neurologic disorders due to a deficiency of pyridoxine and other B vitamins (pantothenic acid, folic acid, and possibly riboflavin)
8. Vitamin E deficiency polyneuropathy and spinocerebellar degeneration
9. "Alcoholic" cerebellar degeneration

Wernicke-Korsakoff Syndrome

This syndrome, a combination of two clinically distinct diseases (one described by Wernicke and the other by Korsakoff), is due to a chronic thiamine deficiency associated most often with chronic alcoholism. Some combination of diplopia and strabismus (bilateral abducens, horizontal and vertical gaze palsies), nystagmus that is both vertical and horizontal, cerebellar ataxia, and a confusional psychosis is the usual mode of presentation. The latter is often transformed into a relatively restricted Korsakoff amnesic state (see Chap. 21). Some degree of polyneuropathy—weakness, distal and symmetrical sensory loss, and areflexia of the legs—is present in most

378

cases. If, in a severely ill patient, the symptoms pass unnoticed, or if the patient is given IV glucose without the addition of thiamine, death may occur from a nutritional cardiomyopathy or some other undefined effect of carbohydrate loading and the diagnosis is then made at autopsy.

The lesions take the form of bilaterally symmetrical areas of necrosis in the paraventricular regions of the medial thalamus and hypothalamus (especially the mammillary bodies), periaqueductal gray matter, anterosuperior vermis, and structures in the floor of the fourth ventricle.

Treatment consists of the administration of thiamine hydrochloride (50 mg IV and 50 mg IM daily, until the patient is consuming a full diet), *instituted immediately upon recognition or suspicion of the disease.* Such treatment arrests the disease, but because of residual damage, a horizontal and occasionally a vertical gaze–evoked nystagmus, ataxia of gait ("alcoholic" cerebellar degeneration), and an amnesic (Korsakoff) state may persist.

Nutritional Polyneuropathy

This takes the form of a symmetrical loss or impairment of sensory, motor, and reflex function, affecting feet and legs more than hands and arms and the distal parts of the limbs more than the proximal ones. As stated above, this type of neuropathy often accompanies the Wernicke-Korsakoff syndrome (more than 80 percent of our cases), but it also occurs alone, particularly in its most severe form (neuropathic beriberi). Special variants of alcoholic-nutritional polyneuropathy are extremely painful, with burning and either excessive sweating or loss of sweating of the feet and sometimes of the hands as well. The cerebrospinal fluid (CSF) protein is normal or only slightly elevated.

The nerve lesion involves axons primarily but also myelin sheaths, the degenerative process being most pronounced in the distal parts of the longest and largest myelinated fibers ("dying-back" neuropathy). Once the legs become paralyzed, complete recovery requires axonal regeneration, a process that takes many months to a year or more. In time, the paralyzed muscles atrophy but nerve conduction is only moderately slowed.

Seldom can a nutritional polyneuropathy be traced to a deficiency of thiamine alone. Usually the patient is deficient in more than one of the B vitamins. The deficiencies can be corrected by oral vitamin therapy or merely a balanced diet adequate in vitamins and they are prevented by the same measures. Alcohol, of course, is interdicted because it tends to replace normal dietary components.

Deficiency Amblyopia

This is a relatively rare syndrome of subacutely evolving bilateral, but not necessarily symmetrical, central visual loss with pallor of the optic discs (optic atrophy). In the past, alcohol and tobacco were thought to be causative ("tobacco-alcohol" amblyopia), but the disease is now known to be due to vitamin deficiency, predominantly the B vitamins. It overlaps the *Strachan syndrome*, in which the amblyopia is associated with a painful and predominantly sensory polyneuropathy and orogenital dermatitis. A recent outbreak of this disorder affected 50,000 persons in Cuba during the period 1991–1994 (see MMWR report, 1994).

Subacute Combined Degeneration (SCD) and Pernicious Anemia (see also p. 409)

Long-standing deficiency of cobalamin (vitamin B_{12}) has two major effects: (1) a macrocytic megaloblastic (pernicious) anemia and (2) a degeneration of the posterior and lateral columns of the spinal cord (and sometimes of brain and peripheral nerves), which may occur independently and precede the hematologic effects. The neurologic disease has been traced to a failure of a cobalamin-dependent enzyme—methylmalonyl-CoA mutase, which is essential for the maintenance of myelinated fibers.

Clinical findings Distressing and persistent paresthesias of the feet and hands are usually the initial symptoms, followed by other signs of posterior column involvement (imbalance, loss of joint position and vibration senses, Romberg sign) and then by weakness and signs of corticospinal disease. The signs of optic neuropathy, if they appear, occur late in the disease, but there are exceptional cases of early blindness. Disorders of cerebral function (irritability, drowsiness, emotional instability, and confusion) may occur early in the course. With advanced disease, there may be a persistent disorder of cognitive functions (dementia) due to lesions of the cerebral white matter, similar to those of the spinal cord. There is some evidence that the mental disorder can be the only manifestation of vitamin B_{12} deficiency, but this needs verification. The main differential diagnoses are from cervical spondylosis, AIDS and HTLV-1 myelopathy, and multiple sclerosis.

Diagnosis and treatment The chief obstacle to early diagnosis of SCD is the lack of parallelism between the hematologic and neurologic signs. Patients who receive folic acid and some who do not may maintain a normal hematocrit and mean corpuscular volume for an indefinite period, while the neurologic signs worsen. Normal red cell size may also be maintained if there is iron deficiency. In such patients, one must search the blood smear for hypersegmented neutrophils. Serum cobalamin levels of less than 100 pg/mL are usually associated with neurologic symptoms and signs of SCD. Levels below 200 pg/mg associated with symptoms call for further investigation. The two-stage Schilling test is a reliable but not absolute indicator of cobalamin deficiency. The more recently developed assays for serum methylmalonic acid and homocysteine appear to be the most sensitive means of detecting cobalamin deficiency.

A high index of suspicion for and early recognition of SCD are essential, since the extent of neurologic improvement is governed by the duration of symptoms before treatment is instituted. Saturation of tissues depleted of vitamin B_{12} requires that large doses be given initially—1000 μg *IM* weekly for 1 or 2 months. This dosage of B_{12} is then given monthly for the rest of the patient's life. Oral administration is ineffective in the common type of B_{12} deficiency, pernicious anemia, because of the absence of intrinsic factor.

In a few unexplained cases, folic acid deficiency has been reported to cause spinal cord lesions identical to those of vitamin B_{12} deficiency.

Pellagra

This is a chronic deficiency state stemming from a lack of nicotinic acid or tryptophan, its amino acid precursor, and usually other B vitamins as well.

In the western world, pellagra is observed only rarely, probably because of the widespread practice of fortifying breads and cereals with nicotinic acid. In developing countries, the disease is still common. The fully established disease is characterized by dermatitis in areas exposed to sunlight, gastrointestinal disturbances (diarrhea), anemia, and neuropsychiatric symptoms. The latter consist of insomnia, irritability, feelings of anxiety and depression, fatigability, and inattentiveness progressing to mental dullness, apathy, and forgetfulness. Signs of corticospinal disorder and those of polyneuropathy are variably present.

The pathologic changes consist of swelling and central chromatolysis of cortical neurons and a symmetrical degeneration of the dorsal columns and, to a lesser extent, of the corticospinal tracts. The peripheral nerve changes are indistinguishable from those of neuropathic beriberi.

Pyridoxine (Vitamin B$_6$) Deficiency Encephalopathy

There are two types of B$_6$ deficiency encephalopathy. One is related to an inherited deficiency of the enzyme glutamic acid decarboxylase, of which vitamin B$_6$ is a cofactor; this disorder presents as neonatal convulsions. The other is an acquired deficiency of the vitamin, either from simple dietary lack or from the therapeutic use of isoniazid or hydralazine, which forms hydrazone complexes and makes pyridoxal unavailable to the tissues. The latter type is a cause of anemia and polyneuropathy in patients being treated for tuberculosis and hypertension.

Paradoxically, excessive dosage of vitamin B$_6$, taken orally, may induce a ganglionopathy and sensory polyneuropathy.

Pantothenic acid deficiency also produces a sensory polyneuropathy, said to be of painful type.

Vitamin E Deficiency

A spinocerebellar ataxia, associated with a polyneuropathy and sometimes pigmentary retinopathy, has been traced to a deficiency of fat-soluble vitamin E. It is corrected by administration of the vitamin. Several underlying diseases, all of them related to impaired fat absorption, may lead to such a deficiency—nontropical sprue, extensive intestinal resections, chronic cholestatic hepatobiliary disease, and other malabsorptive states. Virtually all of the reported cases have been in children. An inherited form has been described in which the hepatic incorporation of vitamin E into α-tocopherol is impaired.

Alcoholic Cerebellar Degeneration

This term refers to a common disorder in alcoholics characterized by a wide-based stance and gait, instability of the trunk, and ataxia of the legs. Arms are affected to a lesser extent, and dysarthria and nystagmus are distinctly uncommon. The pathologic changes consist of a degeneration of neurons of the cerebellar cortex, particularly the Purkinje cells, restricted to the antero-superior vermis and, in advanced cases, to the anterior parts of the anterior lobes.

These changes are similar in type and distribution to the cerebellar manifestations of the Wernicke-Korsakoff syndrome, and the same syndrome has been observed, albeit rarely, in states of malnutrition unassociated with alcoholism. Adequate diet arrests the process and may be attended by improvement.

Central pontine myelinolysis (see Chap. 40) and *Marchiafava-Bignami disease* (degeneration of the corpus callosum) are rare disorders that are observed most often in alcoholics but are not confined to them. In the latter disease, a dementia of subacute onset is accompanied by prominent grasping and sucking responses. A nutritional cause has been suggested for Marchiafava-Bignami disease but not established.

Numerous vitamin-responsive inherited metabolic diseases have been discovered; many are corrected by large doses of the vitamin (see *Adams and Victor's Principles of Neurology*, 7th ed., for details).

For a more detailed discussion of this topic, see Victor and Ropper: *Adams and Victor's Principles of Neurology*, 7th ed, pp 1205–1232.

ADDITIONAL READING

Allen RH, Stabler SP, Savage DG, Lindenbaum J: Diagnosis of cobalamin deficiency. I: Usefulness of serum methylmalonic acid and total homocysteine concentrations. *Am J Hematol* 34:90, 1990.

Beck WS: Cobalamin and the nervous system. *N Engl J Med* 318:1752, 1988.

Gotoda T, Arita M, Arai H, et al: Adult-onset spinocerebellar dysfunction caused by a mutation in the gene for the α-tocopherol-transfer protein. *N Engl J Med* 333:1313, 1995.

Green R, Kinsella LJ: Current concepts in the diagnosis of cobalamin deficiency. *Neurology* 45:1435, 1995.

Ishii N, Nishihara Y: Pellagra among chronic alcoholics: Clinical and pathological study of 20 necropsy cases. *J Neurol Neurosurg Psychiatry* 44:209, 1981.

Lindenbaum J, Healton EB, Savage DG, et al: Neuropsychiatric disorders caused by cobalamin deficiency in the absence of anemia or macrocytosis. *N Engl J Med* 318:1720, 1988.

Morbidity Mortality Weekly Reports. MMWR 43:183, 189, 1994.

Victor M: Polyneuropathy due to nutritional deficiency and alcoholism, in Dyck PJ, Thomas PK, Lambert EH, Bunge R (eds): *Peripheral Neuropathy*, 2nd ed. Philadelphia, Saunders, 1984, pp 1899–1940.

Victor M, Adams RD, Collins GH: *The Wernicke-Korsakoff Syndrome and Related Neurologic Disorders due to Alcoholism and Malnutrition*. Philadelphia, Davis, 1989.

Victor M, Adams RD, Mancall EL: A restricted form of cerebellar degeneration occurring in alcoholic patients. *Arch Neurol* 1:577, 1959.

Victor M, Mancall EL, Dreyfus PM: Deficiency amblyopia in the alcoholic patient: A clinicopathologic study. *Arch Ophthalmol* 64:1, 1960.

Ethyl alcohol or ethanol, in the form of whiskey, gin, vodka, wine, and beer, is the most widely used and abused of all intoxicant drugs. Its acute effects are known to almost everyone. As with all addictive drugs, tolerance develops with chronic usage and a group of stereotyped symptoms develop upon withdrawal of the drug after a period of chronic abuse (withdrawal or abstinence syndrome).

The essential medical facts about the absorption, distribution, excretion, and metabolism of alcohol and its effects on nonneurologic organ systems are discussed in *Adams and Victor's Principles of Neurology*, 7th ed. Reviewed there also are the pharmacologic effects on the nervous system and the theories of causation of alcoholism. Here, only the common neurologic complications are described. Although acute and chronic intoxication underlies all of them, the mechanisms by which alcohol produces its adverse neurologic effects vary. This is the basis of the classification used here.

The most pervasive and important of the alcohol-related problems, namely that of chronic excessive drinking, or *alcohol addiction*, like other forms of addiction, is not fully understood. A familial disposition has been convincingly demonstrated. Early exposure to alcohol and social and cultural approval are factors in other groups of alcoholics. The use of alcohol to allay the symptoms of manic-depressive or chronic anxiety–depressive illness is well known. A few remarks on the treatment of alcohol addiction appear at the end of this chapter.

CLINICAL EFFECTS OF ALCOHOL ON THE NERVOUS SYSTEM

   I. Alcohol intoxication—drunkenness, coma, rarely excitement ("pathologic intoxication"), "blackouts"
  II. The abstinence or withdrawal syndrome—tremulousness, hallucinosis, seizures, delirium tremens
 III. Nutritional diseases of the nervous system secondary to alcoholism (see Chap. 41)
     A. Wernicke-Korsakoff syndrome
     B. Polyneuropathy
     C. Optic neuropathy ("tobacco-alcohol amblyopia")
     D. Pellagra
     E. Cerebellar degeneration
 IV. Diseases of uncertain pathogenesis often associated with alcoholism
     A. Central pontine myelinolysis
     B. Marchiafava-Bignami disease
     C. Alcoholic cardiomyopathy and myopathy
     D. Alcoholic dementia
     E. Cerebral atrophy
  V. Fetal alcohol syndrome

VI. Neurologic disorders consequent upon alcoholic cirrhosis and portal-systemic shunts
  A. Hepatic stupor and coma
  B. Chronic hepatocerebral degeneration
VII. Pressure palsies and alcohol myopathy (page 467)

ALCOHOL INTOXICATION

The usual manifestations of alcohol intoxication are so common as to require no elaboration. The varying degrees of exhilaration and excitement, loss of restraint, loquacity, irregularity of behavior, slurred speech, incoordination of movement and gait, inattentiveness, drowsiness, stupor, and coma need only be mentioned. The usual forms of alcohol intoxication present little difficulty in diagnosis and management. In certain forms (alcoholic coma, "blackouts," and so-called pathologic intoxication), however, diagnosis may be difficult and urgent treatment is required.

Alcoholic coma The diagnosis of alcoholic coma can be made with confidence only after exclusion of other causes of coma; a flushed face and odor of alcohol are in themselves insufficient diagnostic criteria. The blood alcohol level is a useful but imperfect diagnostic measure. A concentration of 400 mg/dL may prove lethal in a nontolerant individual but cause only mild symptoms of intoxication in a chronic sustained drinker. Relatively low blood levels in a comatose alcoholic (200 mg/dL or less) should always suggest the presence of associated drug intoxication (barbiturate, methyl alcohol), infection (pneumonia, meningitis), liver disease, or head injury.

The main objective in the *treatment* of alcoholic coma is to prevent respiratory depression and its complications and follows along the lines indicated in Chap. 17. Hemodialysis should be undertaken in patients with extremely high blood alcohol levels (> 500 mg/dL), particularly those who are acidotic or have concurrently ingested methanol or ethylene glycol or some other dialyzable drug.

"Blackouts" At a certain stage of alcohol intoxication, an individual may cease to form memories, despite being able to carry out an array of complex activities. Later, when sober, the individual has no memory for these activities, which may have taken place over a period of several hours. These are so-called blackouts, which may be taken as a measure of the severity of intoxication. Their occurrence is not necessarily a predictor for the development of alcohol addiction, as has commonly been assumed.

Pathologic intoxication (complicated intoxication, alcohol paranoid state, atypical intoxication) The boundaries of this syndrome have never been clearly drawn, as one might gather from its diverse designations. Well known are certain idiosyncratic reactions to alcohol, in which a few drinks predictably evoke behavioral abnormalities seemingly alien to the personality of the subject—argumentativeness, assaultiveness, acute paranoia, indiscriminate sexual advances, or criminality. Possibly the disinhibitory effects of alcohol have exposed a latent sociopathic trait.

More often the term *pathologic intoxication* designates an outburst of blind fury with assaultive and destructive behavior, the patient being subdued only with difficulty and massive sedation; later the patient has no memory of the episode. This state needs to be distinguished from temporal lobe seizures and sociopathy, which occasionally take the form of explosive outbursts of rage and violence. A similar paradoxic reaction sometimes follows the administration of barbiturates.

ABSTINENCE OR WITHDRAWAL SYNDROME

This is a symptom complex consisting of tremulousness, hallucinations, seizures, confusion, and psychomotor and autonomic overactivity that *develops within several hours or days after an addictive drinker abstains from alcohol.* The parts of the brain upon which alcohol acts and that come to tolerate increasing amounts of the drug appear to be disinhibited and become overactive when alcohol is withdrawn.

Clinical Features

These are depicted diagrammatically in Fig. 42-1. In effect, there are two syndromes: a minor and a major one.

The *minor* or *early syndrome* is characterized by tremulousness, nausea and vomiting, insomnia, flushed facies, relatively mild diaphoresis, hallucinations (visual and auditory, rarely tactile and olfactory), and convulsive seizures; disorientation and confusion are minimal or absent altogether. These symptoms have their onset within 7 to 8 h after the cessation of drinking, reach their peak intensity within 24 h, and then subside over several days, usually without sequelae. Exceptionally, an alcohol withdrawal state that begins as an acute auditory hallucinosis fails to recede and settles into a quiet chronic delusional-hallucinatory psychosis, one that may be mistaken for paranoid schizophrenia. In a relatively small number of patients, the early symptoms of alcohol withdrawal (particularly withdrawal seizures) are a prelude to delirium tremens.

The *major withdrawal syndrome,* traditionally designated as *delirium tremens (DTs),* is characterized by profound confusion, gross tremor and myoclonus, delusions and hallucinations, and signs of autonomic nervous system overactivity (fever, tachycardia, dilated pupils, marked diaphoresis). These symptoms have their onset between 48 and 96 h (peak onset, 72 h) after the cessation of drinking. The major syndrome is much less frequent than the minor one but far more serious, ending fatally in approximately 5 percent of cases. Hyperthermia, circulatory collapse, infection, and serious injury are the conditions usually associated with a fatal outcome. Pathologic study of the brain in these cases has not disclosed any significant histologic abnormalities attributable to the delirium per se.

Withdrawal Seizures ("Rum Fits")

Early in the withdrawal period (7 to 48 h after cessation), there is a marked tendency to convulsion, even in persons with no history or electroencephalographic (EEG) evidence of epilepsy. Stated differently, alcohol withdrawal is an important cause of convulsive seizures occurring for the first time in adult life.

During the period of seizure activity, the EEG may be abnormal and the patient may be unusually sensitive to stroboscopic stimulation, but these abnormalities subside in a few days, even in patients who go on to develop DTs. (In our patients the latter sequence occurred in almost 30 percent with

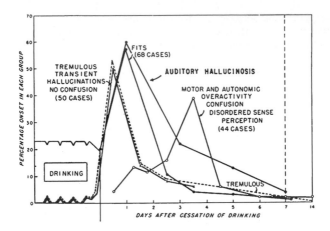

FIG. 42-1   Relation of acute neurologic disturbances to cessation of drinking. The drinking period is greatly foreshortened and not intended to be quantitative. The periodic notching in the baseline represents the tremulousness, nausea, etc., that occur following a night's sleep. The time relations of the various groups of symptoms to withdrawal are explained in the text. *(From Victor and Adams, 1953.)*

withdrawal seizures, but in other series the percentage has been considerably less.) As a rule, such seizures are generalized in type; they may occur singly or, more often, there may be several seizures over a period of several hours; rarely, the seizures take the form of grand mal status epilepticus. It should be noted that focal seizure occurring in this setting indicates the presence of a focal cerebral lesion (most often traumatic) in addition to the effects of alcohol withdrawal.

In patients with idiopathic or posttraumatic epilepsy, seizures may be precipitated by a short period (one evening or a weekend) of drinking, but here also the seizures tend to occur not when the patient is intoxicated but in the "sobering-up" period.

Treatment of Alcohol Withdrawal Symptoms

Minor withdrawal symptoms   The main considerations are replacement of fluids and electrolytes and the judicious administration of sedative drugs. In nutritionally depleted alcoholics, *the use of parenteral glucose solutions carries a special danger, namely the precipitation of Wernicke disease*, and should always be supplemented by B vitamins. Disturbed patterns of electrolytes (hypokalemia, hypomagnesemia, hyponatremia) should be corrected, but the last of these cautiously (see pp. 375–376). A variety of sedative drugs are equally useful in allaying tremor, nervousness, and insomnia. In general, phenothiazine drugs should be avoided because they may reduce the threshold to seizures. Chlordiazepoxide (Librium), lorazepam (Ativan), and diazepam (Valium) are currently the most popular for this purpose. Paraldehyde, for many years a favored drug, is no longer available.

Delirium tremens Treatment of this condition is a more compelling matter than treatment of the minor withdrawal syndrome. It begins with a careful search for an associated injury or infection, particularly cerebral contusions, subdural hematoma, cervical spine injury, pneumonia, and meningitis. A chest film, computed tomography, or magnetic resonance imaging of the head and cervical spine if trauma may have occurred as well as liver function tests should be obtained routinely and a lumbar puncture performed if there is the slightest suspicion of meningitis.

The cornerstones of treatment are the administration of fluids and correction of electrolyte abnormalities. Severe diaphoresis requires the administration of as much as 10 L of fluid daily, of which about one-quarter should be normal saline. The importance of adding B vitamins has been mentioned above. The amounts of glucose and electrolyte to be added are governed by the laboratory findings. Low Na concentrations should be corrected with caution, as already mentioned.

In severe forms of DTs, vital signs need to be recorded frequently, in anticipation of shock and hyperthermia. Shock requires the urgent use of fluids and vasopressor drugs, and hyperthermia requires the use of a cooling mattress in addition to the specific treatment of any infection that may be present.

Drugs must be used circumspectly. The objective is not the absolute suppression of agitation and tremor, which could seriously depress respiration, but simply the blunting of symptoms to the point of facilitating nursing care. Medication usually needs to be given parenterally—diazepam, 10 mg IV and repeated once or twice at 20- to 30-min intervals until the patient is calm but awake; or phenobarbital (120 mg) or haloperidol (1 to 2 mg) may be given at 3- to 4-h intervals. Propranolol and other beta-blocking agents may be useful, but corticosteroids have no place in the treatment of withdrawal symptoms.

Withdrawal seizures In most cases, anticonvulsant drugs are not required, since the seizures occupy only a brief, circumscribed period in the early stages of withdrawal and often have ceased by the time the patient is seen by the physician. The parenteral administration of phenobarbital or chlordiazepoxide early in the withdrawal period may prevent seizures. Phenytoin is generally ineffective in this setting. However, intravenous lorazepam in small doses has been shown to prevent recurrent seizures.

Also, the long-term administration of anticonvulsants is impractical. If the patient remains abstinent, he will suffer no further seizures; if he resumes drinking, he usually abandons his medications.

Status epilepticus due to alcohol withdrawal should be managed like status of any other cause. Focal seizures need to be investigated and managed along the lines indicated in Chap. 16. In patients with idiopathic or post-traumatic epilepsy, drinking is interdicted, and such patients need to be maintained on their anticonvulsant regimen.

Nutritional Diseases of the Nervous System Secondary to Alcoholism

These do not differ in any particular from nutritional diseases in which alcohol plays no part. They have been described in Chap. 41.

Alcoholic Dementia ("Alcoholic Deteriorated State")

These terms are used to designate a supposedly distinctive form of dementia that is attributable to the long-standing toxic effects of alcohol on the brain. However, the clinical picture has been anything but clear, and the descriptions in current textbooks of psychiatry lack consistency. More important, no distinctive neuropathologic changes have ever been described. Such clinical changes as have been attributed to the toxic effects of alcohol are completely reversible.

In our experience and that of others, most of the cases that come to autopsy with the label of "alcoholic dementia" or "deteriorated state" prove to have the lesions of the Wernicke-Korsakoff syndrome. Traumatic lesions are commonly added, as are the lesions of hepatic or anoxic encephalopathy, normal-pressure hydrocephalus, or a variety of diseases unrelated to alcoholism. Practically always, the clinical state can be accounted for by one or a combination of these diseases, and there has been no need to invoke a hypothetical toxic effect of alcohol on the brain.

"Alcoholic Cerebral Atrophy"

This disorder also does not constitute a clinicopathologic entity. The diagnosis is essentially a radiologic one: the lateral ventricles are enlarged and the sulci are widened. The clinical correlates of these findings are quite unpredictable. About 25 percent of patients with the Wernicke-Korsakoff syndrome show dilated lateral and third ventricles and widened sulci, but we have not been able to find a histopathologic basis for these abnormalities. In other alcoholics, the radiologic findings are not associated with any signs of neuropsychiatric disease. Moreover, in alcoholics who remain sober for a protracted period, the radiologic abnormalities are to a large extent reversible, suggesting that a shift of fluids occurred in the brain rather than a true loss of tissue (atrophy). Thus it would be more appropriate to refer to the asymptomatic ventricular enlargement and sulcal widening as such rather than as cerebral atrophy, at least until a consistent pathologic basis for this condition has been established. The attribution of cerebral cortical atrophy and neuronal loss to the toxic effects of alcohol remains to be demonstrated by reproducible and acceptable morphometric techniques.

Nerve and Muscle Disorders

Most of these are focal compression mononeuropathies that arise during an alcoholic stupor. A unique form of alcohol polymyopathy is described in Chap. 51.

Fetal Alcohol Syndrome

Infants born of severely alcoholic mothers who drink throughout pregnancy are often smaller than expected for the duration of pregnancy, are slightly microcephalic, and have short palpebral fissures, epicanthal folds, minor heart abnormalities, micrognathia, and at times cleft palate. At birth, such infants suck and sleep poorly and are irritable and hyperactive. Later in life, at school age, there are signs of psychomotor backwardness and learning difficulty. Developmental anomalies of diverse type have been found in the brain.

Since alcohol readily crosses the placental barrier, it is generally assumed to be the factor that damages the brain. However, the possible toxic effects of acetaldehyde (a breakdown product in the metabolism of alcohol), opiates, smoking, or the contributory role of nutritional deficiency have not been totally excluded. The condition is several times more frequent in African and Native Americans than in whites. It is doubtful that alcoholic fathers produce infants with this syndrome. A genetic predisposition has been suspected, but no clear hereditary pattern or offending gene has been identified.

Treatment of Alcohol Addiction

Following recovery from the acute medical and neurologic complications of alcoholism, the underlying problem of alcohol dependency remains. To discharge the patient at this point and to leave him to his own devices practically assures that he will resume drinking, with a predictable recurrence of medical illness. At a minimum, the physician must inform the patient and his family of the medical and social consequences of continued drinking and of the fact that total abstinence represents the only permanent solution to the problem. To achieve these ends the patient must assume responsibility for his actions. The patient and family must be made aware of the many community resources that are available, including special clinics, "detoxification" centers, hospital units, mental health clinics, and particularly Alcoholics Anonymous—the informal fellowship of recovering alcoholics that has proved to be the single most effective force in the rehabilitation of alcoholic patients.

For a more detailed discussion of this topic, see Victor and Ropper: *Adams and Victor's Principles of Neurology*, 7th ed, pp 1233–1251.

ADDITIONAL READING

D'Onofrio G, Rathlev NK, Ulrich AS, et al: Lorazepam for the prevention of recurrent seizures related to alcohol. *N Engl J Med* 340:915, 1999.

Ferguson JA, Suelzer CJ, Ecjert GJ, et al: Risk factors for delirium tremens development. *J Gen Intern Med* 11:410, 1996.

Goldstein DB: *Pharmacology of Alcohol.* New York, Oxford University Press, 1983.

O'Connor PG, Schottenfeld RS: Patients with alcohol problems. *N Engl J Med* 338:592, 1998.

Schenker S, Becker HC, Randall CL, et al: Fetal alcohol syndrome: Current status of pathogenesis. *Alcohol Clin Exp Res* 14:635, 1990.

Victor M: Neurologic disorders due to alcoholism and malnutrition, in Joynt RJ, Griggs RC (eds): *Clinical Neurology.* Philadelphia, Lippincott, 1986, chap 61.

Victor M: Alcoholic dementia. *Can J Neurol Sci* 21:88, 1994.

Victor M, Adams RD: The effect of alcohol on the nervous system. *Res Publ Assoc Res Nerv Ment Dis* 32:526, 1953.

Victor M, Adams RD, Collins GH: *The Wernicke-Korsakoff Syndrome and Other Disorders due to Alcoholism and Malnutrition.* Philadelphia, Davis, 1989.

43 | Disorders of the Nervous System due to Drugs and Other Chemical Agents

Drugs and other injurious or poisonous substances, customarily designated as toxins, exist in great number. Many of them affect the nervous system directly; some produce their effects secondarily through damage to other organs. The scope of neurotoxicology is vast, and obviously one cannot do justice to it in a few pages. The most that can be done here is to draw attention to the major categories of neurotoxic agents and the manner in which they affect the nervous system.

OPIATES AND RELATED SYNTHETIC ANALGESICS

The term *opiates* refers to the naturally occurring alkaloids of opium; morphine and codeine are the ones used most often. *Opioids* designate all drugs with actions similar to those of opium: (1) chemical modifications of morphine or (2) purely synthetic analgesics. Compounds of the first group include diacetylmorphine or heroin (the most regularly abused opioid), hydromorphone (Dilaudid), hydrocodone (Hycodan), and oxycodone (Percodan). The best-known synthetic analgesics are meperidine (Demerol), methadone (Dolophine or Amidone), and propoxyphene (Darvon). All these drugs have been assigned a "controlled" status because of their highly addictive properties.

Apart from analgesia, the opioids produce a sense of well-being, a state conventionally referred to as *morphine euphoria* or a "high." For this reason, they are sought to allay boredom and misery. Once introduced to the drug, the victim discovers that euphoria is soon followed by dysphoric symptoms—faintness, nausea, and vomiting—which can be alleviated only by repeated self-administration of the drug. This is the genesis of addiction, and the need becomes so compelling that crimes will be committed to relieve it.

Opioid poisoning, the result of a miscalculation of dosage or a suicide attempt, results in varying degrees of unresponsiveness, slow and shallow or periodic breathing, pinpoint pupils, bradycardia, and hypothermia. In the most advanced stage of coma, the pupils are dilated, the skin and mucous membranes are cyanotic, and the circulation fails. Death results from respiratory depression and asphyxia. Survivors may show the effects of hypoxic encephalopathy.

Treatment of opioid poisoning consists of gastric lavage if the intake was oral, maintenance of an adequate airway with a cuffed endotracheal tube, oxygenation, and the administration of naloxone (Narcan), a specific antidote to both opiates and synthetic analgesics. *Naloxone* is given IV in a dose of 0.01 mg/kg, repeated once or twice at 5-min intervals if necessary. If an adequate respiratory response is obtained, 1.0 mg of naloxone IM may then be given and repeated as needed. In cases of minor overdose, however, respiratory support is all that is necessary, thus avoiding the withdrawal reaction that may be precipitated by naloxone (see below).

Addiction to opiates or opioids afflicts more than 600,000 people in the United States, half of them adolescents and young adults in New York City alone. It is characterized by a striking degree of tolerance to increasing doses and the development of typical symptoms and signs when the drug is withdrawn (abstinence syndrome). The latter appear within 8 to 16 h after the last dose of morphine (later with other opioids) and consist of yawning, rhinorrhea, sweating, lacrimation, diffuse pain, dilatation of pupils, waves of gooseflesh, muscle twitching, nausea and vomiting, diarrhea, insomnia, and an increase in temperature, respiratory rate, and blood pressure. These physical changes subside gradually over a period of 7 to 10 days but persist in mild form for several more weeks.

The *diagnosis* of opiate addiction, if history is not available, should be suspected from needle marks on the skin and the finding of opiate derivatives in the urine; it can be confirmed by the administration of naloxone (0.4 mg IV, repeated once if necessary), which induces some of the abstinence symptoms. Clonidine (5 mg/kg bid for a week) counteracts most of the noradrenergic withdrawal symptoms. An alternative method is to stabilize the patient on methadone for 3 to 5 days (10 to 20 mg bid orally) and then to withdraw the latter drug over a similar period.

SEDATIVE-HYPNOTIC DRUGS

There are three main groups: (1) barbiturates, bromides, and chloral hydrate; (2) carbonic acid derivatives (meprobamate is the best known); and (3) the benzodiazepines, the most important of which are chlordiazepoxide (Librium), lorazepam (Ativan), and diazepam (Valium).

Barbiturates

Clinically, these drugs are now used very little. However, their nonmedical and illicit uses are still important causes of suicide, accidental death, and addiction. Pentobarbital (Nembutal), secobarbital (Seconal), amobarbital (Amytal), thiopental (Pentothal), and phenobarbital (Luminal) are the only barbiturates encountered with any regularity, and the first three are the ones most commonly abused.

Acute barbiturate coma Ingestion of 15 to 20 times the oral hypnotic dose of barbiturate induces coma, slow and shallow respiration, and flaccidity of the limbs with diminished or absent tendon reflexes; oculocephalic and oculovestibular reflexes are also muted; however, pupillary light and corneal reflexes are retained (unless asphyxia has occurred). In the early hours of coma, a phase of decerebrate rigidity with hyperactive tendon reflexes and Babinski signs may be present. The pupils become small in extreme overdoses. The *diagnosis*, if history is not available, is established by measurement of barbiturate levels in the blood or by urine toxicology. *Treatment* is directed along the lines indicated in Chap. 17—maintenance of respiration, prevention of atelectasis and infection, and, if coma is profound, hemodialysis.

Chronic barbiturate intoxication   This resembles alcohol intoxication, and the symptoms fluctuate with the time of self-administration of the drug. *Withdrawal* from the barbiturate is followed by insomnia, generalized convulsions, and a confusional state—symptoms similar to those of the alcohol withdrawal syndrome, including seizures. Anxiety states and depression, for which patients may have taken barbiturates, may be uncovered and require psychiatric treatment. Sometimes patients will have abused both alcohol and barbiturates or opioids and barbiturates.

Benzodiazepines

These are among the most commonly prescribed drugs in the world. Chlordiazepoxide, lorazepam, alprazolam, diazepam, and related members of this group are particularly effective in the treatment of anxiety, of insomnia, and (if given parenterally) of delirium, status epilepticus, and the muscle spasms of tetanus and the "stiff-man" syndrome. Flurazepam and triazolam are widely used in the management of insomnia, and clonazepam, in the treatment of tremor and certain types of seizures. Midazolam (Versed) is used for conscious sedation before surgical and other procedures and for treatment of status epilepticus (Chap. 16).

The advantages of the benzodiazepines are their *relatively* low hypnotic effects and low addictive potential and their minimal interactions with other drugs. Despite these attributes, the benzodiazepines are far from ideal. In large doses, they cause drowsiness, unsteadiness of gait, and at times hypotension and syncope, confusion, and impairment of memory, especially in the elderly. Flumazenil partially reverses the effects of diazepines. Also, these drugs can be addictive, and when discontinued, they sometimes give rise to a withdrawal syndrome and seizures much like those due to barbiturates.

ANTIPSYCHOSIS DRUGS (See Also Chap. 58)

This heterogeneous group of drugs, called neuroleptics, includes the phenothiazines, thioxanthines, butyrophenones, rauwolfia alkaloids, molindine, a dibenzoxazepine (loxapine), and newer agents, represented by clozapine, olanzepine, risperidone, and others. The phenothiazines are recognized by their trade names—Thorazine, Sparine, Compazine, Trilafon, Mellaril, Stelazine, and Prolixin. The most familiar of the butyrophenones is haloperidol (Haldol). All these drugs are in common use for the control of psychotic behavior in schizophrenia, manic-depressive disease, and confusional-agitated states that complicate other diseases of the brain (see Chap. 20).

The *side effects* of the phenothiazines and butyrophenones are common and can be serious: parkinsonian syndrome, buccolingual and oromasticatory dystonia and dyskinesia, akathisia, choreoathetosis, the so-called rabbit syndrome (repetitive pouting movements), and other dyskinesias. Some of the movement disorders begin after the drug is discontinued (*tardive dyskinesia*). A severe and often fatal *neuroleptic malignant syndrome* (catatonic rigidity, stupor, unstable blood pressure, high fever, diaphoresis and other signs of autonomic dysfunction, and high creatine kinase levels) may also occur. Dantrolene and the dopamine agonist bromocriptine have been used with some success to treat this syndrome, which otherwise may be fatal (see Chap. 58).

The antipsychosis drugs must be given with great caution, because some of the side effects are worse than the disease for which they are given. One uses the lowest possible dose for the shortest time, interspersing chronic administration with vacation periods. Neuroleptic drugs must be discontinued as soon as the adverse effects are recognized. The parkinsonian syndrome usually resolves under the influence of anticholinergic drugs, but tardive dyskinesia may persist for months or years. The latter is unresponsive to most drug therapy but tends to wane in time. Reintroduction and gradual withdrawal of the medication may be successful; tetrabenazine has also been used with benefit in intractable cases. The newer drugs such as olanzapine, quietapine, and risperidone have found special use because of their minimal extrapyramidal side effects (see p. 511).

ANTIDEPRESSION DRUGS

These are monoamine oxidase (MAO) inhibitors such as isocarboxizide (Marplan), tranylcypromine (Parnate), and phenelzine (Nardil); tricyclic dibenzazepine derivatives such as imipramine (Tofranil), desipramine (Norpramin), and amitriptyline (Elavil); the newer serotonin reuptake inhibitors such as fluoxetine (Prozac), sertraline (Zoloft), paroxetine (Paxil), and numerous others; and lithium. The MAO inhibitors need to be dispensed cautiously and with constant awareness of their potentially serious side effects—restlessness and agitation, insomnia, anxiety, and occasionally muscle twitching, mania, and convulsions. Also, sympathomimetic amines and tyramine (in over-the-counter cold medicines, cheeses, beer, and wine) may induce hypertension, cardiac arrhythmias, pulmonary edema, and even death. The main risks of the tricyclic agents are orthostatic hypotension, especially in the elderly, as well as heart block and atropinic effects such as urinary retention, blurring of vision, and confusion. Either the serotoninergic or the tricyclic antidepressants are preferable for endogenous depression, since they have considerably fewer side effects than the MAO inhibitors. The serotoninergic antidepressants are contraindicated if MAO inhibitors have been used in the prior few weeks.

Lithium is of proven value in controlling and preventing mania. Less certain is its value in treating depression. Diabetes insipidus on a renal tubular basis is a common side effect. Overdosage may result in delirious or confusional states with tremor, myoclonic twitching, dizziness, nystagmus, ataxia, and stuttering speech—symptoms that may persist for a week or two or even longer after cessation of lithium intake. (See Chap. 57 for therapeutic guidelines.)

STIMULANTS

Drugs of this category have relatively limited medical utility. The most important ones are caffeine, amphetamine (Benzedrine), methylphenidate (Ritalin), modafinil (Provigil), and cocaine. Modafinil, methylphenidate, and amphetamine are useful in the treatment of narcolepsy and cataplexy, and methylphenidate, for unexplained reasons, is helpful in controlling the hyperactivity–attention deficit syndrome. The amphetamines also have an appetite-suppressant effect and have been widely and indiscriminately used for the control of obesity as well as for the abolition of fatigue. Cocaine, originally utilized as a topical anesthetic, is now the most common illicitly used stimulant drug in the western world.

Amphetamine and dextroamphetamine The toxic signs consist of restlessness, excessive speech and motor activity, tremor, hallucinations, paranoia, and alterations of thought and affect—a state that at times may resemble paranoid schizophrenia. Chronic usage can lead to a high degree of tolerance and dependence. Withdrawal, after a period of sustained excessive use, is followed by prolonged, predominantly rapid-eye-movement (REM) sleep, from which the patient awakens with a ravenous appetite, muscle pains, and profound fatigue and depression.

Cocaine In chemical structure, cocaine resembles the amphetamines, and its toxic manifestations are also much the same. Typically, cocaine has been taken nasally ("snorting"), but in 1985 a relatively pure and heat-stable form of the drug ("free-base" or "crack"), suitable for smoking, became available. The relative cheapness and ready availability of crack have led to a veritable epidemic of cocaine use; in the United States, an estimated 7 to 8 million people use the drug regularly.

Cocaine induces a state of well-being, euphoria, restlessness, and loquacity. Psychologic dependence or habituation—i.e., an inability to abstain from frequent compulsive use ("craving")—develops readily. Withdrawal, after a period of chronic abuse, is followed by restlessness, anorexia, depression, and signs of dopaminergic hypersensitivity. Severe intoxication causes seizures, coma, and death. Seizures in this setting are best treated with benzodiazepines. Coma requires emergency treatment in an intensive care unit (ICU), along the lines indicated for coma in general (Chap. 17).

With the widespread use of cocaine, serious new medical complications continue to appear—subarachnoid and cerebral hemorrhage, myocardial infarction, cerebral and spinal cord infarction, acute rhabdomyolysis, acute renal failure, and disseminated intravascular coagulation. A diffuse cerebral vasculopathy is another known complication.

The mild adrenergic stimulant phenylpropanolamine (PPA) has been linked to spontaneous cerebral hemorrhages, for which reason it has been removed from over-the-counter cold remedies.

PSYCHOACTIVE DRUGS

This group includes lysergic acid diethylamide (LSD), phenylethylamine derivatives (mescaline and peyote), psilocybin, certain indolic derivatives, cannabis (marijuana), phencyclidine (PCP), ecstasy (MDMA), and others. All are loosely referred to as psychomimetic or psychotogenic drugs, insofar as they can induce a psychosis that in some ways resembles schizophrenia. The psychosis of PCP may last several days or weeks. Widespread use of the monoamine protagonist ecstasy has become a problem among teenagers by producing seizures, cerebral hemorrhages, and psychosis.

Marijuana This is taken by inhaling the smoke from cigarettes. In low doses, its effects are like those of alcohol. With increasing amounts, the effects resemble those of LSD, mescaline, and psilocybin—visual hallucinations, perceptual distortions, feelings of depersonalization, inattentiveness, paresthesias—an experience that some people find pleasing. No definite withdrawal effects and no permanent abnormalities of the brain from excessive or prolonged usage have been documented. The smoking of marijuana has led in some instances to the abuse of other habit-forming drugs in susceptible individuals.

DISORDERS DUE TO BACTERIAL TOXINS

Diphtheria, botulism, and tetanus are the important diseases in this category. They are considered in Chaps. 46, 53, and 55, respectively.

POISONING DUE TO PLANTS, VENOMS, BITES, AND STINGS

Ergotism, which may cause fasciculations, myoclonus, muscle spasms, and seizures, may be a problem in migraine patients who overuse ergotamine compounds. *Mushroom poisoning*, the other important member of this category, is described in *Adams and Victor's Principles of Neurology*, 7th ed.

Neurologically, the most notable disorder resulting from insect bites is *Lyme disease*, which is considered in Chap. 32, with the infectious diseases. The neurotoxic effects of other bites, stings, and venoms are described fully in *Harrison's Principles of Internal Medicine*.

HEAVY METALS

Lead, arsenic, mercury, manganese, bismuth, and thallium each affect the nervous system in special ways. Only plumbism (lead intoxication), the most important of the heavy-metal poisonings, will be described here; the pathogenic properties of the others are summarized in Table 43-1. Restrictions of space preclude consideration of the toxic effects of other heavy metals (iron, antimony, zinc, silver, gold, platinum, etc.), certain nonmetallic elements (phosphorus), and industrial toxins (see suggested reading at the end of this chapter).

Lead poisoning In *young children*, lead poisoning continues to be observed in the slums of large urban centers. The indoor paint in many old houses contains lead, and its sweetish taste appeals to young children, who nibble on it. The ingested lead induces anemia, with stippling of red blood cells, abdominal pain (colic), and, less reliably, deposits in the ends of the metaphyses of long bones, visible in radiographs. Headache, apathy, psychomotor regression, seizures, stupor, and coma are the main central nervous system (CNS) effects. The cerebrospinal fluid (CSF) is under increased pressure as a result of brain swelling, with an elevated protein content and often a low-grade pleocytosis. Lead levels are greatly increased in the blood, usually to 80 μg/dL or more, although acute encephalopathy may occur abruptly and unpredictably at considerably lower levels, and there is increased excretion of coproporphyrin and δ-aminolevulinic acid in the urine.

Once the stage of coma is reached, the child may either die or survive blind and comatose. At autopsy, the brain is swollen and edematous. Deposits of lead salt are seen in the walls of arterioles in association with lymphocytes and perivascular ischemic lesions.

The main elements of *therapy* are (1) establishment of urinary flow, then maintenance of IV fluids at basal water and electrolyte requirements; (2) chelation therapy with BAL and CaNa$_2$-EDTA for 5 to 7 days, followed by a course of oral penicillamine; (3) repeated administration of mannitol for relief of cerebral edema; and (4) use of IV diazepam to suppress seizures.

Lead poisoning is less common *in adults* than in children. Colic and anemia are the common manifestations. Neuropathic syndromes, presenting as bilateral or unilateral radial palsy (wrist drop) or as a polyneuropathy, are now quite rare. Ingestion of water or home-brewed alcoholic concoctions

TABLE 43-1 Heavy-Metal Poisoning

Metal	Source	Clinical effects	Diagnostic tests	Treatment
Lead Children	Lead paint	Anorexia, apathy, vomiting, drowsiness, seizures, stupor, coma	↑ CSF pressure, protein, and cells; basophilic stippling of marrow normoblasts; ↑ blood Pb and urinary coproporphyrin	Chelation with BAL and EDTA; mannitol; IV diazepam for seizures
Adults	H₂O from lead pipes; burning or melting lead; storage batteries	Colic, anemia, wrist drop, polyneuropathy, often asymmetric; delirium from organic lead	As above	As above
Arsenic (inorganic)	Ingestion of herbicides, insecticides, rodenticides, psoriasis skin creams	Encephalopathy, dermatitis, jaundice, Mees lines, sensorimotor polyneuropathy	↑ As levels in blood, urine, hair, nails	Vasopressor agents; BAL
Mercury	Exposure in manufacture of thermometers, mirrors, incandescent lights, x-ray machines, indoor (latex) paints	Tremor, ataxia of gait, confusion, blindness, sensory neuropathy	↑ Hg in blood and urine	N-acetyl-dl-Penicillamine
Manganese	Mining Mn ore	Fatigue, drowsiness, progressive weakness, parkinsonism	Mn in blood and urine	L-Dopa for parkinsonism
Thallium	Rodenticides, insecticides, depilatory agents	Acute polyneuropathy, mainly sensory and may be painful; alopecia	Thallium in urine	KCl orally
Bismuth	Bi subgallate for intestinal disorders	Subacute drowsiness, confusion, tremulousness, myoclonus, twitching, seizures, ataxia	Bi in urine; hyperdense concentration of Bi in cerebral and cerebellar cortices in CT scans	Nonspecific

TABLE 43-2 Neurotoxic Effects of Antineoplastic Agents

Drug	Clinical use	Adverse neurologic effects	Management
Vincristine	Lymphoblastic leukemia, lymphomas, gliomas, some solid tumors	Paresthesias and sensory loss in feet, legs, and hands; slight weakness, loss of tendon reflexes, autonomic effects, and cranial neuropathy may be added	Reduce dose to minimum effective levels or change to another drug
Procarbazine	Hodgkin disease, other lymphomas, bronchogenic cancer, gliomas	Somnolence, confusion, agitation, mild polyneuropathy, orthostatic hypotension	Reduce dosage; avoid alcohol, barbiturates, and narcotics
L-Asparaginase	Lymphoblastic leukemia, multiple myeloma	Drowsiness, confusion, delirium, stupor, coma; cerebral venous thrombosis; other cerebrovascular complications	Discontinue drug
5-Fluorouracil	Ca of breast, ovary, gastrointestinal tract	Dizziness, nystagmus, dysarthria, cerebellar ataxia	Discontinue drug
Methotrexate	Meningeal leukemia or carcinomatosis; chorioepithelioma	Intrathecal use with irradiation may cause focal necrotic lesions of brain or cord; ataxia, dementia, pseudobulbar palsy	Discontinue drug
Cisplatin	Ca ovary, breast; head and neck tumors	Peripheral reuropathy, tinnitus, high-frequency hearing loss, retrobulbar neuritis, seizures	Discontinue drug
Carmustine (BCNU)	Malignant gliomas	Intracarotid injection: orbital and neck pain, focal seizures, transient confusion	Discontinue drug
Cytosine arabinoside (ARA-C)	Acute nonlymphocytic leukemia	Ataxia, dysarthria, nystagmus (usually transient)	Discontinue drug
Paclitaxel (Taxol) and docetaxel	Ovarian and breast Ca	Polyneuropathy (sensory), autonomic neuropathy	Discontinue drug
Thalidomide	AIDS-related aphthous ulcers, vascular tumors, leprosy, erythema nodosum	Sensory neuropathy	Discontinue drug

397

TABLE 43-3 Neurotoxic Effects of Antibiotics and Immunosuppressants

Drug	Clinical use	Adverse effects	Management
Nitrofurantoin	Urinary infections	Polyneuropathy, especially with renal failure	Discontinue drug
Metronidazole	Anaerobic infections, amebiasis, inflammatory bowel disease	Optic neuropathy	Discontinue drug
Imipenem	Mixed bacterial infections	Seizures	Discontinue drug
INH	Tuberculosis	Polyneuropathy	Reduce drug dosage
Ethambutol	Tuberculosis	Optic neuropathy	Discontinue drug
Acyclovir	Herpes encephalitis	Nausea, vomiting, tremor, encephalopathy	Reduce drug dosage
Dapsone	Leprosy	Motor neuropathy	Discontinue drug
Cyclosporin	Transplant rejection, aplastic anemia, immune diseases	Headache, vomiting, confusion, seizures, visual loss, widespread white matter changes on MRI	Discontinue drug
Aminoglycosides	Gram negative infection	Vestibulopathy, cochlear damage, myasthenic syndrome	Discontinue drug

that are conveyed or stored in lead pipes or vessels and inhalation of fumes from the burning or melting of lead are the usual causes of intoxication. In adults, the treatment of inorganic lead poisoning with chelating agents follows along the same lines as in children.

Several studies have shown that long-term exposure of children to lead (with persistent blood levels above 40 µg/dL) may be accompanied by reduced intellectual function and behavioral disorders. Other causative factors have usually not been excluded, however.

ANTINEOPLASTIC AND ANTIBIOTIC AGENTS

Several antineoplastic drugs affect the nervous system adversely, often requiring discontinuation of the drug or modification in its usage. This is also true for several antibiotic and immunosuppressant drugs. Tables 43-2 and 43-3 summarize the most predictable of these complications. A predominantly sensory polyneuropathy has become a common clinical problem after the use of cisplatin, paclitaxel (Taxol), vincristine, and their derivatives, and thalidomide.

For a more detailed discussion of this topic, see Victor and Ropper: *Adams and Victor's Principles of Neurology*, 7th ed, pp 1252–1290.

ADDITIONAL READING

Brust JCM: Drug dependence, in Joynt RJ (ed): *Clinical Neurology*, vol 2. Hagerstown, MD, Harper & Row, 1992, chap. 21.

Goldfrank LR, Flomenbaum NE, Lewin NA, et al (eds): *Goldfrank's Toxicologic Emergencies*, 5th ed. Norwalk, CT, Appleton & Lange, 1994.

Hardman JG, Limbrin LE, Molinoff PB, et al (eds): *Goodman and Gilman's The Pharmacological Basis of Therapeutics*, 9th ed. New York, McGraw-Hill, 1996.

Hollister LE: *Clinical Pharmacology of Psychotherapeutic Drugs*, 3rd ed. New York, Churchill Livingstone, 1990.

Klaassen CD (ed): *Casarett and Doull's Toxicology: The Basic Science of Poisons*, 5th ed. New York, McGraw-Hill, 1995.

LeQuesne PM: Metal neurotoxicity, in Asbury AK, McKhann GM, McDonald WI (eds): *Diseases of the Nervous System*, 2nd ed. Philadelphia, Saunders, 1992, pp 1250–1258.

Mahaffey KR: Exposure to lead in childhood. *N Engl J Med* 327:1308, 1992.

Rosenberg NL: *Occupational and Environmental Neurology*. Boston, Butterworth-Heinemann, 1995.

Rottenberg DA (ed): *Neurological Complications of Cancer Therapy*. Stoneham, MA, Butterworth-Heinemann, 1991.

Spencer PS, Schaumburg HH (eds): *Experimental and Clinical Neurotoxicology*, 2nd ed. New York, Oxford University Press, 2000.

Many disease processes (more than 30 in all) affect the spinal cord predominantly or exclusively and produce a number of distinctive syndromes that relate to the special anatomic features of the cord: its great length compared to width; a predominance of rostrally and caudally directed conductive tracts that course external to the central segmental gray matter; tight enclosure by pia-arachnoid, which renders the cord intolerant to intrinsic edematous lesions; apposition and restriction by the spinal column, allowing compression from adjacent bony and soft tissue masses and making the cord vulnerable to spinal trauma and to diseases of the spine; and a precarious vascular arrangement.

The most commonly observed and important disorders of the spinal cord can be grouped into the following clinical syndromes:

1. Paraplegia or quadriplegia, with sensory loss below a circumferential segmental level, due to complete transverse lesions of the spinal cord
2. Subacute or chronic spinal paraparesis, with or without sensory changes and ataxia
3. Segmental sensory dissociation with brachial amyotrophy (syringomyelic syndrome)
4. Ventral cord syndrome
5. Central cord syndrome
6. Hemicord (Brown-Séquard) syndrome
7. Syndromes of conus medullaris and cauda equina
8. Syndrome of the foramen magnum

PARAPLEGIA OR QUADRIPLEGIA DUE TO COMPLETE TRANSVERSE LESIONS

Spinal Cord Trauma

This is the most widely studied example of complete spinal cord transection and the prototype of several other acute transverse lesions (vascular, demyelinative, compressive) giving rise to paraplegia or quadriplegia with sphincteric paralysis and sensory loss below the level of the lesion. Penetration of the spinal canal by a missile is the common cause in wartime. In civilian life, the usual mechanism is a vertical compression of the spinal column, to which is added the immediate effect of antero- or retrohyperflexion. The resultant tearing of spinal ligaments permits the dislocation of an upper vertebra anteriorly on the one below, often with fracture of the vertebral body or pedicles. The spinal cord is literally crushed. In cases of cervical spondylosis and/or a congenitally narrow canal, an abrupt, forceful extension of the neck can also severely damage the cervical cord.

Clinical effects The immediate effect of an acute transverse lesion is dependent on its level. If at C1–C3, death is immediate unless respiration is supported artificially. If it is lower, there is loss of all motor, sensory, autonomic, and sphincteric functions below the level of the lesion. Or if at first the loss of function is not complete, edema and other secondary changes make it so in a few hours.

The subsequent effects are divided into two stages: the stage of *spinal shock* and the stage of *heightened reflex activity*. Spinal shock is expressed by a loss of all reflex activity below the level of the lesion, an atonic bladder with overflow incontinence, atonic bowel (paralytic ileus), gastric dilatation, and loss of genital reflexes and of vasomotor control. After 1 to 2 weeks, sometimes longer, spinal flexor reflexes (Babinski signs, flexor spasms of the legs) and then tendon reflexes begin to appear in parts of the body supplied by the intact but disconnected lower spinal cord segments. Simultaneously, bladder tone and gastric and bowel function begin to recover. Gradually the tendon reflexes become hyperactive, and the bladder becomes spastic (manifest as frequency and urgency of urination and small capacity of bladder, with automatic emptying). Also, autonomic functions (vasomotor and sweating reactions) become hyperactive. The paralyzed legs tend to remain in flexion or, if the cord lesion is not complete, in extension. In the latter case, there may be some return of motor and sensory function below the lesion. Because gray matter is usually destroyed over two or three spinal segments, the paralyzed arm or hand muscles become atrophic and areflexic (in the case of cervical cord injury); when this effect predominates over that of tract injury, it is referred to as a *central cord syndrome* (see further on).

Injuries of the lowermost thoracic and upper lumbar spine are in a position to damage the spinal cord, cauda equina, or both.

The *treatment* of spine fracture and dislocation is mainly orthopedic—to reduce subluxation and assure fixation of the spine. Whether or not laminectomy and cord decompression are helpful is still a matter of controversy. The value of immediate administration of high doses of corticosteroids is uncertain, but they should be given if the lesion is incomplete. In patients with *complete* spinal cord lesions, the prevailing opinion is against laminectomy.

Nontraumatic Transverse Myelopathies

An acute, complete, or nearly complete transverse cord lesion in the *absence of trauma* should lead to a consideration of the following:

1. Tumor with cord compression (see further on).
2. Hemorrhage into the spinal cord (hematomyelia) from an arteriovenous malformation (AVM) or epidural or subdural hemorrhage (e.g., from anticoagulant drugs), or venous compression of the lower cord by a dural fistula or AVM.
3. Acute postinfectious or infectious necrotizing or demyelinative myelopathy (transverse myelitis, Devic disease). These inflammatory lesions are more often subacute in evolution (see below), but they may strike with such suddenness as to suggest spinal cord infarction. Paraneoplastic necrotizing myclopathy is a rare cause.
4. Epidural abscess. Again, this lesion is more often subacute in evolution.

5. Ischemic infarction of the cord due to occlusion of a major segmental artery arising from a vertebral artery (supplying the cervical cord) or the aorta (supplying the thoracic and lumbar cord). Dissecting aortic aneurysm, arteritis, aortic surgery, and atherosclerosis of the collateral arterial vessels are the usual causes. Rarely, there is thrombosis of the anterior spinal artery itself. Infarction due to fibrocartilagenous embolism (nucleus pulposus material) is a frequently overlooked cause of cord infarction.

The most important of these processes are described below.

SYNDROME OF SUBACUTE OR CHRONIC SPINAL PARAPARESIS WITH OR WITHOUT ATAXIA

This is the mode of presentation of a number of important spinal cord diseases of diverse type. Slowly progressive paraplegia without sensory changes occurs in childhood and adult life as a heredodegenerative disease (familial spastic paraparesis). *Ataxic paraparesis* is a manifestation of the following conditions:

Cervical Spondylosis with Myelopathy

This is perhaps the most frequently observed myelopathy in general practice. It is essentially a degenerative disease of the middle and lower cervical vertebrae in which some combination of degenerating and bulging disc(s), vertebral and facet joint exostoses, and thickening of the posterior longitudinal and yellow ligaments compromise the cervical cord and roots by compression and possibly by reduction of the blood supply. These changes are often engrafted on a congenitally narrow spinal canal.

Clinically, the syndrome consists of a triad of (1) painful stiff neck with limitation of the range of movement; (2) radicular pain and numbness and reduced reflexes in an arm; and (3) symmetrical or asymmetrical spastic paraparesis and ataxia with signs of lateral and posterior column affection. Any one of these features may predominate.

The condition is chronic, and diagnosis is made by magnetic resonance imaging (MRI) or computed tomography (CT) myelography and by the exclusion of other spinal cord diseases (Fig. 44-1). The main differential diagnostic considerations are demyelinative disease and subacute combined degeneration, and there is a superficial resemblance to amyotrophic lateral sclerosis.

In the early stages of the disease, the use of a soft collar may be sufficient to relieve the stiffness and pain in the neck, shoulders, and arms. In cases of advancing myelopathy, a posterior decompressive laminectomy or an anterior approach (if the compression is mainly discogenic) halts progression of the disease and may lead to some improvement.

Lumbar Spondylosis

Lumbar spinal stenosis, due to a congenitally narrow spinal canal, usually combined with varying degrees of arthropathy, may compress the cauda equina. This occurs especially when the patient stands or walks because of the increased lordotic compression in these positions. Pain in the buttocks and legs and numbness and weakness of the legs under these conditions—

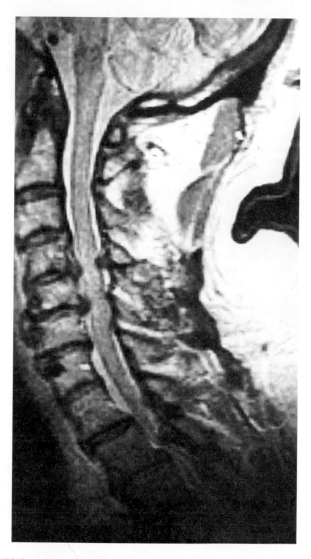

FIG. 44-1   MRI in a patient with symptomatic cervical spondylosis. The spinal cord at C4-5 and C5-6 is flattened on its ventral surface by spondylotic bars and on its posterior surface by ligamentous hypertrophy. Axial images are required to confirm that the cord is truly compressed and that the subarachnoid space (surrounding the cord) is nearly or completely obliterated.

and subsidence of these symptoms when the patient sits or lies with legs flexed—are sometimes referred to as *intermittent claudication of the cauda equina*. Treatment is by decompressive laminectomy over several lumbar segments, but the long-term results are inconsistent.

Transverse Myelitis

This term, introduced briefly in the section on multiple sclerosis (MS), refers to a focal inflammatory lesion of the spinal cord, involving all of its neural elements, more or less, over a short vertical extent. As such, the process is symptomatic of several spinal cord disorders, designated by a variety of names—*acute transverse myelitis, postinfectious myelitis, postvaccinal myelitis, acute multiple sclerosis,* and *necrotizing myelitis.* If the brain is involved simultaneously, it is called *acute disseminated encephalomyelitis* (ADEM).

Days or weeks following an infectious illness, even a mundane upper respiratory syndrome, weakness and numbness of the feet and legs (less often of the hands and arms) develop. The patient is afebrile when these symptoms begin. A sensory level on the trunk, Babinski signs, sphincteric disturbances, and backache mark the disease as a myelopathy. Although usually evolving over several days, in a few instances a complete "transverse" involvement of the cord develops within hours. The CSF typically contains 10 to 100 lymphocytes per cubic millimeter, with slightly raised levels of protein but normal glucose. In milder cases there may be only three or four cells per cubic millimeter, making the inflammatory aspect less clear. The MRI usually shows T2 signal abnormalities and slight gadolinium enhancement extending over two or three spinal segments (Fig. 44-2).

Practically all human viruses have at one time or another been reported to precede acute myelitis, but the large DNA viruses, such as Epstein-Barr and cytomegalovirus, have the greatest tendency to do so. *Mycoplasma* is almost unique as a bacterial trigger. In many instances the connection to a preceding infection is presumed but cannot be proved. In this latter group, fewer than half of patients have shown signs of MS (a lower incidence than following a bout of optic neuritis). A hyperacute form of the disease with petechial hemorrhage and subsequent necrosis occurs independently or as part of Devic's neuromyelitis optica (see Chap. 36).

Once symptoms begin, it is doubtful if any except supportive therapy is of value. High doses of corticosteroids are usually administered, but there is no evidence that they alter the natural course of the illness. Plasma exchange and intravenous immune globulin have been tried in several patients, with uncertain results.

A similar myelitis is known to occur in patients with lupus ("lupus myelitis"), usually in those with antiphospholipid antibodies. Its basis is a minimally inflammatory occlusion of small vessels.

Demyelinative Myelopathy

Among young adults in northern climates, multiple sclerosis is the most frequent cause of symmetrical or asymmetrical paraparesis with hyperreflexia and sensory ataxia. About one-third of patients with multiple sclerosis, including older adults, exhibit this essentially spinal form of the disease. A history of earlier attacks of neurologic disorder and the presence of nonspinal findings referable to white matter (optic atrophy, nystagmus, internuclear ophthalmoplegia, ataxia), oligoclonal bands in the cerebrospinal fluid (CSF), and cerebral white matter lesions on MRI are helpful in diagnosis. This and other forms of demyelinative disease—postinfectious and postvaccinal myelitis and acute necrotizing myelitis—are discussed in Chap. 36.

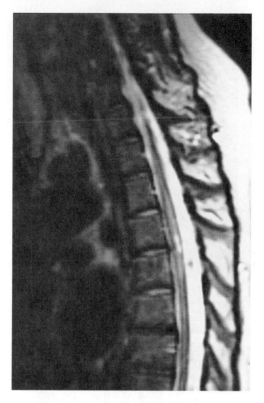

FIG. 44-2   MRI of acute postinfectious myelitis. There is T2 signal change, and other images showed mild enhancement after gadolinium infusion. The cord is slightly enlarged at the involved level.

Spinal Cord Tumors

Conventionally, these are divided into three groups: (1) tumors that lie within the spinal cord (*intramedullary*—e.g., astrocytoma, ependymoma, hemangioblastoma), (2) tumors lying on the surface of the cord and arising from the meninges or from a spinal root (*extramedullary-intradural*, mainly meningiomas and neurofibromas), and most commonly (3) tumors in the epidural space (*extradural*), but in a position to compress the spinal cord. Epidural tumors usually prove to be metastatic carcinomas, lymphomas, plasmacytomas, lipomas, or chordomas. They usually spread from adjacent bone or a paraspinal mass via intervertebral foramina. Nonneoplastic extramedullary tissue masses also occur—extramedullary hematopoiesis, epidural lipomatosis (complicating prolonged steroid therapy), and bacterial or tuberculous abscess (see below). All of these are now identified by MRI (Fig. 44-3) or by CT myelography.

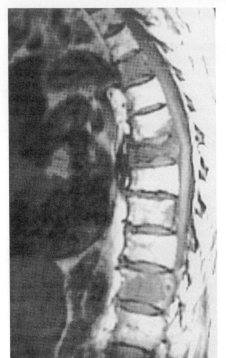

A

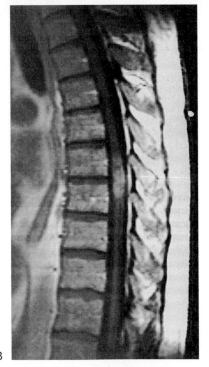

B

Radicular pain in combination with asymmetrical or symmetrical sensory and motor tract involvement and variable sphincteric dysfunction, evolving over weeks or months, constitutes the prototypical syndrome. The pace of the disease varies with the type of tumor. Some of the ependymomas progress slowly over months or years, whereas the time course of epidural lymphomas and metastatic carcinomas is measured in days or weeks. Back pain and percussion tenderness are characteristic of compression by metastatic tumor. Radicular symptoms are prominent with neurofibromas but may occur also with meningiomas and other tumors. Infrequently, an intramedullary tumor induces a frank central or syringomyelic syndrome (see below).

The treatment of most spinal tumors, even the intramedullary ones, is surgical excision and/or radiation therapy. Epidural carcinomas and lymphomas are exceptions; they respond to radiation and high-dose corticosteroids (4 to 10 mg dexamethasone every 4 to 6 h) as well as or better than to surgery. Some lymphomas are so sensitive to radiation that a few exposures, supplemented by steroid therapy, will adequately relieve the cord compression. Cord compression by Paget disease and extramedullary hematopoiesis requires specific therapy.

Spinal Arachnoiditis

This is a relatively rare disorder, characterized by thickening of the arachnoidal membranes and the formation of adhesions between arachnoid and dura, the result probably of a low-grade inflammatory reaction. Arachnoiditis of the thoracic cord presents clinically by a combination of root and spinal cord symptoms, mimicking spinal cord tumor. A few cases can be traced to syphilis or to some other therapeutically resistant chronic meningitis. Others follow the injection of certain chemical agents into the subarachnoid space. In some cases, no preceding event can be identified. Increasingly frequent is the occurrence of a circumscribed lumbar arachnoiditis complicating repeated surgery for lumbar discs. Radicular and low back pain arising weeks or more after the operation are characteristic.

Epidural Abscess

Skin infection, usually but not always in the region of the back, or a bacteremia may permit seeding of the epidural space or a vertebral body, which gives rise to an osteomyelitis with extension to the epidural space. Bacterial endocarditis and drug addictions, associated with injection of infected material, are other common sources of such infections. Rarely, infection is introduced by a lumbar puncture needle or laminectomy. Fever and local pain and tenderness in the back, not necessarily confined to the lumbar spine and

---

FIG. 44-3   *A.* MRI of multiple spinal metastases from carcinoma of the lung. The metastases exhibit low signal intensity on T1-weighted images. An epidural mass is present, compressing the cord. *B.* T1-weighted MRI of an intramedullary thoracic ependymoma, causing expansion of the cord and edema over several segments. There is faint enhancement of the tumor with gadolinium.

sometimes also radicular, are early signs. The pain is usually severe, persistent, and only partially responsive to analgesics and bed rest. Unless an abscess is suspected and surgically drained, sphincteric paralysis and a rapidly progressive paraparesis and sensory loss in the lower parts of the body ensue. Lumbar puncture, if performed, shows a modest pleocytosis and high protein content, with normal glucose. The sedimentation rate is elevated.

The aforementioned clinical findings call for immediate investigation with MRI or CT myelography, followed by laminectomy and drainage and the administration of appropriate antibiotics in high doses. Osteomyelitis, if present, can be dealt with subsequently. If permanent damage to the cord or cauda equina roots is to be avoided, laminectomy must be performed before paralysis becomes established.

Tuberculous spinal osteomyelitis (Pott disease) is a more chronic and bony destructive process that nonetheless often responds to multiple antituberculous antibiotics.

Rheumatoid Arthritis and Ankylosing Spondylitis with Compressive Myelopathy

Usually the spinal canal is wide enough to accommodate these conditions without injury to the spinal cord. The inflammatory process, however, may cause a marked weakness of ligaments that results in frank vertebral dislocation with spinal cord or radicular symptoms. The misalignment arises spontaneously or after even minor trauma. The most dangerous form is an odontoid dislocation, which demands surgical repair to prevent catastrophic cervical cord compression. Other levels of the spine may be similarly involved.

Vascular Malformations of the Spinal Cord and Overlying Dura

These malformations cause both ischemic and hemorrhagic lesions (*hematomyelia*). One of the most clearly delineated types is the *venous angioma* which is located on the dorsal surface of the lower cord and occurs most often in older men. The clinical picture includes acute pain (cramplike, lancinating), usually in a sciatic distribution, occurring in episodes over a period of several days or weeks and sometimes worse in recumbency. Almost always it is associated with weakness or paralysis of one or both legs and numbness and paresthesias in the same distribution. There may be a saltatory progression of symptoms, probably due to thrombotic occlusions of parts of the malformation.

Arteriovenous angiomas tend to involve the posterior parts of the lower thoracic and upper lumbar segments or the anterior parts of the cervical enlargement. The patients are often younger, and the sexes are equally affected. The clinical syndrome may take the form of a slow spinal cord compression, sometimes with a sudden exacerbation; or the initial symptoms may be apoplectic in nature, due either to thrombosis of a vessel or to a hemorrhage. Cavernous angiomas rarely arise in the cord, but they may produce hematomyelia.

Increasingly, it has been recognized that *fistulas* or *arteriovenous malformations of the dura* overlying the spinal cord can cause a myelopathy, sometimes several segments removed from the malformation. The majority are in the region of the low thoracic cord or conus. The clinical effects, presumably the result of ischemia from increased venous pressure, tend to be subacute in evolution, mostly painless, although some are associated with a vague spinal ache, and mimic an intramedullary tumor. Worsening characteristically occurs in progressive steps over a few weeks, quite unlike the case with neoplasm or myelitis.

The diagnosis in these cases is established by selective spinal arteriography that shows the malformation; the most conspicuous finding in true AVMs and fistulas is an enlarged and early draining vein that may, on occasion, be visible on an MRI or myelogram. Otherwise the diagnosis of vascular malformations can be difficult. Endovascular techniques to obliterate the feeding vessels have met with some success in preventing progression of the myelopathy.

Subacute Combined Degeneration (SCD; see also p. 380)

This is the name applied to the spinal cord disease resulting from a deficiency of cobalamin (vitamin B_{12}). It begins with symptoms and signs of posterior column disorder (paresthesias of hands and feet, instability of stance and gait, impaired vibratory and position senses), followed after some weeks by a symmetrical ataxic paraparesis with either increased or decreased tendon reflexes and Babinski signs. The spinal fluid is normal. As noted in Chap. 41, the spinal cord lesion may precede the macrocytic anemia by months or a year or more, particularly in patients taking folic acid or those with iron deficiency.

MS, cervical spondylosis, tropical spastic paraparesis, AIDS myelopathy, syphilitic meningomyelitis, cervical meningioma or AVM, and an unusual combined system disease of non–pernicious anemia type may also cause ataxic paraparesis and must be differentiated from SCD. The diagnosis and treatment of SCD are discussed further in Chap. 41. If the disorder is treated at its onset or soon thereafter, striking improvement may be obtained by cobalamin therapy—hence the overriding importance of early diagnosis.

Radiation Myelopathy

This iatrogenic disease appears many months or a year or more after radiation therapy to viscera in the region of the spine or after direct spinal radiation for an epidural tumor. It takes the form of a transverse myelopathy that develops insidiously and progresses irregularly for several weeks or months. Pathologically there is coagulation necrosis of both gray and white matter extending over several segments of the cord and corresponding with the level of the irradiated zone. An early reversible posterior column injury has also been described. In most cases, these complications can be avoided if the total dose of a given course of radiation is kept below 6000 cGy and is given over a period of 30 to 70 days and if each daily fraction does not exceed 200 cGy.

Myelopathies due to Viral Diseases

A vacuolar myelopathy, clinically and pathologically similar to that of vitamin B_{12} deficiency, may complicate AIDS. Another retrovirus (HTLV-1) has been implicated in the etiology of an endemic spastic paraparesis

observed in tropical and subtropical climates. These and other viral myeli-
tides (poliomyelitis, herpes zoster, etc.) are discussed in Chap. 33.

Friedreich Ataxia and Familial Spastic Paraparesis

These hereditary forms of myelopathy are described with the cerebellar
ataxias in Chap. 39.

SYNDROME OF SEGMENTAL DISSOCIATED SENSORY LOSS WITH BRACHIAL AMYOTROPHY (SYRINGOMYELIC SYNDROME)

This syndrome is usually due to syringomyelia—i.e., central cavitation of
the spinal cord, predominantly cervical, and presumably developmental but
often of undetermined cause. Rarely, it is associated with spinal cord tumor
(especially hemangioblastoma) or occurs as a late complication of spinal
cord trauma or infarction. Clinically, syringomyelia is distinguished by segmental weakness and atrophy of the hands and arms, with loss of tendon
reflexes and a segmental loss of sensation of dissociated type (i.e., loss of
pain and temperature sense and preservation of the sense of touch and pressure) in a "cape" distribution over the neck, shoulders, and arms. Later in the
illness there is weakness and ataxia of the legs from involvement of corticospinal tracts and posterior columns. Pain in the neck and arms, kyphoscoliosis, and lower brainstem signs (syringobulbia) are frequently associated.

There are two main types of developmental syringomyelia: (1) an idiopathic type, which has its onset in early adult life and is not associated with
obstruction at the foramen magnum, and (2) a type that is associated with a
Chiari malformation and signs of obstruction at the foramen magnum. Both
are confined largely to the cervical cord, but they may extend rostrally
(syringobulbia) or caudally. Both the syrinx cavity and the Chiari malformation are readily visualized with MRI (Fig. 44-4).

The treatment of syringomyelia is far from satisfactory. If a Chiari malformation contributes to the clinical picture, unroofing of the upper cervical
canal up to and including the foramen magnum is advisable. Shunting of the
syrinx into the peritoneal cavity or venous system or filleting of the dorsal
cord have given unpredictable results.

OTHER SPINAL CORD SYNDROMES

Ventral (Anterior) Cord Syndrome

With infarction in the territory of the anterior spinal artery (occlusion of the
anterior spinal artery itself or, more often, its extraspinal tributaries), damage is limited to the anterior two-thirds of the spinal cord. Tumor invasion
and inflammatory myelitis may have a similar effect. There is paraplegia or
quadriplegia, bilateral loss of pain and temperature sensation below the
lesion, and sparing of the posterior column (joint position and vibration)
sense.

Central Cord (Schneider) Syndrome

In certain cases of cervical trauma, there is disproportionate damage to the
central gray matter of the cord, clinically duplicating the syringomyelic syndrome. The hands are weakened and have impaired pain sensation, but there
is a relative paucity of long tract signs.

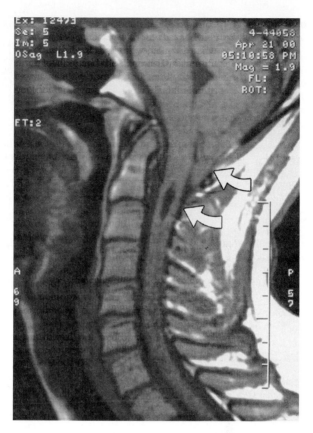

FIG. 44-1 Chiari type malformation and developmental syringomyelia. T1-weighted MRI of the low-lying cerebellar tonsils below the foramen magnum and behind the upper cervical cord (*upper arrow*) and the syrinx cavity within the upper cord (*lower arrow*).

Conus Medullaris and Cauda Equina Syndromes

Pain localized to the low back, severe radicular pain in the legs, loss of bladder and bowel control, laxity of the anal sphincter, and loss of sensation in sacral segments are the principal manifestations; leg weakness, often asymmetrical with upper and lower motor neuron signs, may be added. Metastatic cancer, either of the meninges and roots or compressive from adjacent lumbar vertebrae, viral and demyelinative myelitis, arteriovenous fistulas, and myxopapillary ependymoma are the main causes. Congenital dysraphism syndromes, notably Chiari type II malformations with lumbosacral meningomyelocele, and also a developmental tethering of the cord may affect the conus and cauda equina, with prominent bladder involvement.

Hemicord (Brown-Séquard) Syndrome

Rarely, disease is confined to one side of the spinal cord; pain and thermal sensation are affected on the opposite side of the body and proprioceptive sensation and corticospinal tract function on the same side as the lesion. Not uncommonly, this syndrome is recognizable in the early stages of many types of spinal cord disease that soon involve the cord bilaterally.

Foramen Magnum Syndrome

Progression of spastic weakness from one arm or leg to an adjacent limb (triplegia) and then to the next limb in an "around the clock" pattern is typical. In acutely evolving cases there may be a tetraparesis with muted or normal tendon reflexes, simulating a polyneuropathy. The lower cranial nerves may be implicated.

CONCLUSIONS

In approaching the multitude of diseases that affect the spinal cord, one's primary concern is not to overlook those for which treatment is possible. These are spinal tumors and epidural abscess, subacute combined degeneration due to vitamin B_{12} deficiency, chronic spinal meningitis (syphilitic, tuberculous, fungal), cervical spondylosis, some vascular malformations, and some types of demyelinative myelitis (see Chap. 36). As for the others, diagnosis is advantageous but not crucial, since it does not lead to definitive therapy.

For a more detailed discussion of this topic, see Victor and Ropper: *Adams and Victor's Principles of Neurology*, 7th ed, pp 1293–1345.

ADDITIONAL READING

Aminoff MJ, Logue V: The prognosis of patients with spinal vascular malformations. *Brain* 97:211, 1974

Barnett HJM, Foster JB, Hudgson P: *Syringomyelia*. Philadelphia, Saunders, 1973.

Ebersold MJ, Pare MC, Quast LM: Surgical treatment for cervical spondylotic myelopathy. *J Neurosurg* 82:745, 1995.

Greenberg HS, Kim JH, Posner JB: Epidural spinal cord compression from metastatic tumor. *Ann Neurol* 8:361, 1980.

Katz J, Ropper AH: Progressive necrotic myelopathy: Clinical course in 9 patients. *Arch Neurol* 57:355, 2000.

Reagan TJ, Thomas JE, Colby MY: Chronic progressive radiation myelopathy. *JAMA* 203:128, 1968.

Rossier AB, Foo D, Shillito J: Post-traumatic cervical syringomyelia. *Brain* 108:439, 1985.

Rowland LP: Surgical treatment of cervical spondylotic myelopathy: Time for a controlled study. *Neurology* 42:5, 1992.

Schneider RC, Cherry G, Panter H: The syndrome of acute central cervical cord injury. *J Neurosurg* 11:546, 1954.

Shaw MDM, Russell JA, Grossart KW: The changing pattern of arachnoiditis. *J Neurol Neurosurg Psychiatry* 41:97, 1978.

Sloof JH, Kernohan JW, MacCarty CS: *Primary Intramedullary Tumors of the Spinal Cord and Filum Terminale*. Philadelphia, Saunders, 1964.

PART V | DISEASES OF PERIPHERAL NERVE AND MUSCLE

45 | Physiology of Muscle Contraction and Laboratory Aids in Diagnosis of Neuromuscular Disease

Diseases of nerves and muscle are an integral part of neurology. These structures are of fundamental importance to the organism, since sensory nerves provide information regarding the status of one's own body and of the world and motor nerves and muscles enable motility. Several general remarks are helpful by way of introduction to the group of diseases that affect the neuromuscular apparatus. The human musculature comprises some 30 to 40 percent of the body mass and is disposed in over 600 separate muscles. The muscles also serve as a vast metabolic reservoir. Muscle fibers proliferate under genetic control and arrange themselves during the intrauterine period and grow at a predetermined rate postnatally. They degenerate in several ways during the senium.

Muscle contractility is totally dependent on its nerve supply, without which the muscle becomes immobile and ultimately atrophic. Each anterior horn cell (motor neuron) of the spinal cord and brainstem innervates a large number of muscle fibers; together they form a *motor unit*. If a motor neuron or its axon is destroyed, all muscle fibers within that unit are paralyzed and will atrophy, but some fibers may be adopted by neighboring intact motor units through collateral axonal sprouting. If part of a muscle fiber is injured, the intact parts are capable of restoring the injured fiber; however, a completely destroyed fiber cannot be replaced.

The point of contact between nerves and muscles is the *neuromuscular junction*, which has a special unidirectional conducting property for nerve impulses. The signal from nerve to muscle is effected by the arrival of an electrical impulse, which induces the entry of calcium into the presynaptic side of the junction. This results in release into the junction of the neurotransmitter acetylcholine. The electrical impulse generated by the binding of acetylcholine to postsynaptic receptors spreads over the sarcolemma of the muscle fiber and then to its interior through the transverse tubules and sarcoplasmic reticulum. This impulse in turn releases stored calcium and activates the interaction of actin and myosin filaments, thus shortening the muscle. The enzyme acetylcholinesterase hydrolizes and terminates the action of ACh in the neuromuscular junction. Specialized sensory endings in muscle (spindles and Golgi tendon organs) subserve reflex mechanisms.

The sensory nerves carry information centripetally to the spinal cord and brainstem. Afferent impulses originate in specialized nerve endings for touch, pain, thermal and joint sensation, etc., from which they are conducted in nerve fibers of varying diameters that correspond to the varying thickness of their myelin sheaths. A number of diseases affect preferentially the nerve fiber, the myelin, or the vasculature of the nerve and produce characteristic clinical patterns of neurologic symptoms.

These various aspects of sensation and movement as they are deranged by disease are described in the following chapters, and it will be evident that one may distinguish paralysis and sensory loss due to damage in neurons, nerve fibers, neuromuscular junction, and muscle. The following ancillary tests are helpful in their differentiation.

ALTERED BLOOD CHEMISTRY AND NEUROMUSCULAR DISEASE

Diffuse muscle weakness or muscle twitching, spasms, and cramps may be due to underactivity or overactivity of motor neurons as well as to impaired neuromuscular transmission and muscle activation (contraction and relaxation). The acute occurrence of any such abnormality always raises the question of an alteration of serum electrolytes, which in turn reflects a change in their concentration in the intra- and extracellular fluids. Endocrinopathies are less common causes of such abnormalities.

Abnormalities of Serum Electrolytes

A fall in serum *potassium* below 2.5 meq/L or a rise above 7 meq/L in conjunction with changes in Na and Cl channels results in weakness of limb and trunk muscles or in myotonia. Below a serum concentration of 2.0 meq/L and above 9.0 meq/L, there is almost always complete paralysis of these muscles and later of the respiratory muscles as well. In addition, tendon reflexes are diminished or absent and the reaction of muscle to direct percussion is abolished. In hyperkalemic periodic paralysis and paramyotonia congenita, there is a specific alteration of Na channels that results in either paralysis or myotonia. In myotonia congenita, an abnormality of Cl channels has been identified. In hypokalemic paralysis, in which both water and K enter the muscle fibers, the details of the sarcolemmal pathology are just becoming known (see Chap. 54).

Hypocalcemia of 7.0 mg/dL or less (as occurs in rickets or hypoparathyroidism) or a reduction in the proportion of ionized calcium (as in hyperventilation) causes increased irritability and spontaneous discharge of both sensory and motor nerve fibers—i.e., tetany and paresthesias. Sometimes convulsions result from similar changes in cerebral neurons. These secondary effects upon muscle appear in the electromyogram (EMG) as frequent repetitive discharges and later as prolonged spontaneous discharges.

Hypercalcemia above 12.0 mg/dL (as occurs in vitamin D intoxication, hyperparathyroidism, and metastatic bone disease) causes muscle weakness, lethargy, and confusion, the last two on a central basis.

Hypomagnesemia results in muscle weakness, tremor, tetanic spasms, and convulsions. An increase in plasma Mg also leads to muscle weakness, the result of the depressant action of Mg on lower motor neurons.

Marked *hypo-* or *hypernatremia* is not attended by significant neuromuscular consequences.

Endocrinopathies

Muscle weakness may be a prominent feature of excessive secretion of ACTH (Cushing disease) or prolonged corticosteroid therapy. High and low thyroxin (T_4) levels in the blood are also reflected in diffuse muscle weakness, the result of chemical alterations in the contractile process of muscle fibers. In hyperthyroidism the contraction and relaxation of muscle are abbreviated, and in hypothyroidism they are prolonged.

Changes in Serum Levels of Muscle Enzymes

Release of muscle enzymes into the blood [elevated creatine kinase (CK), aldolase, etc.] is indicative of destruction of muscle fibers, especially if the process is acute. For unclear reasons, however, CK may be elevated in hypothyroidism, in which there is no myonecrosis. For serum CK to be interpretable, one must be certain that it is derived from skeletal muscle and not from heart or brain. The source of these isoenzymes can be determined by qualitative analysis. The MM form of CK is found in highest concentration in striated muscle; in patients with acute destructive lesions (e.g., alcoholic rhabdomyolysis, neuroleptic malignant syndrome, drug-toxic myopathy, polymyositis) it often exceeds 1000 U and may reach 40,000 U. It is raised to lesser degrees in the progressive muscular dystrophies and may be normal in chronic restricted forms of dystrophy.

Myoglobinuria

Red urine is an uncommon but important finding in muscle disease, often being indicative of an acute destructive process. With destruction of muscle fibers, myoglobin, the red pigment, is released into the serum; in sufficient amounts, it will color the urine. Unlike hemoglobin, myoglobin is a small molecule that is rapidly cleared from the serum by the kidneys. Hence, in myoglobinuria, the serum retains its normal color. Approximately 200 g of muscle must be destroyed to color the urine. Smaller quantities, insufficient to color the urine, can be detected spectroscopically or preferably by radioimmunoassay techniques. The commonly used urine dipstick test for hemoglobin will also detect myoglobin because both contain iron. Thus a positive urine Hgb dipstick test in the absence of hematuria should suggest myoglobinuria in the appropriate clinical situation.

ELECTRODIAGNOSTIC TESTS

Muscle weakness and atrophy may be due to a primary disease of muscle (a muscular dystrophy or a myopathy of metabolic, toxic, traumatic, or inflammatory type) or to denervation (from disease of anterior horn cells or peripheral nerves). These causes of weakness can be readily differentiated by electrodiagnostic methods. The two standard procedures are (1) the EMG, which demonstrates, upon the insertion of needle electrodes into muscles, fibrillation and fasciculation potentials and changes in the size and shape of motor unit potentials (MUPs) and (2) the percutaneous stimulation of peripheral nerve fibers and recording of muscle and sensory action potentials (motor and sensory *nerve conduction studies*), expressed as amplitudes [compound muscle action potential (CMAP)], conduction velocities, and distal latencies.

The EMG findings in primary muscle disease are characteristic. During voluntary contraction of muscle, one detects many motor units of small size (short duration and diminished voltage) because the motor units are depleted of their normal quota of muscle fibers (Fig. 45-2D).

In acutely denervated muscle, on the other hand, there is a reduced number of MUPs (decreased recruitment). After several days the individual muscle fibers of motor units, released from nerve control, *fibrillate* independently (Fig. 45-1). Six to eight weeks later, an increased irritability of affected motor nerve fibers or motor neurons that have become reinnervated by preserved adjacent axons may cause *fasciculation* (independent random contraction of all or most of the fibers of a motor unit). After several weeks to months, the remaining MUPs tend to increase in amplitude and duration and become polyphasic, because collateral sprouts from surviving axons reinnervate the denervated muscle fibers (Fig. 45-2). Fibrillations are too small to be visible to the naked eye, except perhaps in the tongue, while fasciculations can be seen as isolated arrythmic twitches of muscle under the skin.

EMG is also useful in demonstrating myotonia and defects in conductance through the muscle membrane electrolyte channels ("channelopathies"; see Chap. 54).

Nerve conduction studies are the other standard procedure in the study of peripheral nerve disease. Slowing of the velocity of nerve conduction, dispersion of the CMAPs, and prolongation of terminal latencies (time from stimulus to onset of contraction) indicate demyelination of the nerve trunk. Motor conduction block is also found in certain demyelinative diseases. In axonal disease, the velocity of nerve conduction is slowed only slightly, because the preservation of only a few large fibers is sufficient to transmit an induced impulse at normal speed. In both demyelinative and axonal types, the amplitude of the elicited CMAP is decreased, the distinction then being made by the needle examination, which shows denervation changes in axonal disease.

Special nerve conduction studies (H reflex and F waves) that utilize the entire length of the nerve and its roots provide information about disease of proximal sensory and motor nerves and roots. Localized slowing or blocks in conduction are particularly useful in the diagnosis of entrapment syndromes—e.g., of the median nerve at the wrist (carpal tunnel) or the ulnar nerve at the elbow—and in localization of the focal lesions in vascular and inflammatory diseases of nerves.

By repetitive stimulation of a motor nerve, defects of presynaptic and postsynaptic neuromuscular transmission can be exposed. In myasthenia gravis, for example, with stimulation at a rate of two or three per second, there is a progressive decrement in the elicited MAPs. By contrast, in the paraneoplastic Lambert-Eaton syndrome and in botulism, there is, with rapid stimulation, an increment in the amplitudes toward the normal level.

BIOPSY PATHOLOGY

Biopsy of muscle and nerve can be of considerable help in differentiating muscle, nerve, and spinal cord disease and sometimes in specifying the disease process.

Both surgical and microscopic techniques must be exacting. The muscle to be studied should be easily accessible; there should be evidence that it has been affected but not too severely damaged, and that it has not been the site of recent injections or needle EMG study.

Myopathies and dystrophies are expressed by random loss of muscle fibers and their replacement by fat and connective tissue. If the sample is

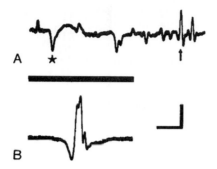

FIG. 45-1 *A.* Fibrillations and positive sharp waves. This spontaneous activity was recorded from a totally denervated muscle—no motor unit potentials were produced by attempts at voluntary contraction. The fibrillations (*above arrow*) are 1 to 2 ms in duration, 100 to 300 mV in amplitude, and largely negative (upward) in polarity following an initial positive deflection. A typical positive sharp wave is seen above the star. *B.* Fasciculation. This spontaneous motor unit potential was recorded from a patient with amyotrophic lateral sclerosis. It has a serrated configuration and it fired once every second or two. Calibrations: 5 ms (horizontal) and 200 mV in *A*; 1 mV in *B* (vertical).

well chosen, one may actually see muscle fibers in the process of degeneration and regeneration. The process does not respect motor units. In the *polymyositides*, inflammatory changes are usually evident. In *denervation atrophy*, there is a great reduction in the size of muscle fibers within affected motor units and an enlargement of intact motor units. This is best demonstrated by grouping of fibers, and by ATPase and other histochemical stains for fiber types, since all the fibers of a motor unit derived from one anterior horn cell are of one histochemical type (so-called fiber-type grouping). Histochemical stains showing an excess of lipid or glycogen within surviving muscle fibers are diagnostic of the lipid and glycogen storage diseases. Mitochondrial diseases of diverse type may be revealed by red staining of clumped mitochondria in Gomori trichrome preparations.

Electron microscopy can be done on specially fixed bits of muscles and will expose some of the characteristic morphologic changes of the mitochondrial and other myopathies (central core, nemaline, myotubular, etc.) and also lipid and glycogen storage products (lipidoses and glycogenoses). Also, by the study of specimens from the innervation point of a muscle fiber, one can find abnormalities that are diagnostic of disorders of the neuromuscular junction (myasthenia gravis, Lambert-Eaton syndrome).

Nerve biopsy is generally of less value but is nevertheless helpful in certain circumstances. Usually the sural nerve is selected, since it is purely sensory, and its interruption results in no disability, only in a patch of sensory loss behind the lateral malleolus and residual pain in a few patients. Light- and electron-microscopic sections may show demyelination, onion bulb formations of Schwann cells, and fibroblasts (reflecting recurrent demyelination), axon degeneration of several types, wallerian degeneration (see p. 422), inflammatory reactions, arteritis, and amyloid deposition. By the

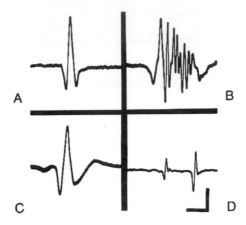

FIG. 45-2   Single voluntary motor unit potentials. *A.* Normal. *B.* Prolonged polyphasic potential seen with reinnervation. *C.* "Giant unit"—normally shaped but of much greater amplitude than normal. *D.* Brief, low-amplitude "myopathic" units. Calibrations: 5 ms (horizontal) and 1 mV in *A* and *B*; 5 mV in *C*; 100 mV in *D* (vertical).

teasing apart of single nerve fibers, the status of myelin and axon and the length of internodal segments can be determined.

Finally, it must be pointed out that none of these laboratory tests is infallible. In biopsy studies there is a prodigious sampling problem, so a bit of nerve or muscle may be normal even though the clinical data indicating disease are indubitable. Also, each procedure is subject to numerous technical errors and the findings may be misinterpreted.

For a more detailed discussion of this topic, see Victor and Ropper: *Adams and Victor's Principles of Neurology,* 7th ed, pp 1346–1369.

ADDITIONAL READING

Aminoff MJ: *Electrodiagnosis in Clinical Neurology,* 4th ed. New York, Churchill Livingstone, 1999.

Asbury AK, Thomas PK (eds): *Peripheral Nerve Disorders,* 2nd ed. Boston, Butterworth-Heinemann, 1995.

Brown WF, Bolton CF (eds): *Clinical Electromyography,* 2nd ed. Boston, Butterworth-Heinemann, 1993.

Engel AG, Franzini-Armstrong C (eds): *Myology,* 2nd ed. New York, McGraw-Hill, 1994.

Fischbeck K: Structure and function of striated muscle, in Asbury AK, McKhann GM, McDonald W (eds): *Diseases of the Nervous System,* 2nd ed. Philadelphia, Saunders, 1992, pp 123–134.

Kuffler SW, Nicholis JG, Martin AR: *From Neuron to Brain,* 2nd ed. Sunderland, MA, Sinauer, 1984.

46 | Diseases of the Peripheral Nerves

The peripheral nervous system (PNS) includes all neural structures lying outside the pial membranes of the spinal cord and brainstem. The optic and olfactory nerves are not included, since they are special extensions of the brain; unlike all other nerves, whose myelin sheaths are enclosed by Schwann cells and supported by fibroblasts, the optic and olfactory fibers lie within oligodendroglia and are supported by astrocytes. The parts of the PNS that are within the spinal canal and are attached to the ventral and dorsal surfaces of the spinal cord are called the *spinal nerve roots* and those attached to the ventrolateral surface of the brainstem, the *cranial nerve roots*. The dorsal (afferent or sensory) roots consist of the central axonal processes of dorsal root ganglion cells; some of them synapse in the dorsal gray matter of the spinal cord and others ascend ipsilaterally in the posterior columns or descend for a few segments, as indicated in Chaps. 8 and 9. Similarly, the central processes of cranial ganglion cells extend into the spinal trigeminal and other tracts in the pons and medulla.

In essence, five categories of neurons are the source of all peripheral axons—spinal anterior and intermediolateral horn cells, cranial motor nuclei cells, dorsal root ganglion cells, and sympathetic and parasympathetic ganglion cells. The peripheral axons of dorsal root ganglion cells are the sensory nerve fibers. They terminate as fine, freely branching fibers or in specialized corpuscular endings in the skin, joints, and other tissues. The ventral (efferent or motor) roots are composed of the emerging fibers of anterior horn cells, which innervate muscle fibers, and of lateral horn cells or special brainstem motor nuclei, which terminate on sympathetic and parasympathetic ganglion cells, respectively. Traversing the subarachnoid space and lacking epineurial sheaths, the cranial and spinal roots are bathed in and susceptible to toxic agents in the cerebrospinal fluid (CSF), the lumbosacral roots having the longest exposure.

Other notable features of the PNS are that (1) the peripheral axons are of different sizes, the larger ones having the thickest myelin sheaths; (2) some axons are myelinated and some unmyelinated, the myelin being produced by Schwann cells adjacent to the axon; (3) all fibers are enclosed in epineurial and perineurial sheaths of fibrous connective tissue; (4) the blood supply is relatively sparse and takes the form of an anastomosing chain of longitudinally oriented nutrient arteries and veins; and (5) most nerves and plexuses are mixtures of motor, sensory, and autonomic fibers.

With these anatomic facts in mind, one can conceptualize the various targets of diseases affecting the PNS. Each type of nerve cell has its special susceptibilities, as do the myelin sheaths, axoplasm, Schwann cells, blood vessels, connective tissue, and spinal-cranial leptomeninges and CSF. The following list gives examples of disease in which each of these elements is affected predominantly:

Anterior horn cells	Poliomyelitis
Dorsal root ganglion cells	Herpes zoster
Intermediolateral horn cells	Shy-Drager syndrome
Sympathetic and parasympathetic ganglion cells	Autonomic polyneuropathy
Presynaptic endings, interfering with acetylcholine transmission at neuromuscular junctions and in autonomic ganglia	Botulism
Myelin sheaths in the most vascular parts of the PNS	Guillain-Barré syndrome; diphtheria
Axons of sensory and motor nerves	Heavy metals (e.g., arsenic)
Myelin sheaths and axons beginning in distal segments ("dying-back" neuropathy)	Alcoholic-nutritional diseases
Blood vessels	Diabetes; polyarteritis
Blood vessels, connective tissue	Connective tissue diseases; amyloidosis
Spinal meninges, CSF, and sensory roots	Tabes dorsalis
Neurotubules within axons	Cisplatin

Pathologic Reactions of Peripheral Nerve

Although more than 100 distinct diseases are known to affect the PNS, there are essentially only four underlying pathologic processes—referred to as wallerian degeneration, segmental degeneration, diffuse demyelination, and axonal degeneration (Fig. 46-1). These processes are not disease-specific but occur in various combinations and topographic patterns in any given disease.

In *wallerian degeneration*, there is degeneration of both the axis cylinder and the myelin sheath, distal to the site of an axonal interruption. Proximal to the site of injury, the motor neuron cell body in the cord becomes rounded and its chromatin disperses (chromatolysis), but the cell remains viable.

In *segmental demyelination*, axons are preserved, so there is no wallerian degeneration and no chromatolysis in nerve cell bodies. Remyelination restores function. This process is most prominent in diphtheritic and inflammatory demyelinating polyneuropathies. Also, there are more diffuse (non-segmental) genetic and metabolic *myelinopathies*—such as Charcot-Marie-Tooth disease, in which the entire myelin sheath is the target of an inherited defect.

Axonal degeneration is characteristic of metabolically determined (including toxic and nutritional) polyneuropathies. Always there is degeneration of myelin as well as axis cylinders, progressing from distal to proximal segments ("dying-back" neuropathy).

One feature of nerve disease to be kept in mind is that both wallerian and axonal degeneration cause muscle atrophy and denervation changes in the electromyogram (EMG), but purely demyelinating processes do not.

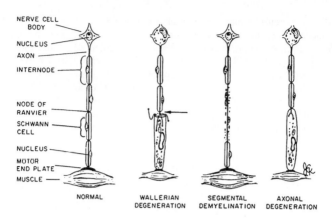

NERVE CELL BODY
NUCLEUS
AXON
INTERNODE
NODE OF RANVIER
SCHWANN CELL
NUCLEUS
MOTOR END PLATE
MUSCLE

NORMAL   WALLERIAN   SEGMENTAL   AXONAL
                DEGENERATION   DEMYELINATION   DEGENERATION

FIG. 46-1   Diagram of the basic pathologic processes affecting peripheral nerves. In wallerian degeneration, there is degeneration of the axis cylinder and myelin distal to the site of axonal interruption *(arrow)* and chromatolysis of the anterior horn cell. In segmental demyelination, the axon is spared. In axonal degeneration, there is a distal degeneration of myelin and axis cylinder as a result of neuronal diseases. Both wallerian and axonal degeneration but not demyelination cause muscle atrophy. Further details in text. *(Courtesy of Dr Arthur Asbury.)*

In addition to these reactions, vasculitic and interstitial inflammation may be present. Ultrastructural studies have revealed a number of more or less specific changes in Schwann cell cytoplasm and axoplasm—e.g., storage products such as amyloid, sulfatide, galactocerebroside, and ceramide. Together, these changes and variations in their time course allow for pathologic differentiation of most peripheral nerve diseases.

Terminology

In discussion of PNS disease, the following terms are conventionally employed: *Polyneuropathy* refers to a bilaterally symmetrical affliction of the peripheral nerves, usually involving the legs more than the arms and the distal segments earlier and more severely than the proximal ones. Involvement of the roots is referred to as *radiculopathy*, and when multiple, *polyradiculopathy*. *Mononeuropathy* designates involvement of a single nerve, and *mononeuropathy multiplex*, the involvement of multiple nerves in an asymmetrical, random distribution. *Plexopathy* denotes involvement limited to the brachial or lumbar plexus. *Sensory ganglionopathy* and *sensory neuropathy* are self-explanatory. The terms *axonal* or *demyelinative* specify the site of principal structural change, but these infrequently occur in pure form.

SYMPTOMATOLOGY

Affliction of the peripheral nerves is expressed by a number of motor, sensory, reflex, autonomic, and trophic symptoms and signs, various combinations of which stand as the clinical criteria for diagnosis.

Most polyneuropathies are marked by weakness and reflex loss and, if chronic and axonal, by denervation atrophy. The pattern of motor loss varies. The common one is a symmetrical involvement of the muscles of the feet and legs followed by those of the hands and arms, because the largest and longest fibers are the most susceptible. This principle does not apply to certain demyelinating neuropathies or to mononeuropathy multiplex, in which any nerve or combination of nerves may be affected. Another pattern, observed in the Guillain-Barré syndrome, is one in which all nerves and roots of the limbs, trunk, and cranial musculature may be involved, leading to respiratory paralysis.

Sensory loss duplicates the pattern of distal motor weakness, but in any given neuropathy it may be more or less severe than the motor affection—hence, sensorimotor or motor-sensory. A loss of proprioceptive fibers gives rise to sensory ataxia and liability to arthropathy; a loss of pain and thermal fibers, to impaired perception of noxious and thermal stimuli; and a loss of autonomic fibers, to paralysis of vasomotor and sudomotor functions and to a number of trophic changes (skin ulcers, bone resorption). The large sensory fibers subserving touch-pressure, vibration, and postural senses are more frequently affected than the small ones subserving pain, temperature, and autonomic functions, but in certain diseases—e.g., amyloidosis and a number of toxic neuropathies—the opposite pertains. Autonomic deficits are manifest mainly by dryness of the soles and palms (sometimes by hyperhidrosis), orthostatic hypotension, impotence, and impairment of pupillary, bladder, and bowel function.

Peripheral nerve diseases not only destroy fibers, leading to sensory, motor, and autonomic deficits, but also may increase the excitability of residual fibers. This is the basis of sensations of numbness, tingling (large fiber damage), burning and pain (small fibers), and pressure and, on the motor side, of fascicular twitching, spasms, and cramps.

The multitude of diseases that cause neuropathy and the principal syndromes by which they present are listed in Table 46-1. Limitations of space permit only a brief consideration of representative and more common examples from each of the major categories.

ACUTE POLYNEUROPATHIES

Guillain-Barré Syndrome (GBS)

This is a nonseasonal, nonepidemic inflammatory polyradiculoneuropathy occurring worldwide at an annual rate of about 1.5 cases per 100,000 population. In about two-thirds of cases, some type of respiratory or gastrointestinal infection precedes the onset of weakness by 1 to 3 weeks. Enteritis due to *Campylobacter jejuni* and infections with Epstein-Barr virus (EBV), cytomegalovirus (CMV), and *Mycoplasma pneumoniae* are the commonest identifiable precedents. The major manifestation is weakness, which evolves more or less symmetrically in all limbs over a period of several days or a week or two. Paresthesias in the toes and fingers accompany the weakness in most cases. Usually, the proximal leg muscles are affected first and then the trunk, intercostal, arm, neck, and cranial muscles, especially the face; occasionally, progression is in the reverse direction. One variant syndrome is characterized by ophthalmoplegia and ataxia (Fisher syndrome). Invariably, tendon reflexes are reduced and then lost. Pain and aching in

TABLE 46-1 Principal Neuropathic Syndromes*

I. Syndrome of acute ascending motor paralysis with variable disturbance of sensory and autonomic function
  A. Acute inflammatory demyelinative polyradiculoneuropathy (Guillain-Barré syndrome)
    1. Acute axonal polyneuropathy
    2. Acute dysautonomic neuropathy
  B. Diphtheritic polyneuropathy
  C. Porphyric polyneuropathy
  D. Certain toxic polyneuropathies (thallium, tick paralysis)
  E. Sepsis and multiple organ failure (critical illness polyneuropathy)
II. Syndrome of subacute sensorimotor paralysis
  A. Symmetric polyneuropathies
    1. Deficiency states: alcoholism (beriberi), pellagra, vitamin B_{12} deficiency, chronic gastrointestinal disease
    2. Poisoning with heavy metals and industrial solvents: arsenic, lead, mercury, thallium, methyl *n*-butyl ketone, *n*-hexane, methyl bromide, organophosphates (TOCP, etc.), acrylamide
    3. Toxic drug effects: cisplatin, paclitaxel, isoniazid, hydralazine, nitrofurantoin and related nitrofurazones, disulfiram, vincristine, amitriptyline, dapsone, thalidomide, clioquinol, amiodarone, etc.
    4. Uremic accelerated polyneuropathy
    5. AIDS-related neuropathies
    6. Some forms of paraneoplastic neuropathy (see III A).
    7. Subacute inflammatory and immune polyneuropathies (CIDP[†])
  B. Asymmetric and multifocal neuropathies (mononeuropathy multiplex)
    1. Diabetes
    2. Polyarteritis nodosa, lupus erythematosus, Churg-Strauss and other vasculitic neuropathies (sometimes symmetrical)
    3. Sarcoidosis
    4. Ischemic neuropathy with peripheral vascular disease
III. Syndrome of early chronic sensorimotor polyneuropathy (*acquired* forms)
  A. Paraneoplastic (carcinoma, myeloma, and other malignancies)
  B. Paraproteinemias (including Waldenström macroglobulinemia)
  C. Uremia (occasionally subacute)
  D. Beriberi (usually subacute)
  E. Diabetes
  F. Hypothyroidism (?)
  G. Connective tissue diseases including Sjögren syndrome
  H. Amyloidosis, systemic type
  I. Leprosy
  J. Lyme disease
IV. Syndrome of chronic (late) polyneuropathy (*hereditary* forms)
  A. Inherited polyneuropathies of predominantly sensory type
    1. Dominant mutilating sensory neuropathy in adults
    2. Recessive mutilating sensory neuropathy of childhood
    3. Congenital insensitivity to pain
    4. Other inherited sensory neuropathies, including those associated with spinocerebellar degenerations and Riley-Day syndrome and the universal anesthesia syndrome

(continued)

TABLE 46-1 *(continued)* Principal Neuropathic Syndromes*

  B. Inherited polyneuropathies of mixed sensorimotor-autonomic types
    1. Idiopathic group
      a. Dominant peroneal muscular atrophy (Charcot-Marie-Tooth), both axonal and demyelinative forms
      b. Dominant hypertrophic polyneuropathy of Déjerine-Sottas, adult and childhood forms
      c. Roussy-Lévy ataxic polyneuropathy
      d. Polyneuropathy with optic atrophy, with spastic paraplegia, with spinocerebellar degeneration, with mental retardation, deafness, or dementia
    2. Inherited polyneuropathies with a recognized metabolic disorder (see also Chap. 37)
      a. Refsum disease
      b. Metachromatic leukodystrophy
      c. Globoid-body leukodystrophy (Krabbe disease)
      d. Adrenoleukodystrophy (myeloneuropathy form)
      e. Amyloid polyneuropathy (Andrade type)
      f. Porphyric polyneuropathy
      g. Anderson-Fabry disease
      h. Abetalipoproteinemia and Tangier disease
V. Syndrome of recurrent or relapsing polyneuropathy
  A. Relapsing Guillain-Barré syndrome
  B. Chronic inflammatory polyradiculoneuropathy
  C. Porphyric polyneuropathy
  D. Certain forms of mononeuritis multiplex
  E. Refsum disease
  F. Tangier disease
VI. Syndrome of mononeuropathy or multiple neuropathies (mononeuritis multiplex)
  A. Pressure, traumatic, and entrapment palsies
  B. Vasculitic neuropathies (see II B 2)
  C. Idiopathic and familial brachial and lumbosacral plexopathies
  D. Hereditary liability to pressure palsies
  E. Immune reaction to serum and vaccines (smallpox, rabies)
  F. Herpes zoster (shingles)
  G. Neoplastic infiltration of roots and nerves
  H. Leprosy
   I. Diphtheritic wound infections with local neuropathy
  J. Migrant sensory neuropathy (Wartenberg disease)

*Primary diseases of motor neurons are excluded from this classification.
†Chronic inflammatory demyelinating polyradiculoneuropathy.

muscles and autonomic disturbances occur frequently but in most patients are relatively mild and evanescent. CSF protein rises after a few days. Conduction block and dispersion of compound muscle action potentials (CMAPs) are characteristic in the EMG. Severe cases result in axonal damage that is reflected by EMG signs of denervation and, in extreme form, by complete electrical inexcitability of some nerves.

GBS is the most rapidly evolving form of polyneuropathy and is potentially fatal (progression to complete paralysis and death from respiratory failure in a few days). For these reasons, it needs to be distinguished from other acute polyneuropathies (diphtheritic, porphyric, polyarteritic, and toxic) as well as from myasthenia gravis and poliomyelitis and from acute cervical myelitis.

All evidence points to an autoimmune, inflammatory, demyelinative disease. Rarely, the axons are the primary target of the immune reaction.

As to *treatment*, the patient needs to be in a unit where intensive respiratory care is available. Respiratory assistance should be instituted at the first sign of dyspnea or atelectasis (arterial Po_2 < 70 mmHg) or markedly reduced vital capacity (< 12 to 15 mL/kg). Patients with rapidly evolving paralysis and those who are too weak to walk without assistance should receive a course of plasmapheresis (250 mL/kg total exchanged volume in 4 or 5 sessions) or IV administration of immune globulin (0.4 g/kg per day for 5 days). Both have been shown to hasten recovery. Controlled studies of the effects of corticosteroids have failed to demonstrate any benefit.

Most patients recover completely or nearly completely (mild motor deficits in the legs may persist), although this may take several months to a year or longer. About 5 percent of patients do not survive, even in the best-equipped hospitals, and 10 percent are left with severe degrees of disability. Another 3 percent suffer one or more recurrences of the disease or fluctuate for a prolonged period of months or years in a pattern described below under CIDP.

Neuropathies Associated with AIDS

These patients are prone to several types of neuropathy, including a predominantly sensory type that may be painful, a restricted lumbosacral polyradiculopathy, cranial and limb mononeuropathies, chronic inflammatory demyelinating polyradiculoneuropathy (CIDP), GBS, and, rarely, a vasculitic mononeuritis multiplex—none of which differs from the idiopathic or conventional varieties of these except that there is more often pleocytosis in the spinal fluid. Unique to the AIDS patient are a CMV cauda equina neuritis and an acute or subacute and painful infiltrative lymphocytic neuropathy—a component of the diffuse infiltrative lymphocytosis syndrome (DILS). Polyneuropathy may also be induced by antiviral agents that are used in the treatment of HIV infection.

Critical Illness Polyneuropathy

An acute or subacute symmetrical polyneuropathy is frequent in critically ill and septic patients, particularly in those with failure of multiple organs. The neuropathy, predominantly of motor type, varies in severity, in its severest form causing quadriparesis with respiratory failure. Usually the cranial nerves are spared and there are no overt dysautonomic manifestations. The disease appears after several days or more of critical illness and is preceded in most instances by a confusional state or a depressed state of consciousness. The polyneuropathy may be recognized days later when it causes difficulty in weaning the patient from the ventilator, even as the underlying medical illness comes under control. The EMG findings of primary axonal degeneration and a normal CSF distinguish it from GBS. The toxic effects of drugs and antibiotics and nutritional deficiency must always be considered in causation of postoperative weakness, but they can rarely be established. Perhaps some of the many systemic mediators of sepsis are toxic to the peripheral nervous system.

This form of polyneuropathy must be distinguished from a poorly understood *acute quadriplegic myopathy* that sometimes complicates critical illness (see Chap. 51). High doses of corticosteroids, particularly in combination with neuromuscular blocking agents, have been implicated. The acute myopathy, which affects both distal and proximal muscles, is usually heralded by an elevation in the serum creatine kinase (CK) concentration and myopathic potentials in the EMG, and there is a unique degeneration of myofilaments.

CHRONIC POLYNEUROPATHIES

Chronic Inflammatory Demyelinating Polyradiculoneuropathy (CIDP)

This disorder is in some respects similar to GBS—both are widespread polyneuropathies and both are characterized by an increased CSF protein (usually without cells), a demyelinative type of nerve conduction abnormality, probable autoimmune pathogenesis, and an inflammatory pathology. However, there are important differences. Whereas GBS is an acute (rarely subacute) monophasic illness, CIDP evolves more slowly, either in a steadily progressive or stepwise manner (sometimes in a slightly asymmetrical pattern) and attains its maximum severity only after weeks, months, or longer, following which it tends to run a relapsing or fluctuating course. A preceding illness is relatively uncommon in patients with CIDP. Also, in distinction to GBS, most cases of CIDP respond favorably to the prolonged administration of corticosteroids, as well as to plasma exchange and, in many cases, to intravenous immune globulin.

Paraproteinemic Polyneuropathies

This heterogeneous group of chronic sensorimotor neuropathies is causally related in some way to a circulating immune protein. There is an excess of a monoclonal immunoglobulin in one of the subclasses (IgG, IgM, IgA paraprotein, or "M spike") that can be identified by immunoelectrophoresis or by immunofixation of the serum. The best-characterized of these neuropathies are associated with IgM antibodies directed against components of myelin: an anti-MAG associated polyneuropathy, which involves predominantly large sensory fibers and gives rise to imbalance and severe loss of proprioceptive and vibration sensibility, and an anti-GM_1 motor neuropathy, which has as its denominative feature multifocal motor conduction block on nerve conduction studies. Multiple myeloma, discussed below, amyloidosis, and Waldenström macroglobulinemia are special instances with unique features, but in contrast to these conditions, the majority of patients with a paraproteinemic neuropathy have lower serum concentrations of the monoclonal protein (less than 3 g/dL). In all these processes, amyloid deposition in nerve may occur as a parallel condition. Treatment is with plasma exchange or immune globulin combined with immunosuppressive drugs, but the long-term results are generally unsatisfactory.

Amyloid neuropathy (acquired and familial types) These are sporadic and less common familial forms of neuropathy characterized by extensive amyloid deposition in nerves. In most cases of the sporadic type, also called primary amyloidosis or AL, the amyloid protein is a light-chain component of a monoclonal paraprotein, either benign or malignant. This is a systemic disease in which deposits of amyloid are found in various organs, especially the liver and kidney. It is mainly a disease of older men, the median age at the time of diagnosis being 65 years.

The neuropathic symptoms and signs are similar to those of hereditary amyloid polyneuropathy, but the progress of the disease is considerably more rapid. The initial symptoms are sensory—numbness, paresthesias, and often acral pain—and the signs are characteristic of involvement of small-diameter sensory fibers (loss of pain and thermal sensation). Weakness follows, initially limited to the feet but becoming more extensive as the disease progresses and eventually affecting the hands and arms. Loss of large fiber–mediated sensation (position, vibratory, touch, and deep pressure sense) may appear later. Twenty-five percent of these patients have a carpal tunnel syndrome from infiltration of the flexor retinaculum.

Involvement of the autonomic nervous system can be severe and becomes evident early in the illness; patients present with disturbances of gastrointestinal motility, especially episodic diarrhea, or with orthostatic symptoms, impotence, and bladder disturbances. The pupils may react slowly, and there may be a reduction in sweating. Death is usually due to the renal, cardiac, or gastrointestinal effects of amyloid deposits, the manifestations of which are already evident in most patients who present with neuropathy. A nephrotic syndrome is particularly characteristic.

Analysis of the serum and urine for an abnormal paraprotein, followed by a microscopic examination of abdominal fat pad, gingival, or rectal biopsy for amyloid, are the most useful initial tests. If a sensory neuropathy or evidence of organ infiltration is evident, biopsy of the sural nerve or the involved viscera has a high diagnostic yield. The liver is positive in all cases and the kidney has amyloid infiltration in about 85 percent. Amyloid is demonstrated in tissue by a green birefringence of the Congo red stain when viewed under polarized light.

The prognosis in AL is poor, and attempts at immunomodulation, immunosuppression (which may help the renal disease), or removal of amyloid by plasma exchange have been only marginally effective. A recent approach has been with stem cell replacement and bone marrow suppression, but the valve of these measures remains to be determined. The pain may become quite severe and is treated with fentanyl patches or with narcotic medications.

The *familial amyloid polyneuropathies*, also termed FA, comprise several distinct clinical groups, all of autosomal dominant inheritance. They do not manifest a circulating paraprotein and have a more chronic course than the acquired type. While a descriptive classification based on the ethnic origin of affected families is still in use clinically, it is now possible to categorize these diseases according to their genetic errors and the corresponding chemical structure of the abnormal protein that is deposited in the tissue as amyloid. In the two most common familial forms, the Portuguese (Andrade) and Indiana-Swiss types, the amyloid is derived from an abnormal transthyretin (formerly called prealbumin). The recent cloning of many more of the amyloid protein genes not only has made possible the detection of the transthyretin gene abnormality but should also make available diagnostic DNA tests for the other types of familial amyloidosis.

Liver transplantation has proved curative of one of the familial amyloid polyneuropathies but obviously has no role in the acquired forms.

Nutritional Polyneuropathy (Neuropathic Beriberi)

In the western world, this form of neuropathy is usually associated with chronic alcoholism and is a common example of subacute sensorimotor polyneuropathy. This and rarer forms of deficiency neuropathy (Strachan syndrome, pellagra, vitamin B_{12} deficiency, and malabsorption syndromes) are described in Chap. 41.

Paraneoplastic Polyneuropathy

A predominantly distal, symmetrical sensorimotor polyneuropathy, affecting first the legs and then the hands and arms and evolving over a period of months, may occur as a *remote effect of carcinoma* and, rarely, of *lymphoma*. A pure sensory ganglionitis-polyneuropathy, with severe ataxia and retention of strength, is a much more distinctive but less common type of paraneoplastic neuropathy. Although this condition is listed here with the chronic polyneuropathies, the onset is often subacute, reaching a maximum state of disability in several weeks. These forms of polyneuropathy are manifest clinically in 2 to 5 percent of all patients with malignant disease, and more than half of them are associated with carcinoma of the lung, the next in frequency being breast and ovarian cancer and lymphoma. More important, the paraneoplastic syndrome may be present for months or longer before the malignant tumor is discovered. Sometimes the polyneuropathy subsides if the primary tumor is effectively treated. The majority of patients with a nondescript paraneoplastic neuropathy, and 90 percent of those with the special sensory ganglionopathy, have circulating antibodies against neuronal nuclear components (called anti-Hu or ANNA-type I). Some of these patients have an associated paraneoplastic encephalopathy (page 264).

Peroneal Muscular Atrophy (Charcot-Marie-Tooth Disease)

This, the most common form of *inherited neuropathy*, is transmitted most often as an autosomal dominant trait. Onset is in late childhood or adolescence, occasionally in later years, with atrophy of muscles of the feet and legs and later of the hands and arms. The early involvement of the peronei and extensors of the toes produces high arches, an equinovarus deformity, and clawfoot. Deep and superficial sensation are impaired, usually to a slight degree, and tendon reflexes are absent in the affected limbs. The illness progresses very slowly, with long periods of stability. Wasting seldom extends above the lower third of the thighs and above the elbows.

Walking difficulty, which is the main disability, is due to a combination of sensory ataxia and weakness. Foot drop and instability of the ankles are additional handicaps; they can be alleviated by arthrodeses and light leg braces.

Genetic testing is now available for the more common types. The EMG is helpful in diagnosis; in the typical form (CMT1A), there is uniform slowing of conduction in all nerves, quite unlike that in any acquired polyneuropathy.

There are several variants of this disorder, particularly an axonal form (CMT2), and others with enlargement of the nerves; in some families signs of spastic weakness or spinocerebellar disease are conjoined (see *Adams and Victor's Principles of Neurology*, 7th ed., for details and for descriptions of the large number of other inherited forms of polyneuropathy).

Diabetic Neuropathies

Neuropathic complications of diabetes mellitus are exceedingly common, particularly in patients over 50 years of age. Several clinical syndromes are recognized, occurring singly or in various combinations. The acute and chronic ones are listed here together for convenience.

1. The most common diabetic neuropathy is the *distal sensory type*. This takes the form of persistent and often distressing pain, numbness, and tingling affecting the feet and lower legs symmetrically. In severe cases, the hands may be affected. The sensory loss contributes to poorly healing foot injuries. Occasionally deep sensation is impaired, with ataxia and bladder atony (*diabetic pseudotabes*) and joint deformities (Charcot joints).

2. *Diabetic ophthalmoplegia*: This is due to infarction of the third or sixth cranial nerve, more often the former. The oculomotor palsy is acute and is accompanied by severe pain around the eye and in the forehead. The pupilloconstrictor fibers, located peripherally in the third nerve, are spared by the infarction, which characteristically affects the central portion of the nerve; hence, pupillary function is usually intact. (Contrariwise, compressive lesions of the third nerve—e.g., aneurysm or temporotentorial herniation—cause pupillary dilatation.)

3. *Acute mononeuropathy and radiculopathy*: Affection of practically all the major peripheral nerves has been seen in the diabetic, but the ones most commonly involved are the femoral and sciatic. The acute peripheral mononeuropathies, like the cranial ones, are presumably due to infarction of nerve; in both, the outlook for ultimate recovery is good.

   Segmental radiculopathy is a relatively uncommon complication of long-standing diabetes, presenting with severe pain, dysesthesia, and superficial sensory loss in a segmental distribution over the chest (intercostal nerve) or abdomen. The EMG changes (fibrillations of paraspinal muscles in multiple myotomes) confirm the presence of a widespread radiculopathy.

4. *Lumbar mononeuropathy multiplex*: This takes the form of a subacutely evolving, painful, asymmetrical or unilateral, predominantly motor neuropathy, affecting multiple lumbosacral nerves. It tends to occur in older people with mild (or unrecognized) diabetes, often at the inception of insulin treatment or as a complication of long-standing diabetes that has been uncontrolled for a short period. Muscle weakness and atrophy are most evident in the pelvic girdle and thigh muscles on one side and the knee jerk is lost, so the condition is sometimes referred to as "diabetic amyotrophy." Recovery is to be expected but may take many months.

6. A second type of *proximal diabetic neuropathy* is characterized by a *symmetrical* weakness and wasting of the pelvic and proximal thigh muscles of insidious onset and gradual evolution. Scapular and upper arm muscles are affected less frequently. Pain is not a consistent feature, and sensory changes, if present, are mild and of the distal symmetrical type.

7. Symptoms of *autonomic neuropathy* include pupillary and lacrimal dysfunction, impairment of sweating and vascular reflexes, nocturnal diarrhea, atonicity of the gastrointestinal tract and bladder, impotence, and postural hypotension. These symptoms are frequently combined with

other forms of diabetic neuropathy, particularly with the distal sensory type.

An endoneurial alteration of nutrient vessels or possibly a metabolic derangement is postulated on uncertain grounds as the basis of all forms of diabetic neuropathy. The CSF protein may be elevated—to 50 to 200 mg/dL and sometimes even higher in diabetics, including in those who do not manifest signs of neuropathy.

As to treatment, strict control of the blood glucose is mandatory. One seldom observes quick improvement, but symptomatic treatment over a period of months usually allows some of the most unpleasant manifestations to recede. Anticonvulsants (e.g., gabapentin), amitriptyline, as well as lidocaine and capsaicin creams and nerve blocks are sometimes helpful in the painful varieties.

DIFFERENTIAL DIAGNOSIS

Once it has been ascertained from existent symptoms and signs that there is disease involving many peripheral nerves, three questions must be answered: (1) Is the disease in question a polyneuropathy, a radiculopathy or polyradiculopathy, or a random affection of multiple nerves (mononeuropathy multiplex)? (2) What is the time course? (3) Is the deficit predominantly due to demyelination or to axonal degeneration?

The features that distinguish polyneuropathy from mononeuropathy multiplex have already been described, and from an inspection of Tables 46-1 and 46-2 it is apparent that the two categories have different causations. The multiple neuropathies usually prove to have a systemic vascular, or arteritic, cause, whereas the polyneuropathies are of inflammatory, paraproteinemic, metabolic, toxic, nutritional, or heredodegenerative nature. The time course provides helpful etiologic clues. Most acute polyneuropathies developing over 2 to 3 days are inflammatory (GBS), vasculitic, or toxic (rare). Those evolving over a period of weeks may be inflammatory or paraneoplastic, but a toxic factor or nutritional deficiency is as likely. Neuropathic diseases evolving over weeks to months tend to be paraneoplastic or metabolic. Any polyneuropathy progressing over 5 to 10 years will probably prove to be a familial, metabolic, or degenerative disease. The only exceptions to this statement are the paraproteinemic and a few of the diabetic polyneuropathies. As already mentioned, many of the subacute or less chronic paraneoplastic polyneuropathies are associated with manifestations of CNS disease (cerebellar ataxia, limbic encephalitis). This is also true of a few of the inherited chronic polyneuropathies.

The most helpful ancillary procedures in differential diagnosis are the electrodiagnostic tests, as described in Chap. 45. They separate a group of slow-conducting motor nerve (demyelinative) diseases from those that are primarily axonal. These tests also yield data concerning multifocality of lesions that reflects demyelination or infarction. The relative degree of involvement of proximal nerves and roots can be determined by testing for H and F responses. The preservation of peripheral nerve sensory conduction in the context of clinical sensory loss also points to a radiculopathy, as described below. Electrical tests also help to exclude primary muscle diseases and diseases of the neuromuscular junctions. CSF examination may be helpful in demonstrating greatly elevated protein levels in the acquired demyelinating polyneuropathies and in some diabetic ones.

TABLE 46-2 Principal Mononeuropathies and Plexopathies

Nerve or plexus	Symptoms and signs	Usual causes
Entire brachial plexus (C4–C8, T1)	All arm muscles paralyzed and tendon reflexes lost; sensation lost to upper third of arm	Vehicular accidents; rare familial forms; carcinomatous invasion
Upper brachial plexus (C5, C6)	Paralysis of deltoid, biceps, brachialis, supinator longus, supraspinatus, rhomboids; hand unaffected	Difficult birth (Erb-Duchenne palsy), idiopathic and familial brachial plexitis ("neuralgic amyotrophy"), radiation damage; less often, carcinomatous invasion
Lower brachial plexus (C7, C8, T1)	Amyotrophy of hand muscles; ulnar sensory loss; sometimes Horner syndrome	Traction on abducted arm (humeral dislocation); apical lung tumor; cervical rib or band; breech delivery (Déjerine-Klumpke palsy); radiation injury or, more often, carcinomatous invasion
Cords of brachial plexus:		
Lateral	Weakness of flexion and pronation of forearm	Dislocation of head of humerus, axillary trauma, cervical rib or band; supraclavicular compression
Medial	Combined median and ulnar palsy	
Posterior	Weakness of deltoid, extensors of elbow, wrist, and fingers; sensory loss on outer surface of upper arm	
Long thoracic nerve (C5, C6, C7)	Winging of medial border of scapula; inability to raise arm over head	Heavy weights on shoulder; brachial plexitis
Suprascapular (C5, C6)	Atrophy of supra- and infraspinatus, weakness of first 15° abduction and external rotation of arm	Part of brachial neuritis; entrapment in spinoglenoid notch
Axillary nerve (**C5**,* C6)	Deltoid atrophy; weakness of arm abduction, between 15 and 90°	Dislocations and fractures of shoulder joint; brachial neuritis
Musculocutaneous nerve (C5, C6)	Wasting of biceps, brachialis, and coracobrachialis; weakness of flexion of supinated arm; ↓ sensation along radial and volar forearm	Fracture of humerus
Radial nerve (C6, **C7**, C8)	Paralysis of extension and flexion of the elbow, supination of forearm, extension of wrist, fingers, abduction of thumb; ↓ sensation over radial aspect of dorsum of hand	Compression in axilla and around humerus; part of brachial neuritis
Median nerve (C5, **C6**, C7, C8, T1)	Weakness of pronation of forearm and flexion of fingers, abduction and opposition of thumb; ↓ sensation over radial aspect of palm and dorsum of distal index and third fingers	Injuries between axilla and wrist; compression at wrist (*carpal tunnel*)

*Bold italics indicate major nerve root contribution.

(continued)

TABLE 46-2 *(continued)* Principal Mononeuropathies and Plexopathies

Nerve or plexus	Symptoms and signs	Usual causes
Ulnar nerve (C8, T1)	Wasting of hand muscles with weakness of ulnar flexor of wrist and abductors and adductors of fingers; hyperextension of fingers at metacarpophalangeal joints and flexion at interphalangeal joints ("claw hand"); ↓ sensation over fifth and ulnar parts of fourth fingers and ulnar border of palm	Fracture-dislocation of elbow with cubitus valgus deformity; compression in cubital tunnel or ulnar tunnel at wrist
Entire lumbosacral plexus (T12, L1–L5, S1–S3)	Amyotrophy of all leg muscles; areflexia; anesthesia from toes to perianal region; warm, dry skin	Carcinomatous infiltration, sarcoid
Upper plexus	Weakness of flexion and abduction of thigh and extension of leg; ↓ sensation anterior thigh and leg	Abdominal and pelvic operations; aortic aneurysm; carcinoma and lymphoma; lumbosacral plexitis; diabetic and other arteritic lesions
Lower plexus	Weakness posterior thigh, leg and foot muscles; ↓ sensation first and second sacral segments	
Lateral cutaneous nerve of thigh (L2, L3)	Paresthesias and sensory loss over anterolateral aspect of thigh	Compression by lateral part of inguinal ligament (meralgia paresthetica)
Obturator nerve (L2–L4)	Weakness of adduction, flexion, internal and external rotation of thigh	Injury by fetal head or forceps; obturator hernia; infarction; carcinoma
Femoral nerve (L2–L4)	Weakness of extension of leg; atrophy of quadriceps; weakness of flexion of leg with proximal lesions; loss of knee jerk	Diabetes; pelvic tumors and operations; bleeding into iliacus muscle (anticoagulation induced)
Sciatic nerve (L4, L5, S1, S2)	Weakness of leg flexors and all muscles below knee. Weakness of gluteal muscles with pelvic lesions; ↓ sensation posterior thigh, posterior and lateral leg, and sole	Fractures of pelvis and femur; lower gluteal injections; compression; diabetes; ruptured discs
Common peroneal nerve (L4–S2)	Weakness of dorsiflexion and eversion of foot and dorsiflexion of toes; ↓ sensation dorsum of foot and lateral aspect of lower leg	Compression or fracture at head of fibula; compartment syndrome; diabetes
Tibial nerve (L4–S2)	Weakness of plantar flexion and inversion of foot and flexion of toes; ↓ sensation over plantar aspect of foot	Diabetes; compression in tarsal tunnel

TABLE 46-3 Tests of Muscle Action

Action tested	Roots*	Nerves	Principal muscles
Cranial			
Closure of eyes, pursing of lips, exposure of teeth	Cranial 7	Facial	Orbicularis oculi
			Orbicularis oris
Elevation of eyelids, movement of eyes	Cranial 3, 4, 6	Oculomotor, trochlear, abducens	Extraocular
Closing and opening of jaw	Cranial 5	Motor trigeminal	Masseters
			Pterygoids
Protrusion of tongue	Cranial 12	Hypoglossal	Lingual
Phonation and swallowing	Cranial 9, 10	Glossopharyngeal, vagus	Palatal, laryngeal, and pharyngeal
Elevation of shoulders, anteroflexion and turning of head	Cranial 11	Spinal accessory	Trapezius, sternomastoid
Brachial			
Adduction of extended arm	*C5*, C6	Brachial plexus	Pectoralis major
Fixation of scapula	C5, C6, C7	Brachial plexus	Serratus anterior
Initiation of abduction of arm	*C5*, C6	Brachial plexus	Supraspinatus
External rotation of flexed arm	*C5*, C6	Brachial plexus	Infraspinatus
Abduction and elevation of arm up to 90°	C5, C6	Axillary nerve	Deltoid
Flexion of supinated forearm	C5, C6	Musculocutaneous	Biceps, brachialis
Extension of forearm	C6, *C7*, C8	Radial	Triceps
Extension (radial) of wrist	C6	Radial	Extensor carpi radialis longus
Flexion of semipronated arm	C5, *C6*	Radial	Brachioradialis
Adduction of flexed arm	C6, *C7*, C8	Brachial plexus	Latissimus dorsi
Supination of forearm	C6, *C7*	Posterior interosseous	Supinator
Extension of proximal phalanges	C7, C8	Posterior interosseous	Extensor digitorum
Extension of wrist (ulnar side)	*C7*, C8	Posterior interosseous	Extensor carpi ulnaris
Extension of proximal phalanx of index finger	*C7*, C8	Posterior interosseous	Extensor indicis
Abduction of thumb	*C7*, C8	Posterior interosseous	Abductor pollicis longus and brevis
Extension of thumb	C6, C7	Posterior interosseous	Extensor pollicis longus and brevis
Pronation of forearm	C6, C7	Median nerve	Pronator teres
Radial flexion of wrist	C6, C7	Median nerve	Flexor carpi radialis
Flexion of middle phalanges	C7, *C8*, T1	Median nerve	Flexor digitorum superficialis
Flexion of proximal phalanx of thumb	C8, T1	Median nerve	Flexor pollicis brevis

(continued)

*Bold italics indicate major nerve roots involved.

435

TABLE 46-3 *(continued)* Tests of Muscle Action

Action tested	Roots*	Nerves	Principal muscles
Opposition of thumb against fifth finger	C8, *T1*	Median nerve	Opponens pollicis
Extension of middle phalanges of index and middle finger	C8, *T1*	Median nerve	First, second lumbricals
Flexion of terminal phalanx of thumb	*C8*, T1	Anterior interosseous nerve	Flexor pollicis longus
Flexion of terminal phalanx of second and third fingers	*C8*, T1	Anterior interosseous nerve	Flexor digitorum profundus
Flexion of distal phalanges of ring and little fingers	C7, *C8*	Ulnar	Flexor digitorum profundus
Adduction and opposition of fifth finger	C8, *T1*	Ulnar	Hypothenar
Extension of middle phalanges of ring and little fingers	C8, *T1*	Ulnar	Third, fourth lumbricals
Adduction of thumb against index finger	C8, *T1*	Ulnar	Adductor pollicis
Flexion of proximal phalanx of thumb	*C8*, T1	Ulnar	Flexor pollicis brevis
Abduction and adduction of fingers	C8, *T1*	Ulnar	Interossei

Crural

Action tested	Roots*	Nerves	Principal muscles
Hip flexion from semiflexed position	*L1, L2,* L3	Femoral	Iliopsoas
Hip flexion from externally rotated position	L2, L3	Femoral	Sartorius
Extension of knee	L2, *L3,* L4	Femoral	Quadriceps femoris
Adduction of thigh	*L2, L3,* L4	Obturator	Adductor longus, magnus, brevis
Abduction and internal rotation of thigh	*L4, L5,* S1	Superior gluteal	Gluteus medius
Extension of thigh	L5, *S1,* S2	Inferior gluteal	Gluteus maximus
Flexion of knee	L5, *S1,* S2	Sciatic	Biceps femoris, semitendinosus, semimembranosus
Dorsiflexion of foot (medial)	*L4,* L5	Peroneal (deep)	Anterior tibial
Dorsiflexion of toes (proximal and distal phalanges)	*L5,* S1	Peroneal (deep)	Extensor digitorum longus and brevis
Dorsiflexion of great toe	*L5,* S1	Peroneal (deep)	Extensor hallucis longus
Eversion of foot	L5, S1	Peroneal (superficial)	Peroneus longus and brevis
Plantar flexion of foot	*S1,* S2	Tibial	Gastrocnemius, soleus
Inversion of foot	L4, *L5*	Tibial	Tibialis posterior
Flexion of toes (distal phalanges)	L5, *S1, S2*	Tibial	Flexor digitorum longus
Flexion of toes (middle phalanges)	*S1, S2*	Tibial	Flexor digitorum brevis
Flexion of great toe (proximal phalanx)	S1, S2	Tibial	Flexor hallucis brevis
Flexion of great toe (distal phalanx)	L5, *S1, S2*	Tibial	Flexor hallucis longus
Contraction of anal sphincter	S2, S3, S4	Pudendal	Peroneal muscles

*Bold italics indicate major nerve roots involved.

436

The predominantly demyelinative polyneuropathies are few—mainly the acute (GBS) and chronic inflammatory polyneuropathy and a subgroup of hereditary polyneuropathies.

Nerve biopsy is undertaken only when etiologic diagnosis remains in doubt, after clinical and electrodiagnostic studies have been completed. Biopsy can be definitive, however, in certain diseases such as vasculitis and amyloidosis of nerve.

RADICULOPATHY AND POLYRADICULOPATHY

The nerve roots are affected to some extent in most polyneuropathies, but certain diseases have a proclivity to attack the nerves proximally, within the spinal subarachnoid space. Radicular disease is indicated clinically by an asymmetry of weakness, affecting adjacent muscles disparately, and by sensory loss and pain in a root distribution. *Single-root patterns*, usually lumbar or cervical, are most often due to ruptured disc and less often to neurofibroma, herpes zoster, or diabetic infarction. Multiple-root disease may have its origin in a degenerative process of the spine or an infiltration of the meninges by carcinoma, lymphoma, sarcoid, or inflammatory disease. Sometimes no cause can be determined. The CSF is invariably abnormal in root disease, and the EMG shows a pattern of denervation that corresponds to involvement of nerve roots; the main findings are the above-mentioned abnormalities of late responses and sparing of the sensory potentials in affected regions because the nerve lesion is proximal to the dorsal root ganglion.

MONONEUROPATHIES AND PLEXOPATHIES

Here the diagnosis rests on the finding of motor, reflex, or sensory changes confined to the territory of a single nerve (or a plexus of nerves) and the presence of other data pointing to the cause. Table 46-2 lists the most frequent entities that make up this category of peripheral nerve disease. Table 46-3 provides a somewhat different perspective—namely, a listing of particular muscle actions, the principal muscles involved in these actions, and their radicular and peripheral innervation.

For a more detailed discussion of this topic, see Victor and Ropper: *Adams and Victor's Principles of Neurology*, 7th ed, pp 1370–1445.

ADDITIONAL READING

Asbury AK, Arnason BGW, Adams RD: The inflammatory lesion in acute idiopathic polyneuritis. *Medicine* 48:173, 1969.

Asbury A, Thomas PK: *Peripheral Nerve Disorders*, 2nd ed. London, Butterworth & Heinemann, 1995.

Dalmau J, Graus F, Rosenbaum MK, Posner JB: Anti-Hu–associated paraneoplastic encephalomyelitis/sensory neuropathy: A clinical study of 71 patients. *Medicine* 71:59, 1992.

Dawson DM, Hallett M, Wilbourn AJ: *Entrapment Neuropathies*, 3rd ed. Philadelphia, Lippincott-Raven, 1999.

Dyck PJ, Thomas PK, et al (eds): *Peripheral Neuropathy*, 3rd ed. Philadelphia, Saunders, 1993.

Feasby TE, Gilbert JJ, Brown WF, et al: An acute axonal form of Guillain-Barré polyneuropathy. *Brain* 109:1115, 1986.

Gorson KC, Allam G, Ropper AH: Chronic inflammatory demyelinating polyneuropathy: Clinical features and response to treatment in 67 consecutive patients with and without monoclonal gammopathy. *Neurology* 48:321, 1997.

Guarantors of Brain: *Aids to the Examination of the Peripheral Nervous System*. London, Baillière-Tindall, 1986.

Henson RA, Urich H: *Cancer and the Nervous System*. Oxford, UK, Blackwell, 1982, pp 368–405.

Kissel JT: Vasculitis of the peripheral nervous system. *Semin Neurol* 14:361, 1994.

Layzer RB: *Neuromuscular Manifestations of Systemic Disease: Contemporary Neurology Series*, vol 25. Philadelphia, Davis, 1984.

Ropper AH, Wijdicks EFM, Truax BT: *Guillain-Barré Syndrome*. Philadelphia, Davis, 1991.

Schaumburg HH, Berger AR, Thomas PK: *Disorders of Peripheral Nerves*, 2nd ed. Philadelphia, Davis, 1992.

Zochodne DW, Bolton CF, Wells GA: Critical illness polyneuropathy: A complication of sepsis and multiple organ failure. *Brain* 110:819, 1987.

47 | Diseases of the Cranial Nerves

The effects of lesions of the olfactory, optic, oculomotor, cochlear, and vestibular nerves have already been described in Chaps. 12 through 15, and certain facial pain syndromes referable to the trigeminal and oculomotor nerves were commented upon in Chap. 10. In this chapter we describe the main disorders of the fifth, seventh, and lower (IX to XII) cranial nerves.

Fifth, or Trigeminal, Nerve

Owing to the wide anatomic distribution of this nerve, complete ablation of both its sensory and motor functions is rarely observed. However, branch lesions, with pain and sensory loss, are common.

Trigeminal neuralgia (tic douloureux) This is the most frequent disorder of the fifth nerve. The idiopathic form occurs mainly in the elderly but also in middle age. It consists of brief paroxysms of stabbing pain in the distribution of the mandibular or maxillary divisions of the nerve; this is so intense that it causes the patient to wince (hence the term *tic*). The paroxysms recur frequently for weeks on end. A characteristic feature of the pain is its initiation by even trivial tactile stimuli to "trigger zones"—face, lips, or gums—or by movement of these parts in chewing, talking, shaving, etc. As a rule, the pain is unaccompanied by sensory loss. The cause of this condition is still unsettled, though the trigeminal nerve root is sometimes found to be compressed by a small tortuous branch of the basilar artery.

Most patients respond favorably to the administration of carbamazepine (Tegretol), which either suppresses the attack or shortens its duration and permits a spontaneous remission to occur; phenytoin, gabapentin, clonazepam, or baclofen may be similarly useful in patients who cannot tolerate carbamazepine. These drugs are administered in the same dosages and with the same precautions as in epilepsy. Severe, intractable pain requires surgery; sterotactically controlled thermocoagulation of the trigeminal ganglion or roots using a radiofrequency generator is a popular procedure, but many neurosurgeons now favor a posterior craniotomy and separation of the trigeminal root from an apposed blood vessel, a procedure that is reported to relieve the pain in more than 80 percent of cases.

Idiopathic trigeminal neuralgia needs to be distinguished from *symptomatic trigeminal neuralgia*, in which paroxysmal facial pain is a manifestation of some other neurologic disease. In this symptomatic type, the neuralgia is usually accompanied by variable degrees of sensory loss and weakness of the muscles of mastication (if the motor division is involved). Branches of the fifth nerve may be compressed by a cerebellopontine angle tumor or by an aneurysm of the basilar or posterior cerebellar artery. A discrete area of infarction or demyelination (multiple sclerosis) at the sensory root entry zone in the pons may give rise to typical tic douloureux; this is a common cause of tic in young women. Trauma (blows to the face) may damage branches of the trigeminal nerve, especially those above and below the orbit. Among inflammatory lesions, *herpes zoster* is the most frequent. Middle ear infections and petrositis may involve the gasserian ganglion and root and also implicate the sixth cranial nerve (Gradenigo syndrome). This and other combined cranial nerve disorders are summarized in Tables 47-1 and 47-2.

Cases of acute or chronic *trigeminal sensory neuropathy*, affecting one or both sides of the face and causing numbness and sometimes pain, are infrequent but well documented. Neoplastic compression and infiltration of branches of the trigeminal nerve is a known metastatic complication of carcinoma of the breast and prostate and of multiple myeloma. The mental nerve is often implicated, causing a patch of sensory loss on the chin. Autoimmune processes such as scleroderma, mixed connective tissue disease, and lupus erythematosus are also known to be causative and tend to involve more than one division of the nerve. In some cases, no cause can be determined. Even less common is a pure trigeminal motor neuropathy; the prognosis for recovery from this disorder is good.

Seventh, or Facial, Nerve

Bell's palsy This is the most common disorder of the facial nerve (annual incidence rate of 23 per 100,000). Formerly considered to be idiopathic, it is now apparent that infection with herpes simplex virus type I may be the cause of most instances of Bell's palsy, which raises the possibility that other viruses and inflammatory processes will be found in the remaining cases. It affects men and women equally and occurs at all ages and at all times of the year. The onset is acute, attaining maximum severity in a few hours or a few days; often it is preceded for a day or two by pain behind the ear.

All the muscles of facial expression on one side are weakened or paralyzed. The eyelids cannot be closed, the corner of the mouth droops, and the forehead does not wrinkle. There is no demonstrable sensory loss, though the affected side of the face may feel "heavy" or otherwise unnatural, a symptom that patients may describe as numbness. Taste will be lost on the anterior two-thirds of the tongue if the lesion involves the facial nerve proximal to the point where it is joined by the chorda tympani. Hyperacusis or distortion of sound indicates involvement of the nerve to the stapedius muscle.

The pathologic changes have not been studied carefully, but the nerve is manifestly swollen and often enhances with gadolinium in magnetic resonance (MR) images of the petrous bone.

About 80 percent of patients recover within several weeks or months. Incomplete paralysis in the first 5 to 7 days is a favorable prognostic sign. Complete and persistent paralysis, indicating structural interruption of nerve fibers, is predictive of a long delay in the onset of recovery (up to 3 months). Recovery in such cases is by regeneration, which may take as long as 2 years and is often incomplete and associated with spasms and contractures of facial muscles and signs of aberrant regeneration of nerve fibers ("crocodile tears," "jaw winking," dyskinesias).

The administration of corticosteroids during the first week is said to speed recovery. Antiviral drugs have been shown in some but not all

TABLE 47-1 Syndromes Involving Cranial Nerves Outside the Brainstem

Site	Cranial nerves involved	Eponymic syndrome	Usual causes*
Sphenoidal fissure	III, IV, ophthalmic V, VI	Foix	Invasive tumors of sphenoid bone, aneurysms
Lateral wall of cavernous sinus	III, IV, ophthalmic (occasionally maxillary) V, VI	Tolosa-Hunt, Foix	Aneurysms or thrombosis of cavernous sinus; invasive tumors from sinuses and sella turcica; sometimes recurrent, benign granulomatous reactions, responsive to steroids
Retrosphenoidal space	II, III, IV, V, VI	Jacod	Large tumors of middle cranial fossa
Apex of petrous bone	V, VI	Gradenigo	Petrositis, tumors of petrous bone
Internal auditory meatus	VII, VIII	—	Acoustic neuroma, tumors of petrous bone (dermoids, etc.)
Pontcerebellar angle	V, VII, VIII, and sometimes IX		Acoustic neuromas, meningiomas
Jugular foramen	IX, X, XI	Vernet	Tumors and aneurysms
Posterior laterocondylar space	IX, X, XI, XII	Collet-Sicard	Tumors of parotid gland and carotid body; primary and metastatic lymph node tumors; tuberculous adenitis, carotid dissection
Posterior retroparotid space	IX, X, XI, XII, and sympathetics (Horner syndrome)	Villaret, Mackenzie	Same as above, and granulomatous lesions (sarcoid, fungi), chordoma
Posterior retroparotid space	X and XII, with or without XI	Tapia	Parotid and other tumors of, or injuries to, or surgery of, the high neck (including carotid endarterectomy)

*Metastatic tumors are possible causes of most of these syndromes.

TABLE 47-2 Intrinsic Brainstem Syndromes Involving Cranial Nerves

Cranial nerves involved	Site	Eponymic syndrome	Tracts and nuclei involved	Signs	Usual causes
III	Base of midbrain	Weber	Corticospinal tract	Oculomotor palsy with crossed hemiplegia	Infarction, tumor
III	Tegmentum of midbrain	Claude	Red nucleus and brachium conjunctivum	Oculomotor palsy with contralateral cerebellar ataxia and tremor	Infarction, tumor
III	Tegmentum of midbrain	Benedikt	Red nucleus, corticospinal tract, and brachium conjunctivum	Oculomotor palsy with contralateral cerebellar ataxia, tremor, and corticospinal signs	Infarction, hemorrhage, tumor
Unilateral or bilateral III	Tectum of midbrain	Nothnagel	Superior cerebellar peduncles	Ocular palsies, paralysis of gaze, and cerebellar ataxia	Tumor, infarction
	Dorsal midbrain	Parinaud	Supranuclear mechanism for upward gaze and other structures in periaqueductal gray matter	Paralysis of upward gaze and accommodation; fixed pupils	Pinealoma, hydrocephalus and other lesions of dorsal midbrain
VII and often VI	Tegmentum and base of pons	Millard-Gubler and Raymond-Foville	Corticospinal tract	Facial and abducens palsy and contralateral hemiplegia; sometimes gaze palsy to side of lesion	Infarction or tumor
X	Tegmentum of medulla	Avellis	Spinothalamic tract; sometimes descending sympathetic fibers, with Horner syndrome	Paralysis of soft palate and vocal cord and contralateral hemianesthesia	Infarction or tumor
X, XII	Tegmentum of medulla	Jackson	Corticospinal tract	Avellis syndrome plus ipsilateral tongue paralysis	Infarction or tumor
Spinal V, IX, X	Lateral tegmentum of medulla	Wallenberg	Vestibular nuclei, lateral spinothalamic tract, descending pupillodilator fibers, spinocerebellar and olivocerebellar tracts, medial longitudinal fasciculus	Nystagmus, ipsilateral V, IX, X, XI palsy, Horner syndrome and cerebellar ataxia; contralateral loss of pain and temperature sense, ipsilateral central facial analgesia, INO*	Occlusion of vertebral or posteroinferior cerebellar artery

*Internuclear ophthalmoplegia.

442

studies to speed recovery. The cornea should be protected with artificial tears or ointment and a patch until recovery allows closure of the lids.

Other causes of facial palsy These are considerably less common than Bell's palsy and are listed below. Descriptions of their characteristic features should be sought in *Adams and Victor's Principles of Neurology*, 7th ed., or other neurology texts.

Lyme disease: This is a cause of facial palsy, often bilateral, in endemic areas and after known tick bite or erythema chronicum migrans.

HIV infection: This virus, even without the manifestations of AIDS, has emerged as a cause of unilateral or bilateral Bell's palsy in the affected population.

Sarcoidosis: The granulomas of sarcoid have a proclivity to affect the seventh nerve more than any other cranial nerve. It is a common cause of alternating or sequential facial palsies. An acute syndrome of fever, enlargement of the parotid gland, and uveitis (Heerfordt syndrome) is a rare but characteristic presentation of sarcoidosis.

Compression of facial nerve by tumor: Schwannoma, meningioma, cholesteatoma, dermoid, carotid body tumor, and mixed tumor of the parotid are the usual ones involved.

Herpes zoster: Inflammation of facial nerve and geniculate ganglion and contiguous ganglia with vesicles on the concha or in the external auditory canal is the usual presentation of this (Ramsay Hunt) syndrome.

Facial diplegia: This is most often due to Guillain-Barré polyneuritis and less often to sarcoid (uveoparotid fever, or Heerfordt syndrome, see above) and Lyme disease.

Melkersson-Rosenthal syndrome: This is a rare disorder of unknown cause characterized by recurrent facial palsy, labial edema, and plication of tongue.

Facial palsy with pontine lesions: These disorders must be distinguished from supranuclear facial weakness. Infarcts, tumors, demyelinative lesions are the usual causes. An associated gaze palsy or ocular abduction palsy is common.

Hemifacial spasm: This disorder is usually idiopathic or may follow Bell's palsy; it responds to periodic injections of affected muscles with botulinus toxin and, in many instances, to intracranial decompression of the nerve root from an adjacent small blood vessel.

Congenital facial palsy: This condition is due to birth trauma or to Möbius syndrome (congenital facial palsy with abducens or horizontal gaze palsy); the latter may be bilateral.

Hemiatrophy of Romberg (pseudofacial palsy): This is a rare one-sided facial lipodystrophy without muscle weakness of unknown cause.

Ninth, or Glossopharyngeal, Nerve

This nerve is seldom affected separately, except possibly in *glossopharyngeal neuralgia*, which consists of severe paroxysmal pain that originates in the tonsillar fossa and is provoked mainly by swallowing but also by talking, chewing, etc. The pain may be localized to the ear or radiate from throat to ear, implicating the auricular branch of the vagus (hence, *vagoglossopharyngeal neuralgia*). Occasionally the pain activates afferent fibers in the ninth nerve, which in turn stimulate brainstem vasomotor mechanisms and induce bradycardia and vasodepressor syncope. The condition should be treated like trigeminal neuralgia—i.e., with carbamazepine or other antiepileptic drugs. If this is unsuccessful, the glossopharyngeal nerve and upper rootlets of the vagus can be interrupted surgically.

More often, cranial nerve IX is compressed together with nerves X and XI by a tumor (neurofibroma, meningioma, plasmacytoma, metastatic cancer, carotid dissection) at the jugular foramen. Then there is hoarseness, difficulty in swallowing, deviation of the soft palate to the sound side (weakness of the stylopharyngeus muscle), anesthesia of the posterior wall of the pharynx, and weakness of the upper trapezius and sternomastoid muscles (see Table 47-1). The causative process is often visible with magnetic resonance imaging (MRI).

The Tenth, or Vagus, Nerve

Complete interruption of one vagus nerve intracranially results in ipsilateral weakness of the soft palate, deviation of the uvula to the normal side, unilateral loss of the gag reflex, hoarse voice and immobile vocal cord on one side, and loss of sensation in the pharynx, external auditory meatus, and back of the pinna. The vagus nerve on one side may be implicated at the meningeal level by tumors, granulomatous disease, and infective processes and within the medulla by vascular lesions (Wallenberg syndrome), by motor system disease, and occasionally by herpes zoster. It may be injured with the other lower cranial nerve by a number of processes including carotid artery dissection.

The left recurrent laryngeal nerve has a longer course in the mediastinum than the right, hooking under the aortic arch, where it may be compressed by an aneurysm of the aorta or a mediastinal or lung tumor. There is no dysphagia with such lesions because the branches to the pharynx leave the vagus nerve more proximally; only the vocal cord is paralyzed. Bilateral vagal lesions occur in some cases of Chiari malformation and syringomyelia (defects on phonation and laryngeal stridor) and Shy-Drager syndrome (multiple system atrophy) and in rare instances of familial hypertrophic and advanced alcoholic-nutritional polyneuropathy. Bilateral destruction of the nucleus ambiguus (motor system disease, poliomyelitis) is probably fatal.

The Eleventh, or Accessory, Nerve

This nerve has two parts: a major spinal one, derived from the anterior horn cells of the upper cervical cord, and a minor medullary one, which issues with the lower bundles of the vagus (vagal-accessory nerve); the latter branch joins the spinal root as it courses through the foramen magnum to exit in the jugular foramen. A complete lesion paralyzes the sternocleidomastoid and upper part of the trapezius muscles. Motor system disease, poliomyelitis, syringobulbia, and Chiari malformation are well-documented causes. Intracranially or extracranially, where it leaves the skull, the eleventh nerve may be affected with cranial nerves IX and X and sometimes with XII (see Table 47-1). An idiopathic accessory nerve palsy akin to Bell's palsy is also a known entity. Polymyositis may affect the trapezius and sternomastoid muscles bilaterally as well as the muscles of the pharynx and larynx and needs to be distinguished from bilateral eleventh-nerve lesions.

Hypoglossal Nerve

Lesions involving only the twelfth nerve are rare. It may be compressed by metastatic or meningeal tumor at or near the hypoglossal foramen, by the bony overgrowth of Paget disease of the clivus, or by a dissection of the carotid artery or in the course of carotid endarterectomy. Complete interruption causes unilateral weakness and atrophy of the tongue, with fasciculations. On protrusion, the tongue deviates to the affected side. Intramedullary lesions—those due to vertebral and anterior spinal artery thrombosis—simultaneously affect the pyramid, medial lemniscus, and hypoglossal nerve; the result is paralysis and atrophy of one side of the tongue together with spastic weakness and loss of deep sensation in the opposite arm and leg.

Multiple Cranial Nerve Palsies

Involvement of multiple cranial nerves may be due to intracranial leptomeningeal carcinomatosis, tumors and granulomas (tuberculous or sarcoid), or lesions of the brainstem (infarcts, tumors, hemorrhages), in which case cranial nerve and long tract signs are conjoined. The extramedullary cranial nerve syndromes are listed in Table 47-1, and the intrinsic brainstem syndromes in Table 47-2.

For a more detailed discussion of this topic, see Victor and Ropper: *Adams and Victor's Principles of Neurology*, 7th ed, pp 1446–1463.

ADDITIONAL READING

Devinsky O, Feldmann E: *Examination of the Cranial and Peripheral Nerves.* New York, Churchill Livingstone, 1988.

Hughes RAC: Diseases of the fifth cranial nerve, in Dyck PJ, Thomas PK, Lambert EH, et al (eds): *Peripheral Neuropathy*, 3rd ed. Philadelphia, Saunders, 1993, pp 801–817.

Jannetta PJ: Posterior fossa neurovascular compression syndrome other than neuralgias, in Wilkins RH, Rengachary SS (eds): *Neurosurgery*. New York, McGraw-Hill, 1985, pp 1901–1906.

Juncos JL, Beal MF: Idiopathic cranial polyneuropathy. *Brain* 110:197, 1987.

Karnes WE: Diseases of the seventh cranial nerve, in Dyck PJ, Thomas PK, Lambert EH, et al (eds): *Peripheral Neuropathy*, 3rd ed. Philadelphia, Saunders, 1993, pp 818–836.

Keane JR: Bilateral seventh nerve palsy: Analysis of 43 cases and review of the literature. *Neurology* 44:1198, 1994.

Lecky BRF, Hughes RAC, Murray NMF: Trigeminal sensory neuropathy. *Brain* 110:1463, 1987.

Murakami S, Mizobuchi M, Nakashiro Y, et al: Bell palsy and herpes simplex virus: Identification of viral DNA in endoneurial fluid and muscle. *Ann Intern Med* 124:27, 1996.

Silverman JE, Liu GT, Volpe NJ, Galetta SL: The crossed paralyses. *Arch Neurol* 52:635, 1995.

Sweet WH: The treatment of trigeminal neuralgia (tic douloureux). *N Engl J Med* 315:174, 1986.

Whitley RJ, Weiss H, Gnann JW, et al: Acyclovir with and without prednisone for the treatment of herpes zoster: A randomized, placebo-controlled trial. *Ann Intern Med* 125:376, 1996.

The symptoms and signs of diseases of muscle, the diagnostic methods utilized in their detection, and the various means of treating them constitute a branch of medicine known as *clinical myology*.

As one would expect from a tissue of uniform structure and function, the symptoms and signs by which diseases of striated muscle express themselves are also relatively uniform and few in number. Weakness, fatigability, limpness or stiffness, spasm, pain, a muscle mass, or change in muscle volume constitute the clinical manifestations. This explains the fact that many different muscle diseases share certain symptoms and syndromes. It is expedient, therefore, first to discuss the symptoms and signs common to all the diseases of striated muscle and in later chapters to specify those peculiar to certain diseases.

Myopathic Weakness and Fatigue

These two symptoms are often confused. While fatigue is a prominent feature of a few muscle diseases, the complaint of fatigue without demonstrable weakness is far more often indicative of anxiety, depression, or an endocrine or other systemic disease (see Chap. 24). To distinguish between weakness and asthenic fatigue, it is necessary to assess the patient's capacity to walk and climb stairs and to arise from a sitting, kneeling, squatting, or reclining position. Difficulty in performing these tasks, either as a single test of peak power or repeatedly in tests of endurance, signifies weakness rather than fatigue. The same applies to difficulty in working with the arms above shoulder level. The demonstration of normal peak power in the action of a muscle but the inability to sustain it for more than a moment or two is typical of asthenia, or nonmuscular weakness. More localized muscle weakness is manifest by drooping of the eyelids; diplopia and strabismus; changes in facial expression and voice; difficulty in chewing and swallowing, closing the mouth, and pursing the lips; and failure of contraction of single muscles or groups of muscles of the limbs. Of course, impairment of muscle function may be due to a neuropathy or to a central nervous system (CNS) disorder rather than a myopathic one, but usually these conditions can be separated by the methods described further on in this chapter and in Chap. 3.

Ascertaining the pattern of muscle weakness, whether restricted or generalized, and its degree requires the systematic testing of the major muscle groups. The actions of the various muscle groups and their innervation have already been considered in relation to the peripheral nerve diseases (Table 46-3).

Grading of Muscle Weakness

Grading of muscle weakness by using a standard scale permits the accurate recording of the severity of weakness and comparison from one examination to another. The most widely used rating scale recognizes the following grades of muscle strength:

0 = complete paralysis
1 = minimal contraction
2 = active movement with gravity eliminated
3 = weak contraction against gravity
4 = active movement against gravity and resistance
5 = normal strength

Finer degrees of weakness can be denoted by a plus or minus sign; e.g., 4+ would represent barely detectable weakness and 4−, easily detectable weakness. This permits the denomination of 10 gradations of muscle power.

Such tests of peak power require the full cooperation of the patient, and the examiner must watch for signs of lack of effort or a "giving way" quality, which has the same significance. Pain during contraction may also hamper tests of strength (antalgic pseudoparesis).

Topography or Patterns of Muscle Weakness

Seldom is a primary disease of muscle the cause of an acute widespread paralysis; the usual cause of such a syndrome is acute polyneuropathy or some spinal cord disease. Nevertheless, in exceptional circumstances certain myopathic disorders can give rise to a rapidly evolving diffuse weakness: botulinum poisoning and rare instances of myasthenia gravis, hypo- or hyperkalemia, toxic myopathy (statin drugs), and the acute myopathy of critically ill patients that is associated with the combined use of high-dose steroids and neuromuscular blocking agents.

Subacutely evolving weakness (over a period of weeks) is attributable to a much wider spectrum of diseases, including some that are clearly myopathic, such as the infective and idiopathic polymyositides, dermatomyositis, and several of the metabolic myopathies. Again, each of the primary muscle diseases exhibits a *particular pattern of involvement*. That is to say, a given pattern of muscle involvement tends to be similar in all patients with the same disease. Thus, the topography or pattern of muscle affection becomes an important diagnostic attribute of myopathic disease, as indicated in Table 48-1.

Qualitative Changes in Muscle Contractility

Apart from simple weakness and proportionate diminution in tendon reflexes, affected muscles undergo a number of special (qualitative) changes in function, mostly in relation to sustained activity. In myasthenia gravis, sustained or repeated muscle contraction rapidly induces increasing weakness and resting restores power. Thus, upward gaze that is held for 2 to 3 min

TABLE 48-1 Patterns of Weakness in Myopathic and Neuropathic Diseases

Pattern of weakness	Causative diseases
1. Bilateral ocular palsies, strabismus, ptosis, and impaired closure of eyelids—diplopia prominent, pupils spared	Myasthenia gravis; oculopharyngeal dystrophy; exophthalmic ophthalmoplegia of thyroid disease; myotonic dystrophy; progressive external ophthalmoplegia; botulism (autonomic symptoms are added)
2. Bifacial weakness—inability to smile, expose teeth, and close eyelids	Myasthenia gravis; myotonic dystrophy; facioscapulohumeral dystrophy; centronuclear, nemaline, and carnitine myopathies; Guillain-Barré syndrome (GBS); Lyme disease, sarcoid, Möbius syndrome
3. Bulbar palsy—dysphonia, dysarthria, dysphagia, amyotrophy of tongue; weak masseter and facial muscles in some	Myasthenia gravis; progressive bulbar palsy (ALS); myotonic dystrophy; botulism; polymyositis or inclusion body myositis, Chiari malformation, and basilar invagination
4. Cervical muscle palsies—inability to lift head or extend neck	Polymyositis; inclusion body myositis; muscular dystrophy; rarely progressive spinal muscular atrophy (motor system disease)
5. Weakness of respiratory and trunk muscles	Motor system disease; acid maltase deficiency; muscular dystrophy; GBS; myasthenia gravis
6. Bibrachial palsy—dangling arms	Motor system disease (ALS); GBS or porphyria; *not* usually a manifestation of muscle disease except scapulohumeral dystrophy
7. Bicrural palsy	Usually a polyneuropathy or motor system disease
8. Limb-girdle palsies	Polymyositis; congenital myopathies; progressive muscular dystrophy
9. Distal limb palsies—foot drop, steppage gait, wrist drop, weak hands	Distal muscular dystrophies; scapuloperoneal syndromes; Welander-Kugelberg amyotrophy
10. Generalized or universal paralysis	Familial polyneuropathies; chronic nonfamilial polyneuropathies *Episodic:* Hypo- or hyperkalemic paralysis *Persistent:* Werdnig-Hoffmann disease (infants); progressive spinal muscular atrophy (children); rarely advanced dystrophy; GBS (acute)
11. Paralysis of single muscles or groups of muscles	Almost always neuropathic or spinal; sometimes inclusion body myositis

causes progressive ptosis, which is quickly relieved by closing and resting the eyes; diplopia and strabismus increase with persistent horizontal or upward gaze; talking for a few minutes causes progressive dysarthria and nasality of the voice. These phenomena, by themselves, establish the diagnosis of myasthenia gravis.

A state of weakness in which a series of successive contractions actually increase the power of a group of muscles (e.g., abduction of the arm) is diagnostic of the *myasthenic syndrome of Eaton-Lambert*.

A fixed shortening of muscle that follows a series of strong contractions, especially under ischemic conditions (BP cuff on arm), is characteristic of McArdle disease (phosphorylase deficiency). This state, referred to as *true contracture*, needs to be distinguished from cramp and from *pseudocontracture* (myostatic contracture—shortening of muscle and tendon), which occurs whenever muscle is immobilized for a long period in a shortened position (spastic states, polyneuropathy, casting).

Slowness and stiffness of contraction and particularly of release of the handgrip ("milkmaid's grip"), which lessen with each contraction, are typical of *myotonia*; the opposite—increasing slowness and stiffness with each contraction (*paradoxical myotonia*)—occurs in some cases of Eulenburg paramyotonia. Forceful voluntary contraction is necessary to evoke myotonia; thus, the eyelids open immediately after an ordinary blink but not after forceful closure, and the hand opens slowly and stiffly after being firmly fisted. Myotonia is characteristic of myotonic dystrophy, paramyotonia congenita, hyperkalemic periodic paralysis, and congenital myotonia. In these conditions, the phenomenon may also be elicited by a sharp tap on the muscle belly (*percussion myotonia*). By contrast, the *myoedema* of cachexia and hypothyroidism is a localized bulge in muscle that appears at the point struck, without contraction of the entire muscle fascicle.

Myotonia needs to be distinguished from neuromyotonia and related disorders (see p. 487) and from the spreading tautness and gradual failure of relaxation that occur in mild or localized tetanus and in a number of rare illnesses characterized by excessive activity of spinal motor neurons that are mentioned below. In the tetany of hypocalcemia, the muscle, once excited in any way, may remain in spasm (cramp) for a protracted period.

Other Features of Muscle Disease

In addition to weakness, denervation of muscle causes a decrease in muscle tone. Infants with *hypotonia* are said to be "floppy." This is an especially valuable finding in infants with muscular and neuromuscular disease, in whom graded tests of voluntary contraction cannot be performed. Fixed contractures of joints in a neonate, called *arthrogryposis*, is indicative of weakness and immobility of affected joints in utero (see Chap. 52).

Diminution or increase in muscle bulk is another useful index of neuromuscular disease. Extreme atrophy (70 to 80 percent loss of bulk) is a mark of muscle dystrophy or of neural denervation. In the former, the atrophy is due to a reduction in the number of muscle fibers and, in the latter, to a reduction in their size. Lesser degrees of atrophy (20 to 25 percent reduction in volume) result from disuse of muscle from any cause (disuse atrophy). Enlargement of muscle may be the result of persistent overactivity (work hypertrophy) or an early sign of certain dystrophies. Usually the enlargement in dystrophy is due to infiltration of fat cells, leaving the muscle in a weakened condition; this is called *pseudohypertrophy*.

Twitches, spasms, and cramps are other natural phenomena that may assume prominence in certain muscle diseases. Fibrillations and fasciculations are described in Chaps. 3 and 45. Cramps are considered in Chap. 55. Fibrillations are an electromyographic (EMG) change and are due to denervation. Fasciculations and cramps are due to hyperexcitability of intact motor units and, though ordinarily benign, become pronounced and widespread in motor system disease. In the latter condition they are always accompanied by weakness, atrophy, and reflex changes. Disinhibition of the inhibitory motor neurons of the spinal cord gray matter is the basis of the frequent and continuous spasms in tetanus and the "stiff-man" syndrome. *Continuous muscle activity*, wherein parts of many muscles or whole muscles are continually twitching, may be due to excessive irritability of motor units and may also be part of the more generalized twitch-myoclonus-convulsive syndrome of renal failure and hypocalcemia.

Pain is a rare complaint in primary muscle disease. Even polymyositis and dermatomyositis are in most cases painless. The pain that follows intense overactivity of unconditioned muscles is probably due to single-fiber necrosis. However, when aching discomfort, especially after every attempt at exercise, is a major complaint, there may be some subtle disorder of muscle contraction, such as one caused by hypothyroidism or by an enzyme deficiency (e.g., a Ca-ATPase deficiency). More often, when pain is associated with evidence of neuromuscular disease, the lesion involves the nerves or blood vessels within muscles or the connective tissue or periarticular structures (e.g., polymyalgia rheumatica, fasciitis, Guillain-Barré syndrome, Lyme disease). Cramps of whatever cause are painful and leave the muscle tender. Most patients who come to muscle clinics complaining only of fatigue and aching muscles will be found to suffer from neurasthenia and depression, although a state of postviral-infection fatigue and the nebulous chronic fatigue syndrome have also been incriminated.

Lumps in muscle are due to hemorrhage, infarction, tumors, discrete extrusions of muscle through a fascial plane, or tendon rupture with balling up of the muscle. In so-called fibromyalgia or fibromyositis, tender nodular areas can be palpated inconsistently, but biopsy seldom reveals a recognizable abnormality.

Diagnosis of Muscle Disease

The findings described in the preceding pages are of diagnostic importance. When they are considered in relation to the age of the patient at the time of onset, to their mode of evolution and time course of the illness, and to the presence or absence of familial occurrence, they enable one to identify all of the more common diseases of muscle. CK elevation is confirmatory of a primary muscle problem. The EMG is of assistance, particularly in differentiating the denervation atrophies from myopathies. One resorts to biopsy to establish the diagnosis firmly.

The clinical recognition of myopathic diseases is facilitated by a prior knowledge of a few syndromes. A description of these syndromes and the diseases of which they are a manifestation form the content of the chapters that follow (Chaps. 49 to 55).

For a more detailed discussion of this topic, see Victor and Ropper: *Adams and Victor's Principles of Neurology*, 7th ed, pp 1464–1479.

ADDITIONAL READING

Adams RD: Thayer lectures: I. Principles of myopathology. II. Principles of clinical myology. *Johns Hopkins Med J* 131:24, 1972.

Brooke MH: *A Clinician's View of Neuromuscular Diseases*, 2nd ed. Baltimore, Williams & Wilkins, 1986.

Engel AG, Franzini-Armstrong C (eds): *Myology*, 2nd ed. New York, McGraw-Hill, 1994.

Fenichel GM, Cooper DO, Brooke MH (eds): Evaluating muscle strength and function: Proceedings of a workshop, *Muscle Nerve* 13(suppl):S1–57, 1990.

Mastaglia FL, Laing NG: Investigation of muscle disease. *J Neurol Neurosurg Psychiatry* 60:256, 1996.

49 | The Inflammatory Myopathies

Infectious and noninfectious inflammatory diseases of muscle are important causes of myopathic weakness. However, much uncertainty attaches to this category of muscle disease. Etiology and pathogenesis of the more common myositides have not been fully established, and at times even definition remains speculative (as in inclusion body myositis).

Infectious Forms of Polymyositis

Of these, only trichinosis is likely to occur with sufficient frequency to be of concern. Mild infections may pass unnoticed. Muscles can also be affected in the course of toxoplasmosis, cysticercosis, trypanosomiasis, and infection with *Mycoplasma pneumoniae* and certain viruses—group B Coxsackie (pleurodynia or Bornholm disease), influenza, Epstein-Barr (EBV), HIV—but other aspects of these infections are usually far more prominent.

Trichinosis results from the ingestion of undercooked pork containing the encysted larvae of *Trichinella spiralis*. Following an initial gastroenteritis, there may be widespread invasion of skeletal muscles, but weakness is limited mainly to the cranial ones—tongue, masseters, and extraocular and pharyngeal muscles. The involved muscles may be slightly swollen and tender and accompanied by conjunctival injection and orbital and facial edema. Other muscles are tender as well. Rarely, in the acute phase of the disease, there may be cerebral symptoms, probably due to embolism from a trichinal myocarditis.

Eosinophilia is the most helpful laboratory finding, peaking in the third or fourth week after infection. Serum antibodies become evident within 3 to 4 weeks after infection. Muscle biopsy is confirmatory but seldom required. There is usually a moderate rise in CK.

Usually the symptoms subside spontaneously, but in severe cases, thiobendazole, 25 mg/kg bid, and prednisone, 40 to 60 mg daily for 10 to 14 days, are recommended.

Idiopathic Polymyositis and Dermatomyositis

These are common diseases in tertiary referral centers. They involve proximal limb and girdle muscles and, to a lesser degree, those of the neck, pharynx, and larynx. If only muscles are involved, the disease is called polymyositis (PM); if skin and muscle, dermatomyositis (DM). If other connective tissue diseases are associated, the designation is PM or DM with rheumatoid arthritis, lupus erythematosus, scleroderma, or mixed connective tissue disease ("overlap group"), as the case may be.

Clinically, PM presents as a symmetrical weakness of the proximal limb and girdle muscles, developing over weeks to months. It affects persons of both sexes and all ages, the middle-aged and elderly and women somewhat disproportionately. Usually there is no pain, fever, or recognizable initiating event. Weakness of the hip and thigh muscles is expressed by difficulty in climbing stairs and arising from a deep chair or from a kneeling or squatting position. Less often, the shoulder and upper arm muscles are affected first—in which case, working with the arms above the head (combing hair, putting objects on a high shelf) becomes increasingly difficult. Lolling of the head (weakness of posterior neck muscles), dysphagia, and dysphonia occur frequently. The affected muscles are not tender, the tendon reflexes are only slightly reduced, and atrophy is not marked. Restricted forms, affecting only the shoulder or pelvic girdle or causing head drop, are well known. Rarely, in the beginning, the symptoms predominate in one limb. Sometimes the myocardium is affected.

In DM, the skin lesions may precede, accompany, or follow the polymyositis. They vary from a few patches of erythematous or scaling eczematoid dermatitis to a diffuse exfoliative dermatitis or scleroderma. A lilac (heliotrope) discoloration over the bridge of the nose, cheeks, and forehead and around the fingernails and mild periorbital and perioral edema are characteristic.

One-third to one-half of our cases of PM and DM have occurred sometime in the course of a connective tissue disease. And in 8 to 30 percent in different series (more in the older age group), PM, and more often DM, has occurred in association with a malignant tumor (most often of lung and colon in males, breast and ovary in females).

A special form of DM is observed in children, in whom, in addition to involvement of skin and muscle, there is pain, intermittent fever, melena and hematemesis, and sometimes perforation of the gastrointestinal tract due to vasculitis of the bowel. Flexion contractures and subcutaneous calcification occur in the late stages of the disease.

Serum concentrations of CK, transaminase, and aldolase are increased. The sedimentation rate may or may not be elevated. An antibody to RNA synthetase, anti-Jol, is found in up to one-quarter of patients with PM and DM and is specific to these diseases. Tests of rheumatoid factor and antinuclear antibodies are positive in fewer than half of the cases. Eosinophilia and neutrophilic leukocytosis are usually absent. The electromyogram (EMG) shows myopathic changes in 85 percent, but there are also fibrillation potentials reflecting damage to the terminal motor axon twigs. One should keep in mind that cancer may be present and an appropriate evaluation should be considered, although routine studies often fail to detect it for some time.

Pathologic findings Muscle biopsy in PM discloses widespread infiltrates of lymphocytes, mononuclear cells, and plasma cells and scattered muscle fibers undergoing necrosis and regeneration. Perivascular lymphocytes are mostly B cells, and those around necrotic fibers, T cells. Because of the limitations of biopsy sampling, the observed proportions of inflammation and necrosis vary widely. DM is characterized by a number of additional changes (degeneration and atrophy of perifascicular muscle fibers and tubular aggregates in endothelial cells). In *childhood DM*, vasculitis and occlusion of intramuscular vessels by fibrin thrombi are prominent changes, accounting for zones of muscle infarction.

As to *pathogenesis*, there is considerable evidence that an autoimmune mechanism is operative—predominantly a humoral response directed against intramuscular vessels in DM and a T cell–mediated attack on the muscle fiber in PM (see *Myology* in the list at the end of this chapter for details).

Treatment The following regimen for PM and DM has been adopted in most centers: *Prednisone* is given in doses of 60 mg daily. Once recovery begins, as judged by an increase in muscle power and a decrease in serum CK, the dose is reduced in increments of 5 mg every 2 to 3 weeks. When prednisone has been reduced to 20 mg daily, administration of 40 mg every other day is preferred. A dose of 7.5 to 20 mg/day needs to be continued for 6 to 12 months or longer. If relapse occurs, the dose is again increased.

In patients who do not respond to steroids alone, *methotrexate*, 25 to 30 mg IV each week, or oral *azathioprine*, 150 to 300 mg/day combined with a low dose of prednisone, may be successful. The latter combination may be given as the initial treatment, the advantage being that a lower dose of steroids can be used. Plasmapheresis or IV immune globulin often prove effective for a brief period. *Physiotherapy*—in the form of gentle massage, passive movement, and stretching of muscles—is useful in preventing fibrous contractures.

With treatment prognosis is favorable except in those with malignant tumors. Approximately 20 percent of our patients have recovered completely. Most of the others experience improvement and are more or less functional but may need continuous therapy.

Inclusion Body Myositis (IBM)

This is a special type of degenerative and inflammatory muscle disease of unknown cause. It is characterized by an increased incidence in males, a disproportionate weakness of the distal limb muscles—often of single muscles such as quadriceps and forearm muscles (particularly the finger flexors), rarity of dysphagia, and a lack of response to corticosteroids. Practically all instances of this disease are sporadic, but inherited forms (usually autosomal recessive) have been reported.

The serum CK is usually elevated to levels lower than typical for PM and DM; approximately 20 percent of patients have normal values. The muscle biopsy findings are distinctive: intranuclear and intracytoplasmic inclusions, composed of masses of filaments and subsarcolemmal whorls of membranes, combined with fiber necrosis, mild cellular infiltrates, and signs of regeneration. The responsible gene for the rare hereditary form has been mapped to chromosome 9. Whether this hereditary myopathy is truly a form of IBM or represents an as yet undefined myopathy has not been established. The *treatment* for inclusion body myopathy is far less satisfactory than that for PM and DM. Corticosteroids, plasma exchange, and immune globulin are usually tried but with limited effect. Indeed, this disease should be suspected in cases of apparent PM that are resistant to corticosteroids.

Necrotizing Polymyopathy (Rhabdomyolysis) and Myoglobinuria

Any disease that results in rapid destruction of muscle tissue may cause myoglobin to enter the bloodstream and discolor the urine. It may be detected with a "dipstick" of the type that is usually used to detect occult blood in the urine. The muscles become painful, tender, and weak, and serum CK is greatly elevated. In most cases, recovery occurs spontaneously within a few days or weeks, but severe degrees of myoglobinuria may damage the kidneys and lead to acute renal tubular damage.

The following conditions may give rise to rhabdomyolysis and myoglobinuria:

1. Extensive crushing, compression, or infarction of muscle.
2. Excessive use of certain muscles, especially those in the tight pretibial compartment. Infarction of muscles within tight fascial compartments, as occurs occasionally in diabetics, does the same.
3. PM and DM when necrosis is exceptionally severe.
4. *Alcoholism* is a common cause of rhabdomyolysis. It is described in Chap. 51, with the other toxic myopathies.
5. Ingestion of drugs, especially the "statin" group of cholesterol-lowering agents, AZT, toxins such as are contained in poisoned fish, and particularly *alcohol* in some people (see below and Chap. 51).
6. Several *hereditary disorders of muscle glycolysis* have been incriminated, all of them rare: myophosphorylase deficiency (McArdle disease), phosphofructose kinase deficiency (Tarui disease), lipid storage myopathy, palmitoyl transferase deficiency, and phosphoglycerate kinase deficiency. The first two of these diseases have other myopathic features, tabulated in Chap. 51; the others are so rare that the reader should turn to textbooks on myology for details.
7. *Paroxysmal myoglobinuria* (Meyer-Betz and related diseases), a recurrent disorder in families with or without chronic myopathy or dystrophy. Usually the episodes of myoglobinuria occur under conditions of intense physical activity, often associated with infection or fasting.
8. *Malignant hyperthermia* is essentially an accident of anesthesia in patients with an inherited (autosomal dominant) metabolic muscle defect that renders them sensitive to certain agents, particularly the volatile anesthetics and succinylcholine. A sudden stiffening of the masseters and other muscles and severe hyperthermia (up to 42° to 43°C), with circulatory collapse and failure of brainstem reflexes, are the main clinical features. Unless the anesthesia is discontinued and the body cooled, patients may die. Dantrolene given intravenously may be lifesaving. There is widespread muscle fiber necrosis and a dramatic rise in serum CK (see p. 484 for further discussion). The *neuroleptic malignant syndrome* (Chaps. 43 and 58) has many similar features.
9. *Critical illness myopathy* is discussed on p. 466 with the corticosteroid-induced myopathies, to which it has a close relationship.

For a more detailed discussion of this topic, see Victor and Ropper: *Adams and Victor's Principles of Neurology*, 7th ed, pp 1480–1492.

ADDITIONAL READING

Banker BQ, Victor M: Dermatomyositis (systemic angiopathy) of childhood. *Medicine* 45:261, 1966.

Dalakas MC: Polymyositis, dermatomyositis, and inclusion-body myopathy. *N Engl J Med* 325:1487, 1991.

Dalakas MC: Progress in inflammatory myopathies: Good but not good enough. *J Neurol Neurosurg Psychiatry* 70:569, 2001.

Engel AG, Hohlfeld R, Banker BQ: The polymyositis and dermatomyositis syndromes, in Engel AG, Franzini-Armstrong C (eds): *Myology*, 2nd ed. New York, McGraw-Hill, 1994, pp 1335–1383.

Garlepp MJ, Mastaglia FL: Inclusion body myositis. *J Neurol Neurosurg Psychiatry* 60:251, 1996.

Mikol J, Engel AG: Inclusion body myositis, in Engel AG, Franzini-Armstrong C (eds): *Myology*, 2nd ed. New York, McGraw-Hill, 1994, pp 1384–1398.

Sigurgeirsson B, Lindelof B, Edhag O, Allander E: Risk of cancer in patients with dermatomyositis or polymyositis. *N Engl J Med* 326:363, 1992.

50 | The Muscular Dystrophies

The *muscular dystrophies* are progressive, hereditary degenerative diseases of striated muscle. They affect primarily the muscle fibers and leave the spinal motor neurons, muscular nerves, and nerve endings intact. Features common to all of these diseases are the symmetrical distribution of muscle weakness and atrophy in particular patterns, intact sensation, relative preservation of tendon reflexes, and heredofamilial occurrence.

By consensus, a number of other primary degenerative diseases of muscle, traceable either to a hereditary metabolic disorder (e.g., myophosphorylase deficiency) or to a congenital and relatively nonprogressive disorder with distinctive morphologic features (e.g., central-core myotubular, nemaline malformations), are referred to respectively as metabolic and congenital myopathies and considered separately from the dystrophies in Chap. 52.

In Table 50-1 are listed the known types of progressive muscular dystrophy, classified according to conventional clinical categories and patterns of mendelian inheritance as well as to the locus of the abnormal gene and gene product, as far as these are known. Only the most common dystrophies are described below.

Duchenne Muscular Dystrophy (Severe Generalized Muscular Dystrophy of Childhood)

This type of dystrophy begins in early childhood or even in infancy and progresses to complete incapacity and death by early adult life. The incidence ranges from 13 to 33 per 100,000 male births annually. It is inherited as a sex-linked recessive trait and is transmitted to male children by the mother, who is usually asymptomatic but, on careful examination, displays subtle signs of muscle involvement (see below).

The clinical presentation varies somewhat. Most of the boys will have begun to walk or even run before it is noticed that they have trouble climbing stairs and arising from the floor. The pelvifemoral muscles are affected before those of the shoulder girdle. Almost invariably, the calf muscles and sometimes the quadriceps and deltoids are enlarged and firm, but soon they become weaker than normal (pseudohypertrophy). Other muscles of the thighs and pelvic and shoulder girdles undergo early atrophy. Characteristically, the gait is waddling because of weak gluteal support of the hips. The lower back becomes lordotic and the abdomen protuberant; later, weakness of the paravertebral muscles results in kyphoscoliosis (Fig. 50-1). The tendon reflexes diminish in proportion to muscle weakness; Achilles reflexes are usually retained because of the relative escape of calf muscles. The weakness of respiratory muscles and the kyphoscoliotic deformity become a threat to life once the patient becomes bedfast. Some of the patients are slightly mentally impaired. Cardiac muscle is usually involved late in the course of the illness, leading to enlargement of the heart, conduction defects, and congestive failure.

Table 50-1 The Muscular Dystrophies

Disease	Pattern of inheritance	Chromosomal locus	Altered gene product
Duchenne/Becker	Sex-linked recessive	Xp21	Dystrophin
Emery-Dreifuss	Sex-linked recessive	Xq28	Emerin
Myotonic dystrophy (dystrophia myotonica)	Autosomal dominant	19q13.2–19q13.3	Myotonin protein kinase
Proximal myotonic myopathy (PROMM)	Autosomal dominant	—	—
Congenital muscular dystrophy (CMD)			
Classic merosin-positive CMD	Autosomal recessive	—	—
Classic merosin-negative CMD	Autosomal recessive	6q22	Laminin α-2 (merosin)
Fukuyama CMD	Autosomal recessive	9q31–33	—
Walker-Warburg syndrome	Autosomal recessive	9q31–33	—
Muscle-eye-brain disease	Autosomal recessive	—	—
Facioscapulohumeral	Autosomal dominant	4q35	—
Scapuloperoneal	Autosomal dominant	12	—
Limb-girdle muscular dystrophy (LGMD)			
LGMD 1A	Autosomal dominant	5q22.3–5q31.3	—
LGMD 1B (Bethlem myopathy)	Autosomal dominant	21q22.3	—
LGMD 1C	Autosomal dominant	3p25	Caveolin
LGMD 2A	Autosomal recessive	15q15.1–15q21.1	Calcium-activated neutral protease (calpain, or CANP3)

LGMD 2B	Autosomal recessive	2p 13–16	Dysferlin
LGMD 2C (SCARMD)	Autosomal recessive	13q12 (pericentromeric)	γ-Sarcoglycan, 35 kDa
LGMD 2D (SCARMD)	Autosomal recessive	17q12–q21.33	α-Sarcoglycan, 50 kDa (adhalin)
LGMD 2E (SCARMD)	Autosomal recessive	4q12	β-Sarcoglycan, 43 kDa (hetarosin)
LGMD 2F	Autosomal recessive	5q33–34	γ-Sarcoglycan
Distal myopathies			
Late adult type 1 (Welander)	Autosomal dominant	14	—
Late adult type 2 (Marksberry)	Autosomal dominant	—	—
Early adult type 1 (Nonaka)	Autosomal recessive	—	—
Early adult type 2 (Miyoshi)	Autosomal recessive	2p12–14	Dysferlin
Oculopharyngeal	Autosomal dominant	14q11.2–14q13	—

Key: LGMD, limb-girdle muscular dystrophy; SCARMD, severe childhood autosomal recessive muscular dystrophy.

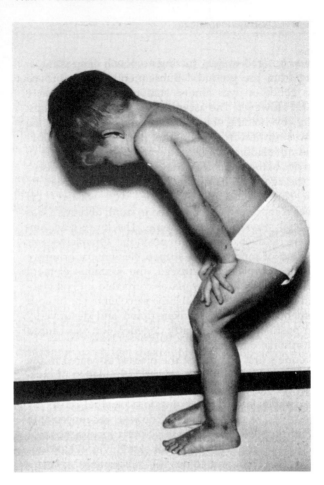

FIG. 50-1 Photograph of a 4-year-old boy with Duchenne dystrophy attempting to extend his hips after rising from the ground. Note hypertrophy of calf and lateral thigh and atrophy of scapular muscles. *(From Engel AG, Yamamoto M, Fischbeck KH: Dystrophinopathies, in Engel AG, Franzini-Armstrong C (eds): Myology, 2nd ed. New York, McGraw-Hill, 1994, p. 1140.)*

Laboratory findings The serum CK concentrations are invariably elevated, and this may precede manifest muscle weakness. The electromyogram (EMG) is myopathic. The female carrier can be identified in almost all cases by a slight enlargement of calf muscles, a mild degree of muscle weakness, elevation of serum CK values, and mild abnormalities in the EMG and muscle biopsy.

Muscle biopsy discloses a loss of muscle fibers in a random distribution (i.e., without respect to motor units) and their replacement by fat cells and fibrous tissue; some of the remaining fibers are hypertrophied. In less affected parts of the muscle, one can observe many contraction bands, indicating irritability of muscle fibers, and single or small groups of fibers in various stages of degeneration and attempted regeneration.

Becker-Type Muscular Dystrophy

This is another form of male sex–linked dystrophy, considerably less common and less severe than the Duchenne type. The incidence rate is 3 to 6 per 100,000. It causes weakness and hypertrophy of the same muscles as are affected in Duchenne dystrophy, but the age at onset is much later (mean age 11 years; range 5 to 45 years), and long survival is the rule. Cardiac and mental disturbances are hardly ever observed.

Etiology of Duchenne-Becker dystrophy An important advance in our understanding of these dystrophies has been the discovery of the abnormal gene that is shared by these two disorders at a specific locus on the short arm of the X chromosome and its protein product. In Duchenne dystrophy, the gene product, called *dystrophin*, is absent; in the Becker type, it is greatly reduced and structurally abnormal. In intermediate phenotypes, the amount of dystrophin in muscle falls between those of the classic types. These findings permit diagnosis by analysis of the patient's DNA and by quantifying the staining of dystrophin in a muscle biopsy.

Unfortunately, these new findings have given no direction to therapy. Early in the course of Duchenne dystrophy, exercise and perhaps the daily administration of prednisone may retard the progress of the disease. Otherwise, only supportive measures such as nighttime mechanical ventilation are helpful. It is desirable to maintain activity for as long as possible.

Emery-Dreifuss Muscular Dystrophy

Another relatively benign sex-linked dystrophy, slightly different in topography and lacking hypertrophy but causing contractures at the elbows and knees, is that described by Emery and Dreifuss. Cardiac involvement (conduction defects and cardiomyopathy) may be severe in this form of dystrophy.

Facioscapulohumeral (Landouzy-Déjerine) Dystrophy

Like that of many dominantly inherited diseases, the onset of this form of dystrophy is during late childhood or adolescence and rarely in early adult life. Usually the first manifestations are difficulty in lifting the arms above the head and winging of the scapulae, although bifacial weakness may have been present since early childhood. The eyelids cannot be closed firmly, and the lips are loosely pursed. The atrophy and weakness affect mainly the muscles of the shoulder girdle (trapezii, pectorals, sternomastoids, serrati, rhomboids) and the proximal arm muscles. The forearm muscles are spared, giving a "Popeye" appearance. As a general rule, pelvifemoral muscles are involved later and to a lesser degree. In one subvariety of this disease, the facial muscles are spared; in another, the pelvic and proximal lower limb muscles are disproportionately involved.

The disease is slowly progressive and may appear to be arrested for long periods; many of the patients therefore attain an advanced age. Cardiac function and mentation are unaffected. Serum CK is slightly elevated and the EMG is myopathic. The gene abnormality has been localized to chromosome 4q.

Restricted Ocular and Oculopharyngeal Myopathies

The best-known form is *progressive external ophthalmoplegia (PEO)*, described in the nineteenth century by Graefe and Fuchs. Conventionally included with the dystrophies, it is now clear that most or all instances are due to a defect in the mitochondrial genome. There is symmetrical paralysis of all the external ocular muscles, usually without diplopia, beginning in childhood and progressing slowly. Paralysis of the levator muscles of the eyelids is an early and troublesome symptom. In middle and late life, other muscles become affected, usually to a slight degree. Inheritance can be autosomal recessive or dominant, but in most instances it is mitochondrial (maternal). The ophthalmoplegia—if combined with retinitis pigmentosa, short stature, elevated cerebrospinal fluid (CSF) protein, and heart-block— is called the *Kearns-Sayre syndrome*, which, like PEO, is essentially a widespread disorder of mitochondria.

Oculopharyngeal dystrophy is inherited as an autosomal dominant trait and is unique in respect to its late onset, usually after 45 years of age, and the restricted muscular weakness, which is *initially manifest as ptosis and dysphagia*. Blepharoplasty and cutting of the cricopharyngeus muscles provide symptomatic relief for variable periods, but progression is inexorable, involving other extraocular muscles and then shoulder and pelvic muscles as well. As in other relatively mild and restricted myopathies, serum CK and aldolase levels are normal, and the EMG is abnormal only in the affected muscles.

Myotonic Dystophy (Steinert Disease)

In this, the most frequent of all types of muscular dystrophy, there are variable degrees of myotonia in association with dystrophic changes in tissue other than skeletal muscle. Slight mental retardation may also be present, and often the heart is affected. A particular type of cortical cataract, frontal balding, and, in the male, hypogonadism are common. The distribution of the muscle weakness and atrophy is unlike that in other dystrophies. The thin, narrow face, temporal atrophy, drooping eyelids, and thin sternomastoid muscles reflect the cranial muscle involvement and, together with the frontal baldness, impart a diagnostic physiognomy. The weak pharyngeal and laryngeal muscles give the voice a soft, monotonous nasal quality. In the limbs, the distal muscles are mainly affected, aligning the condition with the distal dystrophies but differing from them and all the other muscular dystrophies with respect to myotonia. Mild, incomplete forms run in certain families. In general, progression is slow.

A distinctive and potentially lethal form of this disease may be present at birth (*congenital myotonic dystrophy*). The affected parent is almost always the mother, who need not be severely affected but often displays myotonia. The facial and jaw muscles are especially weak. Drooping eyelids, tented upper lip ("carp mouth"), and open jaw allow recognition of the disease in the newborn infant; arthrogryposis may be present. Difficulty in sucking and swallowing, bronchial aspiration, and respiratory distress are present in varying degrees of severity. In surviving infants, delayed motor and speech development and mental retardation are common. The myotonia does not become evident until later in childhood.

The myopathology is characterized by long rows of central sarcolemmal nuclei and sarcoplasmic masses and many circular arrangements of myofibrils in addition to the usual dystrophic changes. Serum CK is slightly elevated. The EMG is diagnostic because of the combination of myopathic changes and myotonic discharges. The mother of an affected infant should be evaluated for the presence of myotonia by EMG examination.

There is no specific treatment. The myotonia can be relieved to some extent by quinine, 0.3 to 0.6 g, or by procainamide, 0.5 to 1.0 g, four times daily. Androgens may offer symptomatic benefit when gonadal deficiency is apparent. Cataracts can be managed surgically. The common complications of all dystrophies—notably fractures, pulmonary infections, and cardiac arrhythmias—need to be treated symptomatically.

The defective gene segregates as a single locus on chromosome 19. This DNA fragment is a CTG trinucleotide repeating segment that may increase in size in successive generations, in parallel with the earlier occurrence and increasing severity of the disease—thus explaining the clinical phenomenon of anticipation. Although there is no specific treatment for myotonic dystrophy, DNA testing makes possible the prenatal recognition of the disease and family counseling.

Other Forms of Muscular Dystrophy

These comprise the limb-girdle dystrophies, late-onset distal dystrophies, and scapuloperoneal and congenital dystrophies of nonmyotonic types. These forms are less common than the ones described above.

The *limb-girdle dystrophies* are characterized by involvement of the shoulder girdle or pelvic girdle musculature or both, beginning in late childhood or early adult life and affecting both sexes. Lacking are the hypertrophy of calves and other muscles and involvement of facial muscles. The status of this group is being steadily eroded; at least nine limb-girdle syndromes have been defined on genetic grounds in the past decade (see Table 50-1). In *scapuloperoneal muscular dystrophy*, there is a distinctive pattern of weakness and wasting involving the muscles of the neck, shoulders, upper arms, and tibial-peroneal compartments; autosomal dominant inheritance is likely. The *distal muscular dystrophies* comprise a group of slowly progressive myopathies involving the distal segments of the limbs and beginning principally in adult life; inheritance may be autosomal recessive or dominant, and the course is relatively benign. *Congenital muscular dystrophy* is defined as a muscle dystrophy already present at birth, often with contractures of the limbs (arthrogryposis) and a wide range of other retinal and central nervous system (CNS) malformations. Comprehensive accounts of these and other dystrophies can be found in *Myology*, 2nd ed., the Engel and Franzini-Armstrong monograph. A recent listing of the diagnostic criteria of all the primary muscle diseases can be found in the monograph published by the European Neuromuscular Centre (Emery).

For a more detailed discussion of this topic, see Victor and Ropper: *Adams and Victor's Principles of Neurology*, 7th ed, pp 1493–1511.

ADDITIONAL READING

Bushby KMD: Making sense of the limb girdle muscular dystrophies. *Brain* 122:1403, 1999.

Emery AEH (ed): *Diagnostic Criteria for Neuromuscular Disorders*, 2nd ed. London, Royal Society of Medicine Press, 1997.

Engel AG, Franzini-Armstrong C (eds): *Myology*, 2nd ed. New York, McGraw-Hill, 1994.

Griggs RC, Mendell JR, Miller RG: *Evaluation and Treatment of Myopathies*. Philadelphia, Davis, 1995.

Harper PS: *Myotonic Dystrophy*. Philadelphia, Saunders, 1979.

Hoffman EP, Fischbeck KH, Brown RH, et al: Characterization of dystrophin in muscle-biopsy specimens from patients with Duchenne's or Becker's muscular dystrophy. *N Engl J Med* 318:1363, 1988.

Rowland LP: Dystrophin: A triumph of reverse genetics and the end of the beginning. *N Engl J Med* 318:1392, 1988.

Victor M, Hayes R, Adams RD: Oculopharyngeal muscular dystrophy: A familial disease of late life characterized by dysphagia and progressive ptosis of the eyelids. *N Engl J Med* 267:1267, 1962.

Walton JN, Karpati G, Hilton-Jones D (eds): *Disorders of Voluntary Muscle*, 6th ed. Edinburgh, Churchill Livingstone, 1994.

51 | The Metabolic and Toxic Myopathies

There are three classes of metabolic-toxic disease of muscle. In one, striated muscle fibers are affected by an endocrine disorder—thyroid, parathyroid, pituitary, or adrenal. In the second, the polymyopathy is based on a primary biochemical abnormality of the muscle cell. A third group is associated with a wide variety of toxins and drugs. The most frequent and representative examples are described here.

ENDOCRINE MYOPATHIES

Thyroid Myopathies

These are (1) chronic thyrotoxic myopathy, (2) exophthalmic ophthalmoplegia (infiltrative ophthalmopathy), (3) hyper- or hypothyroidism with myasthenia gravis, (4) periodic paralysis associated with hyperthyroidism, and (5) muscle hypertrophy and slow muscle contraction and relaxation associated with hypothyroidism.

Thyroxine influences the contractile mechanism of the striated muscle fiber but has no influence on nerve fiber conduction, neuromuscular transmission, or propagation of impulse over the sarcolemma (muscle cell membrane). In *hyperthyroidism*, the duration of the contractile process is somewhat reduced, and the effect is a diminution of muscle power and an increased fatigability. In *hypothyroidism*, the duration of muscle contraction and relaxation is prolonged. The speed of the contractile process is thought to be related to the quantity of myosin ATPase, which is increased in hyperthyroidism and decreased in hypothyroidism. The speed of relaxation depends on the rate of release and reaccumulation of calcium in the sarcoplasmic reticulum.

In *chronic hyperthyroid* or *thyrotoxic myopathy*, there is a progressive weakness and wasting of muscles, particularly those of the thighs (Basedow paraplegia) and shoulders. This may progress to a degree that suggests a diagnosis of motor system disease—especially when tremor and twitching during contraction are prominent. Yet there are no fasciculations at rest, and serum levels of muscle enzymes are not increased. Muscle biopsy discloses slight atrophy of types I and II fiber groups. The electromyogram (EMG) is usually normal. Full recovery follows treatment of the thyrotoxicosis.

In *exophthalmic ophthalmoplegia* (Graves ophthalmoplegia), the eye muscles become thickened and infiltrated by lymphocytes, monocytes, and lipocytes, and many of the muscle fibers degenerate. There is strabismus and diplopia, most prominent on upward gaze, because of disproportionately greater thickening and shortening of the medial and inferior recti. These muscle abnormalities, which can be seen in ultrasonograms or computed tomography (CT) scans of the orbit, are thought to be due to the formation of serum antibodies that react with connective tissue components of eye muscles (glucosaminoglycans). The exophthalmia, which may affect both eyes, sometimes to an unequal degree, is due to thickening of the orbital tissues and needs to be distinguished from tumor and pseudotumor of the orbit.

In hyperthyroidism, an autoimmune disease, there is an increased incidence of *myasthenia gravis*. The latter is the typical autoimmune, prostigmine-responsive form of the disease (Chap. 53). Either the hyperthyroidism or the myasthenia gravis may appear first; each may pursue an independent course and each must be treated separately.

Hypokalemic periodic paralysis, appearing for the first time as the patient develops hyperthyroidism, is particularly frequent among Asians. Correction of the thyroid dysfunction relieves the patient of periodic paralysis as discussed in Chap. 54.

In *hypothyroidism*, *myxedema*, and *cretinism*, the muscles enlarge and movements become slow, stiff, and clumsy. The tongue partakes of the muscle enlargement, resulting in dysarthria. Slowness in the relaxation phase of the tendon reflexes is readily demonstrable, but contraction is slowed as well. Myoedema and spreading myospasm may sometimes be elicited. Serum CK is elevated. Muscle action potentials in the EMG may be myopathic, but the biopsy shows no consistent abnormality.

Corticosteroid Myopathy

Weakness and atrophy of girdle and proximal limb muscles, particularly those of the lower limbs, complicate Cushing disease and the prolonged use of corticosteroids. Climbing stairs, arising from a chair, and using the arms above the shoulders are difficult, and thigh and leg muscles become soft and thin. Yet the serum CK and aldolase levels are normal, and the muscle biopsy discloses only slight thinness and increased variation in size of muscle fibers. Type IIB fibers are the most affected. Discontinuation of steroids or a reduction in their dosage and treatment of the underlying Cushing disease lead to improvement and recovery.

An *acute* and more severe polymyopathy occurs in patients with protracted critical illnesses who have been treated with high doses of corticosteroids (*acute quadriplegic myopathy; critical illness myopathy*). Concurrent use of neuromuscular blocking agents probably contributes to the genesis of this unique myopathy in which myofilaments are destroyed. There is usually an elevation of the serum CK concentration, and the muscle biopsy discloses the characteristic disruption of the thick myosin filaments.

Other Endocrine Myopathies

A proximal myopathy, with weakness and fatigability, is a reported complication of hyperparathyroidism, hypophosphatemia (e.g., induced by hyperalimentation), and the late stages of acromegaly.

PRIMARY METABOLIC MYOPATHIES

Glycogen Storage Myopathies

There are several entities in which glycogen accumulates in muscle fibers and weakens their contractile power. Each is a manifestation of an enzymatic defect that blocks one step in the conversion of intramuscular glycogen to glucose and its further metabolism. Because of the rarity of these diseases, only a tabular summary of their main features is provided (see Table 51-1).

Mitochondrial Myopathies

This interesting group of hereditary myopathies, first recognized in hypotonic infants, has been expanded in recent years to include syndromes that involve the extraocular muscles, retinae, peripheral nerves, brain, and viscera. In the *Kearns-Sayre* syndrome, which is characterized by short stature, weakness of eye muscles, retinitis pigmentosa, cardiomyopathy, and afflictions of other organs, there is a great increase in mitochondria and storage of lipid in muscle fibers. Oxygen transport through the cytochrome oxidative system may be blocked at any of several points in the cycle. In a number of the mitochondrial disorders, muscle biopsies, using the Gomori trichrome stain, show masses of subsarcolemmal mitochondria (appearing as "ragged-red fibers"). Current efforts toward a rational classification of the mitochondrial diseases, based on their genetic and biochemical defects, are summarized in Chap. 38 in *Adams and Victor's Principles of Neurology*, 7th ed., and in the writings of DiMauro and colleagues (see "Additional Reading," below).

MYOPATHIES DUE TO DRUGS AND TOXINS

A vast number of drugs and other chemical agents have been identified as myotoxic. The most important of these are categorized and their main features listed in Table 51-2. The most common causative agents in current practice are the cholesterol-lowering agents ("statins"). If sufficiently severe, virtually all of these intoxications result in myonecrosis (rhabdomyolysis) and myoglobinuria, a subject already considered in Chap. 49. Two other noteworthy conditions characterized by myonecrosis and myoglobinuria are malignant hyperthermia and acute alcohol intoxication.

Alcoholic Myopathy

Alcoholism is complicated by several types of muscle disease. One type is a focal compressive *ischemic myopathy* of buttock, leg, or shoulder muscles, the result of lying on them, when the patient is immobile and insensate for a prolonged period. Severe degrees of hypokalemia (< 2 meq/L), due to diarrhea and vomiting, may develop in the course of a prolonged drinking bout and give rise to a painless and predominantly proximal weakness of limb musculature. Another myopathic syndrome occurs acutely at the height of a prolonged drinking bout and is manifest by severe pain, tenderness, and edema of muscles of the limbs and trunk, accompanied in severe cases by myoglobinuria and renal damage. The muscle affliction may be focal, giving the appearance of a deep venous thrombosis. This syndrome is among the most common forms of rhabdomyolysis seen in a general hospital (the other one being that resulting from the statin drugs mentioned above). Diabetes, by causing muscle infarction, produces a similar syndrome. A short period of fasting after a prolonged period of drinking appears to be the factor that precipitates the myonecrosis. Yet other patients, in the course of a sustained drinking bout, develop muscle cramps and mild diffuse weakness, for which there is no apparent explanation.

The subacute or chronic evolution of painless weakness and atrophy of the proximal muscles of the lower limbs, commonly referred to as "chronic alcoholic myopathy," is probably due to a polyneuropathy.

Table 51-1 The Glycogenoses Affecting Skeletal Muscle*

Glycogenosis type (proper name)	Defective enzyme	Chromosomal locus	Onset of disease†	Hypotonia	Exercise intolerance (myalgia, cramps, stiffness, ±myoglobinuria)	Early fatigue and second wind	Myopathy ±atrophy	Severe respiratory muscle weakness	Contractures	Organomegaly	Myoglobinuria	Positive ischemic exercise test	Enzyme-deficient cells for assay	Membrane-lined vacuoles with glycogen	Increased glycogen in subsarcolemma and intermyofibrillar areas	Intra- and extravacuolar acid phosphatase
II (Pompe)	Acid maltase	17q23	I	+			+	-		+			Muscle, WBC, chorionic villus, amniotic fluid	+	+	+
II	Acid maltase	17q23	C				+	+					Muscle	+	+	+
II	Acid maltase	17q23	A				+	+					Muscle	+	+	+
III (Cori-Forbes)	Debrancher	1p21	C-A	+	+				+	±	+		Muscle, WBC, fibroblasts		+	
IV (Andersen)	Branching		I-C	+			+		+	+			Muscle, WBC, fibroblasts, amniotic fluid		+	+
V (McArdle)	Myophosphorylase	11q13	C, Ad, A		+	+	+		+		+		Muscle, WBC		+	

468

Type	Enzyme	Locus	Types†								Tissue		
VII (Tarui)	Phosphofructo-kinase	1q cent-q32	C-A	+	+	+	+	+		+	Muscle, RBC	+	+
VIII	Phosphorylase B kinase	16q12-q13; 7p12	I, C, Ad, A	+	+	+		+	+	+	Muscle	+	+
IX	Phosphoglycerate kinase	Xq13	I, C-A	+	+	+	+	+	+	+	Muscle, RBC	+	±
X	Phosphoglycerate mutase	7	A	+					+	+	Muscle	+
XI	Lactic dehydrogenase	11	Ad-A	+	+			+	+	+	Muscle	+

*All types: elevated CK; myopathic EMG, with increased irritiability and myotonia.

†I, infancy; C, childhood; Ad, adolescence; A, adult.

Additional features (not charted above): feeding difficulties, II Pompe; retarded growth, III; neurologic abnormalities, II Pompe, IX; hypoglycemic seizures, III; jaundice, VII, IX; cirrhosis, IV; generalized scaling erythema, XI; firm consistency of muscle, II Pompe; elevated serum aspartate aminotransferase and lactic dehydrogenase, II; elevated serum bilirubin, VII, IX; failure of LDH to rise proportionally to elevation of CK, X; fasting hypoglycemia, III; hemolytic anemia and reticulocytosis, VII, IX; hemoglobinuria, IX; excessive rise in serum pyruvates during ischemic exercise test, XI.

Table 51-2 Features of Drug- and Toxin-Induced Myopathies

Myopathic syndrome	Agent	Risk factors
Necrotizing myopathy (rhabdomyolysis)	1. Alcohol abuse 2. Clofibrate, gemfibrozil 3. ε-Aminocaproic acid 4. Lovastatin, pravastatin, simvastatin 5. Hypervitaminosis E 6. Organophosphates 7. Snake venoms 8. High-dose corticosteroids in critical illness 9. Mushroom poisoning (*Amanita phalloides*) 10. Cocaine	1. Cyclosporine/gemfibrozil 2. Renal failure 3. Therapy duration > 4 weeks 5. Uncontrolled self-medication 6. Accidental insecticide exposure
Myoglobinuria	Wide variety of agents	
Steroid myopathy	1. Acute 2. Chronic	High IV steroid doses, ventilated patients on pancuronium 2. Daily prednisone >10 mg
Hypokalemic myopathy	1. Diuretics 2. Laxatives 3. Licorice, carbenoxolone 4. Amphotericin B, toluene 5. Alcohol abuse	Fasting, exercise
Amphiphilic cationic drug myopathy (lysosomal storage "lipidosis")	1. Chloroquine, hydroxychloroquine, quinacrine, plasmocid 2. Amiodarone 3. Perhexiline	1. Daily chloroquine dose > 500 mg
Impaired protein synthesis	Ipecac syrup, emetine	Eating disorders > 600 mg in 10 days
Antimicrotubular myopathy	1. Colchicine 2. Vincristine	1. Chronic renal failure
Inflammatory myopathy	1. D-Penicillamine 2. Procainamide 3. Cimetidine	
Fasciitis, perimyositis, microangiopathy	1. Toxic oil syndrome 2. Eosinophilia-myalgia syndrome	1. Rapeseed oil, Spain, 1981 2. Tryptophan products, 1989
Mitochondrial myopathy	1. Zidovudine 2. Germanium	
Various	1. Cyclosporine 2. Labetalol 3. Anthracycline antibiotics 4. Rifampin, amiodarone	
Myopathy due to IM injections	1. Acute: IM injection of various drugs—e.g., cephalothin, lidocaine, diazepam 2. Chronic: Repeated IM injections—e.g., pethidine, pentazocine, intravenous drug abuse, antibiotics (in children)	 Genetic factor?

*CK (serum creatine kinase): ↑ (mild), ↑ ↑ (moderate), ↑ ↑ ↑ (marked) elevations; myoglobinuria: +/− (may be present).
Adapted from Victor M, Sieb JP: Myopathies due to drugs, toxins, and nutritional deficiency, in Engel AG, Franzini-Armstrong C (eds): *Myology*, 2nd ed. New York, McGraw-Hill, 1994, pp 1697–1725.

Clinical features	Pathology	Laboratory findings*
Acute/subacute painful proximal myopathy; tendon reflexes usually preserved	Necrosis, regeneration	CK ↑ ↑, myoglobinuria +/−
5. Painless	5. Paracrystalline inclusion bodies	
6. Severe, acute intoxication		
	8. Loss of myosin	
Severe muscle pain, swelling flaccid, quadriparesis, areflexia possible, acute renal failure	Severe necrosis, regeneration	CK ↑ ↑ ↑, myoglobinuria + + +
Severe proximal and distal weakness	Types I and II fibers; vacuolar changes, regeneration,	CK ↑ ↑, myoglobinuria +
2. Proximal atrophy, weakness	2. Type II fiber atrophy	Blood lymphocytosis
Weakness may be periodic, reflexes may be depressed or absent, rarely severe myoglobinuria	Necrosis, regeneration, vacuolization	CK ↑ ↑, myoglobinuria +/−, hypokalemia
Proximal muscle pain and weakness, sensorimotor neuropathy, cardiomyopathy	1. Chloroquine: vacuole formation, optically dense structures	CK ↑
Myalgia, proximal weakness, cardiomyopathy	Focal mitochondrial loss, vacuoles	CK ↑
Proximal weakness, peripheral neuropathy; CK may be normal	Vacuolar myopathy (rimmed vacuoles)	CK ↑
Proximal muscle pain, weakness, skin changes possible	Inflammation, necrosis, regeneration	CK ↑, myoglobinuria +/−
Myalgia, skin changes, peripheral neuropathy, other systems also affected	Vasculitis, connective tissue infiltration	Eosinophilia
Proximal myalgia and weakness	1. Ragged-red fibers, necrosis, regeneration	CK normal or ↑
3. Humans: only cardiomyopathy		
Local pain, swelling, sometimes abscess formation	Focal necrosis	CK ↑
Induration and contracture of injected muscles	Marked fibrosis and myopathic changes	Normal

For a more detailed discussion of this topic, see Victor and Ropper: *Adams and Victor's Principles of Neurology*, 7th ed, pp 1512–1528.

ADDITIONAL READING

DiMauro S (ed): Symposium: Mitochondrial encephalomyopathies. *Brain Pathol* 2:111, 1992.

DiMauro S, Tonin P, Servidei S: Metabolic myopathies, in Rowland LP, DiMauro S (eds): *Handbook of Clinical Neurology*, vol 18, rev ed, *Myopathies*. Amsterdam, Elsevier Science, 1992, pp 479–526.

Engel AG, Franzini-Armstrong C (eds): *Myology*, 2nd ed. New York, McGraw-Hill, 1994.

Gorson KC, Ropper AH: Generalized paralysis in the intensive care unit: Emphasis on the complications of neuromuscular blocking agents and corticosteroids. *J Int Care Med* 11:219, 1996.

Haller RG, Drachman DB: Alcoholic rhabdomyolysis: An experimental model in the rat. *Science* 208:412, 1980.

Lacomis D, Giuliani MJ, Van Cott A, Kramer DJ: Acute myopathy of intensive care: Clinical, electromyographic, and pathological aspects. *Ann Neurol* 40:645, 1996.

Layzer RB: *Neuromuscular Manifestations of Systemic Disease*. Philadelphia, Davis, 1985.

Victor M, Sieb JP: Myopathies due to drugs, toxins, and nutritional deficiency, in Engel AG, Franzini-Armstrong C (eds): *Myology*, 2nd ed. New York, McGraw-Hill, 1994, pp 1697–1725.

52 | The Congenital Neuromuscular Disorders

Like all cells and tissues, muscle is subject to complex sequences of growth and development as well as aging. Derangements of these sequences give rise to a number of characteristic neuromuscular disorders, usually at an early age.

NORMAL DEVELOPMENT AND AGING OF MUSCLE

The commonly accepted view of the embryogenesis of muscle, in its briefest form, is that muscle fibers are derived from mesenchymal cells; these cells are transformed into primitive myoblasts, which in turn fuse to form myotubes, and the latter gradually acquire the properties of fully constituted muscle fibers. Each of these steps is under genetic control, as are the varying numbers of fibers that come to constitute each muscle. These numbers vary widely from one person to another, accounting for the variation in size of muscles.

A localized embryologic failure at one point in development may result in the *congenital absence of a muscle*, often occurring in association with aplasia of other tissues (e.g., absence of a pectoral muscle and a mammary gland; agenesis of an abdominal muscle with a defect in the ureters, bladder, or genital organs). Inherent faults in the fine structure of the muscle fiber—such as smallness (hypoplasia), persistence of the myotubular state, central nucleation, or central-core or nemaline body formation—retard the natural growth processes. Defective maturation of motor innervation will also impair the growth of one or another of the muscle fiber types.

Once the full complement of muscle fibers has been reached, presumably by the middle trimester of intrauterine life, the main process then is one of fiber growth (volumetric increase) in each muscle fiber. This follows a predictable time scale up to adult years. At puberty, the growth of certain muscles in the male is greater than in the female.

During late life, there occurs a gradual loss of anterior horn cells, amounting to 30 percent of the lumbar motor neurons between the sixth and ninth decades. This leads to group atrophy, which is observed in 90 percent of gastrocnemii in people more than 60 years of age. In addition, hypotrophy from inactivity (disuse atrophy) and increasing accumulations of lipofuscin and signs of degeneration of single muscle cells are seen. A few of the remaining fibers undergo hypertrophy, so there is greater than normal variation in the fiber size. These aging processes, occurring before their expected time (a kind of presenile polymyopathy), may be part of a generalized organ failure and even contribute to such late-life muscle diseases as oculopharyngeal dystrophy and the late stages of poliomyelitis. This subject is elaborated in *Adams and Victor's Principles of Neurology*, 7th ed.

CONGENITAL FIBROUS CONTRACTURES OF MUSCLES AND JOINT DEFORMITIES

Infants may be born with fixed deformities of discrete parts of the body (e.g., clubfoot or congenital torticollis) or more widespread fixation and deformity of joints (*arthrogryposis*). Sometimes both joints and muscles are affected. The underlying developmental defect may be purely spinal or muscular. If certain groups of anterior horn cells fail to develop or are otherwise developmentally disorganized (as in spinal muscular atrophy), the muscles that they would normally innervate retain their fetal size and are powerless. The unopposed actions of the normally innervated antagonist muscles may then lead to fixed deformities. This is the most common basis of arthrogryposis multiplex, which is often associated with a variety of developmental anomalies of the brain and mental retardation. However, a primary muscular defect, such as the polymyopathies described below and the muscular dystrophies, may have more or less the same effect. Congenital polyneuropathy and Prader-Willi syndrome are other causes, though rare.

THE CONGENITAL POLYMYOPATHIES

In these diseases, which are usually recognized in infancy and early childhood, there is a structural abnormality of muscle from the time of embryogenesis. Their identification has been made possible by the histochemical study of frozen (cryostat) sections of muscle biopsies and by electron microscopy. In most instances, the affected infant shows less than the usual power of muscle contraction, hypotonia (floppiness and lack of resistance to passive movement of the limbs), and delay in the attainment of the milestones of motor development. With growth, there is some improvement, but always a degree of muscular subnormality remains. In many cases, a slight increase in the motor deficit occurs later in life, for unknown reasons. Fiber degeneration is not found by biopsy and the CK levels are usually normal, but the EMG is likely to be myopathic.

The other members of this group of relatively nonprogressive congenital myopathies are central-core myopathy, nemaline myopathy, the mitochondrial myopathies (with "ragged-red fibers"), and other, even rarer types (reducing body, fingerprint, zebra body, sarcotubular). In all these the weakness tends to be proximal in limbs and trunk; eye muscles are involved in central core and mitochondrial myopathies. An account of the distinguishing features of the congenital myopathies, many of them still problematic, cannot be undertaken here. They are considered in detail by Fardeau and Tomé in the Engel and Franzini-Armstrong monograph *Myology*, 2nd ed., and in Emery's monograph (see "Additional Reading," below).

THE SPINAL MUSCULAR ATROPHIES OF INFANCY AND CHILDHOOD

Brief reference to this nonmyopathic group of degenerative anterior horn cell diseases has already been made in relation to the motor system diseases (Chap. 39). A longer description is added here because, with the polymyopathies mentioned above, the spinal muscular atrophies are the main consideration in the diagnosis of the weak or limp infant or child.

The effects of an inherited (usually autosomal recessive) degeneration of anterior horn cells may be apparent at birth (by hypotonicity and occasionally by arthrogryposis) or in the first month or two of life and may terminate life from respiratory failure. More indolent forms express themselves somewhat later in infancy or in early or even late childhood. Progressive enfeeblement of movements of the limb, trunk, and cranial muscles (excepting ocular) interferes with motor development. Tendon reflexes are absent, but sensation, perception, and various cognitive acquisitions remain intact.

In the common early-life, autosomal recessive form of spinal muscular atrophy (*Werdnig-Hoffmann disease*), the child seldom survives more than 2 or 3 years, owing to involvement of the bulbar muscles and resultant dysphagia, inanition, and respiratory insufficiency. Usually such children never attain the capacity to sit, stand, or walk. The EMG reveals fibrillation potentials and reduced numbers of motor units. Serum CK is normal, and the muscle biopsy discloses group atrophy of both fiber types. Some patients, with onset in late infancy or early childhood, may survive to adolescence or to early adult life.

An even milder form of inherited spinal muscular atrophy, in which the onset is between 2 and 17 years and walking is still possible in adult life, was described by Wohlfart and associates and by Kugelberg and Welander (see Chap. 39). These cases and some beginning even later in life affect mainly the proximal muscles or cranial muscles (Fazio-Londe). Yet another form of progressive bulbar and spinal muscular atrophy becomes manifest in the fourth and fifth decades of life (Kennedy syndrome); it is inherited as a sex-linked recessive trait and is associated with testicular atrophy and low androgen levels (page 368).

Only supportive measures are available.

For a more detailed discussion of this topic, see Victor and Ropper: *Adams and Victor's Principles of Neurology*, 7th ed, pp 1529–1535.

ADDITIONAL READING

Banker BQ: Congenital muscular dystrophy, in Engel AG, Franzini-Armstrong C (eds): *Myology*, 2nd ed. New York, McGraw-Hill, 1994, pp 1275–1289.

Byers RK, Banker BQ: Infantile muscular atrophy. *Arch Neurol* 5:140, 1961.

Emery AEH: *Diagnostic Criteria for Neuromuscular Disorders*, 2nd ed. London, Royal Society of Medicine Press, 1997.

Fardeau M, Tomé FMS: Congenital myopathies, in Engel AG, Franzini-Armstrong C (eds): *Myology*, 2nd ed. New York, McGraw-Hill, 1994, pp 1487–1532.

Kakulas BA, Adams RD: *Diseases of Muscle*: The *Pathological Foundations of Clinical Myology*, 4th ed. Philadelphia, Harper & Row, 1985.

Considered in this chapter is a group of diseases in which the fundamental abnormality is one of neuromuscular transmission. The most important member of this group by far is myasthenia gravis. The essential clinical feature of this disease is a fluctuating weakness and fatigability of certain muscles. Usually, some degree of weakness of these muscles is present at all times, but it is worsened strikingly by activity.

MYASTHENIA GRAVIS (MG)

This disease occurs sporadically in people of all ages and both sexes, although the form of the illness in young women differs somewhat from that in older men. Characteristically, the contractile power of affected muscles is easily exhausted by repeated or sustained activity (e.g., drooping of eyelids on upgaze) and is restored by rest, though not to a normal level. As indicated in Chap. 48, the pattern of muscle involvement is unique—the ocular, facial, and bulbar muscles bear the brunt of the disease (hence its old name—myasthenic bulbar paralysis). Drooping of the eyelids, diplopia and strabismus, dysphonia, dysarthria, and dyphagia occur in various combinations. Only in advanced cases are limb and trunk muscles weakened, the proximal limb muscles more than the distal ones. There is no atrophy or loss of tendon reflexes. The onset is usually insidious and progression is subacute, over a period of weeks. The course of the illness varies. In most patients the symptoms resolve to varying degrees with treatment; in a few, however, weakness progresses to the point where the patient is bedfast and in need of respiratory support.

The clinical types of MG vary in respect to the pattern and severity of muscle involvement. The following classification, introduced by Osserman, has proved to be useful in judging the prognosis and in treating the disease.

I. Ocular myasthenia (may persist in isolation in older men)
II. A. Mild generalized myasthenia with slow progression; no crises; responds well to drugs
    B. Moderate generalized myasthenia; severe bulbar and some skeletal involvement, but no crises; response to drugs less than satisfactory
III. Fulminant myasthenia; rapid progression to a state of severe weakness with respiratory crises and poor drug response; high incidence of thymoma; high mortality
IV. Late-onset severe MG; same degree of weakness as III, but with progression over 2 years from class I to II

The close relationship of MG to the thymus gland is another important but incompletely understood feature of the disease. In children, adolescents, and young adults, thymic hyperplasia is usually found. Later in life, 10 percent of patients are found to have a malignant thymoma that may precede the appearance of MG by years.

Not infrequently, the younger myasthenic suffers from some other type of autoimmune disease—thyrotoxicosis, rheumatoid arthritis, lupus erythematosus, or polymyositis. These diseases are also more frequent in first-degree relatives of patients with MG. However, familial occurrence of MG is rare.

The course of the illness is extremely variable. In mild form, it may remain stationary for years. In the early stage of the disease, spontaneous remission and relapse are quite common. A special form of transient MG due to passive transplacental transfer of antibodies and lasting several weeks occurs in infants born of myasthenic mothers (see below).

Pathology and pathogenesis Aside from the thymic pathology, the only definite abnormality is at the neuromuscular junction, where there is a simplification of and reduction in the surface area of the postsynaptic region and a widening of the primary synaptic cleft. The number and size of the presynaptic vesicles and their quanta of acetylcholine (ACh) neurotransmitter are normal. However, on the postsynaptic side of the neuromuscular junction, the number of ACh receptor (AChR) sites is greatly decreased and immune complexes (IgG and complement components) are deposited on the postsynaptic membrane.

Antibodies to AChR protein are found in approximately 85 percent of patients with generalized MG, although the level of serum antibodies does not correlate precisely with the severity of weakness. These antibodies, transferred across the placenta from the myasthenic mother, also account for the transient weakness in infants with transient neonatal MG. Exactly where these antibodies are formed, what stimulates their formation, their relation to the thymus, and how they damage the receptor surface of the end plate are incompletely known.

Diagnosis The electromyogram (EMG) reveals a highly characteristic decrementing response in the amplitude of compound muscle action potentials during 3-per-second nerve stimulation. And in single-fiber EMG recordings, there is an increased variability in the usually precise timing of firing of individual muscle fibers of a motor unit ("jitter") when the muscle is activated. Equally diagnostic is the edrophonium (Tensilon) test. Initially, 2 mg of Tensilon is injected intravenously with 0.6 mg atropine; if this dose is tolerated and no improvement in strength occurs after 45 s, another 4 to 8 mg of edrophonium is given. A positive test consists of an *objective* improvement in muscle contractility, particularly in eyelid, ocular, neck, and respiratory muscles, usually lasting for 4 to 5 min. The combination of clinical findings (particularly the myasthenic fatigue of small cranial muscles and rapid recovery with rest), typical EMG response, positive Tensilon test, and presence of AChR antibodies in the serum leaves little doubt as to the diagnosis.

The failure to find receptor antibodies in apparent instances of MG may be attributable to methodologic deficiencies, or possibly to the presence of an unusual type of antibody, or to an absence of antibodies, as in the nonimmune congenital myasthenic syndromes (see below). Thymic tumors and hyperplastic enlargement of the thymus can be visualized by CT scan or MRI.

Treatment This varies with the severity and pattern of muscle weakness. For patients in class I (see above), anticholinesterase drugs—neostigmine (Prostigmin) and pyridostigmine (Mestinon)—are prescribed. The oral dose of neostigmine varies from 7.5 to 45.0 mg every 2 to 6 h, and the average maintenance dose is 150 mg/day. The doses of pyridostigmine are twice these amounts. Overdosage may cause a *cholinergic crisis* (nausea, vomiting, pallor, sweating, colic, diarrhea, sometimes coupled with increasing weakness); these symptoms should be treated by the slow intravenous injection of atropine sulfate, 1 mg.

Thymectomy is now recommended for all patients with thymic tumors and for all class II and III patients (who will show mainly hyperplasia without tumor). The remission rate in thymectomized patients is about 35 percent, and an equal or larger percentage demonstrate improvement to a variable extent, but the effect is delayed for months or years and generally parallels a fall in antibody levels.

In patients who fail to respond to anticholinesterase drugs and thymectomy, especially elderly patients, corticosteroids are recommended. The usual daily oral dose of prednisone is 40 to 45 mg, or twice this dose every other day. Corticosteroid treatment should generally be initiated in the hospital because a slight exacerbation of myasthenic symptoms is to be expected unless the starting dose is small. Anticholinesterase drugs and potassium supplements are given simultaneously. The dose of steroids is gradually reduced as the patient's condition improves. Azathioprine (Imuran, 150 to 300 mg daily) is a useful adjunct to prednisone and is sometimes effective alone, but its effect becomes evident only after several months. Plasma exchange and intravenous immunoglobulin are reserved for patients with severe MG who do not respond adequately to any of the other methods of therapy and for those with rapid respiratory or bulbar decompensation (myasthenic crisis).

Myasthenic-Myopathic Syndrome of Lambert-Eaton

This is a special form of myasthenia in which the muscles of the shoulders, neck, trunk, and pelvic girdle gradually become weak and easily fatigable. The oculomotor muscles and eyelids are affected far less frequently than in MG, and almost never as an early manifestation. Whereas weakness increases with activity, stamping the condition as myasthenic, there is usually a slight but definite augmentation of power during the first few voluntary contractions. The tendon reflexes are often diminished or absent, raising suspicion of a polyneuropathy. Other symptoms are paresthesias, aching discomfort, and autonomic disturbances such as dryness of the mouth, constipation, impairment of bladder function, and impotence.

The EMG, in contrast to that in MG, records the augmentation in amplitude of action potentials at rapid (10 Hz or higher) rates of nerve stimulation (incrementing response). The basic defect is in the release of quanta of ACh at the *presynaptic* side of end plates, similar to the defect that occurs in botulism. Most cases are associated with an oat-cell carcinoma or other lung tumor, which suggests that the tumor cells elaborate a substance that interferes with ACh release at the neuromuscular junctions and in sympathetic ganglia. Recently this substance was found to be an antibody that alters the presynaptic voltage-sensitive calcium channels. The associated tumors are typically small and sometimes inevident but as many as 25 percent of cases are sporadic, unassociated with malignancy. Removal of the tumor, if found, effects a cure.

Guanidine hydrochloride (20 to 30 mg/kg per day) or the less toxic 3,4-diaminopyridine (20 mg, 5 times per day), in conjunction with pyridostigmine (Mestinon) or prednisone, relieves the symptoms. These drugs have been most effective in nontumoral cases.

Other Myasthenic Syndromes

Several types of congenital and familial nonimmunologic myasthenia, all of them rare, have been described by Engel. A deficiency of pseudo-cholinesterase, either genetic or acquired, may result in prolonged weakness and apnea when succinylcholine or some other depolarizing muscle relaxant is administered in the course of general anesthesia. Aminoglycoside antibiotics and other drugs of similar type may, in some patients, impair release of neurotransmitters by interfering with Ca ion fluxes at nerve terminals. Penicillamine may produce a myasthenic syndrome. These drugs pose a particular danger in patients with MG.

For a more detailed discussion of this topic, see Victor and Ropper: *Adams and Victor's Principles of Neurology*, 7th ed, pp 1536–1552.

ADDITIONAL READING

Drachman DB: Myasthenia gravis. *N Engl J Med* 330:1797, 1994.
Engel AG: Acquired autoimmune myasthenia gravis, in Engel AG, Franzini-Armstrong C (eds): *Myology*, 2nd ed. New York, McGraw-Hill, 1994, pp 1769–1797.
Engel AG: Myasthenic syndromes, in Engel AG, Franzini-Armstrong C (eds): *Myology*, 2nd ed. New York, McGraw-Hill, 1994, pp 1798–1835.
Fink ME: Treatment of the critically ill patient with myasthenia gravis, in Ropper AH (ed): *Neurological and Neurosurgical Intensive Care*, 3rd ed. New York, Raven Press, 1993, pp 351–362.
Vincent A, Palace J, Hilton-Jones D: Myasthenia gravis. *Lancet* 357:2122, 2001.

The Hereditary Myotonias and Periodic Paralyses (Channelopathies)

Grouping of the hereditary nondystrophic myotonias with the periodic, or episodic, paralyses is a new development in the classification of muscle disease. This has come about through the discovery that the diseases in both these categories are caused by gene mutations encoding the calcium, sodium, and chloride channels in muscle fiber membranes. The main features of these *ion channel diseases*, or *channelopathies*, as they are generally called, are summarized in Table 54-1. The more important members of the group are indicated below.

CHLORIDE CHANNEL DISEASES

Myotonia Congenita (Thomsen Disease)

This is a remarkable hereditary disease beginning in early infancy and persisting throughout the patient's lifetime. It is inherited as an autosomal dominant trait. Tonic spasms (*myotonia*) develop after every forceful muscle contraction and are most pronounced after a period of inactivity. Blinking is normal, but a strong voluntary closure of the eyelids initiates a myotonic contraction of the orbicularis oculi that takes seconds to overcome; the same is true in taking the first step after sitting or in making a fist. Repeated contractions of the same muscles alleviate the stiffness; rarely, the converse is observed—i.e., myotonia increasing with each voluntary contraction (myotonia paradoxica). During rest the muscles are soft. In advanced cases, all the musculature is involved. Tapping a muscle with a reflex hammer throws the entire muscle into a contraction that persists for several seconds (percussion myotonia). The muscles may undergo work hypertrophy and reach herculean size.

Microscopic sections of muscle reveal only hypertrophied fibers filled with myofibrillae. Central rowing of sarcolemmal nuclei, so prominent in myotonic dystrophy, is seldom seen. The electromyogram (EMG) exhibits high-frequency repetitive discharges and a characteristic "dive-bomber" sound on the audio monitor. Electron microscopy discloses no change in any of the organelles. Reduction in chloride conductance and, to a lesser degree, in potassium conductance has been found in myotonia congenita but not in myotonic dystrophy.

Mexiletine is effective if the myotonia is severe. Quinidine sulfate, 0.3 to 0.6 g, and procainamide, 250 to 500 mg tid, are clearly beneficial in alleviating the myotonia. Phenytoin, 100 mg tid, has similar but lesser effects.

Other Forms of Myotonia Congenita

Myotonia levior is the name applied to a dominantly inherited form of myotonia congenita in which the symptoms are milder and of later onset than those of Thomsen disease. Yet another form of myotonia is inherited as an autosomal recessive trait (Becker type). In the latter, myotonia does not become manifest until 10 to 14 years of age and tends to be more generalized and severe than in the dominant type. Both forms of myotonia are caused by an allelic mutation of the gene encoding the chloride ion channel of the muscle membrane.

SODIUM CHANNEL DISEASES

Included in this category are the following hereditary muscle disorders: *hyperkalemic periodic paralysis*, *normokalemic periodic paralysis*, *paramyotonia congenita*, *myotonia fluctuans*, *myotonia permanens*, and *acetazolamide-responsive myotonia*. All of them have been mapped to chromosome 17q and are due to mutations in the gene encoding the alpha subunit of the sodium channel in skeletal muscle. The three first-named disorders are the best known; the last three have been defined only in recent years and are included on the basis of shared clinical and molecular defects.

Hyperkalemic Periodic Paralysis

The pattern of inheritance is autosomal dominant, with onset in infancy and childhood. Attacks of severe generalized weakness tend to occur at rest, 20 to 30 min after exercise, affecting first the legs and then the arms; they generally last 15 to 60 min. Respiratory muscles are usually spared. Myotonia may coexist but usually can be detected only electromyographically. During an attack, the serum K rises above a critical point (5.0 to 6.0 meq/L); keeping the level of serum K below this concentration by giving hydrochlorothiazide, 50 to 100 mg daily, prevents the attacks; the addition of acetazolamide (250 to 1000 mg daily) may be beneficial. Giving 2 g of KCl orally will provoke an attack.

Normokalemic periodic paralysis This rare form of episodic paralysis resembles the hyperkalemic form except for the fact that serum K does not increase, even during the most severe attacks. Some patients with normokalemic periodic paralysis are sensitive to potassium loading, but there are kindreds that are not. Inheritance is autosomal dominant, and the genetic defect has been traced to the same mutation as the one responsible for hyperkalemic periodic paralysis.

Paramyotonia Congenita (Eulenberg)

In this form of disease, attacks of weakness are associated with myotonia and are characteristically induced by exposure to cold. Once started, the weakness persists for several hours, even after the body is rewarmed. The myotonia may be paradoxical; i.e., it worsens with exercise. As with hyperkalemic periodic paralysis, serum K is usually increased. Each patient appears to have a critical level of serum K, which, if exceeded, will be associated with weakness. Administration of KCl, raising serum K to or just above 7 meq/L, a level that has no effect on normal persons, invariably induces an attack in the patient.

Table 54-1 Inherited Myotonias and Periodic Paralyses (Channelopathies)

Channelopathy	Chloride	Chloride	Chloride	Sodium	Sodium
Disease	Myotonia congenita (Thomsen)	Generalized myotonia (Becker)	Myotonia levior (DeJong)	Hyperkalemic periodic paralysis	Normokalemic periodic paralysis
Inheritance	Dominant	Recessive	Dominant	Dominant	Dominant
Gene locus	7q32	7q32	7q32	17q	17q
Gene	CLCN1	CLCN1	CLCN1	SCN4A	SCN4A
Channel protein	CLC1	CLC1	CLC1	α subunit	α subunit
Myotonia (electrical)	++	++	+	+/−	+/−
Myotonia (clinical)	++	+++	+	+/−	+/−
Paramyotonia (clinical)	—	—	—	+/−	+/−
Episodic paralysis	—	—	—	+++	+++
Onset	Congenital to late childhood	Late childhood or earlier	Adolescence	First decade	First decade
Precipitating factors					
Appears during exercise	—	—	—	—	—
Increases with exercise	—	—	—	—	—
Appears after exercise	++	++	+	++	++
Fasting	—	—	—	+	—
Carbohydrate load	—	—	—	—	—
Potassium load	—	—	—	++	+/−
Cold	—	—	—	++	+
Emotional stress	+	+	—	++	+
Pregnancy	+	+	—	++	—
Anesthetics (halothane, succinylcholine)	—	—	—	—	—
"Warmup" phenomenon	++	++	+	+	+
Transient weakness following myotonia	+	++	—	—	—
Persistent weakness following myotonia	—	—	—	—	—
Exercise-induced myalgia	—	—	—	—	—
Involvement of cranial muscles	+	+	—	—	+/−
Lid lag and blepharospasm	+	+	—	—	—
Muscle hypertrophy	+	++	—	—	+
Permanent myopathy	—	—	—	+	+
Serum CK during attack	Normal to borderline	Increased 2 to 3 times	Normal	Increased	Increased
Serum K during attack	Normal	Normal	Normal	Increased	Normal
Serum K between attacks	Normal	Normal	Normal	Normal	Normal
Significant myopathology (vacuolar myopathy)	—	—	—	++	++
Treatment	Mexiletine if required	Mexiletine if required	No treatment necessary	During attack, glucose; for prevention, high-CHO, low-K diet	Large doses of Na

Sodium	Sodium	Sodium	Sodium	Calcium	Calcium
Paramyotonia congenita	Myotonia fluctuans	Myotonia permanens	Acetazolamide-responsive myotonia	Hypokalemic periodic paralysis	Malignant hyperthermia
Dominant	Dominant	Dominant	Dominant	Dominant	Dominant
17q	17q	17q	17q	1q31-32	1q13.1
SCN4A	SCN4A	SCN4A	SCN4A	DHP receptor	RYR1
α subunit	α subunit	α subunit	α subunit	Dihydropyridine α subunit	Ryanodine receptor
++	++	+++	++	—	—
—	+	+++	++	—	—
+++	+	|||	+	—	—
+/–	—	—	—	+++	—
Paramyotonia at birth	Adolescence	Early childhood	First decade	Early childhood to third decade	All ages
+++	—	+++	+	—	+
+++	—	++	+	—	+
—	+	+	+	+	—
—	—	—	+	—	—
—	—	—	—	+	—
+/–	++	++	++	—	—
+++	+/–	+/–	+/–	+	—
+	+	+	—	+	—
++	+/–	—	—	+	—
++	++	++	—	—	++++
—	++	—	+	+	—
++	—	+	—	—	—
++	—	+	—	—	—
+	+	—	++	—	—
+++	++	++	+	+	++
+	—	++	—	—	—
—	—	+++	—	—	—
—	—	++	—	+	—
Increased 5 to 10 times	Increased 2 to 4 times	Increased	Increased	Normal to slightly increased	Markedly increased
Normal	Normal	Normal	Normal	Decreased	Normal
Normal	Normal	Normal	Normal	Normal	Normal
—	—	++	—	++	Rhabdomyolysis cores
Mexiletine if needed	Mexiletine if needed	Procainamide, mexiletine	Acetazolamide, carbohydrates	KCl during and acetazolamide between attacks	Intravenous dantrolene

In all forms of hyperkalemic periodic paralysis, there are definable abnormalities in Na channels of the muscle membrane. However, in practical terms, the therapeutic effort is directed to controlling serum K, using hydrochlorothiazide and acetazolamide, as mentioned above. Procainamide in doses of 400 to 1200 mg daily is useful in the treatment of myotonia. Mexiletine, 200 mg tid, is the preferred drug since it prevents both cold- and exercise-induced myotonia.

CALCIUM CHANNEL DISEASE: HYPOKALEMIC PERIODIC PARALYSIS

This, the hypokalemic form, is the best known of the periodic paralyses. The usual pattern of inheritance is autosomal dominant, with reduced penetrance in women. Onset of the disease is generally in late childhood or adolescence. Typically, after a day of unusually heavy exercise or a meal rich in carbohydrate, the patient retires, only to awaken unable to move. Diurnal attacks also occur. The muscles most likely to escape are those of the eyes, face, tongue, pharynx, larynx, diaphragm, and sphincters. Attacks tend to occur every few weeks.

During the attack, serum K levels fall to as low as 1.8 meq/L without an increase in urinary excretion of K. Presumably, K ions enter the muscle fibers, which in biopsy specimens are markedly vacuolated with increase in water (hydropic change). The serum K returns to normal with recovery. Muscle action potentials virtually disappear during the paralysis.

The daily administration of 5 to 10 g of KCl orally in aqueous solution prevents attacks in many of the patients. If it does not, a low carbohydrate, low-salt, high-K diet may be effective. In an attack, 10 g of KCl or other K salt will restore power. Hypokalemic weakness may also be a manifestation of aldosteronism. In all types of periodic paralysis, hypo- or hyperkalemic, frequent attacks may be followed in later life by a mild persistent weakness and proximal wasting.

A special form of this disease occurs with thyrotoxicosis in young individuals of Asian extraction.

MALIGNANT HYPERTHERMIA

This is a syndrome of rapidly rising body temperature and muscle rigidity observed during general anesthesia, particularly with halothane and with the use of the muscle relaxant succinylcholine. This disorder occurs approximately once in 50,000 general anesthetics and has a high mortality if not treated promptly.

Some patients at risk for this condition exhibit certain myopathic and musculoskeletal abnormalities—central core myopathy, Duchenne-Becker muscular dystrophy, and the King-Denborough syndrome (myopathy and multiple congenital musculoskeletal anomalies). The basic defect is thought to be in the ryanodine receptor, a protein component of the calcium channel. Treatment consists of discontinuation of anesthesia at the first hint of masseter spasm or rise in temperature and intravenous administration of dantrolene, which inhibits the release of calcium from the sarcoplasmic reticulum.

The *malignant neuroleptic syndrome*, which occurs as an idiosyncratic reaction to neuroleptic drugs, is clinically and pathologically almost indistinguishable from malignant hyperthermia (see also Chaps. 43 and 58).

> For a more detailed discussion of this topic, see Victor and Ropper:
> *Adams and Victor's Principles of Neurology*, 7th ed, pp 1553–1565.

ADDITIONAL READING

Ackerman MJ, Clapham DE: Ion channels—Basic science and clinical disease. *N Engl J Med* 336:1575, 1997.

Cannon SC, Brown RH Jr, Corey DP: A sodium channel defect in hyperkalemic periodic paralysis: Potassium-induced failure of inactivation. *Neuron* 6:619, 1991.

Denborough M: Malignant hyperthermia. *Lancet* 352:1131, 1998.

Frank JP, Harati Y, Butler JJ, et al: Central core disease and malignant hyperthermia syndrome. *Ann Neurol* 7:11, 1980.

Lehmann-Horn F, Engel AG, Ricker K, Rüdel R: The periodic paralyses and paramyotonia congenita, in Engel AG, Franzini-Armstrong C (eds): *Myology*, 2nd ed. New York, McGraw-Hill, 1994, pp 1303–1334.

McFadzean AJS, Yeung R: Periodic paralysis complicating thyrotoxicosis in Chinese. *BMJ* 1:451, 1967.

Ptácek LJ, Tawil R, Griggs RC, et al: Sodium channel mutations in acetazolamide-responsive myotonia congenita, paramyotonia congenita, and hyperkalemic periodic paralysis. *Neurology* 44:1500, 1994.

Quane KA, Healy JMS, Keating KE, et al: Mutations in the ryanodine receptor gene in central core disease and malignant hyperthermia. *Nature Genet* 5:51, 1993.

Streib EW: Paramyotonia congenita: Successful treatment with tocainide. Clinical and electrophysiologic findings in seven patients. *Muscle Nerve* 10:155, 1987.

55 | Disorders of Muscle Characterized by Cramps, Spasm, and Localized Masses

In addition to the commonplace states of spasticity, rigidity, and dystonia, which are due to disinhibition of spinal motor mechanisms or to extrapyramidal motor diseases, there are forms of muscle stiffness and spasm in which the basic abnormality can be traced to a disturbance of function of spinal interneurons, lower motor neurons, or the sarcolemma of the muscle fiber. Muscles may go into spasm because of an unstable depolarization of motor axons, sending volleys of impulses across neuromuscular junctions—as occurs in myokymia (waves of seemingly spontaneous contractions), hypocalcemic tetany, pseudohypoparathyroidism, and so-called stiff-man syndrome. In other cases, the innervation is normal, but there is persistence of contraction despite attempts at relaxation, as in myotonia congenita (Chap. 54). In the physiologic contracture of McArdle disease and other glycogenoses, the muscle lacks the energy to relax so that once contracted, it is locked into a shortened state (Table 51-1).

In each of these conditions, the complaint is one of cramp or spasm, which is variably painful and interferes with free voluntary activity. Morphologic study provides little or no clue to the nature of the altered contractile process. The best evidence comes from electrophysiologic study of nerve and muscle activity. Each of the aforementioned states of muscle hyperactivity may sometimes be the main characteristic of a particular nerve or muscle disease, so clinical recognition is important.

MUSCLE CRAMPS

Everyone has at times experienced muscle cramps, usually in the foot or leg, after a period of strenuous activity or as a response to a strong voluntary or postural contraction. Such cramps are most frequent at night. The muscle is knotted and extremely painful, and one seeks relief by rubbing and stretching the muscle. Extremely hard cramping can injure muscle, leaving it tender and sore for days. Another variety occurs in athletes after prolonged activity and heavy sweating.

The mechanism is obscure. Low levels of myoadenylate deaminase and release of some unknown metabolite into the perineural spaces are current hypotheses. Quinine, in doses of 300 mg, diphenhydramine (Benadryl) 50 mg, or procainamide 0.5 to 1.0 g reduces the tendency to cramp and, if taken at bedtime, may prevent nocturnal cramping. Maintenance of adequate salt and fluid intake helps to prevent the type of cramping that occurs in athletes.

Repeated cramping during all manner of physical activity should always suggest hypocalcemia (tetany) or hypomagnesemia. The total serum Ca concentration may be normal, but the amount of ionized Ca may be lowered in nervous subjects by hyperventilation. There are also instances of unexplained *malignant cramp syndrome*, in which strong contraction of any muscle group induces cramp (pseudotetany); this disorder, the nature of which is obscure, may run in certain families. In patients with peripheral nerve disease (and in some otherwise normal persons), there may be a sensation of muscle cramping without palpable muscle contraction (illusory cramp). Here the electromyogram (EMG) is helpful, for during a true cramp there are bursts of high-frequency action potentials.

STATES OF PERSISTENT FASCICULATION, CONTINUOUS MUSCLE ACTIVITY, MYOKYMIA, NEUROMYOTONIA, AND THE STIFF-MAN SYNDROME

A few fascicular twitches occurring in muscles that are otherwise normal are very common and nearly always benign. These are frequent in the orbicularis oculi, abductor pollicis brevis, quadriceps, and sternomastoid and are mistaken by anxious patients (particularly physicians) for serious disease. Fasciculations that persist for hours or days in one muscle ("live flesh") represent a benign state that usually appears and disappears without explanation. Only if weakness and atrophy of muscle are associated should fasciculations be considered as manifestations of neurologic disease such as amyotrophic lateral sclerosis (ALS). A state of extremely marked generalized fasciculations, often associated with fatigue and slight weakness and slowing of distal motor latencies in some cases, probably represents a distal motor axonopathy of obscure origin. Eventual recovery can be expected. Phenytoin and carbamazepine have been beneficial in some cases.

Continuous muscular activity (also called Isaacs' syndrome) has been described; the entire musculature is continuously twitching, even when the patient is fully relaxed. This activity is not abolished even by spinal anesthesia and not always by procaine block of nerves. Presumably motor axons and their terminal endings are persistently hyperexcitable.

In the so-called *stiff-man syndrome*, a disorder similar to tetanus gradually develops during adult life and may persist for years, partly or totally disabling the patient. The back, neck, and limb muscles are affected. In most patients there are serum antibodies to glutamic acid dehydrogenase and sometimes to pancreatic islet cells, resulting in diabetes, but otherwise no explanation has been found. Diazepam or other benzodiazepine drugs, in large doses, control the disease. A few cases have benefited temporarily from plasma exchange and intravenous immunoglobulin.

Generalized muscle stiffness and continuous muscle fiber activity also occur as part of a rare, inherited (autosomal recessive) form of dwarfism, the Schwartz-Jampel syndrome.

The continuous rippling and more or less tonic contraction of muscles, called *myokymia*, is closely related to the state of continuous muscular activity as well as to benign fasciculations and cramps. It appears after reinnervation of muscle in recovery from neuropathy (e.g., Guillain-Barré syndrome, Bell's palsy). It is probably similar to *neuromyotonia*, a term that has been applied to a state of stiffness, fasciculatory activity, and delayed relaxation of muscle that is sometimes observed in patients who are recovering from a polyneuropathy. Apparently, the regenerating motor neurons pass through a stage of hyperexcitability. The EMG distinguishes this state from a true myotonia.

In *tetanus*, spinal inhibitory neurons (Renshaw and other cells) are suppressed, leaving anterior horn cells overactive. Activities that normally excite these inhibitory neurons—reflex postural and volitional movements—evoke violent involuntary spasms, which are especially prominent in jaw muscles (trismus), perioral muscles (risus sardonicus), and extensors of the neck and back. The EMG shows the expected interference pattern of fully contracted muscles.

LOCALIZED MUSCLE MASSES

Masses in one or many muscles are found in a variety of clinical settings. *Muscle rupture*, most often of the biceps and soleus muscles, is usually caused by a violent strain, attended by an audible snap and then a bulge. Surgical repair is required. Painful localized *hematomas* follow trauma or complicate the use of anticoagulants, bleeding diseases, or excessive running.

Desmoid tumor is a benign growth of fibrous tissue, observed most often in parturient women and at the site of surgical incision. Closely related are *pseudotumorous* growths, sometimes massive, which are made up of interlacing muscle fibers and fibroblasts and may follow injury. Rhabdomyosarcoma and liposarcoma are the common malignant tumors.

A special type of *muscle infarction* occasionally involves the anterior thigh or other large muscles in patients with diabetes mellitus. Abrupt onset of pain and swelling with the formation of a tender, palpable mass is the characteristic clinical presentation. Occlusion of many medium-sized muscle arteries is the pathologic basis of the infarction. Treatment consists of immediate immobilization of the limb, since early ambulation may cause bleeding into the infarcted tissue. Muscle biopsy in an anticoagulated patient may have the same effect.

Excessive marching or similarly vigorous exercise in poorly conditioned persons may give rise to painful swelling of the anterior tibial muscles (*pretibial compartment syndrome*). The tight pretibial compartment confines the swollen leg muscles, which leads to ischemic necrosis and myoglobinuria. Incision of the pretibial fascia is required to prevent permanent weakness.

Myositis ossificans—deposition of bone within the substance of a muscle—is of two types. A *localized type* follows a muscle tear or a severe blow or repeated minor trauma to a muscle. The injured tissue is gradually replaced by cartilage and, in 4 to 7 weeks, by a solid mass of bone that can be readily palpated and seen in radiographs. The *generalized form* is of an entirely different order. It is probably inherited as an autosomal dominant trait and is frequently accompanied by other congenital anomalies. There is widespread bone formation along the fascial planes of muscles, beginning in infancy and childhood; the process may progress slowly but inexorably or may stabilize for many years at any stage of the disease. Administration of a diphosphonate or prednisone is said to be helpful in some cases.

For a more detailed discussion of this topic, see Victor and Ropper: *Adams and Victor's Principles of Neurology*, 7th ed, pp 1566–1576.

ADDITIONAL READING

Banker BQ, Chester CS: Infarction of thigh muscle in the diabetic patient. *Neurology* 23:667, 1973.

Barker RA, Reeves T, Thom M, et al: Review of 23 patients affected by the stiff man syndrome: Clinical subdivision into stiff trunk (man) syndrome, stiff limb syndrome, and progressive encephalomyelitis with rigidity. *J Neurol Neurosurg Psychiatry* 65:633, 1998.

Burns RJ, Bretag AH, Blumbergs PC, Harbord MG; Benign familial disease with muscle mounding and rippling. *J Neurol Neurosurg Psychiatry* 57:344, 1994.

Kakulas BA, Adams RD: *Diseases of Muscle: Pathological Foundations of Clinical Myology*, 4th ed. Philadelphia, Harper & Row, 1985.

Layzer RB: Muscle pain, cramps, and fatigue, in Engel AG, Franzini-Armstrong C (eds): *Myology*, 2nd ed. New York, McGraw-Hill, 1994, pp 1754–1768.

Moersch FP, Woltman HW: Progressive fluctuating muscular rigidity ("stiff-man syndrome"): Report of a case and some observations in 13 other cases. *Mayo Clin Proc* 31:421, 1956.

Newsom-Davis J, Mills KR: Immunological associations of acquired neuromyotonia (Isaacs' syndrome). *Brain* 116:453, 1993.

Solimena M, Folli F, Aparisi R, et al: Autoantibodies to GABA-ergic neurons and pancreatic beta cells in stiff-man syndrome. *N Engl J Med* 322:1555, 1990.

Spaans F, Theunissen P, Reekers AD, et al: Schwartz-Jampel syndrome: 1. Clinical, electromyographic, and histologic studies. *Muscle Nerve* 13:516, 1990.

Valli G, Barbieri S, Stefano C, et al: Syndromes of abnormal muscular activity: Overlap between continuous muscle fiber activity and the stiff-man syndrome. *J Neurol Neurosurg Psychiatry* 46:241, 1983.

PART VI | PSYCHIATRIC DISORDERS

In the three remaining chapters, we consider several diseases that fall mainly in the specialty of psychiatry. The justification for their inclusion in a manual of neurology has been set forth in *Adams and Victor's Principles of Neurology*, 7th ed. In brief, we state that neurologic medicine embraces all conditions that are based on a pathologic process in the nervous system. It matters not whether the lesion is obvious, like a tumor or infarct, or impossible to detect with the light or even the electron microscope, like manic-depressive disease or the encephalopathy of delirium tremens. In all instances, whether visible or invisible, the pathologic process is traceable to some genetic, chemical, or structural factor acting on the brain and deranging its function. Even the visible lesion represents only the most advanced and irreversible stage of a morbid process.

We take pains to separate these cerebral disease states, which are of concern to both neurologists and psychiatrists, from peculiarities of personality and social behavior, and from a patient's reactions to troubling life experiences—disorders that fall almost exclusively in the domain of psychiatry. Discerning the patient's constitutional peculiarities, tracing his reactions to the circumstances that evoked them, and teaching the patient how better to cope with them are the more practical aims of psychotherapy. The psychosomatic diseases are a special category, once a favored topic in psychiatry. All of them have proved to have a medical basis with possible aggravating psychologic factors.

It is of interest that contemporary psychiatry has gradually adopted this point of view. Schizophrenia, endogenous depression and manic-depressive disease, childhood autism, anxiety, phobic and obsessive-compulsive neuroses, and hysteria—even the sociopathies and paranoia—are being given the status of diseases of the nervous system. As with all diseases, the neuropsychiatric ones are being defined increasingly by explicit criteria without which there can be little focused research or precision of diagnosis and prognosis. With the discovery of more and more specific drug therapies, accurate diagnosis becomes a matter of prime practical importance.

In the following discussion, we emphasize the biologic aspects and particularly the diagnostic features of the common neuropsychiatric diseases—those that should be known to every neurologist and indeed to all physicians.

56 | The Neuroses and Personality Disorders

THE NEUROSES

Encompassed by the term *neuroses* is a diverse group of mental disorders, traditionally designated as anxiety states, neurasthenia, phobic neurosis, obsessive-compulsive neurosis, hysteria, hypochondriasis, neurotic depression, and depersonalization. Originally, Freud referred to these states as the *psychoneuroses*, and their genesis was explained in terms of psychoanalytic theory. Subsequently, biologically oriented psychiatrists abbreviated this term to the *neuroses*, and more recently it has been replaced by the term *neurotic disorders*. The latter include any mental disturbance with the following characteristics: (1) symptoms that are distressing to the patient and regarded by him as unacceptable or alien; (2) intactness of reality testing (i.e., capacity for the rational analysis of one's reactions); (3) behavior (in relation to symptoms) that does not seriously violate social norms, although social functioning may be considerably impaired; (4) disturbances that are enduring, not transitory reactions to stressful situations; and (5) absence of a recognizable organic cause. Not included among the neuroses are the so-called psychosomatic disorders, in which it was formerly alleged that a stressful life situation or an emotional upset played an important role in the causation of a wide range of medical diseases. A large segment of the profession still adheres to this idea.

Each of the syndromes described below is clinically identifiable and separate from others when it occurs in pure form. However, many patients experience symptoms of more than one type; i.e., they have a "mixed neurosis." For this reason, the most recent edition of the *Diagnostic and Statistical Manual of Mental Disorders* (DSM-IV) subdivides these syndromes into two large groups: (1) *anxiety disorders* (which include panic states and the phobic and obsessive-compulsive neuroses) and (2) the *somatoform disorders* (comprising conversion disorder, hypochondriasis, and somatization disorder, or hysteria).

Anxiety Neurosis

This term and its many synonyms (neurasthenia, soldier's heart, etc.) refer to a syndrome consisting of general irritability, anxious expectation, frank anxiety attacks (panic attacks), and the autonomic-visceral accompaniments of anxiety. The syndrome may occur in relatively pure form or be part of another psychiatric disease—such as depression, schizophrenia, hysteria, and phobic neurosis. Its closest link is with depression, which it resembles in another respect—namely, in having a strong hereditary basis. The family history in patients with anxiety neurosis discloses a similar illness in 50 percent of first-degree relatives, although a mendelian pattern of inheritance has not been defined. The average age at onset is 25 years (range 18 to 40), and it occurs twice as frequently in women as in men.

Anxiety neurosis is a chronic disease punctuated by periods of more intense anxiety with or without attacks of panic. In the periods of anxiety—which may appear without warning and last for weeks, months, or a year or more in varying intensity—the patient has feelings of dread and foreboding. Often a sense of apprehension and fear of imminent death (angor animi) or of losing one's mind or self-control brings the patient to the physician. There may be complaints that the surroundings seem strange or unreal (depersonalization or derealization). Dizziness is another common symptom and may be associated with a vague sense of visual distortion or disorientation. Palpitation, pain in the chest, and difficulty in taking a deep breath are other common complaints. In an acute panic attack (which is rarely witnessed by the physician), the heart races or beats forcefully, breathing comes in rapid gasps, the pupils are dilated, and the patient sweats and trembles. A cardiologist may be called because of the prominence of palpitation and feeling of suffocation. Consciousness is retained. After 15 to 30 min the symptoms abate, leaving the patient shaken, tense, perplexed, and often embarrassed. Fear of subsequent attacks is characteristic and may evoke agoraphobia (see below).

Hyperventilation is often a prominent feature of an anxiety attack. Hyperventilation itself, by reducing P_{CO_2}, reproduces the giddiness of an attack and often paresthesias of lips and fingers—and even frank tetany—but these symptoms constitute only the last part of the panic attack.

Such attacks, which are as stereotyped and unique as a faint or seizure, may be the opening phase of a period of illness or may arise on a background of anxiety and chronic worry, easy fatigue, hypochondriasis, and mild depression. Once the attacks appear, they may recur infrequently or several times a day or during the night. Panic attacks have reportedly been induced by infusion of lactate in patients with anxiety neurosis. In the chronic phase of the illness, there is poor tolerance of exercise, with dyspnea and palpitation. The physical examination of such patients yields only a few nonspecific findings: slight tachycardia, sighing respirations, frequent yawning, tremor, and brisk tendon reflexes. Intolerance of hyperventilation is another manifestation.

A 20-year follow-up study of a large group of patients with anxiety disorder showed that symptoms were still present in over 80 percent, but there had been long periods of relative freedom. Severe disability had occurred in only 15 percent.

Figuring prominently in the differential diagnosis are hyperthyroidism, menopausal symptoms, temporal lobe seizures, adrenal tumors, myocardial disease, pulmonary insufficiency, and depression. In thyroid and adrenal disorders, many of the autonomic manifestations of anxiety appear without the mental components. A variety of drugs—including psychostimulants, xanthines, and sympathomimetics—may also induce parts of the syndrome.

Treatment consists of reassuring the patient and teaching tolerance of the symptoms until a remission occurs, as it will within 6 months in over half of the patients. Intensive psychotherapy has not improved the remission rate. Antianxiety drugs such as alprazolam and lorazepam, and, if depressive symptoms are present, a serotonin reuptake inhibitor without activating effects (paroxitine, sertraline), tricyclic agents (imipramine, amitriptyline, nortriptyline), or a monoamine oxidase (MAO) inhibitor may be beneficial. See Chaps. 43 and 57 for descriptions of these antidepressant drugs.

Phobic Neurosis

In this condition there is a preternatural fear of some situation, disease, animal, or object. Among the most common is *agoraphobia*, a fear of open spaces, which results in a homebound state. It is usually associated with a chronic anxiety disorder. While acknowledging that there are no rational grounds for these fears, the patient is powerless to suppress them and becomes panic stricken and incapacitated when put in a situation that evokes the phobia. The resulting symptoms are those of panic. The condition develops in adolescence or early adult life. Many patients are able to intelligently adjust their affairs so as to avoid situations that evoke the phobic reaction and in this way may be able to function quite well. For example, one accedes to a phobia of leaving one's neighborhood or city by working near or at home. Depression may periodically decompensate the adjustment, and antianxiety or antidepressant medication is then required to restore the patient to a functional state. The same drugs also alleviate or prevent the symptoms of panic. In some patients, behavioral modification techniques are helpful.

Obsessive-Compulsive Disorder (OCD)

Like phobic states, OCD begins in adolescence and early adult years, and often there is a family member with an obsessional personality. *Obsessions* are imperative and distressing thoughts and impulses that intrude themselves into the patient's mind despite a desire to resist and be rid of them. Most disturbing are obsessive fears of harming a family member. *Compulsions* are single acts (e.g., hand washing) or series of acts or rituals, such as repeatedly checking a series of door locks, or a stove for gas, that the patient feels compelled to carry out.

Studies by magnetic resonance imaging and single photon emission computed tomography have implicated the caudate nuclei in OCD, and a familial tendency has also been noted. The condition overlaps with the multiple tic disorder of Gilles de la Tourette syndrome. Clomipramine and other nontricyclic drugs, such as fluoxetine, are recommended. When depression causes a worsening of the patient's condition; antidepressant medications similar to those mentioned above for the treatment of anxiety have been helpful in alleviating symptoms.

HYSTERIA (HYSTERICAL NEUROSIS, CONVERSION DISORDER, BRIQUET DISEASE)

The terms *hysteria* and *hysterical* have several different meanings, and one must be certain about how they are being used. One use of the term is to designate a *personality disorder* of special type, characterized by immaturity, egocentricity, emotional instability, and histrionic and "seductive" behavior. Such a personality disorder may be a lifelong source of difficulty in social functioning, but there is no evidence that it is a determinant in the development of a hysterical neurosis. Even the occurrence of certain unexplained symptoms—such as amnesia, paralysis, and aphonia, which mimic neurologic disease ("conversion")—should not in itself be equated with the disease hysteria. In the authors' opinion, the term *hysteria* should be reserved for a *disease* with a distinctive gender predilection, age at onset, natural history, characteristic somatic symptoms and signs (which typically include so-called conversion symptoms), and prognosis.

There are two main types of hysteria: In one, the patient, practically always an adolescent girl or a young woman, presents with a variety of simulated manifestations of disease (usually of neurologic type), often with variable degrees of anxiety; in the other (malingering), which occurs in either sex, various symptoms and signs of disease are feigned for the purpose of obtaining compensation, influencing litigation, avoiding military service or incarceration, etc. Cases of both types are seen regularly in hospitals and are found more often on neurologic than on psychiatric wards.

Classic, or Female, Hysteria (Briquet Disease)

Onset is usually in late childhood, adolescence, or early adult life. Once the ailment has started, various symptoms recur intermittently, though with lessening frequency in adult years. Schooling and later social life, work, and marriage are interrupted repeatedly by violent headaches, simulated seizures, trancelike states, paralyses, intractable vomiting or regurgitation, abdominal crises, unexplained fever, blindness, urinary retention, aphonia, and bizarre unsteadiness of gait. Typical examples are young women who appear in the emergency department with complete amnesia for the past, even of personal identity. Most cases of so-called multiple personality are examples of classic hysteria. Often the illness that is adopted mimics one that was recently observed in some member of the family or in a friend. Many of the complaints center around sexual difficulties—claims (often unsubstantiated) of childhood sexual abuse, severe dysmenorrhea, frigidity, dyspareunia, and vomiting throughout pregnancy. Frequently one notes some one of these somatic symptoms in the course of a neurologic examination of a highly suggestible but otherwise normal person.

A notable feature of this illness is the patient's professed unawareness of the nature of her illness. In this respect, it has been likened to the behavior of a person under the influence of hypnosis. Indeed, most hysterics are hypersuggestible. The validity of this distinction between unconscious and conscious motivation continues to be debated.

Other syndromes include hysterical pain (abdominal, back, atypical facial and limb); trances, fugues, and pseudoseizures; paralyses (monoplegia, hemiplegia, paraplegia); tremors; and urinary retention. Nonneurologic manifestations of hysteria include unexplained hyperpyrexia; factitious ulcers and dermatitis; repeated hospitalizations and surgical operations for vague symptoms, mainly abdominal; and the excessive use of drugs prescribed by physicians.

Compensation Neurosis (Hysteria in Men and Women, Malingering)

As stated above, hysterical-type symptoms do occur in men, but in most instances in those trying to avoid legal difficulties or military service or to obtain disability payments, veterans' pensions, or compensation following injury. Unless such a factor is present, the diagnosis of hysteria in the male should be made with great caution (although a sociopath, for unexplained reasons, may sometimes present with such an illness). The symptoms may be much the same as those listed under female hysteria, but often the patient is monosymptomatic, complaining only of "seizures" or of chronic pain that is confined to the low back, neck, head, or arm.

The *differential diagnosis* of both types of hysteria includes a host of neurologic and medical diseases. A history of repeated illnesses of this type is helpful, but often the patient appears to have forgotten major medical problems and hospital admissions of the past. More often one must depend on the "discrepancy method"—one is unable to elicit the usual neurologic abnormalities that characterize a genuine paraplegia, hemiplegia, or seizure state. Other clues to the presence of a hysterical paralysis are an inconstant ("giving way") quality of muscle contraction, a failure to activate muscles that fixate the trunk or the contralateral limb, and a cocontraction of agonist and antagonist muscles. This method, however, may mislead the novice who has limited experience with neurologic and medical disease. Lack of laboratory corroboration is a third criterion—e.g., a normal electroencephalogram during a frank seizure or a normal sedimentation rate and WBC count with high fever.

There has been much debate concerning *etiology*. In classic female hysteria, there is a high incidence of hysteria in other female relatives (20 percent of first-degree relatives) and an increased incidence of sociopathy in male relatives. This suggests that female hysteria is the equivalent of male sociopathy, neither of which is fully understood.

In *treatment*, one is faced with two problems—the correction of the long-standing basic neurotic disorder and the management of the recently acquired physical symptoms. As to the former, little can be done; long-term psychotherapy has not proved to be effective. However, the acute symptoms of a particular attack nearly always subside with firm reassurance that recovery is imminent and optimistic persuasion (with the help of a physiotherapist) that hour by hour, day by day, function is returning. Hypnosis or suggestion under the influence of amytal or lorazepam, while often effective, is usually unnecessary. If symptoms of anxiety are prominent, antianxiety and antidepressant drugs should be utilized. No success is to be gained by attributing the disease to nerves or neurosis or stating that "it's all in your imagination." Compensation hysteria is managed best by determining the degree of injury, confidently stating the prognosis, urging the settlement of litigation, and using simple medical measures.

HYPOCHONDRIASIS

The term *hypochondriasis* refers to a morbid preoccupation with bodily functions and with sensations of physical signs, leading to the fear or belief of having serious disease. In most instances it is a manifestation of an underlying depression, as discussed in the next chapter. Other instances are associated with schizophrenia or neurosis. Whenever a young person develops hypochondriacal symptoms that are not related to transient episodes of stress, one should suspect an underlying psychiatric disorder. In only about 15 percent of hypochondriacal patients does there appear to be no associated psychiatric illness (*primary hypochondriasis*). Many neurotic persons become depressed at some time, and opinion differs on whether the hypochondriacal symptoms are a reaction to the neurosis or are part of a depressive illness (see Chap. 57).

PERSONALITY DISORDERS

The development of personality has already been discussed in Chap. 28. There it was pointed out that *personality* is the most inclusive of all psychologic terms, encompassing all the physical and psychologic *traits* that distinguish one person from every other one.

Pertinent to this chapter are two generally accepted assumptions about personality traits. One is that certain traits, or types, are characteristic of a particular type of neurosis or psychosis. In one group of personality types—paranoid, schizoid, cyclothymic, and obsessive-compulsive—such a relationship seems to pertain. A second consideration is that in approximately 15 percent of persons, certain personality traits are so indelible and maladaptive as to cause significant functional impairment and subjective distress—in which case they constitute *personality disorders*.

DSM-IV recognizes 10 specific patterns of personality disorder, as follows:

Paranoid—distrust and suspiciousness such that others' motives are interpreted as malevolent

Schizoid—detachment from social relationships and a restricted range of emotional expression

Schizotypal—acute discomfort in close relationships, cognitive or perceptual distortions, and eccentricities of behavior

Antisocial—disregard for, and violation of, the rights of others

Borderline—instability in interpersonal relationships, self-image, and affect as well as marked impulsivity

Histrionic—excessive emotionality and attention seeking

Narcissistic—grandiosity, need for admiration, and lack of empathy

Avoidant—social inhibition, feeling of inadequacy, and hypersensitivity to negative evaluation

Dependent—submissive and clinging behavior related to an excessive need to be taken care of

Obsessive-Compulsive—preoccupation with orderliness, perfectionism, and control

Personality Disorder Not Otherwise Specified is a category applicable to two situations: (1) the features of several different personality disorders are present, but the criteria for any specific one are not met, or (2) the individual's personality pattern meets the general criteria for a personality disorder, but one that is not included in the above tabulation (e.g., "passive-aggressive," "inadequate," "immature").

Antisocial Personality (Sociopathy)

This disorder, known long ago as "moral insanity" and later as psychopathic personality or constitutional psychopathy, is the best defined of all abnormal personality types and the one most likely to lead to trouble in the family and community. Sociopathy is a chronic state that affects mainly males and, unlike most psychiatric disorders, is fully manifest by the age of 12 to 15 years. The most frequent antisocial activities are theft, fire setting, truancy, running away from home, associating with undesirable characters, physical aggression and assault, abuse of drugs and alcohol, precocious and indiscriminate sexual activity, and vandalism. Repeatedly apprehended, the sociopath exhibits no remorse, profits little or not at all from discipline or past experience, and is unable to empathize with family and friends. Restlessness and impulsivity are prominent. School and work performance is erratic and failure almost invariable. This deviant behavior naturally places the sociopath in trouble with the law, and many such persons end up in reform school or jail. The female sociopath differs only in having a higher incidence of hysterical symptoms.

Little is known about the cause. Alcoholism or sociopathy in the father and lack of parental discipline are the most closely related factors but cannot be regarded as causal. It appears that the development of social intelligence and adaptation is delayed. In the classic study of L. N. Robins, more than half of the deviant children lost most of their sociopathic traits in adult life. However, of those who did not become adult sociopaths, the large majority developed other psychiatric illnesses, particularly alcoholism. Psychotherapy has been unsuccessful.

Explosive Disorder and Aggressive Violence

The principal feature of this condition is the occurrence of repetitive, unpredictable outbursts of violent, aggressive behavior out of all proportion to the provocative situation. In some instances such behavior is associated with mental retardation, schizophrenia, epilepsy, or alcohol and drug abuse, but the typical case is seen in otherwise normal but temperamentally excitable individuals. Most of the subjects are male. Propranolol and phenytoin are said to be helpful in controlling such outbursts.

For a more detailed discussion of this topic, see Victor and Ropper: *Adams and Victor's Principles of Neurology*, 7th ed, pp 1583–1607.

ADDITIONAL READING

Andreasen NC, Black DW: *Introductory Textbook of Psychiatry*, 2nd ed. Washington, DC, American Psychiatric Association, 1995.

Berthier ML, Kulisevsky J, Gironell A, et al: Obsessive-compulsive disorder associated with brain lesions: Clinical phenomenology, cognitive function and anatomic correlates. *Neurology* 47:353, 1996.

Diagnostic and Statistical Manual of Mental Disorders, 4th ed (DSM IV). Washington, DC, American Psychiatric Association, 1994.

Goodwin DW, Guze SB: *Psychiatric Diagnosis*, 5th ed. New York, Oxford University Press, 1996.

Gorman JM: Anxiety disorders, in Sadock BJ, Sadock VA (eds): *Kaplan and Sadock's Comprehensive Textbook of Psychiatry*, 7th ed. Philadelphia, Lippincott Williams & Wilkins, 2000, pp 1441–1444.

Keane JR: Hysterical gait. *Neurology* 39:586, 1989.

Lazare A: Current concepts in psychiatry: Conversion symptoms. *N Engl J Med* 305:745, 1981.

March JS: Cognitive-behavioral psychotherapy, in Sadock BJ, Sadock VA (eds): *Kaplan and Sadock's Comprehensive Textbook of Psychiatry*, 7th ed. Philadelphia, Lippincott Williams & Wilkins, 2000, pp 2806–2813.

Purtell JJ, Robins E, Cohen ME: Observations on clinical aspects of hysteria. *JAMA* 146:902, 1951.

Robins E, Purtell JJ, Cohen ME: Hysteria in men. *N Engl J Med* 246:677, 1952.

Robins LN: *Deviant Children Grown Up: A Sociological and Psychiatric Study of Sociopathic Personality*. Huntington, NY, Kreiger, 1974.

Wheeler EO, White PD, Reed EW, Cohen ME: Neurocirculatory asthenia (anxiety neurosis, effort syndrome, neurasthenia): A twenty-year follow-up of one hundred and seventy-three patients. *JAMA* 142:878, 1950.

57 | Grief, Reactive Depression, Endogenous Depression, and Manic-Depressive Disease

The illnesses listed in the chapter title above have one trait in common—a depressed or dysphoric mood. However, the different settings in which the depressive illness occurs, certain variations in the clinical picture, and the fact that each requires somewhat different management make their separation important. Taken together, they constitute the most frequent of all mental illnesses, accounting, for example, for an estimated 50 percent of psychiatric admissions and 12 percent of all medical admissions to one tertiary referral center. It has been stated that of the adult population of the United States, 20 percent of women and 10 percent of men will have a depressive illness at least once in their lifetime.

There are three main forms of depressive illness with which every physician should be familiar.

1. Grief and other forms of reactive or secondary depression in relation to a personal loss or medical disease
2. Dysthymia (chronic mild depression)
3. Endogenous or primary depression (with or without agitation and anxiety) and manic-depressive disease

The essential clinical features of depression are also described in Chap. 24.

Grief Reaction

This, the most common form of depressive reaction, follows the loss of someone who is particularly close and dear to the patient. It is a natural response, to be expected in every thoughtful and sentient person. The grief reaction—an intense subjective sensation of mental pain accompanied by a feeling of exhaustion—alters the usual pattern of behavior. Often there is a preoccupation with the image of the deceased person, a sense of guilt concerning the relationship to the deceased, and sometimes an unwarranted hostility toward friends and relatives. The mood disturbance and the sense of exhaustion and disorganization of daily activities are the only aspects of this reaction for which the authors can vouch.

As a rule, the grief reaction begins to abate after 4 to 12 weeks, but there are wide individual variations in its duration and intensity. It tends to be prolonged in the elderly. Also, patients who have had a previous depression may remain in mourning for a year or more, and it is then impossible to distinguish between a grief reaction and an endogenous depression.

In treating a grief reaction, one attempts to help the patient to a realistic acceptance of the loss and the changes that may be required as a result of it.

A circumscribed course of sedative-hypnotic drugs may be prescribed—flurazepam, 15 to 30 mg at bedtime, or diazepam, 5 mg tid.

If the grief reaction is abnormally prolonged or severe, the assistance of a psychiatrist should be sought to determine the correctness of the diagnosis and the proper management.

Other Reactive Depressions

Often a medical or neurologic disease will be compounded by complaints of undue weakness and fatigue, a loss of interest in and pleasure from the patient's usual activities (anhedonia), inability to concentrate, or inexplicable pain. The presence of nervousness, irritability, pessimism, loss of appetite, and poor sleep may be admitted only on questioning. These should be recognized for what they are—the symptoms of a "masked" depression.

Certain diseases more than others are known to be associated with reactive depression. These are summarized in Table 57-1. Also, there is said to be an increased incidence of depressive reaction with left frontal strokes. A variety of drugs—particularly propranolol, cimetidine, interferon, sedative drugs of any kind, and the phenothiazines—may evoke a depressive reaction (Table 57-1).

The first step in management is recognition of the depressive symptoms and their separation from the symptoms of the underlying illness. The patient is then assured that such reactive symptoms are to be expected and are medically treatable. Most patients with a reactive depression ultimately recover, even without medical assistance or pharmacologic intervention, but the toll taken by the depression in terms of mental suffering and prolongation of convalescence may be significant. In these circumstances one can safely use tricyclic antidepressants (except during the early convalescence from myocardial infarction) or fluoxetine or other drugs of the same class.

Dysthymia

An extremely chronic and unremitting but relatively mild depressive illness ("I have been depressed all my life") is now usually classed as dysthymia. Prevailing opinion is that it responds only to psychotherapy if at all, and that antidepressant drugs are of little use. This generalization does not hold in all cases and some dysthymic patients may respond to antidepressant therapy. Psychologic support—i.e., explanation and reassurance—is helpful but probably does not alleviate the illness.

Endogenous Depression and Manic-Depressive Disease

These are ubiquitous hereditary diseases that occur in cycles lasting several months or longer. Current nomenclature recognizes two types of these diseases: *unipolar or depressive disorder*, in which only endogenous depression occurs, and *bipolar disorder*, in which mania occurs, often alternating with depression. The occurrence of episodic mania without depression is well known but is relatively infrequent.

A *depressive episode* may occur without provocation, but often there is a history of some stressful situation or loss in the preceding months. The patient feels low in spirits, sad, or depressed and expresses feelings of deep pessimism and hopelessness. With this affective disturbance there is a loss of interest in one's affairs and capacity for enjoyment, a lack of energy,

TABLE 57-1 Depression Secondary to Neurologic, Medical, and Surgical Diseases and Drugs

1. *Neurologic diseases*
   a. Neuronal degenerations—Alzheimer, Huntington, and Parkinson disease
   b. Focal CNS disease—strokes, brain tumors and trauma, multiple sclerosis
2. *Metabolic and endocrine diseases*
   a. Corticosteroids, excess or deficiency
   b. Hypothyroidism, rarely thyrotoxicosis
   c. Cushing syndrome
   d. Addison disease
   e. Hyperparathyroidism
   f. Pernicious anemia (vitamin B_{12} deficiency)
   g. Chronic renal failure/dialysis
   h. B-vitamin deficiencies
3. *Myocardial infarction, open heart surgery, and other operations*
4. *Infectious diseases*
   a. Brucellosis
   b. Viral hepatitis, influenza, pneumonia
   c. Infectious mononucleosis
5. *Cancer, particularly pancreatic*
6. *Parturition*
7. *Medications*
   a. Analgesics and anti-inflammatory agents (other than steroids)
   b. Sedative and antipsychosis drugs
   c. Antibiotics, particularly cycloserine, ethionamide, griseofulvin, isoniazid, nalidixic acid, and sulfonamide
   d. Antihypertensive drugs—clonidine, propranolol, reserpine
   e. Cardiac drugs—digitalis, procainamide
   f. Corticosteroids and ACTH (when instituted or withdrawn)
   g. Chemotherapeutic agents
   h. Beta-interferon
8. *Alcoholism*

mental and physical fatigue, disturbed sleep (often early-morning wakening), loss of appetite, weight loss, waning of sexual interest, and pain of various types including headache. Agitation and anxiety are present in many patients, especially the elderly. Psychomotor retardation characterizes others. Self-deprecation, feelings of worthlessness or guilt, suicidal ideation, and preoccupation with some medical condition (dermatologic, rheumatic, etc.) are common accompaniments. Excessive complaints of physical deterioration or poor memory may be mistaken by the physician for an occult medical condition or early dementia.

A *manic attack* expresses itself by an elevation of mood and hyperactivity (excessive amount and speed of speech and all psychomotor activities). With the euphoria, little sleep is required. When the attack is severe, thought may become incoherent. One plan after another is initiated and abandoned. Judgment is faulty. The patient lacks insight into his problem and may embark on impractical schemes that jeopardize his social and financial condition. Despite the patient's lively and expansive state, he often tolerates frustration poorly and his euphoria is mixed with irritability. Some patients are frankly paranoid and hostile. A special problem is posed by the patient who exhibits both depressive and schizophrenic symptoms—the so-called schizoaffective state. Most such patients prove to have manic-depressive disease.

As to *etiology* of this disease, most neurologists and psychiatrists agree that genetic factors are most important. While stress and other environmental changes may be provocative, studies of families show a high incidence of either unipolar or bipolar disease and a concordance rate of 75 percent in monozygotic twins—clear evidence of a genetic basis. Attempts to investigate the mechanism by measurements of serotonin, norepinephrine, corticosteroids, dopamine, or their metabolic products have not yielded consistent results.

Depression is now being managed with reasonable success by pharmacotherapy. For unipolar disease, one of the serotoninergic agents or tricyclic antidepressants is the usual first line of therapy. The former agents are now favored because of fewer side effects. If these drugs are unsuccessful, one of the MAO inhibitors is tried. In the patient with a manic attack, a neuroleptic agent (e.g., Haldol, Thorazine, olanzapine) may be necessary in the acute episode, and lithium carbonate may afford relief from future attacks. Other drugs, under the direction of an experienced psychiatrist, should be tried in the 20 percent of patients who fail to respond to the program outlined above. Medications may need to be given for several weeks before improvement is apparent and then continued for 6 to 12 months. In using any of these drugs, one should be familiar with all the side effects and cross-reactions with other drugs (see Chap. 43).

Electroconvulsive therapy (ECT) is reserved for patients who do not respond to or cannot tolerate antidepressant drugs. ECT is most effective in the treatment of agitated or catatonic depression in middle and late life and can also be used to interrupt a manic episode. The main drawback of ECT is that it causes an impairment, usually transient, of retentive memory. ECT should not be used in the presence of increased intracranial pressure or severe hypertension.

Suicide

Manic-depressive psychosis, endogenous unipolar depression, reactive depression (life-threatening disease, catastrophic financial loss), pathologic grief, and depression in an alcoholic or schizophrenic patient all carry a significant risk of suicide. One of every five suicidal persons with one of these conditions will commit suicide without having made medical contact. In many of the remaining patients, the presence of a depressive illness and potential for suicide will not be recognized by the physician at the time the patient ends his life. Between 20,000 and 35,000 suicidal deaths are recorded annually in the United States, and about 10 times this number of people attempt suicide. The incidence rises with age.

In the evaluation of suicide risk, a previous suicide attempt or a history of suicide in a parent is an important warning. Chronic illness, alcoholism, cancer, disabling heart disease, and progressive, incurable neurologic disease all contribute to the risk. Declared fear of death, devout Catholicism, and avowed devotion to family are deterrents. The only rule of thumb is that depressed patients should be asked about their intentions in a forthright manner and all suicide threats should be taken seriously. If there is a suspicion of risk, the family should be warned, a bed should be obtained in a hospital (preferably in a well-supervised psychiatric ward), and a psychiatrist should be consulted. Precautions against suicide should be taken with the help of the nursing staff. If the patient has already attempted suicide, hospital admission is imperative and the patient should be placed under surveillance.

Anorexia Nervosa and Bulimia

Anorexia nervosa (AN) is a disease of unknown cause, the core of which is excessive voluntary weight loss. It occurs almost exclusively in previously healthy adolescent girls and young women. Anorexia in boys and men is usually linked genetically and clinically to an endogenous depression; hence there is no impropriety in appending the description of the anorectic states to this chapter.

AN is culturally predicated, being prevalent mainly in social groups with free access to food and deeply embedded ideas about body habitus. Many of the patients are depressed, impatient, and irritable. Often as much as 30 percent of the patient's body weight will have been lost by the time medical help is sought. In young women, menses cease. To hasten weight loss, the patient may resort to exercise and purging. The cachexia may reach such proportions as to end fatally. For this reason, treatment is mandatory. This is most effectively carried out in the hospital, where food intake can be strictly supervised. Intake is increased gradually to 3500 to 4000 calories per day. Tube feedings are needed if the patient resists. Once weight is gained, the loss of appetite tends gradually to correct itself. Imipramine, 150 mg/day, has been a helpful adjunct in the therapeutic program, even though patients may not exhibit the typical picture of depression. A relationship between depression and AN is suggested by the unusually high incidence of depression in first-degree relatives of patients with AN. Relapse is frequent in early adult life, and the therapeutic program in most cases needs to be continued for 3 to 4 years.

Bulimia is an eating disorder characterized by massive binge eating followed by induced vomiting and the use of laxatives. It is probably a variant of AN. The authors are attracted to the view that bulimia, like AN, is a manifestation, peculiar to the female, of a deranged appetite-satiety mechanism in the hypothalamus. At present, proof of this hypothesis is lacking.

For a more detailed discussion of this topic, see Victor and Ropper: *Adams and Victor's Principles of Neurology*, 7th ed, pp 1608–1623.

ADDITIONAL READING

Anderson AE: *Practical Comprehensive Treatment of Anorexia Nervosa and Bulimia.* Baltimore, Johns Hopkins University Press, 1985.

Becker AE, Grinspoon SK, Klibanski A, Herzog DB: Eating disorders. *N Engl J Med* 340:1092, 1999.

Cassidy WL, Flanagan NB, Spellman M, Cohen ME: Clinical observations in manic-depressive disease. *JAMA* 164:1535, 1957.

Diagnostic and Statistical Manual of Mental Disorders, 4th ed (DSM-IV). Washington, DC, American Psychiatric Association, 1994.

Gabbard GD: Mood disorders: Psychodynamic aspects, in Sadock BJ, Sadock VA (eds): *Kaplan and Sadock's Comprehensive Textbook of Psychiatry*, 7th ed. Philadelphia, Lippincott Williams & Wilkins, 2000, pp 1328–1338.

Goodwin DW, Guze SB: *Psychiatric Diagnosis*, 5th ed. New York, Oxford University Press, 1996.

House A, Dennis M, Warlow C, et al: Mood disorders after stroke and their relation to lesion location. *Brain* 113:1113, 1990.

Mann JJ: The neurobiology of suicide. *Nature Medicine* 4:25, 1998.

Pirodsky DM, Cohn JS: *Clinical Primer of Psychopharmacology: A Practical Guide*, 2nd ed. New York, McGraw-Hill, 1992.

Robins E: *The Final Months: A Study of the Lives of 134 Persons Who Committed Suicide*. Oxford, UK, Oxford University Press, 1981.

Whooley MA, Simon GE: Managing depression in medical outpatients. *N Engl J Med* 343:1942, 2000.

Winokur G: *Mania and Depression: A Classification of Syndrome and Disease*. Baltimore, John Hopkins University Press, 1991.

58 | The Schizophrenias and Paranoid States

Schizophrenia is the most serious of all unsolved psychiatric disorders: The historical events that led to our present view of schizophrenia and the epidemiology of the disease are elaborated in *Adams and Victor's Principles of Neurology*, 7th ed. Uncertainty of diagnosis, especially of borderline (pseudoneurotic) cases, has thwarted efforts to accumulate vital statistics, since there is no way of proving that a patient is schizophrenic except by the use of clinical criteria. Schizophrenia is defined in DSM-IV as an illness that has lasted for at least 6 months, beginning during adolescence and early adult life, and consisting of delusions, hallucinations, and disordered thought (looseness of associations and tangential thinking) and verbal communication, all of which result in a deterioration from a previous level of functioning. Of diagnostic importance are absence of depression, mania, dementing brain disease, and mental retardation. To these we would add a positive family history of a mental disturbance of similar nature.

In most cases, eccentricity of personality and behavior (a tendency to be solitary and withdrawn socially) is evident in adolescence and may precede frank psychosis by many years. Then, usually during adolescence and practically always before the age of 40, the patient becomes disturbed and is unable to continue school or work. When first examined, the patient expresses bizarre fears and ideas and suspicions of the motives of family members or of others. Often there are frank hallucinations, delusions, and fantasies about controlling the thoughts of others or having one's own thoughts controlled. Notably absent are primary disturbances of memory, perception, orientation, etc., which are the identifying features of dementing brain diseases and confusional-delirious states. Such episodes of illness occur repeatedly until the patient finally settles into a condition in which delusions and hallucinations are denied but for unclear reasons continuation of education and effective work are impossible. Unfortunately, suicides or, rarely, unprovoked irrational homicides may occur and are unpredictable. Some patients recover, but in such cases there is always the question of reliability of diagnosis (see below).

The traditional subdivision of schizophrenia into simple, hebephrenic, catatonic, and paranoid types is not always helpful. *Catatonia*, in which the patient lies in a dull stupor—mute, negativistic, and apathetic—is a syndrome more closely related to a retarded form of depression than to schizophrenia, and paranoid schizophrenia is considered by many European psychiatrists to be a mental illness of diverse origin, some examples clearly not being schizophrenic.

Bleuler classified the basic psychologic disturbances of schizophrenia into two groups: the first included the "four As"—loose associations, flat affect, ambivalence, and autism; the second were considered secondary phenomena—delusions and hallucinations. The modern view of Liddle and

Barnes, more in conformity with neurologic thought, separates positive (hallucinations and delusions) from negative features (psychomotor retardation, inadequate thinking, and passivity). Others have made a distinction between the thought disorder and disturbances of reality. Even if these distinctions prove not to have neurologic meaning, they facilitate the study of the behavioral aspects and illogical thought processes of the disease.

Acute psychosis in a previously well-adjusted person (called "brief reactive psychosis") is probably not a form of schizophrenia. In 75 to 80 percent of such patients admitted to a mental hospital as schizophrenic, the illness is reversible within a few months; often the family history is one not of schizophrenia but of manic-depressive disease, and the patient responds to anti–manic-depressive medication. Thereafter, the mental disorder is likely to pursue the course of manic-depressive disease rather than of schizophrenia. Brief illnesses (2 weeks or less) with schizophreniform symptoms often have the characteristics more of a confusional state than of schizophrenia; probably an illness of this type lasting less than 6 months is also unlikely to be schizophrenia (possibly they are examples of some type of metabolic disease). There is still much debate about the existence of a childhood form of schizophrenia, which must be distinguished from autism in high-functioning patients (Asperger syndrome).

Even in the group of patients conforming to the diagnostic criteria for schizophrenia, not all patients are alike. Some have suggestive thalamic–frontal lobe signs such as inattentiveness, difficulty in shifting cognitive attention from one task to another, poor function on continuous-performance tasks, and poorly sustained initiative and drive. Also, impairment of smooth ocular pursuit movements, paroxysmal saccadic eye movements, episodic lateral deviation of the eyes, reflex asymmetries, and slight lowering of IQ are recorded in some. In others, delusions, hallucinations, and a disorder of communication dominate. The symptomatology incriminates different parts of the frontal and temporal lobes, a topography now being verified by functional imaging studies. The electroencephalogram (EEG) is abnormal in a nondescript way in many cases. Finally, some patients have slightly enlarged third and lateral ventricles, unrelated to the duration of the illness and medication. These findings, taken together, have led to the notion that schizophrenia is a syndrome, not a single disease, and that within the syndrome there is a genetic core disease that might be called true schizophrenia, as well as other diseases that simulate schizophrenia (i.e., schizophreniform).

A consistent neuropathology for schizophrenia has been singularly elusive. Crude neuronal destruction and gliosis have not been found. Yet quantitative studies are beginning to reveal decreased neuronal populations in certain structures such as the cingulate gyri, nucleus accumbens, globus pallidus, and other parts of the limbic system. Some MRI studies have demonstrated ventricular enlargement and sulcal widening in chronic schizophrenics and a volumetric reduction of the hippocampal formation and superior temporal gyrus on the left side. Studies with positron emission tomography also point to the medial part of the left temporal lobe and related limbic and frontal areas as the focus of a developmental abnormality.

Etiology The evidence favors a genetic origin. The siblings of schizophrenic patients have a higher incidence of schizophrenia (10 percent) than is expected in the general population (0.9 percent). The concordance rate in monozygotic twins is three to six times greater than in dizygotic twins. If children of schizophrenic parents are placed in a foster home with normal parents, the children have the same liability to schizophrenia as if raised by their biologic parents. The exact pattern of inheritance—whether dominant with incomplete penetrance or polygenic—is not settled.

The major pathophysiologic hypothesis is that an abnormal gene or genes cause a hyperfunctional dopamine system. Supporting this concept is the observation that drugs blocking dopamine receptors are potent therapeutic agents. Recently, serotoninergic mechanisms have also been implicated.

A number of other hypotheses have been offered, including a developmental disorder that is induced during intrauterine development, perhaps by a viral infection. On the other hand, psychodynamic explanations of the disease have failed to provide useful insight and have largely been discarded.

Treatment Frank psychotic episodes usually require that the patient be admitted to a psychiatric hospital, especially if there is danger of injury to self or others. In the florid stage of the disease, antipsychotic medication (a phenothiazine, such as thioridazine or fluphenazine, haloperidol, or one of the newer drugs, risperidone, olanzapine, quetiapine, and clozapine) is administered. Anxiety and insomnia, if present, should be controlled by anxiolytic drugs (benzodiazepine). With the use of antipsychotic drugs, there is always the danger of developing tardive dyskinesia, parkinsonian rigidity, or the neuroleptic malignant syndrome (Table 58-1). In this respect, the use of the newer antipsychotic drugs represents a major advance in the treatment of schizophrenia; these drugs are weak dopamine receptor agonists and are infrequently associated with tardive dyskinesia (Table 58-2). Electroconvulsive therapy (ECT) has successfully terminated psychotic episodes in patients refractory to drugs. Some patients continue to deteriorate despite treatment.

Paranoia and Paranoid States

Patients who have fixed suspicions, persecutory delusions, or grandiose ideas that are false but logically elaborated are said to be paranoid. They often display other traits that are indicative of schizophrenia and are then classified as paranoid schizophrenics. However, there is a group whose conduct is formally correct, whose emotional reactions are adequate, and whose train of thought is entirely coherent. To them the term *pure paranoia* is applicable. Mild degrees of the latter are found among eccentric persons of every community. Only when their behavior becomes overtly bizarre or socially unacceptable and annoying to others do they come to the attention of legal authorities or a physician. In some cases, neuroleptic drugs have been helpful.

A few of our alcoholic patients have developed a chronic delusional-hallucinatory state as a sequela to an attack of acute auditory hallucinosis. Acute or chronic drug intoxication (amphetamines, cocaine, phencyclidine) accounts for episodes of paranoid behavior in others.

Puerperal (Postpartum) and Endocrine Psychoses

These are complex problems. Postpartum depression of mild degree and short duration is a frequent and well-known phenomenon. Severe prolonged depression in this setting differs in no particular way from a monophasic

TABLE 58-1 Neurologic Side Effects of the Neuroleptic-Antipsychotic Drugs

Reaction	Clinical features	Period of maximum risk	Proposed mechanism	Treatment
Acute dystonias	Spasm of muscles of tongue, face, neck, back	1–5 days	Dopamine excess? Acetylcholine excess?	Antiparkinson agents are diagnostic and curative (IM or IV, then PO)
Parkinson syndrome	Bradykinesia, rigidity, masked facies, shuffling gait, variable tremor	5–30 days (may persist)	Dopamine blockade	Antiparkinson agents (PO); dopamine agonists risky?
"Rabbit" syndrome	Perioral tremor; flexed posture; usually reversible	Months or years	Unknown	Antiparkinson agents: reduce dose of neuroleptic
Akathisia	Motor restlessness with anxiety or agitation	1–60 days (commonly persists)	Adrenergic excess?	Reduce dose or change drug; low doses of propranolol*; antiparkinson agents or benzodiazepines may help
Neuroleptic malignant syndrome	Catatonia, stupor, fever, unstable pulse and blood pressure, myoglobinemia, elevated CPK†; can be fatal	Weeks	Unknown	Stop neuroleptic; antiparkinson agents usually fail; bromocriptine and dantrolene often help; expert supportive care crucial, ICU best
Tardive dyskinesia	Oral-facial dyskinesia, choreoathetosis, often slowly reversible, rarely progressive	6–24 months (worse on withdrawal)	Dopamine excess?	Treatment unsatisfactory; slow, spontaneous remission; tetrabenazine

Abbreviations: IM, intramuscularly; IV, intravenously; PO, per os (orally); ICU, intensive care unit.
*There may be an increased risk of hypotension on interaction between high doses of propranolol and some antipsychotic agents; clonidine may also be effective at doses of 0.2–0.8 mg/day but carries a high risk of hypotension, and tolerance (loss of efficacy) may develop.
†CPK, creatine-phosphokinase in serum, released from hypertonic muscle.
Adapted from Baldessarini and Cole, by permission.

TABLE 58-2 Newer Antipsychotic Drugs with Limited Extrapyramidal Side Effects

Medication	Brand name	Initial dose	Target or maximal dose	Potential side effects*
Olanzapine	Zyprexa	5 mg	10 mg	Orthostatic hypotension, transaminase elevatior, hyperprolactinemia
Quetiapine	Seroquel	25 mg bid	300 mg	Orthostatic hypotension, cataracts, transaminase elevation
Clozapine	Clozaril	12.5 mg bid	300 mg	Agranulocytosis, transient fever, anticholinergic activity, hyperglycemia
Risperidone	Risperidol	1 mg bid	3 mg bid	Orthostatic hypotension

*All have the potential to cause tardive dyskinesias and neuroleptic malignant syndrome (Table 58-1), but these complications are thought to be less frequent than with phenothiazines and haloperidol.

endogenous depression and should be treated as such. It is of interest that some patients with depression have lapsed into this state only in the postpartum period, being normal at all other times.

An acute confusional-delusional psychosis, unlike any of the previously described psychiatric illnesses, may also appear during the postpartum period. Here, major affective changes are mixed with delusional ideas, disorientation, and clouding of the sensorium. The new mother may reject or even kill her baby. Recovery takes weeks or months, but the outlook in general is better than for schizophrenia. Careful exclusion of drug psychosis and diseases such as postpartum cerebral venous thrombosis is part of the neurologic investigation. In some instances, a frank schizophrenic break can occur in the postpartum period. The treatment of this type of syndrome must be undertaken in a psychiatric hospital, and antipsychotic medication is usually needed.

The *endocrine psychoses* are also difficult to classify, for they vary widely in symptomatology (Chap. 40). An acute onset of confusion, insomnia, mood elevation or depression, hallucinosis, and delusional thinking in some combination has been reported with large doses of steroids or ACTH, Cushing disease, and hyperthyroidism. Control of the endocrine disease usually restores the patient to normality.

For a more detailed discussion of this topic, see Victor and Ropper: *Adams and Victor's Principles of Neurology*, 7th ed, pp 1624–1644.

ADDITIONAL READING

Andreasen NC: Symptoms, signs, and diagnosis of schizophrenia. *Lancet* 346:477, 1996.

Baldessarini RJ, Cole JO: Chemotherapy, in Nicholi AM Jr (ed): *The New Harvard Guide to Psychiatry*, 2nd ed. Cambridge, MA, Harvard University Press, 1988, pp. 481–533.

Buchanan RW, Carpenter WT: Schizophrenia: Clinical features, in Sadock BJ, Sadock VA (eds): *Kaplan and Sadock's Comprehensive Textbook of Psychiatry*, 7th ed. Baltimore, Lippincott Williams & Wilkins, 2000, pp. 1096–1110.

Carpenter WT, Buchanan RW: Schizophrenia. *N Engl J Med* 330:681, 1994.

Kane JM, Marder SR: Psychopharmacologic treatment of schizophrenia. *Schizophr Bull* 19:287, 1993.

Liddle PF, Barnes TRE: Syndromes of chronic schizophrenia. *Br J Psychiatry* 157:558, 1990.

Marder SR: Schizophrenia: Somatic treatment, in Sadock BJ, Sadock VA (eds): *Kaplan and Sadock's Comprehensive Textbook of Psychiatry*, 7th ed. Baltimore, Lippincott Williams & Wilkins, 2000, pp. 1199–1210.

Pearlson GD: Neurobiology of schizophrenia. *Ann Neurol* 48:556, 2000.

Winokur G: Delusional disorder (paranoia). *Compr Psychiatry* 18:511, 1977.

Index

Note: Page numbers in *italics* refer to figures; those followed by the letter *t* indicate tables.